Principles and Practice of Nursing Research

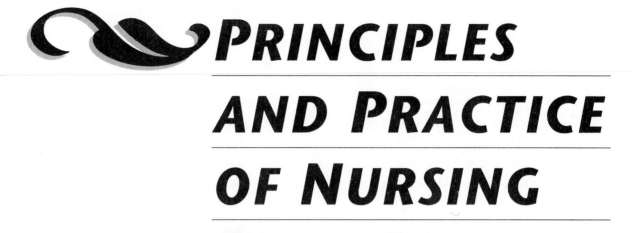

PRINCIPLES
AND PRACTICE
OF NURSING
RESEARCH

Laura A. Talbot, RN, C, PhD

Assistant Professor
Texas Christian University
Harris School of Nursing
Fort Worth, Texas

Lieutenant Colonel, United States Air Force Reserves
Chief, Nursing Services
Tinker AFB, Oklahoma

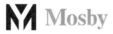 Mosby

St. Louis Baltimore Boston Carlsbad Chicago Naples New York Philadelphia Portland
London Madrid Mexico City Singapore Sydney Tokyo Toronto Wiesbaden

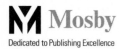
Mosby

Dedicated to Publishing Excellence

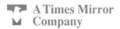 A Times Mirror
Company

Publisher: Nancy L. Coon
Executive Editor: N. Darlene Como
Senior Developmental Editor: Laurie Sparks
Project Manager: Barbara Bowes Merritt
Editing, Production, and Design: University Graphics
    Production Services
Manufacturing Supervisor: Betty Richmond
Cover Design: The Composing Room

Printed in the United States of America
Composition by University Graphics, Inc.
Printing/binding by RR Donnelly and Sons, Inc.

Mosby-Year Book, Inc.
11830 Westline Industrial Drive
St. Louis, Missouri 63146

International Standard Book Number 0-8016-6450-0

94 95 96 97 98 / 9 8 7 6 5 4 3 2 1

CONTRIBUTORS

Ivo L. Abraham, RN, PhD, FAAN, CS
Professor of Nursing and Associate Professor of
    Psychiatric Medicine,
Co-director, Center on Aging and Health,
University of Virginia,
Charlottesville, Virginia;
Adjunct Professor of Public Health,
Catholic University of Leuven,
Leuven, Belgium

Patricia Hayden Allen, EdD, (c), MSN, RN
Assistant Professor,
College of Nursing,
University of Oklahoma,
Oklahoma City, Oklahoma

Janalou Blecke, RN, PhD
Professor and Assistant Dean,
College of Nursing,
Saginaw Valley State University,
University Center, Michigan

Janet L. Blenner, PhD, RN
Professor,
School of Nursing,
College of Health and Human Services,
San Diego State University,
San Diego, California

Suzanne H. Brouse, PhD, RN
Associate Professor,
University of Louisville School of Nursing,
Louisville, Kentucky;
Nurse Researcher,
Louisville Veterans Administration Medical
    Center,
Louisville, Kentucky

Gail C. Davis, RN, EdD
Professor of Nursing,
Harris College of Nursing,
Texas Christian University,
Fort Worth, Texas

Patricia A. Davis-LaGrow, PhD, RN
Associate Professor,
Department of Nursing,
University of Central Oklahoma,
Edmond, Oklahoma

Sally Decker, PhD, RN
Professor of Nursing,
College of Nursing,
Saginaw Valley State University,
University Center, Michigan

Geri Dickson, RN, PhD
Assistant Professor,
College of Nursing,
Rutgers, The State University of New Jersey,
Newark, New Jersey

v

Agatha M. Gallo, RN, PhD
Associate Professor,
College of Nursing,
University of Illinois at Chicago,
Chicago, Illinois

Joan P. Garity, RN, EdD
Assistant Professor,
College of Nursing,
University of Massachusetts at Boston,
Boston, Massachusetts

Audrey G. Gift, PhD, RN, FAAN
Associate Professor,
School of Nursing,
University of Pennsylvania;
Assistant Director,
Center for Nursing Research;
Research Facilitator,
Hospital of the University of Pennsylvania,
Philadelphia, Pennsylvania

Kathleen A. Knafl, PhD
Professor and Associate Dean for Research,
College of Nursing,
University of Illinois at Chicago,
Chicago, Illinois

Renee Leasure, PhD, RN, CCRN
Assistant Professor,
College of Nursing,
University of Oklahoma,
Oklahoma City, Oklahoma

Carla Mariano, RN, EdD
Director, Advanced Education in Nursing Science,
Master's Degree Programs,
Division of Nursing,
New York University,
New York, New York

Anne Griswold Peirce, RN, PhD
Director of Doctoral Studies,
School of Nursing,
Columbia University,
New York, New York

Carolyn J. Pepler, RN, BNSc, MScN, PhD
Consultant for Nursing Research,
Royal Victoria Hospital;
Associate Professor,
School of Nursing,
McGill University,
Montreal, Quebec, Canada

Maryann F. Pranulis, RN, DNSc
Director of Nursing Research and Education,
University of California at San Diego Medical Center,
San Diego, California

Barbara M. Raudonis, PhD, RN
Assistant Professor,
Harris College of Nursing,
Texas Christian University,
Fort Worth, Texas

Michael C. Robinson, PhD
Assistant Professor of Psychology,
Texas Christian University,
Fort Worth, Texas;
Assistant Professor of Psychology,
Texas Wesleyan University,
Fort Worth, Texas

Karen Kelly Schutzenhofer, EdD, RN, CNAA
Consultant in Nursing Education,
St. Louis, Missouri

Barbara S. Thomas, PhD
Professor,
College of Nursing,
University of Iowa,
Iowa City, Iowa

Inez Tuck, PhD, RN
Associate Professor,
College of Nursing,
University of Tennessee—Knoxville,
Knoxville, Tennessee

B. Gayle Twiname, PhD, RN, CS
Associate Professor,
Department of Nursing,
Lamar University,
Beaumont, Texas

Lynn I. Wasserbauer, MS, RN
Doctoral Candidate, School of Nursing;
Research Associate, Center on Aging and Health,
University of Virginia,
Charlottesville, Virginia

To Bill
for his constant love, support, and encouragement;

To Mark, Paul, Christopher, and Lauren
for their unconditional love;
and

To my parents,
Joseph and Therese Meyers,
who instilled the fundamental values
and principles necessary in life.

PREFACE

As the United States health care delivery system shifts its focus from the treatment of disease to the promotion of health and places greater emphasis on outcomes and cost effectiveness, nursing is also in a state of change. As the largest group of health care professionals, nurses have the potential to make the greatest impact on health care. Research is crucial to meeting this challenge. Use of the research process and research findings in clinical settings fosters critical thinking and leads to the discovery of new ways of improving patient care as well as the discovery and exploration of alternative types of care. Research can also help nurses demonstrate their major contribution to cost-effective health care.

Nursing research is important to nursing practice because it can lead to improved patient care and/or decreased costs. At the same time, the use of research assures the public that the care provided is empirically based and that the nursing profession is striving to provide the highest possible standard of care. To assure credibility and accountability, nursing practice must be based on research findings that are obtained through the use of scientific research methods. More important, nurses must know how to locate and read research reports, to evaluate them critically, to apply the findings to practice, and to participate in the research process. Thus it is vital for nurses, regardless of their level of educational preparation, to understand the research concepts.

Principles and Practice of Nursing Research is a comprehensive text covering concepts of nursing research, steps in the research process, evaluation of nursing research, and use of research in practice. Written for students learning to conduct as well as understand and use nursing research, the text introduces and clearly defines basic research terminology and leads the student through the research process. At the same time it contains enough detail to prepare the student to conduct nursing research.

The text is organized into six parts. Part I, Research and the Profession of Nursing, discusses the historical development of nursing research and its importance to

ix

practice, the relationship between theory and research, and the legal and ethical issues relevant to research. It also provides an introduction to the research process and a discussion of qualitative and quantitative approaches to research. Part II, Preliminary Steps in the Research Process, describes the early stages of the research process, with emphasis on those aspects common to both quantitative and qualitative research. Part III discusses the quantitative research process in detail, whereas Part IV discusses the qualitative research process in detail. Part V, Using Research in Practice, provides the reader with a foundation for evaluating and critiquing research for its applicability to practice, along with guidelines for implementation of research findings. Part VI, Conducting Nursing Research, discusses other aspects of the research process, including writing a proposal, using computers, and disseminating the findings.

In recent years qualitative research methods have gained greater acceptance among nurse researchers and scholars. A unique feature of this text is a full unit devoted to this important type of research. This unit explores the theoretical foundations of qualitative research, the research methods, and the qualitative research process. The final chapter in the unit discusses the integration of qualitative and quantitative research.

To facilitate planning and conducting each phase of the research process, "steps" boxes summarizing key elements of the research process are included where appropriate. Examples of actual published research illustrate the steps of the research process, to give the reader practice in reading and evaluating published research.

To effectively implement research findings in practice, nurses must become proficient at critically evaluating published research studies. To assist in acquiring this skill, each chapter contains a section discussing evaluation of that stage of the research process. Boxes summarizing factors for evaluation are also included.

Critical thinking guides the student to use independent judgment and evaluation based on reasoned appraisal of material presented. A section titled "Facilitating Critical Thinking" is included at the end of each chapter. Exercises assist the reader in developing critical thinking skills and in applying the concepts discussed in the chapter.

Accompanying the text is an *Instructor's Resource Manual* written by Renee Leasure, Patricia Allen, and Patricia Davis-LaGrow. It is designed to assist the instructor in planning and implementing class activities. It includes learning objectives, teaching strategies, suggested learning activities for classroom use, critical thinking questions, test questions, and student worksheets. Instructors may copy and hand out these worksheets for students to complete. In addition to these chapter-by-chapter activities, transparency masters are included for approximately 25 of the illustrations in the text.

I wish to acknowledge Darlene Como, Executive Editor, who supported my initial conceptualization of this book and then provided guidance and support throughout this process. I also extend special appreciation to Laurie Sparks, senior developmental editor, whose hard work and expertise were a significant driving force for completion of this project. Her understanding, encouragement, advice, editing, and sustained support coupled with a "can do" attitude were invaluable in completing this book.

Laura A. Talbot

CONTENTS

PRINCIPLES
AND PRACTICE
OF NURSING
RESEARCH

PART I

RESEARCH AND THE PROFESSION OF NURSING

CHAPTER 1

THE ROLE OF RESEARCH IN NURSING

LAURA A. TALBOT

One of the first issues of the *American Journal of Nursing* describes the technique of using a mustard tub bath to reduce the temperature of a child with pneumonia.

> A child's tub is filled three-fourths full with tepid water. Mustard in the proportion of one heaping tablespoonful to a gallon is added. The patient is given stimulant before being placed in the tub; ice is kept on the head and constant gentle friction is applied during immersion (Hitchcock, 1902, p. 172).

Today's nurse would not accept such advice unquestioningly. The practicing nurse would ask: What is the age or size of the child this procedure is designed to treat? How hot is tepid? What kind of mustard is used? What effect does the mustard have on fever control? What is appropriate stimulant? Why is ice placed only on the head? What is the purpose of gentle friction? Where is the friction applied?

In the past, nursing procedures were based on customs or traditional practice, not on research. Today a mustard tub bath is not used in fever control. What became of the mustard tub bath? Probably through the years it was found on a trial-and-error basis to be ineffective. However, there is no documentation on the use of this procedure in our professional literature to confirm this conjecture.

The above example demonstrates the need to conduct research. The use of the trial-and-error method is not only ineffective, it is inefficient in terms of time and energy. In addition it is vulnerable to the differing skill levels of each practicing nurse. Research methods provide a process for discovery and validation of practices that are much less vulnerable to diversity among practitioners. This process facilitates building a scientific knowledge base so that nurses will know if specific procedures actually have positive outcomes for the patient.

WHAT IS NURSING RESEARCH?

Nursing research is a systematic approach to examining phenomena important to nursing and nurses. Since nursing is a practice-based discipline, the purpose of nursing research is to create and maintain a strong scientific basis for nursing practice. This is accomplished through generating and validating knowledge that promotes better patient care outcomes. Without a scientific basis, the nursing profession is prone to repetition of useless behaviors and procedures that neither promote patient well-being nor contribute to effective nursing practice. This is why it is important for nurses to examine the application of nursing knowledge and to evaluate its effects through research.

THE IMPORTANCE OF RESEARCH TO NURSING

The future of nursing hinges on the quality and quantity of nursing research for several reasons: (1) It validates nursing as a profession; (2) it provides a scientific basis for nursing practice; and (3) it demonstrates accountability of the profession.

VALIDATION AS A PROFESSION

Research is often considered part of the criteria for distinguishing nursing as a profession rather than a service occupation. To meet the criteria for a profession, nursing must be based on a well-defined body of specialized knowledge. Critics assert that nursing does not have a specialized body of knowledge but borrows from other disciplines such as education, psychology, sociology, and medicine. This is partially true, as it is of some other professions such as social work, counseling, and education, which deal with problems of human existence. In the past nurses have received advanced degrees in a variety of disciplines other than nursing, especially in the social sciences. These researchers, trained in the philosophies of other disciplines, have been an asset to nursing, for they have brought relevant elements of those disciplines into nursing. The primary argument against using theories borrowed from other disciplines is that information has not been tested for its relevance to nursing. A scientific knowledge base unique to nursing needs to be developed to validate nursing as a discipline. We are challenged to identify those elements that are unique to nursing and to build our scientific base around them.

SCIENTIFIC BASIS FOR PRACTICE

Research also provides a scientific basis for nursing practice. A common misconception is that because a nurse does the research it is nursing research. There has been discussion as to what is the difference between research in nursing and nursing research. Research in nursing is broad in nature. Research in nursing studies the nursing profession or characteristics of the nurse, whereas nursing research focuses on the practice of nursing. Briones and Cecchini (1991) clarified nursing research by stating: "If the research focus of these nurse scientists is within the theoretic orientation of nursing and the findings they generate contribute to nursing's body of knowledge, then their work is considered nursing research" (p. 206).

ACCOUNTABILITY OF THE PROFESSION

Research demonstrates accountability of the profession. To the consumer accountability implies a duty or obligation to clients to provide quality patient care with predictable outcomes. Predictable outcomes are determined through research.

Research assists the nurse in making rational decisions. Nursing research improves the standards of nursing care by providing the basis for sound nursing action, particularly planning, predicting, and controlling patient care outcomes. Research is critical for improving nursing practice and is the only way a profession can consistently improve over time.

↬ DEVELOPING NURSING KNOWLEDGE THROUGH THEORY AND RESEARCH

Nursing practice can acquire a scientific body of knowledge through theory development and research. Theories are used to categorize and organize the phenomena of interest. The most sophisticated theories describe, explain, and predict properties of a phenomenon. Theories in development may describe how a phenomenon exists at a certain time; or they may explain past occurrences with the ultimate aim of predicting future occurrences.

Theories are important, for they provide the map to achieving specific nursing outcomes. As nurses we want to avoid a haphazard approach to practice. We want to be able to describe and explain nursing phenomena as well as predict outcomes. Theories provide the means to manage practice and shape patient outcomes.

Concepts are abstract ideas. They are the basic elements of a theory. Theories take these concepts and organize them systematically, showing the abstract nature of their relationships to explain and predict a phenomenon. Research takes these abstract notions and applies them to real-life situations in the context of the scientific method. Systematic inquiry is used to examine these conceptual relationships. Once these abstractions are tested, the results are used to validate elements of the theory.

One purpose of research is to formulate theory. The researcher whose purpose is to formulate theory identifies, describes, and specifies the nature of relationships among phenomena. The first step is to identify and define the elements, properties, or events related to the phenomenon. The next step is to define specific characteristics of the phenomenon. Finally the researcher describes relationships between concepts or ideas. An example of research that formulates theory is seen in a phenomenological study that explored the meaning of stressful life experiences among children 9 to 11 years old (Jacobson, 1994). Fourteen children were interviewed in their homes. Using the phenomenological approach, the researcher explored the meaning of the children's experiences from their perspective. Data were analyzed by the researcher through reading the interview transcripts many times.

> When the researcher had a general sense of the child's whole statement, the interview text was read again, with the specific aim of discriminating "meaning units" that focused on the phenomena being studied. . . . The researcher then synthesized the transformed meaning units into a constituent statement regarding the subject's experience. . . . Seventeen categories of situations related to children's stressful life experiences were extracted from the interview transcripts. After these categories were identified, they were found to be concentrated within three principal dimensions: feelings of loss, feelings of threat to self, and feelings of being hassled (Jacobson, 1994, p. 97).

Feelings of loss were associated with "loss of a significant person, pet or space, such as home, school, friends or familiar neighborhood" (p. 97). Feelings of threat to self involved "disapproval by a regarded adult, lack of regard or respect for feelings and actual or potential threat to self-esteem" (p. 97). Feelings of being hassled evolved around situations such as forgetting classroom homework, siblings' disagreements, the household chores, or, more threatening, disagreements with a parent or friend. The results of this study identified a conceptual framework centered around new knowledge of a child's stressful life experiences.

Another purpose of research is to test theory. Research used to test theory seeks to provide empirical evidence about proposed relationships derived from the theory. An example of theory testing is demonstrated in Ahijevych and Bernhard's (1994) research concerning health-promoting life-style behaviors of African American women. The research was based on Nola Pender's (1987) health promotion framework. This conceptual framework defines health and presents models for understanding the benefits of healthy behaviors and barriers to the selection of health-promoting life-style behaviors. Due to the limited knowledge of health behaviors in ethnic and racial communities, this researcher selected African American women as the focus of the study. To test the theory, the Health-Promotion Lifestyle Profile (HPLP) developed by Walker, Sechrist, and Pender (1987) was administered to 187 participants. This instrument measured the probability of engaging in health-promotion behaviors. HPLP subscales measured "self-actualization, health responsibility, exercise, nutrition, interpersonal support, and stress management" (Ahijevych and Bernhard, 1994, p. 87). The results showed self-actualization and interpersonal support ranked the highest, followed by stress management, nutrition, and health responsibility. Exercise ranked last among the subscales. When compared to prior studies of

ethnic and racial communities, African American women scored next to the lowest on the HPLP, with Hispanic participants ranking last. These findings added a new dimension to the health promotion framework. Assessing health promotion in all ethnic and racial communities is important in identifying barriers to the selection of health-promoting life-style behaviors and in focusing on each specific group's needs. Based on the study results and health promotion framework, there appears to be a need to direct health intervention and health promotion resources to ethnic minority communities. More research-based knowledge is needed to examine other ethnic groups to further validate the health promotion framework.

COMPARING THE NURSING PROCESS TO THE RESEARCH PROCESS

The nursing process is a systematic method of problem solving used by nurses to organize patient care. The research process and the nursing process are very similar in that both are systematic methods of examining a problem. The two are compared in Table 1-1.

The nursing process consists of five steps: assessment, diagnosis, plan, implementation, and evaluation. In the nursing process the nurse conducts an assessment based on subjective and objective data elicited from the patient and other available sources. Based on the assessment a nursing diagnosis is formulated. Specific patient outcomes are identified and goals established as means of measuring these outcomes in relation to the nursing diagnosis. A plan of care is derived to meet the goals based on scientific principles and theories. Implementation is putting the plan of care into action. Evaluation examines

Table 1-1
Comparison between the Nursing Process and the Research Process

Nursing Process	Research Process
Assessment	Identify phenomena
Diagnosis	Research problem
Goal/patient outcomes	Hypotheses
Plan	Study design
	Review of literature
	Theoretical/conceptual framework
Implementation	Data collection
Evaluation	Analysis of results
	Recommendations and implications for further research

the patient's response to the interventions and the extent to which the goals have been met. Patient care outcomes are evaluated in relation to each goal set by the nurse and patient. The plan of care is then revised based on the patient's immediate need and the development of new needs.

The research process is similar in its approach. Based on data from various sources, the researcher identifies a researchable problem in nursing. The problem can be one of a practical nature needing resolution or one of a theoretical nature associated with a particular theory. Much like the goal in the nursing process, the hypothesis is a prediction of outcomes related to the problem. A study design is the overall plan for the study. It specifies how the study will be put into action. The rationale for the study and its design is based on the literature and the theoretical/conceptual framework. Data collection is the actual implementation of the study. Data are analyzed and conclusions drawn, providing evidence for support or failure to support the hy-

pothesis. Recommendations are then made for further research based on the results of the research study.

HISTORICAL PERSPECTIVE OF RESEARCH IN NURSING

Looking at the historical perspective of research in nursing provides a basis for understanding nursing and its present problems and successes. Understanding how historical issues influenced modern health care provides a basis for building for the future. Knowledge of history provides nurses with a sense of origin. By exploring the origin of a given issue, one can see how it has shaped nursing practice and research. If analyzed, historical knowledge can provide insight into the past, thus leading to resolution of present and future issues in nursing. The historical evolution of research in nursing is discussed in the following section and summarized in the box on the next page.

FLORENCE NIGHTINGALE: NURSE RESEARCHER

Florence Nightingale (1820-1910) is considered the founder of professional nursing; she is also considered the first nurse researcher. She was born into an upper-class, aristocratic English family during the male-dominated Victorian era. She received an education equal to or better than that of most men of her social class. She was learned in art, mathematics, and statistics; this was unusual for a woman in Victorian England.

Nightingale understood the importance of the scientific method and tracking. During the Crimean War she kept meticulous records and statistics of mortality rates among sick and wounded British soldiers. She demonstrated that as a result of her nursing efforts an overall drop in the mor-

HISTORICAL EVOLUTION OF NURSING RESEARCH

1820   Florence Nightingale, the first nurse researcher, is born.

1854   Nightingale at military hospital in Scutari during the Crimean War.

1858   Nightingale's *Notes on Matters Affecting the Health, Efficiency and Hospital Administration of the British Army* and *Notes on Hospitals* published in London by Harrison and Sons.

1858   Nightingale made a fellow of the Royal Statistical Society.

1859   *Notes on Nursing* published.

1860   Nightingale Training School opens at St. Thomas's Hospital, London.

1896   Nurses' Associated Alumnae of the United States and Canada organized.

1900   *American Journal of Nursing* first published.

1903   North Carolina first state to pass permissive licensure law.

1907   Nutting's "The Education and Professional Position of Nurses," Nutting and Dock's *A History of Nursing.*

1923   Goldmark Report sponsored by the Committee for the Study of Nursing Education.

1924   Yale University offers first degree in nursing.

1924   Teachers College, Columbia, offers first doctoral program for nurses, granting an EdD.

1932   The Association of Collegiate Schools of Nursing is organized.

1934   NYU offers first PhD in nursing.

1936   Sigma Theta Tau awards first grant for research in the United States.

1948   Ginzberg Report published.

1948   Brown Report prepared for the National Nursing Council.

1949   Murdock Report published.

1952   *Nursing Research,* the official research journal of the ANA, is published.

1952   Mildred Montag publishes *Community College Education for Nursing.*

1953   Institute of Research and Service in Nursing Education at Teachers College in Columbia University.

1955   The American Nurses' Foundation is formed.

1956   Committee on Research and Studies formed by the ANA.

1957   Western Interstate Commission on Higher Education (WICHE), Southern Regional Educational Board (SREB).

1963   Surgeon General's Consultant Group on Nursing (*Toward Quality in Nursing,* 1963).

1964   *International Journal of Nursing Studies* is published.

1966   *International Nursing Index* published.

1967   *IMAGE* (Sigma Theta Tau publication) is first published.

1970   Lysaught report titled *An Abstract for Action.*

1976   ANA Commission on Nursing Research publishes *Preparation of Nurses for Participation in Research.*

1978   *Research in Nursing and Health* published.

       Advances in Nursing Sciences published.

1979   *Western Journal of Nursing Research* published.

1981   ANA Commission on Nursing Research publishes *Research Priorities for the 1980s* and *Guidelines for the Investigative Function of Nurses.*

1985   ANA Cabinet on Nursing Research publishes *Directions for Nursing Research: Toward the Twenty-first Century.*

1986   Establishment of the National Center for Nursing Research at the National Institutes of Health.

1988   *Nursing Scan in Research* published.

1989   Clinical Practice Guidelines published by the Agency for Health Care Policy and Research.

1992   *Healthy People 2000* published by Department of Health and Human Services.

1993   National Center for Nursing Research renamed the National Institute of Nursing Research.

tality rate, from 42% to 2.2%, occurred within a 6-month period.

Palmer (1977) described Nightingale the researcher as having an

> . . . extraordinary capability to maintain detailed and copious anecdotal notes and records on a wide variety of occurrences and events, her gift for expressive communication, her aptitude for ordering and codifying her observations, her talent in using statistics, her skill in graphic portrayal of data, and her ability to extrapolate. Her outstanding capacity to conceptualize, infer, analyze, and synthesize was revealed time and again as she reviewed multiple sources of complex data and abstracted meaningful information, related data to a larger universe, and explained it clearly (p. 88).

She used statistics to support her argument for reform in medical care in military and civilian hospitals (Nightingale, 1858). These recommendations for hospital changes were based on meticulously tabulated statistics on the outcomes of hospitalized patients.

In 1858 she was made a fellow of the Royal Statistical Society and presented a paper titled "Miss Nightingale's Scheme for Uniform Hospital Statistics" at the Statistical Congress of 1860. She received honorary membership in the American Statistical Society in 1874. Her famous book *Notes on Nursing* (Nightingale, 1859) was based on the data collected during the Crimean War and the years preceding its publication in 1859.

AFTER NIGHTINGALE

In the United States Florence Nightingale was well known for her system of training women for nursing. The Nightingale system of preparing women for the profession of nursing was adopted in several American schools, but her beliefs on data collection and statistical analysis were not. There was an increase in the number of hospitals and with that an increase in the need for nursing services. It was quickly discovered that the best way to staff hospitals with nurses was to establish a nursing school. From the late 1800s until the early 1950s, the majority of nursing care in hospitals was done by student nurses. Graduates from the early programs worked as private-duty nurses, superintendents in hospitals, nurse-instructors for schools of nursing, or visiting nurses. Some went into the newly developing field of public health nursing. The climate was not conducive for research, based on the overall concept of nursing and the conditions nurses worked under at that time. The profession was still dominated by physicians.

At the time it was felt that nursing practice could be improved through the education of qualified nurses, not through nursing research. There was no uniformity in nursing education. Students were given certificates of completion, but programs varied in length from 6 weeks to 3 years. The quality of education was dependent on which program the nurse attended. Licensure to measure minimum competency did not come into play until 1903, when the state of North Carolina passed its permissive licensure law. By 1923 all 48 states had enacted permissive licensure laws.

Preparation after the completion of the basic nurse curricula had usually been for those seeking to teach in schools of nursing or to take administrative positions. Postgraduate education then was not clearly defined. It usually meant any organized study offered by a recognized school for graduates of diploma programs. In the first issue of the *American Journal of Nursing* an article discussed the "Course in Hospital Economics" offered by Columbia University, Teachers College. The purpose of the course was "to fit persons who are already trained nurses for the responsible duties of superintendents of hospitals and principals of training-schools for nurses" (Robb, 1900, p. 29). It was specifically designed for the graduate nurse with a specific curriculum or course of study directed by the Members of the Hospital Economics Committee.

THE EARLY TWENTIETH CENTURY

The American Nurses' Association was organized in 1896 under the name of Nurses' Associated Alumnae of the United States and Canada. The *American Journal of Nursing* was first published in October 1900 as the official organ of the American Nurses' Association.

From 1900 to 1909, Carnegie (1976, p. 6) identified five articles based on research conducted by nurses that appeared in *AJN*. The first appeared in March 1902. Fulmer (1902) surveyed 53 visiting nurses' associations in the United States. She did a comparative analysis of each association's establishment date, mission, funding, and staffing, plus future recommendations for the direction of visiting nurse associations. Hitchcock (1902) gave the morbidity and mortality statistics of pneumonia for 1901 in Nurses' Settlement in New York as well as the usual home care provided by the visiting nurse. Goler (1904) compared the mortality statistics of young children who drank contaminated or "dirty" milk before the establishment of nurse-run summer milk stations and the decrease in mortality rate after its founding. In January 1906 the journal published a description of Emily Richards' invention of an appliance for surgical beds that she patented with the U.S. Patent Office. Mac-Donald (1906) sent a questionnaire to 50 representative hospitals questioning "the average requirements for the same purposes of surgical materials in common use"

(p. 677). Conclusions were then presented based on the responses received.

Two of the earliest studies of nursing and nursing education are Nutting's (1907) "The Education and Professional Position of Nurses" and Nutting and Dock's (1907) *A History of Nursing*. These studies documented the need for reform in nursing and nursing education so as to establish the discipline as a valued profession.

In the 1920s the *American Journal of Nursing (AJN)* began publishing case studies. (A case study is a research method that provides a detailed analysis of a single individual, group, institution, or problem of interest.) By the 1930s case studies were regularly featured in *AJN*. Marvin (1927), in an article from *AJN* titled "Research in Nursing: The Place of Research and Experimentation in Improving the Nursing Care of the Patient," discussed the need for research in nursing in the clinical area so that "every nursing procedure will be scientifically tested with the results measured . . ." (p. 334). Research priorities were listed as was the identification of the need for organized and directed research by competent, trained people. She also identified the need for a journal to publish the results of the nursing research.

At the end of World War I, the Committee on Nursing and Nursing Education conducted a nationwide study of nursing education with Josephine Goldmark, Ph.D., as the trained investigator and with funding provided by the Rockefeller Foundation. It came to be known as the Goldmark Report (1923). Included in the survey were schools of nursing, public health groups, and private-duty nurses. Based on the study results, the committee recommended a reorganization of nursing education and the establishment of more university schools of nursing. From these recommendations came the founding of Yale University School of Nursing, offering a baccalaureate program in nursing. It was the first independent collegiate school of nursing offering a degree in nursing. A Master of Nursing degree followed in 1929.

Graduate schools with degrees in nursing grew slowly. Advanced programs many times referred to a baccalaureate program that was pursued after completing a diploma nursing program. These baccalaureate programs focused on specialization in teaching, administration, or a clinical track. Both baccalaureate programs and master's programs were listed under the general category of "post-graduate programs," making it difficult to determine the number of master's programs in the United States until 1956, when they were cataloged separately (Brown, 1978).

Initially, doctoral programs in nursing were primarily in the field of education. Their goal was to prepare nurses to teach in a college setting. Teachers College, Columbia University, offered the first doctoral program for nurses in 1924. It was offered through the School of Education and nurses were awarded the Ed.D. degree. In 1934 New York University offered the first Ph.D. program in nursing, again in the School of Education.

In 1932 the Association of Collegiate Schools of Nursing was organized. This organization promoted research in nursing education and practice and later sponsored the journal *Nursing Research.*

Despite these advances, it was not until 1936 that the first grant in the United States was awarded for research in nursing. The award was for $600 and was funded by Sigma Theta Tau, the national honor society of nursing (Sigma Theta Tau International, 1990).

WORLD WAR II

World War II brought a shortage of nurses to care for the civilian population. This continued through the postwar years. In 1948 three research studies were conducted to evaluate the nursing shortage. They were the Murdock Report, the Ginzberg Report, and the Brown Report. Nursing organizations turned to researchers from other fields who held doctoral degrees to direct the studies.

The Murdock Report came from a Committee to Study the Nursing Problem in the United States and was supported by the American Medical Association. Thomas P. Murdock, an M.D., was chairman of the committee. The committee's recommendations were to have two groups of nurses, the trained practical nurse and

the professional nurse which was to be subdivided into (a) collegiate and (b) clinical nurses. The collegiate nurse should have college credit before, during, or after her basic nursing training; her chief function would be nursing education. The clinical nurse would be the present hospital school graduate . . . (Murdock, 1949, p. 439).

The Ginzberg Report was inaugurated by the Committee on the Function of Nursing (1948), Division of Nursing Education, Teachers College, Columbia University. Eli Ginzberg, Associate Professor of Economics, Columbia University, was the chairman. The recommendations were for the 4-year professional collegiate nurse, a 2-year prepared technical nurse, and a 1-year practical nurse. It emphasized the use of nursing teams consisting of all preparation levels of nurses.

The Brown Report was funded by the Carnegie Foundation. Esther Lucille Brown, a social anthropologist, reported the results of the study in her book *Nursing for the Future* (Brown, 1948). It pointed out serious weaknesses in the current education of nurses. Recommendations were to have basic schools of nursing brought to the university or college setting with a 4-year curriculum. In addition, patient care would be given by a team approach consisting of the professional nurse, the trained practical nurse, and other subsidiary care providers.

THE 1950s

The 1950s saw an increase in nurses with advanced degrees, an increase in federal funding for research in nursing, and the American Nurses' Association instituting the American Nurses' Foundation devoted exclusively to the promotion of research in nursing. The ANA Committee on Research and Studies was formed in 1954. In order to facilitate the dissemination of research findings, a journal devoted exclusively to research in nursing, *Nursing Research,* was established. Sponsored by the Association of Collegiate Schools of Nursing, *Nursing Research* was first published in June 1952. During the beginning years of the journal, more than half the authors were not nurses but psychologists and sociologists studying nurses. There were very few articles on clinical nursing practice. The focus was nursing education and specific characteristics of nurses (e.g., attitudes, behaviors, roles).

The Conference on Graduate Nurse Education in 1952 passed a resolution to phase out specialized baccalaureate programs and shift specialization and research to the master's programs. The baccalaureate degree would then be reserved for basic nursing education. In 1956 the Department of Baccalaureate and Higher Programs of the NLN elected to accredit diploma, baccalaureate, and master's programs in nursing, further affirming this resolution.

The 2-year associate degree nursing program was implemented based on applied research. Mildred Montag (1959) published her research in *Community College Education for Nursing.* She demonstrated that in a community college setting qualified students could be adequately educated in less than the traditional 3 years and be competent in basic bedside nursing. Her findings were the basis for implementation of the associate degree program in nursing.

In 1953 the Institute of Research and Service in Nursing Education was established at Teachers College, Columbia University. This was the first university system to establish an institute for research in nursing. In addition, two major regional programs were established in 1957 that promoted research, its dissemination, and a research-based curricula: Western Interstate Commission on Higher Education (WICHE) and Southern Regional Educational Board (SREB).

It was not until 1954 that the University of Pittsburgh offered a Ph.D. in maternal-child nursing. This brought a change in the focus of doctoral preparation, from an educational focus to a clinical specialty. In 1960 Boston University offered a Doctorate of Nursing Science (D.N.S.) in psychiatric nursing. In 1964 the University of California, San Francisco, also offered a Doctor of Nursing Science, but instead of a nursing specialty the curriculum was comprehensive in scope with several specialty options.

THE 1960s

The 1960s brought a reordering of research priorities. The focus was to target practice-oriented research to improve the quality of patient care. This was seen in the recommendations from the Surgeon General's Consultant Group on Nursing (*Toward Quality in Nursing,* 1963). This report strongly supported research in nursing and recommended increased funding for that research.

In 1965 the American Nurses' Association took an official position on the educational preparation of the licensed nurse. The ANA stated that "Education for those who work in nursing should take place in institutions of learning within the general system of education" (p. 5). This was controversial for the ANA because at that time the majority of practicing nurses were diploma graduates with no advanced preparation in a college or university setting. With this statement was also the recognition of a need for research in nursing and for educating nurse researchers.

In August 1967 the National Commission for the Study of Nursing and Nursing Education (NCSNNE) was first convened, and Jerome P. Lysaught was appointed director. The focus of the group was to study nursing education as recommended by the Surgeon General's Consultant Group on Nursing.

The final report, titled *An Abstract for Action,* was published in 1970. It is commonly called the Lysaught Report. Priority recommendations were to increase research in nursing practice and nursing education; to use research-based educational systems and curricula; and to increase financial support for research in nursing practice and nursing education.

A series of three articles published in *Nursing Research* presented an overview of 178 nursing research studies funded in part by the Division of Nursing, National Institutes of Health, from 1955 to 1968. Based on this review, research priorities for nursing were identified for the 1970s (see box).

THE 1970s

A content analysis of articles published in *Nursing Research* from 1970 to 1975 showed "a shift from research in nursing being conducted by a large number of members of

---

RESEARCH PRIORITIES IN NURSING FOR THE 1970s

- Studies of clinical problems related to nursing practice, especially descriptive studies of physiological and behavioral responses of patients with various diagnoses in varied settings
- Studies to develop instruments to measure patient care directly
- Studies to identify the criterion measures needed to study the effect of nursing care
- Studies to develop models and theories of nursing practice
- Studies of effects of technological advances on the functions of nursing service personnel
- Studies of patient care systems; hospital systems
- Studies to develop tools to measure effectiveness of health services
- Studies of ways to standardize medical and nursing records for computerization

- Studies of patient care using monitoring systems and computer-aided diagnosis
- Studies of organization patterns of extra-hospital based facilities
- Studies of communication of nursing information in relation to organization patterns of nursing service in the hospital, home, and community
- Studies of methods of incorporating new scientific and technological advances into the nursing curriculum
- Studies to develop criteria of job performance and measures for evaluation
- Studies to define success in nursing and to develop tools to measure this
- Studies to explore the concept of career ladders in nursing
- Historical research in nursing

Abdellah, F: Overview of nursing research 1955-1968, part 1, *Nursing Research, 19*(1), 6, 1970.

other disciplines, especially the social sciences, to that being conducted almost exclusively by nurses themselves" (Carnegie, 1976, p. 23). This increase was attributed to the increase in doctorally prepared nurses.

Along with the increase of nurse researchers came a change in research focus. Clinical practice research came to the forefront. Prior research had focused primarily on nursing education, administration, and nurses themselves. The focus on clinical practice research served as the basis for much of what nurses do in practice today.

The number of doctoral programs in nursing increased dramatically during the 1970s. "In 1960 only 4 doctoral programs in nursing existed; by 1980 this number had grown to a total of 21" (Grace, 1983, p. 146). The primary purpose of the doctoral programs in nursing was to complete a piece of original research with the intent of developing and testing new nursing knowledge.

In 1976 the American Nurses' Association Commission on Nursing Research published guidelines for the academic preparation of nurses for participation in research and its utilization in *Preparation of Nurses for Participation in Research*. These guidelines stated that at the undergraduate level "education for research should prepare the nurse to read research critically and to determine its value to practice" (p. 1). The graduate student "builds upon a previously gained background of knowledge, assumes development of an advanced knowledge base and includes advanced study of methods in research" (p. 3). There was no distinction made in the document between the master's and doctoral level student's preparation.

The 1970s also saw an increase in nursing research journals: *International Journal of Nursing Studies* (1964), *Advances in Nursing Sciences* (1979), *Research in Nursing and Health* (1978), *Western Journal of Nursing Research* (1979), and *Annual Review of Nursing Research* (1983). Specialty journals with a focus in nursing research soon followed, such as *Heart & Lung, American Journal of Critical Care, Journal of Burn Care & Rehabilitation, Journal of Cardiopulmonary Rehabilitation,* and *Nursing Diagnosis.*

THE 1980s

In 1981 the American Nurses' Association Commission on Nursing Research again published guidelines for the academic preparation of nurses for participation in research and its use (ANA, 1981). This publication delineated guidelines for all four levels of nursing: associate degree, baccalaureate degree, master's degree, and doctoral degree. It was expressed that all levels of nursing preparation will have an "active role in the processes of developing scientific knowledge and incorporating that knowledge into practice" (pp. 1-2).

April 18, 1986, marked the establishment of the National Center for Nursing Research (NCNR) at the National Institutes of Health (NIH) under the Health Research Extension Act of 1985 (Public Law 99-158). This historic move has several benefits to the profession of nursing. First, it provides the security of a stable funding base for research in nursing. Second, it increases opportunities for nurse researchers to augment with other biomedical disciplines. Collaboration with other disciplines is encouraged with the availability of cofunding for research projects. Third, it promotes the generation of multidisciplinary knowledge within the health science structure of NIH. Research in nursing can be mainstreamed into the biomedical and behavioral research structure of NIH. The National Center for Nursing research was renamed the National *Institute* of Nursing Research in 1993. This name change further validates the National Institutes of Health's political efforts toward promoting research in nursing.

Specialty groups are making strides to support research in nursing. On November 15, 1989, Sigma Theta Tau, the national honor society for nursing, dedicated the International Center for Nursing Scholarship at the Indiana University-Purdue University campus in Indianapolis, Indiana. The center symbolizes a commitment to the perpetuation of nursing scholarship and excellence in nursing. Former Sigma Theta Tau president, Sr. Rosemary Donley, expressed this sentiment by stating: "By accepting the Center for Nursing Scholarship, we celebrate a return from exile, or more explicitly, a coming home" (Sigma Theta Tau International, 1989, p. 3).

During the 1980s two significant events for the improvement of research in nursing occurred: an increase in new journals designed for reporting research in nursing and theory development, and a significant growth in the number of graduate schools in nursing, particularly doctoral programs.

Publications begun in the 1980s include those that scan research journals and present abstracts to their readers for application in clinical practice. *Nursing Scan in Research: Application for Clinical Practice* reviews 114 research journals for each issue. Specialty groups sponsored research scans, including *AACN: Nursing Scan in Critical Care, ONS: Nursing Scan in Oncology, ENA: Nursing Scan in Emergency Care,* and *NAACOG: Nursing Scan in Woman's Health.*

THE 1990s

The 1990s bring the promise of closing the gap between practice and research. The publication of *Healthy People 2000* in 1992 by the Department of Health and Human Services stresses the national health agenda for the future. This document set the tone for research priorities. For example, nursing administration research priorities were based on *Healthy People 2000* (see Table 1-2). Health promotion, disease prevention, and primary care delivered in a community-based health care delivery system will be the focus of the future.

ROLE OF THE NURSE IN CONDUCTING RESEARCH

Nurses at all levels of educational preparation have an obligation to assist in the development of nursing knowledge and its use in practice. The nurse can take on the role of research participant, advocate, evaluator, implementer, and investigator.

One role of a nurse is as a research participant. Nurses have participated in research efforts since the turn of the century. Clara Maass (1876-1901) gave her life during the Spanish-American War. She volunteered to be a participant in a research study whose purpose was to isolate the vector mosquito and develop an immunization for yellow fever. She was deliberately bitten by an infected mosquito and, at the age of 25, died of the disease. In memory of her efforts a U.S. stamp was commemorated in her honor (Forrester and Grandinetti, 1992).

Nurses also act as advocates for the rights of those participating in a research study. Participants must be made aware of their rights. These include obtaining informed consent to be a participant in the study, knowledge of the risks and benefits associated with the study, assurance of confidentiality and anonymity, and freedom to withdraw from the study at any time without penalty. It is the nurse's responsibility as advocate to be sure that codes of ethics are followed.

In 1976 the American Nurses' Association published "guidelines for the prepara-

Table 1-2
Nursing Administration Research Priorities Based on the *Healthy People 2000* Report

Level I Priorities	Level II Priorities
Further develop classifications and linkages among nursing problems, interventions, and outcomes relevant to promotion and prevention at both individual and community levels.	Develop and test strategies to increase the diversity in nursing and nursing administration.
Identify group level outcomes sensitive to the delivery of nursing care in various settings and with various types of delivery systems.	Identify models for health care delivery that provide the most effective and efficient primary, secondary, and tertiary patient care.
Develop models of effective and efficient interaction between client communities and provider systems that help to build community capacity.	Evaluate the cost-effectiveness of community-based nurse-run centers.
Develop and use a standardized management data set to help build large data bases and means to evaluate clinical strategies employed to promote health.	Identify the role of the nurse administrator in the reformed healthcare system.
Develop nurse-sensitive outcomes for the continuum of care across acute-care, community, long-term, and home health settings.	Develop target group outcomes related to health prevention, protection, and promotion.
Determine the most clinically and fiscally effective intervention strategies for at-risk populations.	Develop structures to shift provider behavior to health promotion, disease prevention, and protection.

Supported by grant HS 07519-01 from the Agency for Health Care Policy and Research.
Lynn, M. S., & Cobb, B. K. (1994). Changes in nursing administration research priorities: A sign of the times. *Journal of Nursing Administration, 24*(4S), 12-18.

tion of nurses for participation in and utilization of research" (1976, p. 1). These guidelines defined the researcher's role according to educational preparation (ANA, 1976; 1981; 1984).

The role of nurses with an Associate Degree in Nursing (ADN) is to assist in identifying areas where research is needed. They also assist in the research process through data collection. To be able to do these tasks, the ADN must have an appreciation of research in nursing.

The Baccalaureate Nurse (BSN) should be able to read the research report critically and evaluate it for its relevance to nursing practice. The BSN should then be able to utilize established research findings in their practice and share those findings with col-

leagues. For example, if a study had involved only a small number of participants and had not been replicated successfully, the nurse may conclude that more evidence is needed before the results should be implemented in practice. In support of the research process, the BSN may identify research topics, may participate in the collection of data, and may be an active participants in implemention of the study.

With a Master's Degree in Nursing, the practitioner identifies nursing practice problems, then analyzes and reformulates the problem for research inquiry. The master's nurse acts as an expert in the clinical area to facilitate research investigations. The practitioner conducts research to monitor quality of nursing practice in a clinical area, then assists in the integration of knowledge into nursing practice.

The ANA distinguishes between doctoral degrees with a clinical focus and those with a research-oriented role. Graduates of a practice-oriented program are leaders in integrating knowledge for the advancement of the profession. Their research focus is to evaluate client outcomes based on nursing interventions by developing methods to measure quality nursing practice.

The graduate of a research-oriented program develops a theoretical framework to explain phenomena related to nursing. Methods are developed to measure nursing phenomena, and preexisting knowledge is analyzed to discover new nursing knowledge. The doctorally prepared nurse is an independent investigator and collaborator in large, complex studies promoting theory testing and theory development in the profession.

∾ FUTURE DIRECTIONS FOR THE YEAR 2000

In 1985 the American Nurse's Association Cabinet on Nursing Research stated priorities for research in nursing in its publication *Directions for Nursing Research: Toward the Twenty-first Century* (see box). To ensure

---

PRIORITIES FOR NURSING RESEARCH

THE CABINET ON NURSING RESEARCH OF THE AMERICAN NURSES' ASSOCIATION

- Promote health, well-being, and ability to care for oneself among all age, social, and cultural groups.
- Minimize or prevent behaviorally and environmentally induced health problems that compromise the quality of life and reduce productivity.
- Minimize the negative effects of new health technologies on the adaptive abilities of individuals and families experiencing acute or chronic health problems.
- Ensure that the care needs of particularly vulnerable groups, such as the elderly, children with congenital health problems, individuals from diverse cultures, the mentally ill, and the poor, are met in effective and acceptable ways.
- Classify nursing practice phenomena.
- Ensure that principles of ethics guide nursing research.
- Develop instruments to measure nursing outcomes.
- Develop integrative methodologies for the holistic study of human beings as

they relate to their families and lifestyles.
- Design and evaluate alternative models for delivering health care and for administering health care systems so that nurses will be able to balance high quality and cost-effectiveness in meeting the nursing needs of identified populations.
- Evaluate the effectiveness of alternative approaches to nursing education for the kind of practice that requires broad knowledge and a wide repertoire of skills, and for the kind of practice that requires specialized knowledge and a focused set of skills.
- Identify and analyze historical and contemporary factors that influence the shaping of nursing professionals' involvement in national health policy development.

American Nurses' Association Cabinet on Nursing Research (1985). *Directions for nursing research: Toward the twenty-first century.* Kansas City, Mo.

progress toward meeting the nursing research priorities by the year 2000, goals and strategies were developed by the Cabinet on Nursing Research with suspense dates of 1990 and 1995.

The National Institute for Nursing Research, in collaboration with the National Advisory Council on Nursing Research and the nursing scientific community, is involved in the development of a National Nursing Research Agenda (NNRA) to set long-range research priorities and to assist in defining and guiding nursing research priorities already set. At the 1988 June meeting of the Council for Nursing Research, seven priorities were identified. These areas of special concern are listed in the box below.

Other specialty organizations have since followed, publishing their research priorities. The American Association of Critical Care Nurses focuses on both clinical practice research and the "context within which critical care nursing takes place" (see box on p. 19). Sigma Theta Tau priorities

for the 1990s (see box on p. 20) focus on its commitment to knowledge, development, dissemination, and utilization.

Professional nursing organizations agree that research is necessary to build a scientific knowledge base for the advancement of nursing practice. To meet this challenge organizations are using research techniques to help set their research priorities. The 1991 Oncology Nursing Society research priorities listed quality of life and symptom management as their highest priority items based on a simple descriptive survey design (Mooney et al., 1991). The Society of Gastroenterology Nurses and Associates (SGNA) used a questionnaire to identify its membership's research interests and needs. Areas of greatest interest were patient care, procedural issues, and nursing care related to endoscopy (Biddle, 1990).

The Agency for Health Care Policy and Research (AHCPR) is an agency of the U.S. Department of Health and Human Services. Established in December 1989, its mission is to support and conduct health services

---

RESEARCH PRIORITIES FROM THE NATIONAL CENTER FOR NURSING RESEARCH

Low birthweight: mothers and infants—includes prevention of premature delivery and care of low-birthweight infants

HIV infection: prevention and care—includes ethical issues, and physiological, psychosocial, and systems factors relating to care of persons with HIV infection.

Long-term care for older adults—includes such issues as quality of care, continuity of care, and family caregiving.

Symptom management—includes biopsychosocial parameters of pain and other symptoms, and measures for symptom assessment and management.

Information systems—includes development of standardized data sets to document nursing care across settings and a taxonomy to classify nursing phenomena.

Health promotion for children and adolescents—includes psychosocial mechanisms underlying health promotion behaviors.

Technology dependency across the lifespan—includes individual and family responses to technology dependency and prevention of complications.

NCNR. (1992). National Center for Nursing Research (basic brochure). Bethesda, Md.: The Center.

AACN RESEARCH PRIORITIES

Priorities for clinical practice research in critical care nursing are:
- Techniques to optimize pulmonary functioning and prevent pulmonary complications
- Weaning of mechanically ventilated patients
- Effect of nursing activities/interventions on hemodynamic parameters
- Techniques for real-time monitoring of tissue perfusion and oxygenation
- Nutritional support modalities and patient outcomes
- Interventions to prevent infection
- Pain assessment and pain management techniques
- Accuracy and precision of invasive and noninvasive monitoring devices
- Effect of nursing activities, environmental stimuli, and human interactions on intracranial and cerebral perfusion pressure

Priorities for research on the context within which critical care nursing takes place are:
- Incorporation of research findings into critical care nursing practice
- Levels of nursing competence (e.g., certification) and the effect on patient outcomes
- Occupational hazards (e.g., HIV, noise, substance abuse, premature delivery)
- Ethical issues related to initiation, maintenance and withdrawal of life support technology (e.g., living wills)
- Patient care delivery models for critical care
- Collaboration and communication among health care professionals
- Role of critical care nurses in decisions regarding resuscitation status of critically ill patients

(From *AACN Announces Research Priorities* Aliso Viejo, Calif, November 21, 1991, American Association of Critical-Care Nurses.)

research, including the formulation of clinical practice guidelines. These practice guidelines were developed by a panel of interdisciplinary experts through an intensive review of research findings. Using scientific literature, recommendations were made for the effective and appropriate care of specific clinical conditions such as urinary incontinence, pain, and pressure ulcers (see box on p. 22). The Clinical Practice Guidelines provides an example of the validation of practice through intensive review of research findings and research synthesis.

SUMMARY

- Nursing research is a systematic approach used to examine phenomena important to nursing and nurses. Its purpose is to create a strong scientific basis for nursing practice.
- Research is important to the profession of nursing in that (1) it validates nursing as a profession, (2) it provides a scientific basis for nursing actions, and (3) it demonstrates accountability of the profession.
- The historical development of nursing research has been a slow process.
  - Florence Nightingale (1820-1910) is considered the first nurse researcher. Her system of training women for nursing was well accepted in the United States, but her beliefs on data collection and statistical analysis were basically ignored. Education was

SIGMA THETA TAU: ACTIONS FOR THE 1990s

I. Knowledge Development

A. Foster an environment conducive to development of nursing knowledge through
1. forums/conferences
2. development of scholarly outreach
3. recognition of scholarly achievement
4. research grants
5. publications
6. development of a lexicon and taxonomy for categorizing nursing knowledge
7. attraction of funds for research and development

B. Continue to expand the body of nursing knowledge through
1. grants to support research
2. state-of-the-science conferences
3. collaborative and interdisciplinary research
4. development of data bases and electronic retrieval systems necessary to facilitate and promote networks of nursing scholars worldwide
5. development of a program to facilitate collaborative international research

C. Create research partnerships with others in nursing and in other disciplines through
1. research roundtables
2. collaborative health service/research studies
3. joint meetings with honor societies in other fields and other nursing research groups
4. co-sponsored research conferences

II. Knowledge Dissemination

A. Increase access to nursing knowledge through
1. development of the nursing library
2. support for scholars, fellows, and lectureship programs
3. publications
4. conferences and forums
5. networking across chapters

B. Apply the technology of information management and improve nurses' skills in information management

C. Develop a plan for an international electronic bulletin board, which can serve as an information clearinghouse

D. Communicate research findings to multiple audiences (e.g., scholars, practitioners, other health care disciplines, the general public)

E. Develop models for dissemination and utilization of new knowledge

F. Increase access to general health knowledge

G. Enhance the public's understanding of nursing and nursing knowledge through
1. public relations, programs/campaigns, news releases, and public service programs
2. media awards, honorary membership in Sigma Theta Tau International, and public receptions
3. programs for high school students and counselors

H. Establish an International Nurse Consultant list

III. Knowledge Utilization

A. Encourage appropriate use of nursing knowledge in practice through
1. conferences
2. research utilization awards
3. development of mechanisms to make available the data base for practice
4. synthesis of research findings in IMAGE, *Reflections,* monographs, and other publications
5. interfaces with the National Library of Medicine and other health-

---

SIGMA THETA TAU: ACTIONS FOR THE 1990s—cont'd

care related data bases
B. Increase utilization of nursing knowledge to influence health-promoting public policy through
1. publicity for research findings
2. specialized surveys
3. development of other mechanisms to communicate with policy makers
4. development of policy-making skills of nurses
C. Develop mechanisms to guide/assist decision-making related to knowledge utilization (i.e., ethical/social change) through
1. IMAGE articles, monographs, other publications
2. debates/discussions, special programs/forums
3. ethics conferences
D. Encourage the synthesis of knowledge for practice through
1. Arista conferences and monographs
2. Distinguished Nurse Scholars/Scholars in Residence Programs
3. integrated reviews

IV. Resource Development
A. Promote the growth of Sigma Theta Tau International membership through
1. maximization of opportunities for qualified individuals, especially minorities, to join
2. continued participation of active members
3. member reinstatement incentive programs
4. publicity for renewal opportunities
5. worldwide information programs on the purposes and activities of Sigma Theta Tau International
6. increased participation of members and chapters outside the United States.
B. Promote growth of Sigma Theta Tau chapters through
1. mentor chapter programs
2. continued development of chapters
3. networks across chapters
4. support to chapters in financial management
C. Develop human resources within nursing through

1. information on the range of career options open to individuals and the requirements for each
2. information programs on available financial support and mechanisms for personal professional development
3. enhancement of nurses' understanding of career development and development of the potential of others
D. Recognize achievements of individuals and groups
E. Increase interdisciplinary collaboration
F. Attract necessary resources through
1. links with appropriate foundations and corporations
2. programs to foster fundraising skills development
3. use of development or resource committees and advisory boards (making full use of the energies of retired members)

Sigma Theta Tau. (1990). Sigma Theta Tau International's "Actions for the 1990s: will lead the Society into the next century," *Reflections, 16*(1), 2.

---

viewed as the means of improving the practice of nursing.
• American Nurses' Association was organized in 1896 with the *American Journal of Nursing* as the official organ of the organization.

• Two of the earliest studies of nursing and nursing education are Nutting's (1907) "The Education and Professional Position of Nurses" and Nutting and Dock's (1907) *A History of Nursing.*
• After World War I the Goldmark Re-

CLINICAL PRACTICE GUIDELINES

Acute Pain Management Guideline Panel. (1992). *Acute pain management: Operative or medical procedures and trauma.* Clinical practice guideline (AHCPR Publication No. 92-0032). Rockville, Md.: Agency for Health Care Policy and Research, U.S. Public Health Service, U.S. Department of Health and Human Services.

Pressure Ulcers Guideline Panel (1992). *Pressure ulcers in adults: Clinical practice guideline.* (AHCPR Publication No. 92-0047). Rockville, Md.: Agency for Health Care Policy and Research, U.S. Public Health Service, U.S. Department of Health and Human Services.

Urinary Incontinence Guideline Panel. (1992). *Urinary incontinence in adults: Clinical practice guideline.* AHCPR Pub. No. 92-0038. Rockville, Md.: Agency for Health Care Policy and Research, U.S. Public Health Service, U.S. Department of Health and Human Services.

These and other clinical practice guidelines can be obtained through the AHCPR Clearinghouse. Its toll-free number is 1-800-358-9295 or write to: AHCPR Publications Clearinghouse, P.O. Box 8547, Silver Spring, MD 20907.

---

port (1923) studied the nursing shortage and nursing education.

- Three research studies were conducted with the purpose of evaluating the nurse shortage after World War II. They were the Murdock Report, the Ginzberg Report, and the Brown Report.
- *Nursing Research,* first published in 1952, was devoted exclusively to research in nursing.
- *An Abstract for Action* was published in 1970. It is commonly called the Lysaught Report.
- In 1976 the American Nurses' Association Commission on Nursing Research published guidelines for the academic preparation of nurses for participation in research and its utilization in *Preparation of Nurses for Participation in Research.*
- The 1970s saw an increase in journals designed to report research in nursing.

- The 1980s saw continued increase in new journals designed for reporting nursing research and theory development and significant growth in the number of graduate schools in nursing.
- Future directions for the 1990s are increased research priorities by specialty organizations and more doctorally prepared nurses to generate new nursing knowledge.

FACILITATING CRITICAL THINKING

1. This chapter described a controversy in nursing. Some nursing experts feel all research that involves any aspect of nursing is nursing research. Proponents feel that only clinical research is nursing research. Take a position on the controversy and argue your point.
2. Florence Nightingale is considered the first nurse researcher. Do you think she

would have been surprised at the slow development of research in nursing? Explain your answer.

3. Based on your clinical experiences in nursing, what do you feel nursing's research priorities should be?

4. The American Nurses' Association stated guidelines for each level of educational preparation. Do you agree with their recommendations? How would you modify their guidelines?

References

SUBSTANTIVE

BROWN, J. (1978). Master's education in nursing, 1945-1969. In M. Louise Fitzpatrick (Ed.), *Historical studies in nursing,* New York: Teachers College Press.

DONAHUE, M. P. (1985). *Nursing, the finest art: An illustrated history.* St. Louis: C.V. Mosby.

FORRESTER, D. A., & GRANDINETTI, P. M. (1992). Nurses on stamps: A distinguished history. *American Journal of Nursing, 92*(5), 62-65.

HINSHAW, A., & MERRITT, D. (1988). Moving nursing research to the National Institutes of Health. In National League for Nursing (Ed.), *Perspectives in nursing: 1987-1989.* New York: The League.

KALISH, P., & KALISH, B. (1986). *The advance of American nursing.* Boston: Little, Brown and Company.

LYNN, M. S., & COBB, B. K. (1994). Changes in nursing administration research priorities: A sign of the times. *Journal of Nursing Administration, 24*(4S), 12-18.

SIGMA THETA TAU INTERNATIONAL. (1990). Sigma Theta Tau research . . . A rich history. *Reflections, 16*(3), 32.

SIGMA THETA TAU INTERNATIONAL. (1989). The dedication. *Reflections, 15*(4), 1-3.

CONCEPTUAL

BRIONES, T., & CECCHINI, D. (1991). Nursing versus medical research. *Heart & Lung: Journal of Critical Care, 20*(2), 206-207.

PENDER, N. (1987). *Health promotion in nursing practice* (2nd ed.). Norwalk, Conn.: Appleton & Lange.

METHODOLOGICAL

AHIJEVYCH, K., & BERNHARD, L. (1994). Health-promoting behaviors of African American women. *Nursing Research, 43*(2), 86-89.

BIDDLE, W. (1990). Survey results: Identification of research interests and needs in SGNA. *Society of Gastroenterology Nurses and Associates, 13*(2), Fall supplement, 12S-16S.

JACOBSON, G. (1994). The meaning of stressful life experiences in nine- to eleven-year-old children: A phenomenological study. *Nursing Research, 43*(2), 95-99.

MOONEY, K., FERRELL, B., NAIL, L., BENEDICT, S., & HAVERMAN, M. (1991). 1991 Oncology Nursing Society Research Priorities Survey. *Oncology Nursing Forum, 18*(8), 1381-1388.

WALKER, S., SECHRIST, K., & PENDER, N. (1987). The health-promoting lifestyle profile: Development and psychometric characteristics. *Nursing Research, 36,* 76-81.

HISTORICAL

ABDELLAH, F. (1970). Overview of nursing research 1955-1968, Part 1. *Nursing Research, 19*(1), 6-17.

AMERICAN NURSES' ASSOCIATION. (1984). *Standards for professional nursing education.* Kansas City, Mo.: The Association.

AMERICAN NURSES' ASSOCIATION CABINET ON NURSING RESEARCH. (1985). *Directions for nursing research: Toward the twenty-first century.* Kansas City, Mo.: The Association.

AMERICAN NURSES' ASSOCIATION COMMISSION ON NURSING RESEARCH. (1981). *Guidelines for the investigative function of nurses.* Kansas City, Mo.: The Association.

AMERICAN NURSES' ASSOCIATION COMMISSION ON NURSING RESEARCH. (1976). *Preparation of nurses for participation in research.* Kansas City, Mo.: The Association.

AMERICAN NURSES' ASSOCIATION'S FIRST POSITION ON NURSING EDUCATION. (1965). *American Journal of Nursing, 65,* 106-107.

BARRITT, E. R. (1973). Florence Nightingale's values and modern nursing education. *Nursing Forum, 12*(1), 7-47.

BROWN, E. L. (1948). *Nursing for the future, a report prepared for the National Nursing Council.* New York: Russell Sage.

CARNEGIE, M. E. (1976). *Historical perspectives of nursing research* (Presented to the Eastern Conference on Nursing Research). Boston: Nursing Archives.

COMMITTEE FOR THE STUDY OF NURSING EDUCATION. (1923). *Nursing and nursing education in the United States.* New York: Macmillan.

COMMITTEE ON THE FUNCTION OF NURSING. (1948). *A program for the nursing profession* (Ginzberg Report). New York: Macmillan.

COMMITTEE ON THE NURSING PROBLEM. (1948). Report of Committee on Nursing Problems (Murdock Report). *Journal of the American Medical Association, 137*(10), 878-879.

FULMER, H. (1902). History of visiting nurse work in America. *American Journal of Nursing, 2*(6), 411-426.

GOLER, G. W. (1904). Nurses' work in milk stations. *American Journal of Nursing, 4*(6), 417-423.

GRACE, H. (1983). Doctoral education in nursing: Dilemmas and directions. In Norma Chaska (Ed.), *The nursing profession: A time to speak.* New York: McGraw-Hill.

HITCHCOCK, J. E. (1902). Five hundred cases of Pneumonia. *American Journal of Nursing, 3*(3), 169-174.

LYSAUGHT, J. (1970). *An abstract for action.* New York: McGraw-Hill.

MACDONALD, M. V. (1906). Economy in the use of surgical supplies. *American Journal of Nursing, 6*(10), 676-685.

MARVIN, M. (1927). Research in nursing: The place of research and experimentation in improving the nursing care of the patient. *American Journal of Nursing, 27*(5), 331-335.

MONTAG, M. (1959). *Community college education for nursing: An experiment in technical education for nursing; report.* New York: McGraw-Hill.

MURDOCK, T. P. (1949). A physician's view point. *American Journal of Nursing, 49*(7), 439-441.

NIGHTINGALE, F. (1969). *Notes on nursing: What it is and what it is not* (pp. 9-10, 131-133). New York: Dover Publications, Inc. (originally published, 1859).

NIGHTINGALE, F. (1946). *Notes on nursing: What it is, and what it is not/by Florence Nightingale.* Philadelphia: Lippincott.

NIGHTINGALE, F. (1859). *Notes on nursing: What it is, and what it is not.* London: Harrison and Sons.

NIGHTINGALE, F. (1858). *Notes on matters affecting the health, efficiency and hospital administration of the British Army, founded chiefly on the experience of the late war,* presented by request to the Secretary of State for War. London: Harrison and Sons.

NUTTING, M. A. (1907). The education and professional position of nurses. In *Report of the Commissioner of Education for the year ending June 30, 1906.* Washington, D.C.: U.S. Government Printing Office, 155-205.

NUTTING, M. A., & DOCK, L. L. (1907). *A history of nursing.* New York: G.P. Putnam's Sons.

PALMER, I. (1977). Florence Nightingale: Reformer, reactionary, researcher. *Nursing Research, 26*(2), 84-89.

RICHARDS, E. H. (1906). Richards' invention. *American Journal of Nursing, 6*(1), 232-236.

ROBB, I. (1900). Hospital economics. *American Journal of Nursing, 1*(1), 29-36.

Toward quality in nursing: Needs and goals. (1963). Report of the Surgeon General's Consultant Group on Nursing. U.S. Public Health Service, Washington D.C., U.S. Government Printing Office.

U.S. DEPARTMENT OF HEALTH AND HUMAN SERVICES. (1992). *Healthy People 2000: Summary Report* (Publication No. PH591-50213). Boston: Jones & Bartlett.

CHAPTER 2

DEVELOPING NURSING KNOWLEDGE

LAURA A. TALBOT

Angela Clark is a researcher who has studied extensively in the area of endotracheal (ET) suctioning (Dyer 1993). One aspect of ET suctioning that has received little attention is what this experience means to the patient. When questioned, ICU patients will readily state that endotracheal suctioning is one of the worst experiences they have encountered; still, physiologic changes experienced by the patient during suctioning have never been related to the patient's fear level. While writing an article on oxygenation, a completely different topic, the notion of fear evolved. This researcher then postulated that part of the physiologic changes experienced by a patient during ET suctioning might be related to fear.

As this example shows, ideas rarely come from "out of the blue." Usually an individual is contemplating a situation or problem. When the solution does not come readily, we usually move on to other issues. Then, suddenly it comes—"Ah ha! Eureka! I've got an idea that might solve the problem." In fact, ideas come at the most un-

predictable times, such as while exercising, reading, or dreaming. Providing time for free thinking and the creative inspiration of new ideas is part of promoting the creative process and brings newly discovered possibilities to reality.

KNOWLEDGE DEVELOPMENT

Knowledge is information, and discovery is the creative process of obtaining new knowledge. The researcher seeks new knowledge. Concurrently, the goal of knowledge generation is its development into usable information. Nurses are creative and are known for cultivating new ideas and generating possibilities. Since scientific discovery is a creative process, nurses must use their creative abilities.

Creativity is often stifled when limitations are placed on the initial role of discovery in the research process. Placing narrow, precise, and standardized rules on researchers limits their freedom to consider new possibilities and cultivate new ideas.

25

Discovering new knowledge requires more than collecting facts or making observations. Creativity is not a standardized process that occurs by blindly following predetermined rules. Yet discovery is more than a chance occurrence, guesswork, or luck. A balance is needed in which attention is paid to detail, but in which imagination and daring ideas are used in the search for solutions.

Promoting natural curiosity, cultivating creative freedom, and being open to new ideas are methods vital to understanding, accessing, and implementing creativity. To develop new knowledge the nurse must be willing to take risks by making some good, imaginative guesses. The researcher uses the creative process to identify the problem and brainstorm possible solutions. Then follow-up is needed, since even the best idea is worthless unless it is acted on.

ᘒ THE IDEA: FORMAL AND INFORMAL DISCOVERY OF KNOWLEDGE

Kindling the creative spirit to promote nursing knowledge is a new challenge. In the past, nursing has followed the scientific method of problem solving to generate knowledge. While the scientific method clearly has merit, it is not without limitations, and these will be addressed later in the chapter. Other sources of nursing knowledge include informal sources such as intuition, trial and error, ritual and tradition, and input from experts; and formal sources such as observations and experience, acquisitions from other disciplines, and logical reasoning.

INTUITION

Intuition is an informal method of discovery. In Western society it has seldom been granted legitimacy as a sound approach to research, because intuition is hard to pin-point. Researchers prefer phenomena to be directly measurable or amenable to rigorous analytic thought processes. Instead, intuition is spontaneous and emotion based.

Yet one's first judgment about a new idea is often intuitive. It is the intuitive flash that makes the individual stop and say, "I've got it!" Too often the novice perceives the best way to approach knowledge as occurring through the rigors of the scientific method, focusing on quantification and objective reasoning, keeping biases, emotions, and opinions from contaminating the findings. Yet it is through intuitive imagination that new knowledge is discovered and through logical reasoning that its worth is proven.

Walker and Avant (1988) acknowledge that intuition is a valid method of theory generation and propose a comprehensive set of strategies to facilitate the intuitive processes that theorists already use in forming concepts, statements, and theories. These approaches are analysis, synthesis, and derivation. Analysis is used to clarify or refine concepts, statements, or theories. Synthesis is used with data-based information, seemingly unconnected, to construct new concepts, statements, or theory. Derivation involves the technique of analogy to transpose and redefine concepts, statements, or theory (Walker and Avant 1988). Their strategies have been used as guidelines by many theorists in the development of theory, statement, and concept. Yet they acknowledge that these strategies are not a substitute for the creative work required of the theorist.

TRIAL AND ERROR

Another informal method of knowledge acquisition is the use of trial and error. When a solution does not exist, the researcher conducts multiple trials to test various possibilities until error is adequately decreased. Clinical problems bring special challenges in the search for new ideas. For example, a stoma product that works for one individual might be completely inappropriate for another. The nurse could test a series of products until the one that works best is found.

This approach has been common in nursing, where observation and experience rather than theory have guided practice. Many call this the "school of hard knocks," in which years of practical knowledge and the use of the human senses make a seasoned professional of great value.

EXPERT IN THE FIELD

An expert in the field possesses not only experiential knowledge but theoretical understanding in a specific area. The combination of these two sources of knowledge fully describes an expert. By using this repertoire of information, experts act as a resource and catalyst in guiding the development of nursing knowledge.

Experts are used in research to contribute information in their area of expertise or to validate an instrument of measurement. Experts are asked to use their knowledge to review written material for publication. In a referred journal, manuscripts are sent to experts in the field to analyze and make recommendations for publication.

To evaluate an instrument of measurement, a panel of experts is used to determine content validity. The panel evaluates each item on the questionnaire to see if it indeed measures the content being assessed. Information is provided to the researcher so the instrument can be modified to reflect the construct of interest.

RITUAL/TRADITION

Rituals and traditions are another informal method of knowledge development. Many, including detailed procedural methods, have been passed down from generation to generation without rigorous testing. Re-

search is needed to determine which of these rituals are indeed valid and should be continued, so that high-quality nursing care is delivered in a cost-effective manner.

ACQUISITION FROM OTHER DISCIPLINES

Another informal method of generating new knowledge is to take an idea or theory from another discipline and examine it from a new perspective. The use of creativity allows one to look at a presumably understood phenomenon and see something that no one else has seen, to look at old knowledge in a new way. Noted nursing theorist Martha Rogers (1970) used this method to develop her conceptual model of unitary man. Four concepts basic to her theory are energy fields, open system, pattern and organization, and four-dimensionality. Taking from other disciplines, she refined these concepts within a nursing framework, developing a specific knowledge base for nursing practice, research, and theory development. For example, energy, pattern, and organization originated from physics; the concept of system came from von Bertalanffy's (1968) general systems theory; and four-dimensionality was originally proposed by Einstein.

LOGICAL REASONING

New knowledge may be developed formally through the use of logical reasoning. Two methods of logical reasoning are deductive and inductive reasoning. Deductive reasoning is the process of making assumptions or predictions based on reasoning from the general to the specific. It involves drawing inferences from principles that are already known. Deductive reasoning is used to generate a hypothesis from a conceptual framework. The researcher selects a specific relationship or proposition to test that has been deduced or partially derived from an existing theory.

Coffman, Levitt, and Brown (1994) used

deductive reasoning in their study testing Levitt's (1991) theoretical model of support expectations between a couple after childbirth. The primary focus was on changes in close relationships during a couple's transition into parenthood. From the theory, three hypotheses were deduced to test the theoretical propositions centering around the vulnerability of a couple experiencing the major life transition of parenthood. The result of this transition is an increase in support needs and a test of the individual's expectations.

Inductive reasoning is the process of making generalizations based on reasoning from the specific to the general. The researcher observes emerging patterns from the examination of specific events. Inductive reasoning is used when specific ideas generate identification of concepts that progress to theoretical propositions. The process of analytic induction in qualitative research involves the identification of variables that generate theory.

Inductive reasoning was used in Price's (1993) phenomenologic study exploring healthy and chronically ill adults' understanding of their own body awareness termed *body listening*. An example to describe this experience is a diabetic describing hypoglycemia. "I usually know it's coming on. My blood feels effervescent" (p. 38). Colaizzi's (1978) method of data analysis saw repetitious statements from informants emerge into specific patterns and themes. Significant patterns and themes were then integrated into an exhaustive description, resulting in a new body paradigm.

∾ THE SCIENTIFIC PROBLEM-SOLVING APPROACH

The scientific approach to problem-solving is a systematic, objective method of discovery that uses empirical evidence and rigorous control. The researcher applies this approach to a specific problem, adding to the scientific knowledge base through discovery of new knowledge, expansion and validation of existing knowledge, and the reaffirmation of previous knowledge.

Fundamental to the scientific method is control. Control is achieved by holding conditions constant and varying only the phenomena under study. The strengths of the scientific method are also its limitations: structure and control. The rigors of the scientific method focus on structure and control to establish a cause-and-effect relationship. This is conducive to theory testing, but limits theory generation. The amount of structure yields specific information obtained with only a fraction of the theory examined. A loosely structured research method is also needed to generate theory to show the totality of the human experience of the phenomenon under study.

∾ APPROACHES TO RESEARCH

Research may be categorized in many ways, depending on its purpose, setting, time involved, degree of control exerted, and specific design used. This section discusses various categories of research, including basic vs applied research, laboratory vs field research, retrospective vs prospective research, cross-sectional vs longitudinal research, experimental vs nonexperimental research, and quantitative vs qualitative research. It is important to remember that these are not mutually exclusive categories; all studies will fall somewhere within each of the categories discussed. For example, a study may be basic, retrospective, cross-sectional, nonexperimental, quantitative field research.

BASIC VS APPLIED RESEARCH

Basic research, sometimes called pure research, focuses on the development of new knowledge by developing, testing, and expanding theory. It is the pursuit of new knowledge for its own sake. Any practical application of the research is secondary to knowledge generation. Using this knowledge, a theory is developed, tested, expanded, and evaluated. Creative processes are promoted in the pursuit of theory development. Research conducted to test or expand theory is done within a unifying conceptual framework to validate the theory, building on past research. Testing theoretical propositions and performing a concept analysis are examples of basic research. Other examples of basic research are some of the studies done by NASA. Research conducted in space is many times a pursuit of new knowledge in the hope of future application.

Applied research seeks knowledge to solve a specific problem. Applied studies generate research-based knowledge to address issues in nursing practice, education, and administration. Theory is also the basis of applied research. Applied research emphasizes the use of theory in predicting future occurrences of the problem.

An example of applied research is a study by Miller and Bodie (1994) in which they observed that commercially prepared patient education materials were often written at the ninth-grade reading level. The assumption was "that the last grade level completed equals literacy skill . . ." (p. 118). Because they were not convinced of this assumption, their research conducted at a Department of Veterans Affairs medical center determined that 80% of the veterans in their sample were partially illiterate, indicating that the comprehension level of that patient group was below the ninth-grade reading level. This study has immediate application to the development of education materials, suggesting that the reading level of much current patient literature is too high and should be rewritten at a lower level.

Both basic and applied research are necessary and form a reciprocal relationship in generating nursing knowledge. Applied research will generate theoretical questions that will be tested by basic research. Reciprocally basic research generates theory that is validated in practice through applied research.

LABORATORY VS FIELD RESEARCH

Research may occur in many different settings. Laboratory research takes place in a sterile or highly controlled environment in which every aspect of that environment is accounted for by the researcher. A simulated environment would also be considered a form of laboratory research. This is an environment that is constructed to imitate the appearance, form, or sound of an actual situation or setting. Areas that would be controlled are: temperature, lighting, size of the room or cage, and furniture arrangement. Even the color of the walls should be taken into account as it could influence the results of the study. An example of such a simulated study would be investigating the relationship between music played in the operating room and staff errors. Simulated research could not be conducted during an actual surgery, so the situation and setting could be constructed to measure staff errors when a variety of music is played.

Laboratory research is frequently criticized because it creates an artificial situation from which it is difficult to generalize the findings of the study to other populations. In addition, laboratory research frequently uses laboratory animals as subjects and generalizes those results to humans. The goal of laboratory research is to minimize the artificiality of the environment while maximizing environmental control.

Often laboratory experiments are not conducive to answering the researcher's questions. The researcher needs to study the subjects in the natural setting of the occurrence. Field research is then conducted. It is a research study conducted in a "real life" setting. Most nursing studies involve research in the field. For example, to study interactions between preterm infants and their mothers in a neonatal intensive care unit (NICU), a field study would be conducted in the NICU area.

RETROSPECTIVE VS PROSPECTIVE STUDIES

A researcher may study a phenomenon as it is occurring or after it has occurred. Retrospective (or ex post facto) studies are those in which the phenomenon of interest has already occurred. The researcher then looks for other factors in an attempt to identify what may have contributed to the phenomenon occurring. One example is to identify individuals with chronic obstructive pulmonary disease (COPD) and look for common factors that are related to COPD, such as a history of smoking.

In prospective studies (also called longitudinal studies), an independent variable is identified. Subjects are then observed over time for the occurrence of the dependent variable. For example, a researcher might identify individuals who smoke (independent variable) and follow them over a period of time to evaluate the effects of smoking on their health (dependent variable) compared to the health of a group of non-smokers.

CROSS-SECTIONAL VS LONGITUDINAL STUDIES

Studies differ in the way they collect data over time. Two approaches are cross-sec-tional and longitudinal (also called prospective studies). They allow us to examine age-related changes. For example, age-related changes associated with physiologic aging have been examined quite extensively. Both the cross-sectional and longitudinal approaches have been used to describe body changes as we age. When using the cross-sectional approach, the researcher takes a representative sample of different age groups: a 20-year-old group, a 50-year-old group, and an 80-year-old group. Body make-up is described at the same time for all the groups. Then physical changes for each age group are compared. For example, kyphosis, an exaggeration of the posterior thoracic curve of the spine, is a common development in older adults. When a cross-sectional study is conducted, the researcher can assess the degree of spinal curvature seen in each age group and compare the differences at one point in time.

Longitudinal studies follow the same person over time. Subjects are examined at least twice, usually with a number of years between each examination. In the above kyphosis example, subjects would be followed over a period of time, and the angle of spinal curvature would be measured at age 20, again at age 50, and finally at age 80. Any changes in the angle of spinal curvature would be compared as they occurred over time.

The advantage of the cross-sectional approach is that only one testing period is needed. The disadvantage is that because different groups are studied the researcher cannot be sure if personal differences, culture, educational background, and values are being measured rather than age-related changes.

The advantage of the longitudinal study is that the same individuals are used throughout the study. The researcher can be certain that personal factors are the same. The disadvantage is that the research takes years to complete, and participants may drop out of the study. In addition, the effects of testing may influence the results.

A caution should be interjected when generalizing study findings from cross-sectional research. Changes seen in cross-sectional studies may be related to cohort differences instead of age-related changes. A difference seen in a cross-sectional study needs to be replicated using a longitudinal design to validate these differences and assure they are truly age-related.

EXPERIMENTAL VS NONEXPERIMENTAL RESEARCH DESIGNS

Research is also categorized by the actions taken by the investigator. An experimental design is one in which the researcher actively manipulates the subjects in some way in order to show a cause-and-effect relationship. The experimental design's ability to demonstrate causality depends on the degree to which the effects of the treatment (the cause) can be detected by measurement of the dependent variable (the effect).

The three critical elements in experimental research are randomization, manipulation, and control. *Randomization* is the assignment of subjects to conditions within the experiment. This occurs after subjects are randomly selected for the study. They are randomly assigned into an experimental or control group, giving each an equal and independent chance of being included in either group. The independent variable is then *manipulated* for the experimental group only. The data solicited from the control and experimental groups are then compared to determine whether differences exist. *Control* is achieved by screening out extraneous variables and by holding constant all factors other than the independent variable. Because of these features, experimental research is considered the most powerful research method.

The focus of nonexperimental research

is to describe how a phenomenon exists in nature *without* manipulation. Since the researcher does not manipulate or control the variables, a cause-and-effect relationship cannot be demonstrated. Random assignment is not used because members of the group are included in the study based on the characteristics or traits they possess. For example, if a researcher was studying factors associated with breast cancer, one group would consist of individuals with breast cancer and the other would consist of individuals without breast cancer. The researcher would solicit information hoping to discover differences between the groups that could possibly be associated with breast cancer; for example, increased age or family history.

QUALITATIVE VS QUANTITATIVE RESEARCH

Qualitative and quantitative research are two distinct approaches to conducting research. The researcher chooses the method based on the current level of knowledge about the phenomenon and the problem to be studied. Qualitative research explores phenomena about which little is known and that cannot easily be quantified or categorized. Quantitative research examines specific concepts and their relationships to test theory.

A qualitative approach is chosen when the phenomenon of interest is not easily quantifiable and little is known about the domain but the researcher suspects a phenomenon exists. Qualitative research focuses on identifying and describing new phenomena. It does not prove or disprove a hypothesis. The study sample is usually small and nonrepresentative. Using data collection techniques of open-ended interviews and participant observations, the researcher takes the participant's perspective when describing a phenomenon. Experimental controls are not placed upon the phenomenon being studied. The method is flexible and evolves as the study progresses. To accomplish this the research is conducted in a naturalistic setting. The researcher inductively discovers patterns or themes within the context of the research design used; for example, phenomenology, grounded theory, ethnography, or historiography.

In contrast, the quantitative approach is chosen when the phenomenon is easily quantified or classified. The researcher uses a deductive approach by selecting the theory, defining the concepts, hypothesizing variable relationships, collecting the data, statistically analyzing the data, and interpreting the findings. The hypotheses are then accepted or rejected and the theory supported or modified based on the findings. The study sample is usually large and representative of the population. Whenever possible, intervening variables are controlled so causality may be explained and accurate predictions about the variables are possible.

LEVELS OF RESEARCH

The four levels of research are exploratory, descriptive, correlational, and experimental. The level chosen will depend on how much knowledge exists about the phenomenon of interest.

Exploratory research identifies and describes concepts related to the phenomenon under study. It is used in the early stages when little is known. Both qualitative and quantitative approaches to research can be used to gather data.

Descriptive research allows a researcher to systematically describe a phenomenon as it occurs in its natural environment. This level is used when the phenomenon has been identified but little else is known about it. The researcher accumulates data

that are solely descriptive and does not seek to explain, predict, or control the variables. The purpose of descriptive research is to describe the identified phenomena with clarity and refinement to generate relationships for further research or theory modification.

When a phenomenon has been described but relationships or propositions between variables are not understood, correlational research is undertaken to explore relationships. Correlational research seeks to discover if there is a relationship among the variables and/or the degree to which that relationship exists. Cook and Campbell (1979) use the term *passive observation* to describe correlational research, because the design is a nonintrusive observational study (without manipulation) in a natural setting. Quantification of the data is necessary so that a correlation coefficient can be statistically calculated to show a relationship between the variables. The variables are not manipulated because the purpose is still to describe them as they exist in their natural setting.

Once a phenomenon has been described and relationships explored, experimental research can be used. A theory that predicts relationship is then needed so cause and effect can be established. The data are quantifiable, requiring quantitative methods. With experimental research the researcher manipulates one variable (the independent variable) to study its effect on another (the dependent variable). Control is used to eliminate all other factors that might influence the dependent variable.

SUMMARY

- Developing knowledge involves the use of creative thinking and idea generation techniques.
- Informal methods for the discovery of

new knowledge include intuition, trial and error, expert consultation, ritual/tradition, and acquisition from other disciplines. While they are less rigorous than formal methods, they are equally valid.

- The scientific approach to problem solving is a formal method of discovery. It is a systematic, objective approach to problem solving that uses empirical evidence and rigorous control.
- Logical reasoning is a formal approach that includes inductive and deductive reasoning. Inductive reasoning involves generalizations from specific incidents, while deductive reasoning involves specific predictions based on general principles.
- Conceptual dichotomies in approaches to research techniques include basic vs applied research, laboratory vs field research, retrospective vs prospective studies, cross-sectional vs longitudinal studies, nonexperimental vs experimental studies, and qualitative vs quantitative research.
- Exploratory, descriptive, correlational, and experimental are four levels of research. The level chosen depends on the current level of knowledge of the phenomenon under study. Exploratory research identifies and describes concepts; correlational research explores relationships between variables; and experimental research tries to ascertain a cause-and-effect relationship.

FACILITATING CRITICAL THINKING

Be a creative thinker. Conceptualize an idea or problem by using these steps to seek a creative solution:

1. State the problem or idea of interest.
2. Write down as many aspects of the problem/idea as you can, using the entire paper. Write in a linear, circular, or hierarchical mode to try to see the problem and its relationships on the paper. (Some people refer to this brainstorming procedure as mind mapping.)
3. Now use arrows to connect the flow of the conceptual aspects of the problem/idea.
4. Next circle various groupings or themes and place them into several dominant categories.
5. Finally write down various solutions to the problem to see what new resolutions evolve.

References

SUBSTANTIVE

COFFMAN, S., LEVITT, M., & BROWN, L. (1994). Effects of clarification of support expectations in prenatal couples. *Nursing Research, 43*(2), 111-116.

DYER, J. (1993). Putting critical care research into practice. *American Journal of Nursing, 93*(7), 51-56.

LEVITT, M. J. (1991) Attachment and close relationships: A life span perspective. In J. L. Hewirtz and W. F. Kurtines (Eds.), *Intersections with attachment* (pp 183-206). Hillsdale, NJ: Erlbaum.

MILLER, B., & BODIE, M. (1994). Determination of reading comprehension level for effective patient health-education materials. *Nursing Research, 43*(2), 118-119.

PRICE, M. (1993). Exploration of body listening: Health and physical self-awareness in chronic illness. *Advances in Nursing Science, 15*(4), 37-52.

THOMPSON, C. (1992). *What a great idea! Key steps creative people take.* New York: Harper Perennial.

CONCEPTUAL

ROGERS, M. (1970). *An introduction to the theoretical basis of nursing.* Philadelphia: F.A. Davis Company.

VON BERTALANFFY, L. (1968). *General system theory.* New York: George Braziller, Inc.

WALKER, L., & AVANT, K. (1988). *Strategies for theory construction in nursing.* Norwalk, Ct: Appleton-Century-Crofts.

METHODOLOGICAL

SARNECKY, M. (1990). Historiography: A legitimate research methodology for nursing. *Advances in Nursing Science, 12*(4),1-10.

HISTORICAL

CAMPBELL, D., & STANLEY, J. (1963). *Experimental and quasi experimental designs for research.* Chicago: Rand McNally.

COLAIZZI, P. (1978). Psychological research as the phenomenologist views it. In R. Vale and M. King (Eds.), *Existential-phenomenological alternatives for psychology* (pp. 48-71). New York: Oxford University Press.

COOK, C., & CAMPBELL, D. (1979). *Quasi-experimental: Design and analysis issues for field settings.* Chicago: Rand McNally.

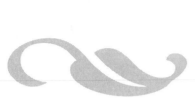

CHAPTER 3

ETHICS IN RESEARCH

JOAN GARITY

- A well-respected clinical nurse specialist fabricates the data in a national pain study.
- A faculty member from a prestigious school of nursing publishes multiple articles from the same research study listing co-authors who did not make significant contributions.
- A nurse administrator embellishes the statistics on cost-effectiveness in the annual report of a top-ten teaching hospital.

All of the above scenarios are fictitious, but consider the following, which are true:

- A prominent cardiac physician fabricated data for several years, which were first published, later retracted, in a national medical journal (Relman, 1983).
- A hospital psychiatrist from a world-renowned university resigned after multiple examples of plagiarism were observed in four papers written years earlier in his career (McDonald, 1988).
- Two scientists were found guilty of falsely conducting and reporting scientific research at a major West Coast university (Palca, 1990).

If the above examples are happening in the biomedical sciences, could they just as easily take place in nursing? If so, how? If not, why? What ethical principles exist to guide nurses conducting research? In today's complex and highly technological health care system, which ethical codes of conduct can be employed to protect human subjects, secure their informed consent, and maintain their confidentiality as participants in a research study? When reading a research article or study, how can the nurse detect fraud or misconduct? In designing a research study, how can the principal nurse investigator protect the most vulnerable populations: the elderly, the HIV-infected, and the cognitively impaired? What cultural differences exist that may affect obtaining informed consent? The answers to these and other relevant ethical questions in nursing research are fully explored in this chapter.

REVIEW OF ETHICAL PRINCIPLES

Ethics is a form of philosophic inquiry used to investigate morality (Fry, 1991). It is based on scientific ethical principles that are used to justify actions and assist in the resolution of moral dilemmas. According to Beauchamp and Childress (1994) there are four main ethical principles: autonomy, nonmaleficence, beneficence, and justice. These principles, which can help the nurse researcher in carrying out the ethical duties and responsibilities involved in nursing research, are summarized below:

Autonomy: The individual is free to make independent decisions without the coercion of others. This is usually referred to as the self-determination of an individual. It includes the concept of privacy.

Nonmaleficence: The individual neither intends nor permits risk or harm to another person.

Beneficence: The individual acts to prevent harm, remove harmful conditions, and promote positive benefits for others.

Justice: The individual gives to each person what is owed or due.

For a more detailed explanation of each principle, the reader is referred to Beauchamp and Childress (1994).

RELATIONSHIP OF ETHICAL PRINCIPLES TO NURSING RESEARCH

AUTONOMY

Individuals may choose to participate in a research study. This choice must be made free from coercion or the threat of harm. This principle also allows the individual to withdraw from the study at any time without penalty or loss of benefit. Competency of the individual is central to the concept of autonomy, particularly where vulnerability may exist: the elderly, the mentally ill, or the HIV-infected. Competency will be discussed in more detail in this chapter's section on informed consent. Other points of emphasis in autonomy include disclosure, understanding, and voluntariness.

Disclosure

Disclosure of necessary information is needed for a patient to make a decision in a research project (Beauchamp & Childress (1994, pp. 146-163). For example, a patient should be told the known risks and benefits of an experimental treatment. It should be noted that in some studies, however, it is necessary to withhold information that could potentially invalidate the findings. This is called incomplete disclosure. An example would be a double blind study (neither the researcher nor the patient know who is receiving the treatment) of a new drug in which one group of patients receives a placebo while another group receives an experimental drug.

Understanding

The nurse researcher is obligated to facilitate obtaining good decisions based on sound information from the ignorant, sick, frightened, or inexperienced patient (Beauchamp & Childress, p. 157). This includes discussing other available choices and how these may be better or worse than participating in the study.

Voluntariness

This implies that the individual is free of manipulative and coercive influences exerted by others (Beauchamp & Childress, p. 163). For example, students who do not participate in a faculty member's research should not feel that their grades will be adversely affected.

NONMALEFICENCE

This principle states that no harm will come to the subject from participating in the research study. The Department of Health and Human Services (HHS) has defined the risk of harm to a research subject as exposure to injury beyond everyday situations, including physical, emotional, legal, financial, or social harm. The nurse researcher must do everything possible to minimize such risks in a research study. However, risks in a nursing research study may be subtle. For example, increased anxiety and guilt may be found in parents participating in a study questionnaire to elicit "family health issues" after the death of a child from sudden infant death syndrome (SIDS). This type of study would require a debriefing (disclosing information previously withheld) and provision for referral counseling in its protocol. Other examples of potential harm include a 50% risk of receiving ineffective or substandard care or treatment when participating in randomized hospital trials on pain, nausea and vomiting, or infection.

BENEFICENCE

The nurse researcher balances the associated benefits and risks of the subject's participation in the study. The benefits should outweigh any associated risks. Levine (1981) has classified risk into four categories:

Physical: Adverse reaction to an experimental drug or treatment protocol.

Psychologic: An increase in anxiety secondary to being a research subject.

Social: Participation in a sensitive topic study (alcohol or HIV) could result in labeling or loss of privacy for the subject.

Economic: Financial threats such as loss of a job, money, or health insurance if participation in the research study becomes known. These risks will be addressed in more detail later in this chapter's section on research design.

JUSTICE

Samples and populations for a research study should be selected equally from all populations. For example, populations such as the elderly, mentally ill, military, and prisoners should not be used merely for their convenience.

୬ ETHICAL RULES IN PROFESSIONAL-PATIENT RELATIONSHIPS

According to Beauchamp and Childress (1994), the four basic ethical principles can be used to establish related ethical rules of conduct: veracity, privacy, confidentiality, and fidelity. These rules can then be applied in the analysis of the professional relationship that must exist between the research subject and the nurse researcher. These four ethical rules of conduct in the patient-professional relationship are summarized below:

Veracity: Obligation to tell the truth, not to lie or deceive others (Veatch & Fry, 1987). For example, individuals should know the purpose of a study, such as testing a new clinical drug or treatment. The researcher needs to refrain from raising false hopes in the patient about the potential effects of the drug or treatment in this situation.

Privacy: Obligation to maintain the state or condition of limited access to a person, including knowledge or information about the person's body, relationships, or secrets (Beauchamp & Childress, 1994, p. 406). The nurse researcher ensures this by keeping any information obtained in a research study anonymous, including letters, diaries, and school or health records. Privacy can be facilitated by using code numbers for subjects' identity so that even the researcher can not link reported information to the subjects. A master code list should be kept in a separate locked cabinet.

Confidentiality: Obligation not to divulge information learned in treating or caring for a patient to a third party without the patient's permission to do so (Beauchamp & Childress, 1994, pp. 418-429). This is especially important when the information may carry a stigma, such as HIV positive status, or evidence of a prison record. Confidentiality is especially important when the research involves a sensitive topic such as domestic violence. Access to the raw data in these studies should be limited to the principal investigator to decrease any threat of loss of confidentiality.

Fidelity: Obligation to remain faithful to one's commitments, which includes keeping promises, maintaining confidentiality, and demonstrating caring behaviors (Fry, 1991, p. 157). For the nurse researcher this means conducting the research study as outlined in the section on informed consent, following the steps and procedures of the treatment design, reporting data anonymously, and demonstrating through caring behaviors that the patient is more important as a person than the information learned from the study, such as the ef-fects and benefits of a new drug or treatment.

RESEARCH WITH HUMAN SUBJECTS

Formal experimentation with human subjects to improve medical treatment of disease has existed since the late eighteenth century (Adams, 1985). Society began to regulate such research in the middle of the twentieth century as public awareness grew about the increasing numbers of such experiments, and the potential for abuse of subjects' human rights. Recent years have seen the development of professional codes and laws to control the conduct of scientific research (Oddi & Cassidy, 1990).

HISTORICAL CASES OF ABUSES IN HUMAN RIGHTS

It is shocking to consider, but serious violations of the human rights of subjects often took place in the recent past, supposedly to advance the biomedical sciences. Some of the more well-known cases are:

Nazi "Medical" Experiments
Highly qualified Nazi physicians and scientists conducted "medical" experiments with appalling disregard for the human rights of their prisoner subjects. These included, among others, mass sterilization, genetic reengineering, deliberate infection of wounds with gas gangrene, and malaria (Steinfels & Levine, 1976).

The Tuskegee Experiment
Over 400 black Alabama sharecroppers and day laborers were denied treatment for syphilis from 1932 to 1972 in a government study so physicians could study the effects of the untreated disease (Jones, 1981).

LSD

An American soldier was administered lysergic acid diethylamide (LSD) without his knowledge in an United States Army Intelligence Corps experiment conducted between 1955 and 1958. The soldier subsequently suffered hallucinations, periods of memory loss, and episodes of wife-beating (*U.S. v. Stanley*, 1987).

Jewish Chronic Disease Hospital in Brooklyn, 1963

A physician injected hospitalized patients with live cancer cells without their informed consent (Bandman, 1985).

RECENT CASES

- During World War II 732 Navy submariners and 6881 Army airmen received radium treatments to reduce nasal swelling associated with differences in air pressure during training. There have been recent claims by many of these individuals that they were not fully informed about this procedure, and that they believe they are suffering related effects such as throat cancer and thyroid problems (Robinson, 1994).
- During the 1940s, 1950s, 1960s, and 1970s, 45 United States teaching hospitals exposed human test subjects to head-to-toe radiation while conducting research. Whether the research was done for medical science, the government, or both is unclear. President Clinton has appointed a committee to evaluate whether these experiments were medically or scientifically necessary (Whole-body radiation cases cited, 1994).

The reader should consider that most of the above-cited experiments, with the exception of the Nazi war crimes, were conducted with the Nuremburg Code and the Declaration of Helsinki in place and fully operational. Why some scientists act unethically, which is incongruent with the scientific goal to discover truth, is not completely known or understood. Some journal editors, scientists, and professors have identified several reasons: (1) limited guidance for the young scientist (Miskin, 1988; Relman, 1983; Woolf, 1981), (2) the phenomenon of excessive publications (Smith, 1985), (3) pressures of tenure and promotion in academe (Woolf, 1986), and (4) inadequacies and bias in the peer review system (Lock, 1985).

DEVELOPMENT OF ETHICAL CODES OF CONDUCT

THE NUREMBURG CODE

The Nuremburg Code was developed in 1947 to address problems in human experimentation, specifically the revelations of Nazi atrocities conducted during World War II. The core of the Nuremburg Code is protection of human subjects, particularly obtaining their informed consent. Additional principles emphasize that research with human subjects be based on the results of prior animal experimentation, free of unnecessary physical and mental harm to subjects, and conducted for the good of society by qualified researchers (Fromer, 1981). Finally, these principles have shaped the field of biomedical research and are the most highly recognized and developed maxims on research with human subjects.

THE DECLARATION OF HELSINKI

This is a set of ethical guidelines for clinical research developed by the 1964 World Medical Association held in Finland (Silverman, 1983). In addition to reiterating the Nuremburg Code, it added language on the protection of subjects' rights. Periodic up-dates have stressed use of (1) scientific prin-ciples, (2) adequate research design, (3) qualified researchers, and (4) minimal risk to subjects (Curran & Shapiro, 1982). A major contribution of the declaration is the distinction it draws between therapeutic and nontherapeutic research. For example, strong, independent justification is re-quired to allow an investigator to expose a healthy volunteer to substantial harm to gain new information such as in drug and vaccine trials (World Medical Association, 1964).

THE PATIENT'S BILL OF RIGHTS

This document, set forth by the American Hospital Association in 1973 and revised in 1992, addresses informed consent, privacy, and confidentiality within institutional set-tings such as hospitals. Particular emphasis is placed on the right of patients to choose to participate or to choose not to partici-pate in human experimentation in agen-cies.

BELMONT REPORT

The Belmont Report (National Commis-sion, 1978) identified three basic ethical principles of research: respect for persons, beneficence, and justice. These principles can guide the nurse researcher in designing procedures for selecting subjects, develop-ing written consents, and assessing risk/ benefits ratios of proposed research stud-ies.

NURSING CODES

The 1893 Nightingale Pledge can be con-sidered the first code of ethics for the nurs-ing profession (Fowler and Levine-Ariff, 1987). More recently, the American Nurses' Association (ANA) has issued three publica-tions that can help the nurse researcher in exploring ethical concerns that arise in practice and research. These are the Code for Nurses (ANA, 1985), Guidelines for the Investigative Functions of Nurses (ANA, 1981), and Human Rights Guidelines for Nurses in Clinical and Other Research (ANA, 1985). In addition there is an inter-national code of ethics for nursing and an international concord for nursing research (Fowler, 1988).

Code for Nurses

Although the Code for Nurse addresses pri-marily practice issues, it does contain lan-guage that can be applied to research ef-forts. For example, the need to respect human dignity, protect the confidentiality of patient records, and safeguard the public from incompetent, unethical, or illegal practices are all discussed.

Guidelines for Investigative Functions

The Guidelines for Investigative Functions describe research activity for nurses pre-pared at different educational levels: associ-ate degree, baccalaureate, masters, and doctorate levels. Concern for ethics is ex-pressed in statements about the nurse's role in designing and carrying out research (ex-pertise), application of research to the pa-tient situation (benefit to society), and the quality of research-based protocols in the clinical setting (accountability).

Human Rights Guidelines

The Human Rights Guidelines underscore the principles in the Nuremburg Code con-cerned with voluntary participation of sub-jects, such as recruitment of subjects, pro-tection of their human rights, and informed consent. The nurse's role in the collection of data and participation in dou-ble-blind studies (where neither the nurse or the patient knows whether the experi-mental or control treatment is being ad-ministered) are also discussed.

International Code of Ethics

As early as 1953 member nations of the International Council of Nurses adopted a code of ethics for nursing (Grady, 1989). By 1977 the council published descriptive statements of ethical problems in nursing practice developed by nurses from 25 member nations. Examples of these ethical problems are grouped to reflect the five main categories of the International Council of Nurses Code of Ethics: people; practice; society; co-workers; and the profession (Crisham, 1992).

During the 1987 International Congress on Nursing Research, jointly organized by Sigma Theta Tau, the Royal College of Nursing Research Society, and the University of Edinburgh, it became evident that nurses from every part of the globe (33 member nations) were struggling with the same ethical issues: (1) protection of human subjects, and (2) actual conduct of nursing research (Fowler, 1988). Therefore, it was proposed that nursing develop an international concord or agreement for nursing research, which is still in the process of being developed (Fowler, Chaney, Davis, & Flynn, 1987).

∿ INFORMED CONSENT

The essence of the numerous codes of ethics reviewed above is protection of human subjects through informed consent. The following ethical practices govern the nurse researcher in obtaining informed consent. The Code of Federal Regulations (pp. 9-10) is used by most institutional review boards to define informed consent:

> . . . the knowing consent of an individual or his legally authorized representative, under circumstances that provide the prospective subject or representative suffi-

cient opportunity to consider whether or not to participate without undue inducement or any element of force, fraud, deceit, duress, or other forms of constraint or coercion.

For an individual to give informed consent, three elements are needed: (1) adequate information, (2) mental competence, and (3) freedom from coercion and vulnerability. At first glance this might seem to be a fairly easy and open process. Some of the potential difficulties that may arise for the nurse researcher in obtaining informed consent, however, are clearly illustrated by Grady (1989) within an HIV patient framework. For example, the HIV patient may be asked to participate in a research drug protocol that is still highly experimental (lack of adequate information). Since it is estimated that 60% to 70% of patients with AIDS have some degree of associated dementias (Price, et al., 1988), this may raise questions about their mental competence being compromised in regard to making autonomous decisions. Finally, because current available treatment and care options for HIV-infected persons are still limited, some patients may feel coerced in their range of choices.

ADEQUATE DISCLOSURE OF INFORMATION

For individuals to choose freely to participate in a research study, they must be fully informed about the following:

1. Purpose, methods, procedures, and processes of the study revealed in easily understood language. For example, "blood sugar (not glucose) levels will be tested every morning before breakfast."
2. Possible uses of the findings, and potential benefits to the individual and society. For example, "to identify

stressors for caregivers of Alzheimer patients, which will be used to plan follow-up resources and support groups."

3. Potential harms, risks, inconveniences, and discomforts. For example, "the individual may be randomly assigned to the control group, not the experimental group for a new pain medication."
4. Any side effects or results. For example, longitudinal follow-up studies or interviews.
5. Available alternatives. For example, methods of relaxation therapy for pain control.
6. The right to refuse to participate or to withdraw at any time.
7. Identity of the investigator(s) and how to contact.

In addition, the study must be free of deceit or deception. For example, participants should not be told that the study is investigating generalized family behaviors and practices if it really is intended to identify characteristics of wife or husband batterers. Financial compensation offered for the inconveniences (if any) of participating in the study (not as an inducement to participate) should be openly acknowledged. Finally, prospective participants should not be pressured to participate by repeated phone calls and follow-up letters if they have not responded to previous mailed consent forms.

COMPREHENSION

In addition to disclosing sufficient information about the research study, the nurse researcher must also address adequate comprehension of this information by the patient (Sorrell, 1991). According to Silva and Sorrell (1984), nurse researchers usually document disclosure but rarely specify methods of comprehension. This becomes critical based on the following cited in Sorrell (1991):

- Only 10% of subjects recalled discussing possible complications of their cardiac procedures.
- As few as 25% of subjects understood the purposes, risks, and freedom to withdraw from a clinical investigation protocol.
- Fully 50% of patients were confused about whether they consented to the use of a research drug or test.

Two studies by Silva and Sorrell (1984; 1988) identified several factors that influence comprehension of information for informed consent: type of information, method of presentation of information, subject's health patterns of recall, and attitudes toward the consent process. More recently, Sorrell (1991) found that specific writing and speaking strategies with patients in the informed consent process can augment the nurse researcher's efforts to enhance patient comprehension of the information. It should be noted that this study did not support the previously consistent body of research findings from multiple other studies that identified that a higher level of education was a powerful predictor of comprehension (Cassileth, et al., 1980).

Ethical implications raised by Silva and Sorrell (1984) relative to comprehension in informed consent, which should be considered by nurse researchers, are summarized below:

1. A clear, brief, and well-written consent form needs to be developed.
2. Allow a day or longer for subjects to read and digest the information.
3. Be aware that:

a. Individuals with lower educational and vocabulary levels may need more help in processing the consent form.
b. Forgetting may occur with threatening information.
c. Comprehension should be assessed independently of memory (pp. 238-239).

COMPETENCY

Most readers are already familiar with the concept of competency as this relates to nursing judgment in everyday practice; that is, that the patient is "sound enough in mind and body" (*Random House Webster's Dictionary,* 1993) to fully give or make an informed choice about naming a health care proxy, agreeing to surgery, or undergoing a specific test or treatment. Cooke (1986) and Veatch and Fry (1987) state that competence in adults should always be assumed unless careful evaluation, adjudication, or agreement by third parties (including the patient) suggest otherwise.

With respect to nursing research, participants must also be shown to be competent at the time of agreeing to participate in the study. This is particularly true in those studies where there is the threat of potential harm occurring during the course of the study because of sudden or increased vulnerability of the subject. One example of such a population is nursing home residents who begin to experience signs and symptoms of dementia. Another such group is HIV-infected individuals whose mental abilities are compromised secondary to a central nervous system infection. The astute nurse researcher can plan for such eventualities by suggesting the naming in the study's protocol of a designated proxy who will make decisions about the patient's continuance in the research study in the event of incompetence (Grady, 1989).

VULNERABILITY

Levine (1981) defined vulnerable individuals as those who (1) suffer from chronic or disabling illnesses, (2) experience increased feelings of loneliness such as the terminally ill, or (3) lack adequate funds and resources to obtain necessary health care. Recently Good and Fisher (1993) addressed vulnerability in the elderly as an ethical concern in clinical research. Specific questions they raised center around the nurse researcher determining: (1) the actual or potential vulnerability of the older adult, (2) whether or not the older adult still has the societal obligation to participate in such research, (3) the risks and benefits to the individual and the population, and (4) the methods used to assure autonomy and self-determination during informed consent, especially if there is loss of cognitive function.

It should be noted here that the American Bar Association (ABA) Commission on the Mentally Disabled recommended in 1976 that research with subjects who have cognitive disabilities be limited. Further the National Commission for the Protection of Human Subjects of Biomedical and Behavioral Research concluded in 1978 that the proposed research should:

> relate directly to the etiology, pathogenesis, prevention, diagnosis, or treatment of mental disability and only be sought if such information cannot be obtained from other types of subjects. (p. 156)

COERCION AND UNDUE INFLUENCE

The freedom (1) to choose to participate or not to participate in a research study, and (2) to do so free of undue influence or coercion are two important areas usually discussed under the concept of vulnerability. The National Commission for the Protection of Human Subjects of Biomedical and

Behavioral Research (1978) distinguishes coercion from undue influence:

> Coercion occurs when an overt threat of harm is intentionally presented by one person to another in order to obtain compliance. Undue influence, by contrast, occurs through an offer of an excessive, unwarranted, inappropriate or improper reward or other overture in order to obtain compliance. Also, inducements that would ordinarily be acceptable may become undue influence if the subject is especially vulnerable. (p. 14)

An example of undue influence could occur in situations in which the older adult is becoming more dependent on health care providers. For example, Duffy, et al. (1989) found that older veterans' decisions to participate in a research study were related, perhaps either out of loyalty to their caregivers or fear of reprisals, to the amount of veterans benefit income received.

Similarly, patients who are desperate, such as the HIV-infected or terminally ill, may feel coerced into participating in just one more research study with an experimental drug or research protocol for the sake of themselves, their family and loved ones, or their health care providers. Nurse researchers need to be alert for both overt and covert signs of undue influence in the process of obtaining informed consent from such patients.

CULTURAL CONSIDERATIONS

The nurse researcher may encounter cultural differences in the process of obtaining informed consent (Davis, 1990). For example, personhood in Africa is defined by the tribe, village, or social group, not by the individual as is so common in Western culture (De Craemer, 1983). Who then gives consent? In Uruguay the physician normally resolves all issues concerning the patient's health (France, 1988). China places more emphasis on the virtuous character of the health professional than the use of principle-based ethics as in the United States (Unschuld, 1989; Wilson, 1982). For example, China's Ministry of Public Health issued its first practice code in 1988, emphasizing the obligations of health workers', not patients', rights (Davis, 1990).

The above brief overview illustrates some of the differences and challenges that remain in addressing informed consent within different cultures. It is hoped that nurse researchers will begin to examine the ethical process of obtaining informed consent within these cultures in the near future.

Finally, the United States Department of Health and Human Services (1981) regulations provide a very comprehensive format for the nurse researcher seeking informed consent from participants. The box lists the basic elements needed for informed consent by the HHS.

INSTITUTIONAL REVIEW BOARD

Federal regulations require that institutions that receive significant federal funding or conduct drug or medical device research regulated by the Federal Drug Administration (FDA) establish institutional review boards (IRBs). The 1974 Code of Federal Regulations clearly described the activities under the review board's jurisdiction as follows:

> . . . any research, development, or related activities which depart from the application of those established and accepted methods necessary to meet the subject's needs or which increase the risk of daily life. (*Federal Register,* May 30, 1974)

The nurse researcher should obtain a copy of the written guidelines for investiga-

ELEMENTS NEEDED FOR INFORMED CONSENT

1. A statement that the study involves research, an explanation of the purposes of the research and the expected duration of the subject's participation, a description of the procedures to be followed, and identification of any procedures which are experimental;

2. A description of any reasonable foreseeable risks or discomforts to the subject;

3. A description of any benefits to the subject or to others which may reasonably be expected from the research;

4. A disclosure of appropriate alternative procedures or courses of treatment, if any, that might be advantageous to the subject;

5. A statement describing the extent, if any, to which confidentiality of records identifying the subject will be maintained;

6. For research involving more than minimal risk, an explanation as to whether any compensation and an explanation as to whether any medical treatments are available if injury occurs and, if so, what they consist of, or where further information may be obtained;

7. An explanation of whom to contact for answers to pertinent questions about the research subjects' rights, and whom to contact in the event of a research related injury to the subject; and

8. A statement that participation is voluntary, refusal to participate will involve no penalty or loss of benefits to which the subject is otherwise entitled, and the subject may discontinue participation at any time without penalty or loss of benefits to which the subject is otherwise entitled. (pp. 116-117)

From *Code of Federal Regulations*, Title 45, Part 46, Washington, DC, January 26, 1981.

---

tors from the potential institution(s) in which the research study will take place. These guidelines will contain information on how to gain approval, develop the consent form, prepare the protocols for human subjects, and expedite the review process.

The major responsibility of the IRB is to protect human subjects from unnecessary risk or deprivation of personal rights and dignity. The IRB does this by verifying that the wording of the consent form promotes the free self-determination of the potential research subjects. Particular attention is paid to the consent form involving vulnerable populations such as prisoners, minors, fetuses, unconscious patients, psychiatric patients, the mentally retarded, students, fellows, and employees. The nurse should be aware that many IRBs will not approve studies using these populations if similar information can be obtained from other adult subjects (Oddi & Cassidy, 1990). Robb (1983) argues that nurse researchers need to find creative solutions for obtaining written consent or risk losing entire study populations such as the elderly.

SUMMARY

All of the above considerations in informed consent are not meant to discourage but rather to alert the reader to the very real ethical concerns and questions that must be raised when validating that patients have given their informed consent in a nursing research project or study. The nurse researcher can determine this better if the study, its consent form, and related procedures acknowledge that the unique aspects of its population such as age, evidence of dementia, fear, discrimination, lack of adequate support systems, level of comprehension, and voluntariness have been properly addressed.

✎ ETHICAL ISSUES IN RESEARCH DESIGN

The research design is the overall plan for implementing the study. While violations of human rights could occur in any phase of the study, the greatest potential exists in three critical areas: (1) the idea being studied, (2) the selected sample, and (3) the specific type of study design.

IDEA

Ways to strengthen the study's ideas include a literature review, feasibility or case study, and a pilot study to demonstrate the significance and overall need for the research project or study.

SELECTED SAMPLE

One group should not be used disproportionately over another. Neither should the institutionalized elderly, populations of prisoners, or the military be used simply for convenience.

Recently, Lane, Cassell, and Bennett (1990) reviewed 143 articles in six separate journals that published research studies on elderly subjects. These authors found that only seven studies (4.9%) reported institutional review board approval; only 33 (23.1%) mentioned that informed consent was obtained; only 17 (11.9%) discussed the intact decisional capacity of their subjects, and nearly one quarter (25.5%) failed to mention how subjects were recruited.

SPECIFIC TYPE OF STUDY DESIGN

Exploratory, descriptive, and correlational study designs do not administer a treatment. What happens if the nurse re-searcher is working with elderly, terminal, or other compromised groups in a research project and the need for treatment is identified? Remember, the Tuskegee Syphilis Experiment (Jones, 1981) violated human rights because treatment was deliberately withheld to continue this exploratory study. More recently Miller and Evans (1991) eloquently addressed similar concerns in an article on nursing research with nursing home residents.

Quasi-experimental or experimental designs require use of a control group. The experimental group receives the treatment and the control group does not. The risks for each group need to be carefully addressed. This is even more true for double blind studies in which neither the nurse or the patient knows whether the experimental or control treatment is being administered.

An assessment tool for qualifying the risk-benefit ratio in a research study is shown in Figure 3-1. It enables the nurse researcher to assess critically each area described above and determine whether the risk-benefit ratio is balanced in favor of total benefits for the research study participants.

First the nature of each risk-benefit is identified according to the areas of physical, psychologic, social, and economic factors. Next a percentage is assigned as to the probability of occurrence. The percentile range is from 0% to 100%. Last, the degree of the risk-benefit is determined based on a scale of 0 to 5 (0 being the least and 5 being the most).

The scores for each column are added together. First, the total score for the estimated probability of risk is compared to the total score for estimated probability of benefit. The score for the estimated probability of risk should not be greater than the score for the estimated probability of benefit. If the estimated probability of risk score

Risk Benefit Assessment

1. State the nature of the risk/benefit.
2. Indicate in percentile the probability of occurrence.
3. On a scale of 1 to 5 indicate the degree of the risk/benefit.
4. Add the columns to obtain a total score.

	Risks			Benefits		
	Nature of risk	Estimated probability of occurrence	Degree of risk*	Nature of benefit	Estimated probability of occurrence	Degree of benefit*
Physical						
Psychological						
Social						
Economic						
Total score						

*Any injury of inhumane treatment is an automatic disqualification for the research to be initiated.

Figure 3-1. Assessment tool for calculating a risk-to-benefit ratio. (Prepared by Laura A. Talbot, RN, C, PhD.)

is higher, the study needs to be reevaluated to decrease the probability of risks or to increase the probability of benefits.

Next the degree of the risk score is compared to the degree of the benefit score. Again the risk score should not be greater than the degree of the benefit score. If the degree of the risk score is greater than the degree of the benefit score, the study needs to be reevaluated to decrease the degree of risk or increase the degree of benefit. It should be noted that any injury or inhumane treatment to the participant is an automatic disqualification for the research to be initiated.

An evaluation of the risk-benefit ratio should be calculated at the beginning of a research study and periodically throughout. If at any time the risks outweigh the benefits, the study should be terminated until a balance can be maintained.

MODEL FOR DETERMINING THE ETHICAL MERITS OF A RESEARCH STUDY

When determining the ethical merits of a research study, it may be beneficial to use this author's memory device (see box) developed from Wilson's 10 characteristics for judging the ethical merits of a study (1989, pp. 67-69) and Crisham's model for critically analyzing case studies in ethics (1992, p. 21).

ACCOUNTABILITY OF THE NURSE RESEARCHER

DISREPUTABLE SCIENCE
Disreputable science, either through fraud or misconduct, is not new. Examples include astronomers in the second century

EVALUATING THE ETHICAL ASPECTS OF RESEARCH

*E*xamine the study's reported results for evidence of:
- Freedom from bias, fraud, or misconduct.
- Review by an institutional board.
- Full disclosure of all risks, discomforts, and benefits to study participants.

*T*hink reflectively about:
- The Nuremburg Code
- The Declaration of Helsinki
- The Belmont Report
- The Patient's Bill of Rights
- The Code for Nurses
- The International Nurses Council Code of Ethics

*H*elp determine:
- The nurse's role and responsibilities as data collector.

- Acknowledgement of co-workers and work of others.
- Use of research assistants.
- Sources of financial support and other sponsors.

*I*dentify the steps and procedures used for:
- Informed consent
- Protection of human subjects from harm, deceit, coercion, and invasion of privacy
- Confidentiality and anonymity of data

*C*onfirm that there is:
- An adequate research design.
- A qualified nurse researcher.
- Assessment of the risk-benefit ratio.
- Fruitful results for utilization by the discipline of nursing.

and scientists in the seventeenth and twentieth centuries who were accused of exaggerating, falsifying, or using data from others without credit (Broad & Wade, 1982). During the twentieth century a famous British psychologist linked intelligence and heredity with invented data, and an American Nobel Prize winner published only part of his data (Broad & Wade, 1982). More recent examples include the case scenarios cited from the biomedical sciences earlier in this chapter. Finally, the National Institute of Health (NIH) estimates that there are 15 to 20 reported cases of scientific misconduct yearly from a pool of approximately 50,000 scientists (Windom, 1988).

According to Morrison (1990) nurse scientists have not been included in public accusations of scientific misconduct to date. Hawley and Jeffers (1992) agree but cite the potential for its occurrence secondary to increased competition for scarce funding; publication, tenure and promotion pressures, and the use of large research teams.

One way to prevent scientific misconduct from happening in nursing is to continue self-regulation by the profession (Gortner, 1974). Examples of self-regulation, a hallmark of science, recommended by Hawley and Jeffers (1992) include: (1) careful socialization of the young nurse scientist, (2) limiting the number of publications to two for tenure and promotion review, and (3) increasing the number of replication studies that will validate or detect problems with the data of the original study.

Additionally, nurse researchers need to be aware of the following definitions for judging disreputable science:

Fraud: Deliberate falsification, misrepresentation, or plagiarism of data, findings, or ideas of others (Broad & Wade, 1982; Angell, 1986; Miskin, 1988). An example would be to write the literature review portion of a study in which the work of another, such as Selye's work on stress (1976), is portrayed as one's own.

Misconduct: Includes fraud, bias in recording and reporting research data, mishandling of data, and incomplete reporting of results (Relman, 1989; Broad & Wade, 1982). An example would be to inflate a study's data or report only part of its data results, such as the favorable effects of a particular drug or treatment protocol.

Further, in 1989, the NIH defined scientific misconduct as:

. . . fabrication, falsification, plagiarism or other practices that seriously deviate from those that are commonly accepted within the scientific community for proposing, conducting or reporting research. It does not include honest error or honest differences in interpretations or judgements of data. (U.S. Department of Health and Human Services)

AGENCIES RESPONSIBLE FOR INVESTIGATING SCIENTIFIC MISCONDUCT

Anderson (1990) reported that Congressional hearings into alleged scientific misconduct are ongoing. This includes two new reporting and investigating agencies (Hawley and Jeffers, 1992):

1. *The Office of Scientific Integrity Review (OISR)*
   This agency, established within the Public Health Service, establishes and oversees policies and procedures to prevent scientific misconduct by grant recipients and makes recommendations to the Secretary of Health and Human Services when misconduct has been established (U.S. Department of Health and Human Services, 1989).

2. *The Office of Scientific Integrity (OSI)*
   This agency, housed within the NIH director's office, supervises the implementation of the established rules and regulations regarding scientific misconduct and monitors any investigations (U.S. Department of Health and Human Services).

Nurses receiving funds from the National Center for Nursing Research (NCNR), part of NIH, must comply with these reporting mechanisms and criteria for scientific misconduct.

Nurse researchers, especially beginning ones, who may be part of large research teams need to be aware that while much of the current criticism is focused on biomedical colleagues, nursing may be suspect by association in the public's mind (Hawley & Jeffers, 1992). For example, one area in which scientific misconduct could potentially occur is in the use of the nurse as a research assistant (RA) in complex and sophisticated medical or nursing research studies. According to Gift, Creasia, and Parker (1991), research assistants may unknowingly simplify the protocol or distort the findings of a project because they lack the research knowledge base of the principal investigator. These authors suggest scientific guidelines for decreasing the threat of scientific misconduct due to potential incompetence of the RA. These include hiring qualifications, writing a specific contract, and procedures for orienting, supervising, monitoring, mentoring, and evaluating the RA. Finally, nurse researchers must lead the way with accountable and reputable scientific practices if nursing is to continue being known as a trusted profession (McClure, 1978; Morrison, 1990).

✎ FUTURE IMPLICATIONS FOR ETHICAL RESEARCH

This chapter has described the ethical principles, codes, and responsibilities that should guide the conduct of those nurses undertaking research projects or studies. Cassidy (1991) stated that little research related to the ethical responsibilities of nurses has been published despite heightened awareness within the profession about the ethical dimensions of practice and concerns about nurses' ethical decision-making ability. Erlen and Frost (1991) suggested three scientific areas for future research: (1) differences between nurses and physicians' perceived roles in ethical decision-making, (2) identification of variables besides age, education, and work experience that may influence the nurse's role in ethical dilemmas, and (3) strategies to empower nurses who face ethical dilemmas.

Finally, Fry (1991) recommended that nursing review and evaluate the state of ethical inquiry in nursing based on the three main subject matters of ethics: (1) descriptive (phenomena of morality), (2) normative (standards and criteria) (3) metaethics (theories of ethics), and investigate the relationship of the formal teaching of ethics and its effects on the increased moral development of practicing nurses both in terms of performance and client outcomes.

SUMMARY
- The ethical principles relevant to nursing research are autonomy, nonmaleficence, beneficence, and justice.
- The principle of autonomy states that the individual is free to decide independently whether or not to participate in a research study.
- The principle of nonmaleficence states that no harm should come to a subject as a result of participation in research.
- The principle of beneficence states that the benefits attained from participation in the research study should outweigh the risks of participation.
- The principle of justice states that samples and populations for a research study should be selected equally from all populations.
- The four basic ethical principles that can be used to establish ethical rules of conduct are veracity, privacy, confidentiality, and fidelity.
- The principle of veracity is an obligation to tell the truth about the nature of the study.
- The principle of privacy is an obligation to keep all information about a subject anonymous, so that it cannot be linked to an individual subject.
- The principle of confidentiality is an obligation not to divulge information about a subject to a third party without the subject's permission.
- The principle of fidelity is an obligation to remain faithful to one's commitments.
- There have been many cases of human rights abuses, including the Nazi "medical" experiments, the Tuskegee syphilis experiment, and the Jewish Chronic Disease Hospital experiment.
- Codes of conduct that have been formulated to guide researchers in their work include the Nuremburg Code, the Declaration of Helsinki, the Patient's Bill of Rights, the Belmont Report, and the ANA Code for Nurses.
- Informed consent includes the elements

of adequate disclosure (the individual must be given enough information to make a decision), comprehension (the individual must clearly understand the information given), and freedom from coercion and undue influence.

- Institutional review boards are established to protect the rights of human subjects in research.
- The greatest potential for violations of human rights in research are in the idea being studied, the selected sample, and the specific type of study designs.
- When selecting a sample, one group should not be used disproportionately over another. Vulnerable populations should not be used simply because they are convenient.
- When using a nonexperimental design and it is determined that a treatment is needed, the treatment must not be deliberately withheld, as this will harm the patient.
- When using an experimental design, the risks to both the control and experimental groups must be addressed.
- When reading published research, the ethical aspects of the study must be evaluated.
- Self-regulation is needed to prevent scientific misconduct from occurring in nursing.

FACILITATING CRITICAL THINKING

1. Describe the relationship of each of the following ethical principles to nursing research:
   a. autonomy
   b. nonmaleficence
   c. beneficence
   d. justice
2. Define each of the four related ethical rules of conduct:
   a. veracity
   b. privacy
   c. confidentiality
   d. fidelity
3. Give one or two historical case examples where the human rights provision of either the Nuremburg Code or the Declaration of Helsinki were violated.
4. List and define the three critical elements of informed consent.
5. Discuss the difference between scientific misconduct and fraud.
6. Name at least one of the two national agencies responsible for investigating scientific misconduct.

References

SUBSTANTIVE

ANDERSEN, K., & HOLLAND, J. (1992). Maintaining the patency of peripherally inserted central catheters with 10 units/cc heparin. *Journal of Intravenous Nursing, 15*(2), 84-88.

ANDERSON, G. C. (1990). Scientific misconduct: Dingell tries again [news], *Nature, 345,* 195.

CASSIDY, V. R. (1991). Ethical responsibilities in nursing: Research findings and issues. *Journal of Professional Nursing, 17*(2), 112-118.

COOKE, M. (1986). Ethical issues in the care of patients with AIDS. *QRB 12* (10), 343-346.

DUFFY, L. M., WYBLE, S. J., WILSON, B., & MILES, S. H. (1989). Obtaining geriatric patient consent. *Journal of Gerontological Nursing, 15*(1) 21-24.

FRANCE, O. (1988). In Uruguay, an ethic of care for the dying. *Hasting Center Report, 18*(4), 21-22.

GIFT, A. G., CREASIA, J., & PARKER, B. (1991). Utilizing research assistants and maintaining research integrity. *Research in Nursing and Health, 14*(1), 229-233.

GOOD, B. A., & FISCHER, L. (1993). Vulnerability: An ethical consideration in research with older adults. *Western Journal of Nursing Research, 15*(6), 780-783.

GORTNER, S. R. (1974). Scientific accountability in Nursing. *Nursing Outlook, 22*(12), 764-768.

LEVINE, R. J. (1981). *Ethics and regulation of clinical research.* Baltimore-Munich: Urban & Schwarzenberg.

MILLER J., & EVANS, T. (1991). Some reflections on ethical dilemmas in nursing home research. *Western Journal of Nursing Research, 13* (3), 375-381.

PRICE, R., BREW, B., SIDTIS, I., ET AL. (1988). The brain in AIDS: Central nervous system HIV-1 infection and AIDS? complex. *Science, 239-586.*

REILLY, D. E., & BEHRENS-HANNA, L. (1991). Perioperative nursing: Moral and ethical issues in high technology practice. *Today's O.R. Nurse, 13*(8), 10-15.

RELMAN, A. S. (1989). Essay fraud in science: Causes and remedies. *Scientific American, 260* (4), 126.

ROBINSON, M. (1994, July 25). Study of radium testing urged. *The Patriot Ledger* (Quincy, Mass.), p. 4.

SILVA, M. C., & SORRELL, J. M. (1984). Factors influencing comprehension of information for informed consent: Ethical implications for nursing research. *International Journal of Nursing Studies, 21*(4), 233-239.

SILVA, M. C., & SORRELL, J. M. (1988). Enhancing comprehension of information for informed consent: A review of empirical research. *IRB: A Review of Human Subjects Research, 10*(1), 1-5.

SORRELL, J. M. (1991). Effects of writing/speaking on comprehension of information of informed consent. *Western Journal of Nursing Research, 13*(1), 110-122.

Whole-body radiation cases cited (1994, July 25). *The Patriot Ledger* (Quincy, Mass.), p. 2.

WOOLF, P. K. (1986). Pressure to publish and fraud in science. *Annals of Internal Medicine, 104,* 254-256.

WOOLF, P. K. (1981). Fraud in Science: How much, how serious? *Hasting Center Report 11,* 9-14.

World Medical Association (1964). Human Experimentation Code of Ethics of the World Medical Association, Declaration of Helsinki. *British Medical Journal, 2,* 177.

CONCEPTUAL

ADAMS, B. M. (1985). Medical research and personal privacy. *Villanova Law Review, 30,* 1081.

ANGELL, M. (1986). Publish or perish: A proposal. *Annals of Internal Medicine, 104,* 261-262.

BEAUCHAMP, T. C., & CHILDRESS, J. F. (1994). *Principles of biomedical ethics* (4th ed.). New York: Oxford University Press.

CRISHAM, P. (1992). Resolving ethical and moral dilemmas of nursing interventions. In M. Snyder (Ed.), *Independent nursing inventions* (2nd ed., pp. 19-32). Albany, NY: Delmar .

DAVIS, A. J. (1990). Ethical issues in nursing research. *Western Journal of Nursing Research, 10* (3), 413-416.

DE CRAEMER, W. (1983). A cross-cultural perspective on personhood. *Millbank Memorial Fund Quarterly, 61,* 19-24.

ERLEN, N. A., & FROST, B. (1991). Nurses' perception of powerlessness influencing ethical decisions. *Western Journal of Nursing Research, 13,*(3), 397-407.

FOWLER, M. (1988). Ethical issues in nursing research: A call for an international code of ethics for nursing research. *Western Journal of Nursing Research, 10,*(3), 352-355.

FOWLER, M., CHANEY, E. A., DAVIS, A. J., & FLYNN, P. (1987). Toward an international concord for nursing research. Unpublished poster presentation, Edinburgh, Scotland.

FOWLER, M., & LEVINE-ARIFF, J. (1987). *Ethics at the bedside: A sourcebook for critical care nurses.* Philadelphia: J.B. Lippincott.

FROMER, M. (1981). *Ethical issues in health care.* St. Louis: Mosby.

FRY, S. (1991). Ethics in health care delivery. In J. L. Creasia & B. Parker (Eds.), *Conceptual foundations of professional nursing practice,* (pp. 149-164). St. Louis: Mosby.

HAWLEY, D. J., & JEFFERS, J. M. (1992). Scientific misconduct as a dilemma for nursing. *IMAGE: Journal of Nursing Scholarship, 24* (1), 51-55.

MORRISON, R. S. (1990). Disreputable science: Definition and detection. *Journal of Professional Nursing, 15,* 911-913.

Random House Webster's Dictionary (1993). New York: Ballantine Books.

SELYE, H. (1976). Forty years of stress research: Principal remaining problems and misconceptions. *Canadian Medical Association Journal, 115,* 53-56.

UNSCHULD, P. (1989). *Medical ethics in Imperial China.* Berkeley: University of California Press.

VEATCH, R. M., & FRY, S. (1987). *Case studies in nursing ethics.* Philadelphia: J.B. Lippincott.

WILSON, E. (1982). *The wisdom of Confucius.* New York: Crown.

METHODOLOGICAL

American Bar Association Commission on the Mentally Disabled (1976). Statement before the National Experimentation Group. *Mental Disability Law Reporter, 1*(2), 156.

American Hospital Association (1992), A patient's bill of rights. Chicago: American Hospital Association.

American Nurses Association (1985). *Code for Nurses.* Kansas City, MO: The Association.

American Nurses Association (1981). *Guidelines for investigative functions of nurses.* Kansas City, MO: The Association.

American Nurses Association (1985). *Human rights guidelines for nurses in clinical and other research.* Kansas City, MO: The Association.

Code of Federal Regulations. Title 45, Part 46. Washington, D.C., January 26, 1991.

CURRAN, W., & SHAPIRO, E. (1982). *Law, medicine, and forensic science* (3rd ed.). Boston: Little, Brown.

GRADY, C. (1989). Ethical issues in providing nursing care to human immunodeficiency virus-infected populations. *Nursing Clinics of North America, 24*(2), 523-534.

LANE, L. W., CASSELL, C. K., & BENNETT, W. (1990). Ethical aspects of research involving elderly subjects: Are we doing more than we say? *The Journal of Clinical Ethics, 1*(4), 278-285.

National Commission for the Protection of Human Subjects of Biomedical and Behavioral Research (1978). Research involving those institutionalized as mentally infirm (DHEW Publication No. OS-78-006). Washington, D.C.: Author.

National Commission for the Protection of Human Subjects of Biomedical and Behavioral Research (1978). *The Belmont report: Ethical principles and guidelines for the protection of human subjects of research* (revised October 1, 1990). DHEW Publication No. (OS).

ODDI, L. F., & CASSIDY, V. R. (1990). Nursing research in the United States: The protection of human Subjects. *International Journal of Nursing Studies, 27*(1), 21-34.

U.S. Department of Health and Human Services (1989). *Responsibilities of awardee and applicant institutions for dealing with and reporting possible misconduct in science.* National Institute of Health Guide No. 18. Washington, D.C.: Government Printing Office.

WILSON, H. S. (1989). *Research in nursing* (2nd ed.). Reading, MA: Addison-Wesley.

WINDOM, R. E. (1988). Statement before the House Energy and Commerce Subcommittee on Oversight and Investigations, House of Representatives, April 12, 1988. U.S. Department of Health and Human Services.

HISTORICAL

BANDMAN, E. L. (1985). Protection of human subjects. *Topics in Clinical Nursing, 7,* 15-23.

BROAD, W., & WADE, N. (1982). *Betrayers of the truth.* New York: Simon and Schuster.

CASSILETH, B. R., ZUPKIS, R. V., SUTTON-SMITH, K., & MARCH V. (1980). Informed consent: Why are its goals imperfectly realized? *New England Journal of Medicine, 302,* 896-900.

JONES, J. H. (1981). *Bad blood: The Tuskegee syphilis experiment.* New York: Free Press.

LOCK, S. (1985). *A difficult balance.* Philadelphia: ISI Press.

MCCLURE, M. L. (1978). The long road to accountability. *Nursing Outlook, 26,* 47-50.

MCDONALD, K. A. (1988). Noted Harvard psychiatrist resigns post after faculty group finds he plagiarized. *Chronicle of Higher Education, 35,* 1.

MISKIN, B. (1988). Responding to scientific misconduct: Due process and prevention. *Journal of the American Medical Association, 260*(13), 1932-1936.

PALCA, J. (1990). Scientific misconduct cases revealed [news], *Science, 248,* 297.

RELMAN, A. S. (1983). Lessons from the Darsee affair. *The New England Journal of Medicine, 308,* 1415-1417.

ROBB, S. S. (1983). Beware of the informed consent. *Nursing Research, 32,* 132.

SILVERMAN, W. A. (1983). *Human experimentation: A guide step into the unknown.* Oxford: Oxford University Press.

SMITH, J. (1985). Scientific fraud probed at AAAS meeting. *Science, 228,* 1292-1293.

STEINFELS, P., & LEVINE, C. (1976). Biomedical ethics and the shadow of Nazism. *The Hastings Center Report* (Supplement, August), 1-9.

United States v. Stanley, 107 S. CT. 3054 (1987).

CHAPTER 4

INTRODUCTION TO THE RESEARCH PROCESS

RENEE LEASURE • PATRICIA H. ALLEN

Ignaz Semmelweiss, born in Budapest in 1818, received his medical degree in Vienna. Following graduation he worked in the First Maternity Division of an obstetric clinic. Semmelweiss was surprised to learn that approximately 11% of the patients admitted to First Maternity developed the life-threatening disease of "childbed fever." This was especially disconcerting when the adjacent Second Maternity Division experienced only a 3% incidence of the disease.

Semmelweiss explored several possible explanations for this problem. One theory for the cause of childbed fever was that "atmospheric-cosmic-telluric-changes" affected whole regions, causing the death of pregnant women. He rejected this theory on the basis that had this been true the incidence of deaths would have been the same in both the First and Second Maternity Division as well as in the entire city of Vienna. In fact, the fever occurred rarely in Vienna and much more frequently in the First than in the Second Division. Another theory, that of overcrowding, was also rejected. Due to fear caused by the First Division's high mortality rate, women sought placement in the Second Division, which resulted in much more crowding of patients in the Second Division.

Semmelweiss noted that whenever a patient was dying the priest was called to administer last rites in a sick room. He noted that in the Second Division the priest had direct access to the room, whereas in the First Division the priest passed through five wards of women saying the funeral chant and ringing a bell. Semmelweiss tested the theory that the ringing bell terrified the women and caused the fever. He persuaded the priest to enter the First Division silently and unobserved. Unfortunately, Semmelweiss did not witness a decrease in the incidence of fever in the First Division.

Semmelweiss next noted that women in the First Division delivered babies while lying on their back, whereas women in the Second Division delivered babies while lying on their sides. Semmelweiss tested his hypothesis that there would be a difference in incidence of childbed fever in First Division when women delivered on their side rather than on their back. Unfortunately, once again, there was no decrease in the incidence of childbed fever.

Then, early in 1847, a physician on the ward was performing an autopsy. During the autopsy Dr. Kolletschka was cut by a scalpel and subsequently died of an illness that showed many of the same signs and symptoms as childbed fever. The similarity of symptoms led Semmelweiss to hypothesize that Kolletschka had died because "cadaveric matter" had poisoned his blood. For this theory to hold true, the women in First Division must somehow be having contact with "cadaveric matter." Semmelweiss noted that he and the students were sometimes called to the maternity ward directly from the autopsy room. They would only superficially wash their hands. Semmelweiss also noted that the women in Second Division were cared for by nurse midwives whose training did not include dissection of cadavers. Semmelweiss tested his hypothesis that childbed fever was being caused by "cadaveric matter" on the physicians' hands. He had the students wash their hands in chlorinated lime before any examination. The incidence of deaths due to childbed fever promptly declined with the implementation of Semmelweiss's experimental intervention (Sinclair, 1966).

The work of Dr. Semmelweiss illustrates the primary goal of research, the discovery of knowledge. He used both a systematic scientific approach and creativity in finding a solution to the problem of childbed fever.

Research is a very creative yet orderly process. Creativity in research emerges from the spectrum of choices the researcher makes—from the identification and refinement of the research topic, to the design of data collection measures, to the recruitment and retention of research subjects. For example, one researcher investigating diabetes symptomatology in an isolated Native American tribe noted that the subjects valued coffee and souvenirs with a university logo as an incentive to participate. Another researcher found that a study sample of elderly clients had difficulty reading traditionally formatted questionnaires. Therefore the investigator had the questionnaire enlarged to poster size and administered it in person rather than by mail.

The purpose of this chapter is to introduce research terminology and provide an overview of the steps of the research process. Information will be provided pertaining to problem identification, selection of a research approach, subject recruitment and retention, methods of data analysis, and dissemination of findings.

✌ BASIC RESEARCH TERMINOLOGY

Research is a scientific process of inquiry that involves purposeful, systematic, and rigorous collection, analysis, and interpretation of data. The scientific approach to inquiry refers to a set of orderly, disciplined procedures used to acquire useful and dependable information. The rules and assumptions of the study design, sampling methods, and data analysis are crafted to minimize bias, thus allowing the investigator to evaluate the conclusions and implications of the study with some measure of confidence. Basic research terms are defined in the box on the next page.

The two broad categories of research approaches are qualitative and quantitative. *Qualitative design* and analysis involves the collection, integration, and synthesis of nonnumerical narrative data.

BASIC RESEARCH TERMINOLOGY

Assumptions   A statement of principle whose correctness has not been proven but is taken for granted on the basis of logical reasoning.

Concept   A mental or word picture of a phenomenon that is based on the presence or absence of certain behaviors or characteristics.

Conceptual framework   A network of interrelated concepts that provide a structure for organizing and describing the phenomenon of interest.

Construct   A concept that is invented for a specific scientific purpose and that has no empirical meaning unless it is linked to an observational term.

Control   The process of preventing extraneous influences on the dependent variable, which might alter the true effect between the study variables.

Critique   An unbiased and objective critical review of the strengths and weaknesses of a research report.

Data   The pieces of information collected that pertain to the study variables.

Generalizability   The ability to relate the study findings from the sample to a larger population.

Hypothesis   A statement of the expected relationship between the independent and dependent variable.

Limitations   Weaknesses in a study, such as uncontrolled variables, that limit the generalizability of the findings.

Operational definition   The definition or description of a study variable that specifies how it will be measured.

Research   A scientific process of inquiry that involves purposeful, systematic, and rigorous collection, analysis, and interpretation of data to gain new knowledge.

Theory   A set of interrelated concepts that provide a systematic method of organizing, integrating, and conceptualizing a phenomenon.

Theoretical or conceptual definition   The definition or description of a study variable that is drawn from the theoretical or conceptual framework.

Variable   A characteristic or attribute that varies or differs among the persons or objects being studied.

  Attribute variable   A preexisting characteristic or attribute.

  Extraneous variable   A variable present in the research environment that threatens the internal or external validity of the study. Such a variable clouds the results of the study by interfering with the relationship between the study variables.

  Independent variable   The variable that is believed to influence or cause the dependent variable. In an experimental study the independent variable is the treatment or intervention that the researcher manipulates.

  Dependent variable   The outcome or criterion variable that is hypothesized to be caused by another variable.

Predictability   A property of the data collection measurement that characterizes the instrument's dependability or stability in producing consistent results over time.

It is also used for theory generation and formulation of hypotheses. *Quantitative design* and analysis involves the collection, integration, and analysis of numerical data.

✎ THE RESEARCH PROCESS

While the research process consists of many small steps, the overall process may be divided into four major phases. These

STEPS OF THE CONCEPTUAL STAGE

- Problem identification and significance
- Formulating the problem statement and purpose
- Placing the problem in a conceptual/theoretical context
- Reviewing the literature

- Specifying assumptions and limitations
- Formulating the hypothesis/research questions
- Defining the terms
- Ethical considerations

are the conceptual phase, the design phase, the implementation phase, and the analysis and interpretation phase.

THE CONCEPTUAL PHASE OF THE RESEARCH PROCESS

Problem Identification and Significance

Compared to other disciplines, nursing is fairly new in the research arena. As nursing makes strides toward basing practice on research rather than on tradition, we are faced with numerous problems in our need for systematic investigation. Rather than experiencing a dearth of research problems, nurse researchers may be overwhelmed by the great number of problems in need of study. Identification of the topic of the research study is often one of the most difficult and challenging steps of the research process.

Research problems may be derived from a variety of sources. Problems may arise as a result of a clinical situation encountered, an unresolved issue in the literature, a research priority identified by a professional organization, or an issue that you have wondered about and argued about. In the clinical situation we may question why something is being done in a particular way. A nurse working in a critical care area may wish to discover if it is really necessary to add heparin to arterial line flush solutions. The nurse working on a medical-surgical unit may wish to determine whether subjects receiving enteral feedings using a sterile protocol have a decreased incidence of diarrhea compared to patients receiving the traditional clean protocol. Another source of research problems can be the discussion and implications sections of completed research, which generally include suggestions for future research.

Given the limited human and financial resources usually available, coupled with the large number of problems in need of study, several groups have developed research priorities for specific populations. Generally, groups of individuals within the area of interest have synthesized input from a variety of sources, identifying specific areas in need of further research. One example is the research priorities identified by the American Association of Critical Care Nurses. This specialty organization selected nine clinical practice priorities and seven contextual priorities for research (see box on p. 19). These priorities provide a "focus for the research programs of AACN member chapters, and supply guidance to health care agencies setting institutional research priorities" (Lindquist et al., 1993, p. 117).

The large number of problems in need of study and the varied interests of nurse researchers have resulted in a widely scattered body of knowledge (Bloch, 1990). To

NATIONAL INSTITUTE OF NURSING RESEARCH PRIORITIES

1994	Technology dependency	
1995	Community-based nursing model	
1996	Nursing interventions in HIV/AIDS	
1997	Remediating cognitive impairment	
1998	Interventions for coping with chronic illness	

1999 Identify biobehavioral factors and test interventions to promote immuno-competence

National Institute of Nursing Research, National Institutes of Health, unpublished paper, September 23, 1993.

focus research efforts, the National Institute for Nursing Research (NINR) has developed a national nursing research agenda. This agenda provides structure for selecting scientific opportunities and initiatives, promotes depth in developing a knowledge base for nursing practice, and provides direction for nursing research within the discipline (Hinshaw, 1988). Research priorities for the remainder of the century are listed in the box. Another source of research priorities is *Healthy People 2000*. These priorities may provide a direction for researchers seeking to identify research problems and may also give insight into potential sources of funding for research ideas.

Following selection of a primary problem of study, it is important to consider several areas that may influence the ultimate success or failure of the study. Does the researcher have sufficient knowledge of the topic to conduct the study? Are sufficient resources available to conduct the study? Can the problem be empirically investigated? Does a sufficient accessible population exist from which to draw the sample? Is this topic researchable?

Formulating the Problem Statement and Purpose
Writing the research problem statement is not easy. A problem well stated is a research question half answered. The prob-

lem statement may be conveyed in either the declarative or interrogative form. The problem statement typically identifies the study variables and population, and it must explicitly and unambiguously define the problem topic and provide guidelines for the expected answer. It must also express a relationship between two or more variables (Kerlinger, 1986). This initial problem statement typically goes through many revisions as the research proposal is developed and refined.

Through the process of deductive reasoning the problem statement flows from the research topic, and the purpose flows from the problem statement. The problem statement presents the situation in need of investigation; the purpose defines the goal or specific study aim. For example, in a study of women treated for breast cancer, Mock (1993) developed this problem statement: What are the effects of four different types of treatment for breast cancer on body image in women? The purpose was to compare body image as a component of self-concept in four groups of women following treatment for breast cancer (Mock, 1993).

Placing the Problem in a Conceptual/Theoretical Context
A *theory* is a set of interrelated concepts that provide a systematic method of orga-

nizing, integrating, and conceptualizing a phenomenon. *Concepts,* the building blocks of theory, are a mental or word picture of a phenomenon that is based on the presence or absence of certain behaviors or characteristics. A *construct* is a concept that is invented for a specific scientific purpose and that has no empirical meaning unless it is linked to an observational term. In research studies the concepts and constructs frequently are the study variables. A theory describes, explains, or predicts a phenomenon. The outcome of a qualitative study may be to generate theory, whereas the goal of a quantitative study may be to test a theory. A *conceptual framework* is a network of interrelated concepts that provide a structure for organizing and describing the phenomenon of interest. Research studies are based on a theoretical or conceptual framework that facilitates visualizing the problem and places the variables in a logical context. Qualitative studies generally use inductive reasoning, developing generalizations from specifics. The purpose of a qualitative study may be to generate a conceptual framework to develop a theory. Quantitative studies often use deductive reasoning, which develops specifics from generalizations, to test theory. Locating a conceptual/theoretical framework congruent with the investigator's approach to guide the research project is time well spent.

Reviewing the Literature

Following problem identification, an extensive review of the literature, using primary sources wherever possible, can be invaluable in narrowing the study focus by refining and redefining the research topic. A *primary source* is a summary report of the study prepared by the researcher who conducted the study. A *secondary source* is a recounting of the findings by someone other than the investigator. A limitation of using secondary sources is that the author may introduce summary bias. By reviewing existing literature the researcher can identify current knowledge of the subject matter, evaluate potential theoretical frameworks, and survey possible data collection measures. The literature search should initially be broad and then narrowed to note gaps in and recommendations of prior studies to justify the need for researching the current subject matter. Typically the review of the literature is organized around three or four subheadings. These subheadings are made up of the concepts and interrelationships of the study variables. The researcher generally provides the organizing framework for the review of the literature in the introductory paragraph and summarizes the salient points in a summary paragraph. The material is organized in such a way as to establish the need for conducting the study.

When writing the literature review, it is important to critique studies as well as report them. A *critique* is an unbiased and objective analysis of the strengths and weaknesses of a research report. Was the sample too small? Were reliability and validity of the measuring instrument established? Was the theoretical framework established? Studies with conflicting findings must be reported as well as those that support the topic at hand. The researcher can point out how the proposed study will differ from the cited study. This is also a time to examine gaps in this area of research.

Specifying Assumptions

Assumptions are those ideas universally accepted as true and that are taken for granted on the basis of logic or reason even though they have not been scientifically tested. Assumptions are the bedrock upon which the study rests.

Assumptions are embedded in the philosophical base of the theory, the study methodology, and data analysis techniques. Theories and instruments are based on assumptions that may or may not be recognized by the researcher. Following an extensive review of published nursing research and other health care literature, Williams (1980) developed a list of assumptions that seem to underlie many nursing research studies (see box below). Although the reader may not agree with the study assumptions, it is important to the integrity of the study that they be specified.

Identifying the Study Variables
A *variable* is a characteristic or attribute that varies or differs among the persons or objects being studied. An *attribute variable* is a preexisting characteristic such as age or gender that is simply noted. An *active variable* is one that the researcher investigates in the course of the study. Depending on the focus of the investigation, an attribute variable may become an active variable and vice versa. *Extraneous variables* are those present in the research environment that

threaten the internal or external validity of the study. They cloud the results of the study by interfering with the true relationship between the study variables.

An *independent variable* is the variable that is believed to influence or create the dependent variable. In an experimental study the independent variable is the treatment or intervention that the researcher manipulates. A *dependent variable* is the outcome or criterion variable that is hypothesized to be caused by the independent variable.

Formulating the Hypothesis/Research Questions
A *hypothesis* is a statement of the expected relationship between the independent and dependent variables that may be stated as (1) directional or nondirectional, (2) simple or complex, or (3) null or research. It is a "tentative proposition set forth as a possible explanation for an occurrence or a provisional conjecture to assist in guiding the investigation of the problem" (Leedy, 1993, p. 76). A *simple hypothesis* is a statement of the causal or associative relationship be-

---

ASSUMPTIONS COMMON TO MANY NURSING STUDIES

1. People want to assume control of their health problems.
2. Stress should be avoided.
3. People are aware of the experiences that most affect their life choices.
4. Health is a priority for most people.
5. People in underserved areas feel underserved.
6. Most measurable attitudes are held strongly enough to direct behavior.
7. Health professionals view health care in a different manner than do lay persons.
8. Human biological and chemical factors show less variation than do cultural and social factors.
9. The nursing process is the best way of conceptualizing nursing practice.
10. Statistically significant differences relate to the variable or variables under consideration.
11. People operate on the basis of cognitive information.
12. Increased knowledge about an event lowers anxiety about the event.
13. Receipt of health care at home is preferable to receipt of care in an institution.

tween one independent variable and one dependent variable. A *complex hypothesis* is a statement of the causal or associative relationship between two or more independent variables and/or two or more dependent variables. A *directional hypothesis* specifies the direction of the relationship between the dependent and the independent variable. A *nondirectional hypothesis* does not specify the direction of the relationship between the independent and dependent variable. While a qualitative study may generate hypotheses, a quantitative study often tests them.

A hypothesis may be stated as either a research or a null hypothesis. The research hypothesis is a statement of the expected causal relationship between the independent and the dependent variable. The independent variable is also called the presumed cause. The null hypothesis is a statement of no difference and is tested statistically. Statement of the null hypothesis allows the investigator to reject or fail to reject the null hypothesis based on the statistical test findings. Acceptance or rejection of a hypothesis is based on what the findings reveal, therefore establishing a relationship of causality between the study variables. Table 4-1 shows how the same concept may be worded as different types of hypotheses.

Many research topics are not amenable to experimental manipulation. For example, because cigarette smoking is harmful, it would be unethical to develop an experimental study that assigned subjects to a smoking or nonsmoking group. Nonexperimental descriptive and correlational study designs ask the research question: What is the relationship between cigarette smoking and the incidence of lung cancer? In this design subjects are not randomly assigned to a smoking or nonsmoking group. Rather, subjects are placed in the smoking

Table 4-1
Examples of Hypothesis and Research Questions

Hypothesis Type	Example
Directional simple hypothesis:	Comatose patients placed on an air bed will have a lower incidence of skin breakdown than those who are not.
Nondirectional hypothesis:	There will be a difference in incidence of skin breakdown between comatose patients who are and are not placed on an air bed.
Null hypothesis:	There will be no difference in incidence of skin breakdown between patients who are and are not placed on an air bed.
Complex hypothesis:	Patients placed on an air bed will have a decreased incidence of skin breakdown and an increased perception of comfort.
Research question:	Is there a relationship between placement on an air bed and incidence of skin breakdown?

or nonsmoking group based upon the presence or absence of a preexisting characteristic, in this case smoking. Although *research questions* flow from the problem statement, they are more specific than the problem statement. For example, a problem statement might be: What are admission predictors of student nurses' ability to successfully complete the NCLEX examination on the first attempt? A research question for this study might be: What is the relationship among entry GPA, science GPA, writing score, and student nurses' ability to successfully complete the NCLEX examination on the first attempt? Research questions investigate associations between variables, whereas hypotheses investigate causality between variables.

Acknowledging the Limitations

Research exists in the real rather than the ideal world. As such, researchers make numerous decisions throughout the development of the conceptual and methodological phases of the research process. *Generalizability* is the ability to relate study findings from the sample to a larger population. *Limitations* are weaknesses in a study, such as uncontrolled variables, that limit the generalizability of the findings. They may be both theoretical and methodological. Limitations occur because of the use of an unrepresentative study sample, lack of control of extraneous variables caused by a faulty study design, use of data collection instruments with questionable reliability and validity, and incorrect statistical analyses. Limitations represent potential threats to the internal and external validity of the study.

Defining the Terms

A *theoretical* or *conceptual definition* of a study variable is one that is drawn from the theoretical or conceptual framework. The *operational definition* represents how the researcher plans to measure the study variable. Qualitative research studies do not generally contain definitions. Rather, the data are collected and analyzed, and the definitions emerge from the data.

An example of theoretical and operational definitions is provided in a study of "Stress at Hospital Discharge after Acute Myocardial Infarction" (Toth, 1993), as shown in Table 4-2.

These definitions make the concepts of this study empirically testable. The theoretical definitions link the study variables to the study framework, whereas the operational definitions specify the activities necessary to measure the concept.

Ethical Considerations

When planning and implementing research concerning human beings and human behavior, it is important to recall the ethical principles of beneficence, nonmaleficence, autonomy, and justice. In essence, the nurse researcher will do good (beneficence), support self-determination (autonomy), and be fair (justice). The researcher accomplishes this by doing no harm to participants (nonmaleficence). Benefits to participants are maximized, while real and potential risks are minimized. The principle of justice is evoked when the researcher maintains privacy and uses fair procedures in identifying and se-

Table 4-2

Relationships among Concepts, Theoretical Definitions, and Operational Definitions

Concept	Theoretical Definition	Operational Definition
Stress	A generalized stimulation of the autonomic nervous system that alerts a person to the presence of stressors arising from an actual or perceived threat	Scores on the Stress of Discharge Assessment tool
Acute myocardial infarction	An acute obstruction in coronary artery blood flow to an area of cardiac muscle resulting in myocardial cellular death	The death of cardiac tissue, documented by cardiac history, ECG changes, and/or elevations in the blood serum level of creatine kinase-MB

STEPS OF THE IMPLEMENTATION PHASE

- Developing a timetable
- Developing a budget and seeking funding
- Recruiting and retaining subjects
- Collecting the data

lecting research participants so that risks and benefits are equally shared. In this way the benefits to the subject outweigh the risks.

The rights of the subject are safeguarded by the researcher's role of limiting risk of harm and providing for full disclosure about the nature, duration, and purpose of the study as well as informing the subject of the methods, procedures for data collection, findings, and inconveniences or discomforts that may occur. The participant must be informed of the right to withdraw at any time during the investigation.

Institutional Review Boards, which are made up of both professionals and the public, are maintained for the purpose of ensuring that the research subjects' ethical rights are not violated. Research proposals are scrutinized with regard to their potential risk. Special attention is paid to protected groups such as children, the elderly, prison inmates, the mentally incompetent, abortuses, fetuses, the pregnant, and the disabled.

THE IMPLEMENTATION PHASE OF THE RESEARCH PROCESS

Developing a Timetable

A very helpful tool for implementing the research project is breaking the project into small steps and estimating how much time will be required to complete each activity. Because almost all research projects operate under some type of deadline, it is helpful in focusing activities to develop some type of timetable that breaks down activities

into small steps. The timetable may also indicate the individual or individuals who are responsible for designated tasks. The types of activities and the amount of time spent on them vary greatly according to the problem under study, availability of subjects, and study design.

Time should be included for seeking approval of involved agencies, including data collection sites and institutional review boards, acquisition of supplies, training of personnel, recruitment of subjects, data collection, data coding, data analysis, preparation of summary reports, and dissemination of research findings. A hypothetical timetable is presented in Figure 4-1. This is an example of a study timetable used for a descriptive correlational study that used questionnaires to collect data.

Developing a Budget and Seeking Funding

Conducting research is costly in both time and money. An ever-increasing number of large and small sources for acquisition of research funds are becoming available. The first step in budgeting is to break down the resources needed, identify the quantity required, and calculate the cost. Resources needed may include personnel, equipment, and supplies. Personnel costs may include consultation with a statistician, secretarial support for transcription of taped interviews, and staff salaries. When calculating the cost of equipment and supplies, it is important to be realistic. To decrease the risk of potential budget shortages, it is gen-

Task	Person Responsible	Nov	Dec	Jan	Feb	Mar	Apr	May	Jun	Jul	Aug
Identify problem and review literature	AL,LH*	▓									
Select design, data collection procedure, and sampling method	LH,AL		▓								
Consent letter written	AL		▓								
Pilot study conducted and revisions made	LH,AL			▓							
Ethical review board approval obtained	LH				▓						
Pilot data entered and reliability estimates calculated, pilot of data analysis completed	AL				▓						
Application for funding submitted	LH,AL					▓					
Approval from data collection sites finalized	LH					▓					
Supplies ordered	LH						▓				
Subject list coded, computer labels generated, study packets assembled and coded	LH,AL						▓				
Initial distribution of study packets. Follow-up of nonrespondents in two weeks	LH							▓			
Data entry	AL								▓		
Data analysis and interpretation	LH,AL								▓		
Implications of study findings and recommendations for future research	LH,AL									▓	
Poster and/or paper presentation and manuscript preparation	LH,AL									▓	▓
Plans developed for next study	LH,AL										▓

Figure 4-1. Sample timetable for a descriptive correlational study.

*Hypothetical initials of persons responsible for tasks.

erally not wise to use a discounted or sale price in calculating costs. It is also prudent to consider inflation if purchases will be made over several years. The more specific the budgetary information, the easier it will be to make modifications should they become necessary.

Next is the identification of potential sources of funding. The researcher's employer may have small quantities of monies available to support research efforts. Another source of monies is Sigma Theta Tau International at both the chapter and national levels. The American Nurses' Association, as well as many specialty organizations, will fund research projects of interest to the group. In addition to professional organizations, many private foundations, such as AARP, may fund studies of interest.

Manufacturers may be willing to donate equipment and supplies. Also, many individuals will donate time and resources to a study. In one study of enteral nutrition the manufacturer donated tube feeding formula, tubing, and feeding pumps. A hospital donated space and telemetry monitoring for an exercise-based research project. These sources of indirect and in-kind funding facilitate the pilot work for many larger studies. If companies are not able to donate equipment, they may permit the researcher to use the equipment on a trial basis at little or no charge.

A letter of inquiry will generally result in receipt of the guidelines for grant application, funding criteria, and submission deadlines. In preparing a research grant application, it is important to clearly justify the significance of the study, the capabilities of the researchers to carry out the proposed investigation, and the appropriateness of the methods to address the proposed study aims. An excellent example of an NIH research grant application is that of Naylor (1990), who used a quantitative study approach. Sandelowski, Davis, and Harris (1989) provide helpful guidelines for preparing a qualitative funding proposal.

The costs of conducting a research study are numerous and can add up very quickly. The ever-increasing sources of money available to fund research efforts are more than offset by the ever-increasing number of individuals applying for the funds. In general, the more funds required, the more competitive the grants review process. Therefore, beginning researchers and those researchers conducting pilot studies may initially be more successful competing at the local and regional level.

Recruiting and Retaining Subjects

The contribution of each study subject is of value in its clarification of the group picture that emerges. Inadequate sampling of subjects and excessive attrition may ultimately affect the validity of the study. Attrition may be categorized as either preinclusion or postinclusion attrition (Given, Keilman, Collins, & Given, 1990). Preinclusion attrition occurs when subjects are not included in the study either through lack of consent on their part or exclusion from the study by the researcher. Support from other health care professionals, the community, and the media are very helpful in recruiting subjects (Diekmann & Smith, 1989). Previous research subjects may also be a very powerful source of support in publicizing the study.

To have the most representative picture possible, it is important to consider numerous measures to encourage as many of the subjects as possible to participate. Nonrespondents have been shown to differ from respondents in fundamental ways. Although a response rate of 100% is the goal, a response rate of 50% or greater is generally considered adequate. During the data collection phase the researchers may wish to follow up with nonrespondents to ascertain reasons for withdrawal from the study. These results may then be reported in the discussion section of the final research report.

In addition to identifying physical measures to encourage completion of the questionnaire, strategies aimed at developing the subjects' commitment to the study have been shown to increase response rate (Gordon & Stokes, 1989). The format of the data collection packet is also important. A cover letter printed on letterhead or a verbal explanation is important in encouraging subjects' participation. Participants are interested in knowing why they were selected to participate in the study, what are the benefits and risks to them, and what participation will entail. If printed data collection tools are used, their appearance should be professional and easily read. In general, a businesslike appearance enhances response rates. An off-white, ecru, or gray background that uses a dark brown, navy, or dark burgundy ink is clearly readable and different from the ordinary printed material received. If you use a printed questionnaire, you can determine from the pilot study if the directions for completion of the questionnaire are clearly and unambiguously stated. The wording of the questions should be geared to the least-educated respondent, and the most sensitive information should be covered at the end of the questionnaire. An equal number of positively and negatively worded questions may help reduce response bias. If respondents will be returning the questionnaires by mail, a stamped, self-addressed return envelope should be included.

Incentives serve as an inducement for participation in the study. They should be items that participants will want and should not be coercive in nature. Incentives include pens, mugs, bags, movie tickets, money, or a summary of the study findings. Analyzing the distinction between incentives versus coercion for participating in a study is carefully evaluated by both the investigator and the institutional review board.

If you use a longitudinal study design, you should also build in retention strategies. Do not underestimate the positive influence of interaction between the study team and the research subjects as a powerful retention strategy. Other retention strategies include periodic incentives, birthday cards, follow-up on each subject's own progress, and a study newsletter (Given, Keilmen, Collins, & Given, 1990; Killien & Newton, 1990; Rudy, Estok, Kerr, Menzel, 1994) Wineman and Durand (1992) found that "the combination of tangible and intangible rewards and incentives, including money, is likely to be most effective in recruiting and retaining subjects and minimizing attrition."

If data will be collected in the hospital, adequate time should be allocated to negotiate the internal approval process. In accessing clinical agencies the researcher may initiate the process with a phone call or letter. The purpose of this query is to determine the policies that will need to be observed prior to access (Barnsteiner, 1989). The time required may vary from several days to several months. In addition to information relevant to the scientific merit and ethical review board approval, clinical agencies may also examine consumption of agency resources. At times denial to the agency is based not on the merits of the study, but on the burden to the clinical agency. Therefore, any strategies the researcher implements to decrease this burden such as the use of research assistants for data collection, some sort of reimbursement to the clinical agency for services, and the development of an open collaborative relationship aids not only the present research project, but also subsequent studies conducted by this and future research teams.

Collecting and Managing Data

The pieces of information collected pertaining to the study variables are referred to as *data* (singular *datum*). Collecting and managing data are often learned through trial and error. One of the purposes of the pilot study may be to examine the data collection and management process. It is helpful to keep a journal or calendar to track study progress and document activities. Data collection packets may be assembled in advance. For example, in one longitudinal study, packets were assembled for each subject. Dividers were used to separate each of the data collection periods for the subject. All files were maintained in one central area. A large wall calendar was used to record the date of each subject's measurements, the data to be collected at that time, and the person responsible for the activity. A data entry file was developed at the beginning of data collection, and a codebook or key to the variables was developed. Entering data near the time they were collected was helpful in clarifying the process of questionnaire scouring and the transfer of non-numerical data to a categorical system.

Questionnaires, physiological measures, and other forms of numerical data may be entered into one of many computer programs. Depending on the size of the data set and the resources available to the study, the data may be entered into either a personal or mainframe computer. There are benefits and drawbacks to using either a personal computer or mainframe computer for data analysis. However, no matter what choice the researcher makes, it is helpful to run a small pilot analysis of data early in the study. Issues such as whether to store longitudinal data by subject number, or by subject number and data collection period, may be decided early in the study, before a great deal of time and energy has been invested in the process. Once data are collected, they are transcribed and coded for reduction and analysis. Taped interviews may be transcribed verbatim for data analysis. Following data entry, the data is analyzed and interpreted.

THE DESIGN PHASE OF THE RESEARCH PROCESS

Selecting a Research Design

The *research design* is the structural framework for study implementation. The design phase includes selection of the research design, data collection methods, sampling framework, and the data entry/analysis plan. It is the blueprint for study implementation that maximizes control over factors interfering with the true relationship among study variables. Both the theoretical and design frameworks are critical to the study. The two interlinked frameworks must complement each other. For example, the researcher wishing to study the concept of caring for the purpose of theory generation would probably use a qualitative design, as this provides broader information. The researcher wanting to compare caring behaviors by nurses in inpatient and outpatient settings would probably use a descriptive correlational study design. In an experimental study design the researcher notes whether there is a difference in caring behaviors of nurses who attend a caring conference and those who do not. Table 4-3 demonstrates the linkage between the research question and the research design.

Research studies may also be described as being either basic or applied. A basic study is implemented to broaden understanding of the phenomenon of interest. Basic re-

_____ **STEPS OF THE DESIGN PHASE** _____

- Selecting a quantitative or qualitative study design
- Identifying a data collection method
- Selecting a sampling plan
- Conducting a pilot study

Table 4-3
Appropriateness of the Design for the Research Question

Research Approach	Research Question
Descriptive	What is?
Correlational	What is the relationship?
Experimental	What is the effect of the independent variables on the dependent variable?

search seeks to discover new knowledge for the advancement of theory. An applied study seeks to find a solution to a problem. Whether your study is basic or applied, there are several mechanisms that the researcher employs to maintain the integrity of the study design—maximizing control, minimizing bias, and controlling threats to validity.

Control involves the imposing of "rules" by the researcher to decrease the possibility of error and thus increase the probability that the study's findings are an accurate reflection of reality. The rules to achieve control are embedded in the design. Through control, the researcher reduces the influence of extraneous variables. Controlling extraneous variables enables the researcher to clarify "true" relationships among the study variables and to examine the true "effect" of one variable on another. Mechanisms for control within a quantitative

study include subject selection, subjects' knowledge of the study, and the research setting.

Bias means to slant away from the truth or the expected. Bias can be thought of "as if it were a numerical discrepancy between the mean of the intended infinite data set and the mean of the actual infinite data set" (Moses, 1985). An important concern in designing a study is to identify possible causes of bias and eliminate or avoid them. Potential sources of bias include the researcher, measurement tools, individual subjects, samples, data, and statistics. The rules of design are developed to reduce the possibility of bias, enabling study findings to represent the truth.

Validity is an examination of the approximate truth or falseness of the propositions from which the study was developed. It is concerned with whether the conclusions about relationships and/or differences drawn from statistical analysis are an accurate reflection of the real world. Internal validity is the extent to which the findings of the study are a true reflection of reality, rather than the result of the effects of extraneous variables. Internal validity is attained in a study when the findings can be shown to result only from the effect of the independent variable. Threats to the internal validity of a study include history, maturation, testing, instrumentation, statistical regression, selection, and mortality (see box on next page). External validity is attained

---

TYPES OF THREATS TO THE VALIDITY OF A RESEARCH STUDY

INTERNAL VALIDITY

History: External events that occur at the same time the independent variable is introduced and affect the dependent variable.

Maturation: Events that occur between the first and second measurement of the variable, which is the result of time rather than the treatment.

Testing: The difference between the scores of study participants who have and have not been previously exposed to the data collection tool.

Instrumentation: Changes in the measuring instrument over time.

Statistical regression: A phenomenon that occurs when participants' scores regress to the mean because of the instability of extreme scores.

Selection: Bias that results from systematic differences in treatment groups through group assignment.

Mortality: Differential loss of subjects in either the treatment or control group.

EXTERNAL VALIDITY

Hawthorne effect: Alteration in participants' behavior because of their awareness of study participation.

Novelty effect: Subjects' behavior is altered by a treatment that is new.

Experimenter effect: Communication of the investigator's expectations to the subjects.

Measurement effect: The results of variation in data collection procedures.

---

when the results can be generalized to situations outside the specific research setting. Threats to the external validity of a study include the Hawthorne effect, novelty effect, experimenter effect, and measurement effect.

Designs are described as being either experimental or nonexperimental.

Experimental designs are the most powerful methods of examining causality (see Figure 4-2). True experimental designs require three components: (1) randomization, (2) control, and (3) manipulation. They are crafted to provide the maximum amount of control to more closely examine causality between variables. To examine cause one must eliminate all factors influencing the dependent variable other than the cause (independent variable) being studied. Other factors that threaten the validity are controlled by selection of subjects, manipulation of the treatment, and reliable measurement of the dependent and

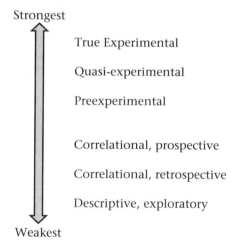

Figure 4-2. Strengths of designs in establishing causal relationships.

independent variable. The study is designed to prevent any other element from intruding into observation of the specific cause and effect that the researcher wishes to examine. Limitations of experimental

---

TYPES OF RESEARCH DESIGNS

QUANTITATIVE STUDY DESIGNS

Descriptive	Describes the variable(s) of interest as it naturally occurs.
Correlational	Examines the relationship between two or more variables.
Preexperimental	Examines the effect of a treatment on a single group.
Quasi-experimental	Examines the effect of a treatment on a group but lacks random assignment or control.
Experimental	Provides the maximum amount of contol in order to examine causality between variables. True experimental designs are characterized by randomization, treatment, and control.

QUALITATIVE STUDY DESIGNS

Phenomenological	Evaluates the human experience.
Grounded theory	Theory building.
Ethnography	Culture exploration.
Historical	Life histories as a person's life experience.

---

study designs occur because many variables are not amenable to manipulation, ethical considerations do not allow for manipulation, impracticality of manipulation, and/or artificiality. When choosing a design, the investigator should strive to select the one offering the maximum amount of control possible within the study situation. Specific experimental designs are discussed in Chapter 13.

The researcher manipulates the independent variable(s) in experimental study designs. Experimental designs include experimental, quasi-experimental, and preexperimental. Quasi-experimental and experimental designs examine causality. Experimental study designs are practical, feasible, and to a certain extent generalizable. Quasi-experimental designs have been developed to control as many threats to validity as possible in a situation where at least one of the three components of true experimental design (randomization, con-

trol groups, and manipulation of the treatment) is lacking. Preexperimental study designs involve examination of the effects of a treatment on a single group; they lack both randomization and control.

Nonexperimental designs do not manipulate a variable. Examples of nonexperimental designs include descriptive and correlational study designs. Descriptive study designs are formulated to gain more information about characteristics within a particular field of study. Their purpose is to provide a picture of situations as they naturally happen. A descriptive design may be used for the purpose of developing theory, identifying problems with current practice, justifying current practice, making judgments, or determining what others in similar situations are doing. The description of the variables leads to an interpretation of the theoretical meaning of the findings and the development of a hypothesis. Correlational study designs are used to examine the relationship or association between two or more variables. The researcher may wish to know if two or more concepts vary directly, if they vary inversely, or if there is no association between the variations in the study concepts. In exploratory, descriptive, and correlational studies no attempt is made to manipulate the study variables. Rather than testing the effects of an intervention, the purpose is to describe a situation as it exists. Studies classified as nonexperimental do not involve manipulation of a variable.

Nonexperimental designs allow exploration of those problems that are not amenable to experimentation. They are strong in reality and an efficient and effective means of collecting a large amount of data about a problem area. Two weaknesses of nonexperimental designs are lack of control and an increased risk of erroneous interpretation of results. Protection against bias is achieved through conceptual and operational definitions of variables, sample selection, and the use of valid and reliable data collection measures.

Determining the Sampling Plan

The term *population* refers to the entire set of individuals or objects that possess specific characteristics that the researcher is interested in studying. The population may be women with heart disease, graduates of NLN-accredited baccalaureate nursing programs, patient records, or serum blood samples. The two types of population considered in research are the target population and the accessible population. The *target population* is the set of individuals or objects for which the researcher wishes to generalize findings. The *accessible population* is the portion of the target population that is available to the researcher.

It is rarely feasible to study the entire population. Therefore a subset of the population, a *sample,* is generally drawn from the accessible population to represent the population of interest. An important consideration in utilizing a sampling method to identify study subjects is to obtain a sample that parallels characteristics of the target population. In doing this the researcher is attempting to minimize sampling error, minimize sampling bias, and maximize representativeness of the sample to the population.

Sampling methods are classified as either probability or nonprobability. *Probability samples* are drawn in a random manner so that every member of the population has an equal chance of being selected. Probability sampling methods include simple random, stratified random, cluster sampling, and systematic sampling. *Nonprobability samples* are drawn utilizing nonrandom methods. Types of nonprobability sampling methods include convenience sampling, quota sampling, purposive sampling, and snowball sampling. Whenever possible, it is preferable to utilize a probability sampling method.

In addition to selecting a sampling approach, the researcher also determines the size of the sample to be drawn for the study. In a qualitative study, where depth of data collection is more important than breadth of information, a smaller sample size is acceptable. When implementing a quantitative study, the researcher generally uses a larger sample. A study may fail to demonstrate differences between groups, not because they did not exist, but because of the small sample size. Larger samples reduce the risk of making a Type II error, or reporting that no difference exists between groups when in fact a difference does exist but is not apparent due to a small sample size. *Power* is defined as the probability that an inferential procedure (statistical test) will support a research hypothesis when it should be supported, or the probability that the inferential procedure (statistical test) will reject the null hypothesis when it should be rejected (Rudy & Kerr, 1991).

However, it is both labor intensive and costly to study an unnecessarily large sample. To draw an appropriately sized sample, sampling tables and computer programs are available that will determine the number of subjects necessary to the study. To determine the sample size the researcher will need to determine the statistical test to be used, the number of study groups, effect size, power, and the level of significance (Cohen, 1988). A conventional standard for power (β) is 0.80 or greater (Polit & Sherman, 1990; Hazard, 1992). This means that the risk of committing a Type II error is 0.20. There is only a 20% risk of rejecting the research hypothesis when it should be accepted. Effect size denotes the degree of the relationship of the research variables. It is a measure of how wrong the null hypothesis is (Polit & Sherman, 1990). In new areas of research, effect sizes are likely to be small. Effect size can be calculated from pilot work, theoretical or clinical information, or from "dummy tables" (Rudy & Kerr, 1991). An alpha of 0.05 is generally the level of significance selected for use in nursing research studies. This means we want to be 95% sure that we did not reject the null hypothesis when the null hypothesis is true. The sampling plan includes the method for obtaining the study sample, type of sampling procedure to be used, and specification of the sample size.

Identifying a Method of Data Collection

Data collection instruments are the link between theoretical and operational definitions. Theoretical concepts are made operational by the data collection methods. The type of study design determines the data collection method and how the study variables are measured. Qualitative data collection methods, which are less structured than those in quantitative designs, collect nonnumerical data through interviews, observational methods, and analysis of written diaries. Qualitative methods of data collection are generally more subjective in nature, as they seek the subjects' view of the phenomenon of interest or description of experiences. Interview data may involve one or more broad questions. The researcher uses communication techniques such as reflection, restatement, and clarification to gather in-depth data from the subject. Qualitative methods usually provide a deeper and broader understanding of the phenomenon of interest. Qualitative data collection methods allow the researcher great freedom in conceptualizing the research problem through a systematic approach to describing events, phenomena, culture, and life experience. Among the weaknesses of these methods are researcher bias and researcher influence.

In contrast, quantitative data collection methods collect numerical data through the use of checklists, questionnaires, and physiological measurements. Quantitative methods are structured in nature and are used for studies involving the testing of hypotheses to measure a particular reality or realities. Quantitative methods of data collection allow the researcher to make comparisons across groups.

The review of the literature is often helpful in identifying possible data collection tools. A phone call or letter to the study's author is often helpful in locating the source of the data collection tool used in that study. The developers of quantitative scales have spent a great deal of time and money developing and testing tools. Usually, they are most willing to share the tool, scoring information, and reliability and validity information. Other sources of data collection tools are listed in Appendix 4-2. There are many advantages to using a data collection tool that has already been tested, one of which is the preestablishment of critical reliability and validity information.

Validity looks at the issue of truth in determining whether the instrument measures what it is supposed to measure. Types of validity include content, construct, and criterion-related validity. Content validity refers to the degree to which the instrument reflects the universe of content. It asks: Does the data collection tool reflect the body of knowledge pertaining to the concept of study? Content validity is established through review of the literature and evaluation by a panel of experts (both professional and lay). Construct validity examines the degree to which the data collection instrument measures the theoretical concepts. "Correlational studies comprise the most widely used approach to construct validation. Examples include simple predictive and concurrent correlational studies, multiple regression/prediction studies, the 'known-groups comparisons' designs, factor analysis studies, and multitrait-multimethod studies (to obtain evidence of convergent and discriminant validities)" (Goodwin & Goodwin, 1991). Criterion-related validity, in general, is the relationship between the measurement tool and some external measure. It can be subdivided into predictive validity and concurrent validity. Predictive validity of an instrument refers to its ability to predict a future behavior on some measure. An example of predictive validity might be the ability of the Mosby AssessTest to predict NCLEX pass rates. Concurrent validity addresses the relationship between two measures of the same concept. An example of this might be the relationship between blood pressure readings using a mercury sphygmomanometer and a Dinamap electronic blood pressure instrument.

As crucial to the evaluation of an instrument's validity is its reliability. A data collection measure cannot be valid if it is not reliable. Reliability explores the issue of reproducibility or consistency. Reliability can be defined as the absence of errors of measurement. When an instrument is used in a sample, the observed score is the true score minus measurement error, and reliability estimates this. Reliability examines errors of measurement through internal consistency (coefficient alpha, split half, kappa coefficient, and KR-20), stability (test-retest), and homogeneity (intrarater and interrater reliability). The focus of reliability is the ability of the instrument to produce these measures on repeated administrations or data collection points. Reliability coefficients vary from 0.0 to 1. A reliability coefficient of 1 indicates that no measurement error exists, whereas a reliability coefficient of 0 indicates that all of the observed variance is due to measurement error. When an instrument is being used for group level comparisons, the reliability coefficient should be at least 0.80 for an established instrument and 0.70 for a new instrument. There is not a single correct way of assessing reliability. Reliability estimates are population dependent. Therefore, the reliability of the tool should be recalculated in the study sample during the data analysis phase.

Conducting a Pilot Study

A pilot study may fulfill many functions and is well worth the time involved. A pilot study generally involves a small sample of subjects drawn from the same population as those from which the study sample will be drawn. A pilot study uses the same tools as those that will be administered during the larger study. It will allow the researcher to determine the reliability of the measuring instruments when used in this population. Other information re-

STEPS OF THE ANALYSIS, INTERPRETATION, AND DISSEMINATION

- Analyzing the data
- Interpreting and evaluating the findings
- Communicating the findings
- Using research findings

garding administration may be clarified, such as the time it will take to complete the data collection protocol, the presence of confusing information, problems utilizing physiological measurements in this population, and projected costs. The researcher may also use data collected at this time to evaluate the data entry and analysis methods that are planned in the larger study. Many proposal review groups look very critically at the preliminary work prior to funding.

THE ANALYSIS AND INTERPRETATION PHASE OF THE RESEARCH PROCESS

Analyzing the Data

Following data entry, the data gathered are analyzed in order to elucidate underlying patterns and relationships. Data analysis differs depending on whether a quantitative or qualitative approach is used.

Quantitative studies generate numerical data that fall into one of four categories. These four rank-ordered categories are: nominal, ordinal, interval, and ratio. The lowest level, *nominal* measurement, is simply assignment of numbers to signify categories. Nominal categories must be exhaustive and mutually exclusive. They are simply a classification scheme for sorting. Examples of nominal level data include: gender, eye color, profession, type of hepatitis, type of contraception used, and blood type. *Ordinal* measurement permits the ordering of attributes according to some hierarchy or relative standing. The ordinal level does not specify equal distance between the relative standing regard-

ing the attribute of interest. Examples of ordinal ranking would be level of education or when caring behaviors are ranked from lowest to highest. At times an ordinal scale may be treated as an interval level scale (Knapp, 1990). *Interval* measurement specifies both rank ordering and equal distance between the rank of the attribute of interest and contains an arbitrary zero. Examples of interval levels of measurement include IQ tests and temperature in Fahrenheit or centigrade. The highest level of measurement is that of *ratio* level. Ratio scales specify rank ordering and equal distance between ranks and specify a rational and meaningful zero. Examples of ratio levels of data include height, weight, blood pressure, hematocrit, cardiac output, and oxygen saturation.

Once the level of measurement of the variables has been identified, quantitative data can be analyzed using descriptive and/or inferential statistical tests. *Descriptive statistics* summarize or describe the characteristic of the sample. Descriptive statistics include frequency distributions, measures of central tendency (mean, median, mode), and measures of dispersion (range and standard deviation).

Inferential statistics are those statistical tests that are used for hypothesis testing. The two types of inferential statistical tests are parametric and nonparametric. *Nonparametric* statistical tests are used with nominal or ordinal data, a small sample size, or when the group is not normally distributed. *Parametric* statistical tests are used when the data are at the interval or ratio

STEPS OF HYPOTHESIS TESTING

1. Formulate the hypothesis
2. Set the level of significance
3. Determine the sample size
4. Calculate the test statistic
5. Accept or reject the null hypothesis

level, the variable being measured in the sample is normally distributed in the population to which you plan to generalize your findings, and the sample size is adequate (size determined by power analysis). While inferential statistical tests measure differences between groups regarding the variable of interest, correlational statistical procedures measure relationships among the variables of interest. Table 4-4 provides an overview of parametric and nonparametric statistical tests. Once the statistical test has been selected, the computations are generally carried out by computer. Following statistical analysis of the data, the study findings are evaluated and interpreted. The steps of hypothesis testing are provided in the box.

Qualitative methods are an accepted means for studying nursing phenomena. In contrast to quantitative studies that specify a relationship between variables, qualitative research questions are broadly stated. Data collection occurs via systematic observation and/or the use of open-ended interviews to generate nonnumerical data, which represents a sample of situations or events. "In analyzing the data, verbatim statements, thoughts, actions, and observations are critically examined to identify patterns, themes, categories or exemplars" (Bull, 1992, p. 378). Qualitative analysts immerse themselves in the culture of those studied in order to better report what the subjects think, feel, and know. The major approaches to qualitative research include grounded theory (development of theory), phenomenology (study of the experience), ethnography (culture exploration), and life histories (a person's life experience). These four inductive approaches to qualitative research are utilized to understand situations, experiences, and cultures of those studied (Bull, 1992). Data analysis generates themes and recurring commonalities and/or patterns. Validation of themes by researchers' sharing and/or triangulation methods is the next phase of data analysis; finally themes is integrated into a whole, providing a framework or model of data discovery.

Qualitative studies collect and analyze nonnumerical data. Data collection and data analysis occur simultaneously. In qualitative research the data are collected until the data begin to repeat. Data are analyzed by emerging patterns, themes, and categories. Ethnograph and Zy-Index are computer software programs designed to analyze qualitative data.

Interpreting and Evaluating the Findings
Interpretation and evaluation of the findings are the final areas of the research process. These sections are concisely and sequentially presented. "The function of these final sections are to interrelate all aspects of the research process and to discuss, interpret, and identify the limitations and generalizations relevant to this investigation, thereby furthering nursing research" (LoBlondo-Wood & Haber, 1994, p. 425).

The interpretation of the findings section is considered to be a data-bound area of the investigation. Interpretation of data sets the stage for later discussion of results; therefore this section should reflect a sequential presentation of data for all hypotheses tested. Data are reported for both the supported and nonsupported hypotheses with no conclusions drawn or inferences made in this presentation. The statistical test used and the results obtained are reported. Tables are very useful for data presentation. This section is for objectivity of thought and not opinions or generalizations. The interpretation section should be stated concisely, logically, and in an organized format.

The discussion and evaluation section evaluates the results of the interpretation section. Here the researcher ties the study findings to the real world. Limitations are noted in regard to the study design, sample, and data collection methods. Findings are generalized to a similar population with caution. The investigator discusses the data in relation to all hypotheses and research questions stated. This is the investigator's opportunity to discuss the logic of the hypotheses posed, the theoretical framework, the methods, and the data analysis. This section concludes with a discussion of recommendations or suggestions for application to clinical practice, current theoretical knowledge, and/or for future research.

Communicating the Findings

The final step in the research process is the dissemination phase. Even the most important study findings will not change practice unless they are communicated to others. The greatest impact will be achieved if the findings are communicated to nurses practicing in the clinical arena and not just to other researchers. Research findings may be presented in the format of a verbal paper presentation, written paper presentation, or poster presentation.

Presenting a poster presentation provides the opportunity for researchers to review ongoing as well as completed research studies. A poster presentation is an opportunity to interact with other professionals who are interested in the research topic. In designing the poster, the researcher should keep in mind that the primary impact will be visual. Therefore, for maximum utility the poster should be eye-catching, simply written, and clearly convey the essential points of the study. Typically, conference organizers will provide a list of guidelines for the poster presentation. This will include the size limitations of the poster, whether the poster will need to be freestanding or attached to a bulletin board, the type of audience anticipated, and the time the poster is to be displayed (Lippman & Ponton, 1989). The poster generally contains the study purpose, sample, procedures for data collection and analysis, study findings, and study implications (Sexton, 1984). During the conference a poster may be overlooked, not because of the quality of the research, but because the poster is not visually appealing or because it contains too much information. The text of the poster should be such that it can be read at a distance of 4 to 6 feet. McDaniel, Bach, and Poole (1993) recommend print of ¼" to ⅜" (24 to 30 point type). Pictures, graphs, or brightly colored symbols are helpful in adding interest to the poster. Handouts with your name and address can be distributed at the time of the presentation to provide more in-depth information on the research project. The actual time of presentation of the poster is a wonderful opportunity to discuss your project with other interested individuals.

Research findings are also disseminated through generally short 10- to 15-minute

Table 4-4
Statistical Tests

Level of Measurement of the Dependent Variable	1 Sample Case	2 Sample Cases—Related	2 Sample Cases—Independent	3 or More Sample Cases—Related	3 or More Sample Cases—Independent	Measures of Correlation
			NONPARAMETRIC STATISTICAL TESTS			
Nominal (mode)	Chi-Square (to test the difference in proportions in two or more groups)	McNemar Change Test (tests the difference in proportions for two paired samples)	Fishers Exact Probability Test Chi-Square for Independent Samples	Cochran Q	Chi-Square for Independent Samples	Contingency Coefficient (measures the association between two variables)
Ordinal (median)	Kolmogorov-Smirnov One Sample Runs	Sign Test Wilcoxon Matched Pairs	Median Test Mann Whitney U Kolmogorov-Smirnov 2 sample test Wald-Wolfowitz Runs Test	Friedman Two-Way Analysis of Variance	Kruskal-Wallis One Way ANOVA	Logistic Regression (measures the association between more than two dichotomous variables) Spearman Correlation (measures the association between two variables) Kenndall Correlation (measures the association between two variables)
Interval (mean)		Walsh Test	Randomization test for two independent samples			

PARAMETRIC STATISTICAL TESTS

Interval or ratio	t test		Repeated Measures ANOVA	ANOVA (tests the difference between three or more groups) ANCOVA (difference between groups after controlling for the influences of another variable) MANOVA (the effect of two or more indep variables on a dependent variable)	Pearson's r (measures the association between two variables) Multiple Regression (examines the effects of two or more independent variables on a dependent variable) Canonical Correlation (2 or more independent variables correlated with 2 or more dependent variables) Path Analysis (tests the strength of the relationship among variables)
	t test (dependent) a single group tested twice	Independent t test—two groups (tests the differences between two groups or two sets of scores)			

(Adapted from Siegel, S. (1956). *Nonparametric statistics for the behavioral sciences.* New York: McGraw-Hill Book Company.)

verbal paper presentations. Audiovisuals, slides, or overhead transparencies are generally used to supplement the oral presentation. There are many commercial presentation packages available, such as Aldus Persuasion and Wordperfect Presentation that can be used to generate visually appealing and clearly readable slides and overhead transparencies. Because of the time limitations associated with the presentation, the researcher may present only a portion of the entire study or briefly cover the major points of the project. Presenters usually begin with the specific aims of the study and its scientific merit, and then discuss the design and data collection phase. The majority of the presentation focuses on the study findings, implications, and recommendations. At the end of the presentation period 2 to 3 minutes are often left for the audience to ask questions. It is beneficial to rehearse the presentation with colleagues before the conference. Feedback received can identify portions of the study that are unclear and validate that the presentation is within the specified time frame.

The final phase of the research process is the publication of research findings. There are numerous research journals that publish data-based articles. The author guidelines can be obtained either from an issue of the journal or by a query letter. The following are some very general guidelines for developing a data-based manuscript. Data-based manuscripts are generally limited to 15 to 20 typed pages. The content of the article is generally concisely written and organized around several headings. The article is often preceded by a brief abstract. The text of the article begins with a review of the problem of study. This is the time when the researcher can catch the attention of the reader by pointing out the importance of this problem of study and discussing the aims of this study. In general, a research-based manuscript follows the steps of the research process.

Dissemination of findings to the clinical audience is equally important to dissemination of findings to the research audience, for if research is not communicated to the people who will utilize it in practice, its value is limited (Tornquist, Funk, & Champagne, 1989). The numerous benefits of communicating research findings include personal and professional recognition, the ability to positively change practice, and the enhancement of the body of nursing knowledge.

Using Research Findings
Using research findings bridges the gap between research and practice. This goal is fulfilled through the collaborative efforts of nurse researchers, nurse educators, and practicing nurses.

Nurse educators can set the stage for the use of research in practice by integrating current research findings throughout the curriculum. Relevant investigations should be incorporated into each lecture, seminar, discussion, or demonstration topic. Gaps in research areas should be emphasized by educators. The nursing student should emerge from the academic learning environment supporting the spirit of inquiry and consistently utilizing the most current valid research findings in practice.

Practicing nurses, both administrators and clinical nurses, then emerge from this environment supporting practice innovations validated by theory and research findings. Continuing education through critique of the latest research findings and attendance at research dissemination meetings are the ultimate goal of nurses invested in the most current nursing research. Practicing nurses should seek nursing systems supporting research use and collaborate with nurse researchers.

Practicing nurses can discover the reward of developing optimum care from scholarly inquiry (Long, 1992).

Nurse researchers bridge the gap between research and practice by becoming active members of hospital, clinic, and/or unit nursing research advisory committees within practice institutions. Nurse researchers should continue with the pursuit of high-quality, focused research, and seek publication and dissemination of research findings via journals and conferences.

SUMMARY

- Research problems may be derived from a clinical situation, an unresolved issue in the literature, or a research priority identified by a professional organization.
- Research studies are based on a theoretical or conceptual framework that allows the researcher to visualize the problem within a logical frame of reference.
- The review of literature is organized around subheadings, which are the concepts and interrelationships of the study variables. The review of the literature is a critical analysis of earlier work that delineates what is and is not known about the research topic.
- Assumptions are those matters that are universally accepted to be true even though they have not been scientifically tested.
- A hypothesis is a statement of the expected relationship between the independent and dependent variables, which may be directional or nondirectional, simple or complex, research or null.
- A theoretical or conceptual definition of a study variable is one that is drawn from the theoretical or conceptual framework. The operational definition represents how the researcher plans to measure the study variable.

- The research design is the blueprint for study implementation that maximizes control over factors that could interfere with the true relationship between study variables. The design phase includes selection of the research design, data collection methods, sampling framework, and the data entry/analysis plan.
- Qualitative research involves the collection, integration, and synthesis of nonnumerical narrative data. It is used for theory generation and formulation of hypotheses. Quantitative research involves the collection, integration, and analysis of numerical data.
- Research designs may be categorized as either experimental or nonexperimental. Nonexperimental designs include descriptive and correlational study designs. Experimental designs may be true experimental, quasi-experimental, and preexperimental. When choosing a design, one should select the design that offers the greatest amount of control possible within the study situation.
- The term *population* refers to the entire set of individuals or objects that possess specific characteristics that the researcher is interested in studying. As it is rarely feasible to study the entire population, a subset, or sample, is drawn to represent the population. Samples may be either probability (random) or nonprobability (nonrandom).
- The data collection methods represent how the study variables are measured. Methods of data collection include observation, interviews, questionnaires, and physiological measures. Data collection measures must be both valid and reliable.
- When collecting data, every effort should be made to recruit and retain as many study subjects from the sample as possible.

- Numerical data can be classified as either nominal, ordinal, interval, or ratio level data. The data collected can be analyzed using either descriptive or inferential statistical tests. Nominal and ordinal level data are analyzed using nonparametric statistical tests. Interval and ratio level data are generally analyzed using parametric statistical tests, providing the sample size is adequate and the variable being measured in the sample is normally distributed in the population to which the findings will be generalized.

FACILITATING CRITICAL THINKING

1. Identify the independent variable, dependent variable, sample, and form of the hypothesis (directional, nondirectional, or null).
   a. Patients in open wards of general hospitals will receive more minutes of nursing care than will patients in private rooms.
   b. There will be no difference in the incidence of lung cancer in adult white males who do or do not smoke.
   c. There will be no difference in attitudes of caring for AIDS patients among junior, senior, and career-ladder baccalaureate nursing students.
   d. There will be a difference in muscle mass between adult solid organ transplant patients who do and do not participate in a structured exercise program.
2. Hypothesis: Premature infants supported by diaper rolls will gain weight faster than unsupported infants.
   a. Write a problem statement for this study.
   b. Write a null hypothesis.
   c. Is this a basic or applied research study? Explain your answer?

   d. Write operational definitions for the study variables.
   e. List an assumption of this study.
   f. Will this study use an experimental or nonexperimental study design?
3. For each of the problems listed discuss whether you think the research problems are examples of basic or applied research.
   a. Is there a difference in stress scores between men and women hospitalized with an acute MI?
   b. Is there a difference in the incidence of diarrhea in patients who receive enteral feedings using a sterile protocol and a clean protocol?
4. For each of the following terms state an operational definition.
   a. Caring
   b. Hypertension
   c. Anxiety
   d. Impaired perfusion
5. Identify whether the following variables would be measured at the nominal, ordinal, interval, or ratio level.
   a. Hematocrit
   b. Income
   c. Gender
   d. Cardiac output
   e. Specialty certification examination score

References

SUBSTANTIVE

MOCK, V. (1993). Body image in women treated for breast cancer. *Nursing Research, 42*(3), 153-157.

TOTH, J. C. (1993). Is stress at hospital discharge after acute myocardial infarction greater in women than in men? *American Journal of Critical Care, 2*(1), 35-40

CONCEPTUAL

BARNSTEINER, J. H. (1989). Accessing clinical agencies: the do's and don'ts. *Nursing Research, 38*(6), 382.

BLOCH, D. (1990). Strategies for setting and implementing the National Center for Nursing Research priorities. *Applied Nursing Research, 3*(1), 2-6.

BULL, M. A. (1992). Using qualitative methods in teaching undergraduate students research. *Nursing in Health Care, 13*(7), 378-381.

CHINN, P. L., & JACOBS, M. K. (1983). *Theory and nursing.* St. Louis: C.V. Mosby.

COHEN, J. (1988). *Statistical power analysis for the behavioral sciences* (2nd ed.). New Jersey: Lawrence Erlbaum Associates Publishers.

DIEKMANN, J. M., & SMITH, J. M. (1989). Strategies for assessment and recruitment of subjects for nursing research. *Western Journal of Nursing Research, 11*(4), 418-430.

GIVEN, B. A., KEILMAN, L. J., COLLINS, C., & GIVEN, C. W. (1990). Strategies to minimize attrition in longitudinal studies. *Nursing Research, 39*(3), 184-186.

GOODWIN, L. D., & GOODWIN, W. L. (1991). Estimating construct validity. *Research in Nursing & Health. 14*, 235-243.

GORDON, S. E., & STOKES, S. A. (1989). Improving response rate to mailed questionnaires. *Nursing Research, 38*(6), 375-376.

HAZARD, B. H. (1992). How many subjects are enough? *Clinical Nurse Specialist, 6*(1), 20.

HINSHAW, A. S. (1988). Evolving clinical nursing research priorities: A national endeavor. *Journal of Professional Nursing, 4*(6), 398, 458-459.

KILLIEN, M., & NEWTON, K. (1990). Longitudinal research—the challenge of maintaining continued involvement of participants. *Western Journal of Nursing Research, 12*(5), 689-692.

KNAPP, T. R. (1990). Treating ordinal scales as interval scales: An attempt to resolve the controversy. *Nursing Research, 39*, 121-123.

LEEDY, P. D. (1993). *Practical research* (5th ed.). New York: Macmillan.

LIPPMAN, D. T., & PONTON, K. S. (1989). Designing a research poster with impact. *Western Journal of Nursing Research, 11*(4), 477-485.

LOBIONDO-WOOD, G., & HABER, J. (1994). *Nursing research: Methods, critical appraisal, and utilization* (3rd ed.). St. Louis: C.V. Mosby.

LONG, R. E. (1992). Research utilization by staff nurses: successful strategies. *Critical Care Nursing Quarterly, 15*(3), 23-28.

MCDANIEL, R. W., BACH, C. A., & POOLE, M. J. (1993). Poster update: getting their attention. *Nursing Research, 42*(5), 302-304.

MOSES, L. E. (1985). Statistical concepts fundamental to investigators. *The New England Journal of Medicine, 312*(14), 890-897.

NAYLOR, M. D. (1990). An example of a research grant application: Comprehensive discharge planning for the elderly. *Research in Nursing and Health, 13*, 327-347.

POLIT, D. F., & SHERMAN, R. E. (1990). Statistical power in nursing research. *Nursing Research, 39*(6), 365-368.

RUDY, E., ESTOK, P., KERR, M., MENZEL, L. (1994). Research incentives: Money versus gifts. *Nursing Research, 43*(4), 253-255.

RUDY, E. B., & KERR, M. (1991). Unraveling the mystique of power analysis. *Heart & Lung, 20*(5), 517-522.

SANDELOWSKI, M., DAVIS, D. H., & HARRIS, B. G. (1989). Artful design: Writing the proposal for research in the naturalist paradigm. *Research in Nursing & Health, 12*, 77-84.

SEXTON, D. L. (1984). Presentation of research findings: The poster session. *Nursing Research, 33*(6), 375-376.

TOURNQUIST, E. M., FUNK, S. G., & CHAMPAGNE, M. T. (1989). Writing research reports for clinical audiences. *Western Journal of Nursing Research, 11*(5), 577-592.

WILLIAMS, M. A. (1980). Assumptions in research. *Research in Nursing and Health, 3*, 47-48.

WINEMAN, N. M. & DURAND, E. (1992). Incentives and rewards for subjects in nursing research. *Western Journal of Nursing Research, 14*(4), 526-531.

WOODS, N. F., & CATANZARO, M. (1988). *Nursing research: Theory and practice.* St. Louis: C.V. Mosby Co.

METHODOLOGICAL

FAWCETT, J., & DOWNS, F. S. (1992). *The relationship of theory and research* (2nd ed.). Philadelphia: F.A. Davis.

KERLINGER, F. (1986). *Foundations of behavioral research* (3rd ed.). New York: Holt, Rinehart and Winston.

KIRKPATRICK, H., & MARTIN, M. (1991). Communicating nursing research through poster presentations. *Western Journal of Nursing Research, 13*(1), 145-148.

KNAFL, K. A., & WEBSTER, D. D. (1988). Managing and analyzing qualitative data: A description of tasks, techniques, and materials. *Western Journal of Nursing Research, 10*(2), 195-218.

HISTORICAL

SINCLAIR, W. J. *(passim),* C. G. HEMPEL, pp. 3-6. In Mannoia, V.J. (1980). *What is science? An introduction to the structure and methodology of science.* Washington D.C.: University Press of America, Inc.

Appendix 4-1
PUBLICATIONS THAT DISCUSS RESEARCH PRIORITIES FOR NURSING SPECIALTIES

ALBRECHT, M. (1992). Research priorities for home health nursing. *Nursing & Health Care, 13*(10), 538-541.

BAYLEY, W. W., CARROUGHER, G. J., MARVIN, J. A., KNIGHTON, J., RUTAN, R. L., & WEBER, B. (1991). Research priorities for burn nursing: patient, nurse, and burn prevention education. *Journal of Burn Care & Rehabilitation, 12*(4), 377-383.

BENEDICT, S. (1990). Nursing research priorities related to HIV/AIDS. *Oncology Nursing Forum, 17*(4), 571-573.

BLOCH, D. (1990). Strategies for setting and implementing the National Center for Nursing Research Priorities. *Applied Nursing Research, 3*(1), 2-6.

BROWER, H. T., & CRIST, M. A. (1985). Research priorities in gerontologic nursing for long-term care. *IMAGE, 17,* 22-27.

BURNS, T. J., BATAVIA, A. I., SMITH, Q. W., & DEJONG, G. (1990). Primary health care needs of persons with physical disabilities: What are the research and service priorities? *Archives of Physical Medicine & Rehabilitation, 71*(2), 138-143.

BUSHY, A. (1992). Rural nursing research priorities. *Journal of Nursing Administration, 22*(1), 50-56.

FITZPATRICK, E., SULLIVAN, J., SMITH, A., MUCOWSKI, D., HOFFMANN, E., & DUNN, P. (1991). Clinical nursing research priorities: A Delphi study. *Clinical Nurse Specialist, 5*(2), 94-99.

HENRY, B., MOODY, L. E., PENDERGAST, J. F., O'DONNELL, J., HUTCHINSON, S. A., & SCULLY, G. (1987). Delineation of nursing administration research priorities. *Nursing Research, 36*(5), 309-314.

HINDS, P. S., NORVILLE, R., ANTHONY, L. K., BRISCOE, B. W., GATTUSO, J. S., & QUARGNENTI, A. (1990). Establishing pediatric cancer nursing research priorities: A Delphi study. *Journal of Pediatric Oncology Nursing, 7*(2), 51-52.

HINDS, P. S., NORVILLE, R., ANTHONY, L. K., BRISCOE, B. W., GATTUSO, J. S., & QUARGNENTI, A. (1990). Establishing pediatric cancer nursing research priorities: A Delphi study. *Journal of Pediatric Oncology Nursing, 7*(3), 101-8.

KNIGHTON, J., CARROUGHER, G. J., MARVIN, J. A., BAYLEY, W. W., RUTAN, R. L., & WEBER, B. (1992). Research priorities for burn nursing: Report of psychosocial issues group. *Journal of Burn Care & Rehabilitation, 13*(1), 97-104.

LINDQUIST, R., BANASIK, J., BARNSTEINER, J., BEECROFT, P. C., PREVOST, S., & RIEGEL, B. (1993). Determining AACN's research priorities for the 90's. *American Journal of Critical Care, 2*(2), 110-117.

MARCHETTE, L., & FAULCONER, D. R. (1986). Perioperative nursing research: A study of priorities. *AORN Journal, 44*(3), 387-394.

MISENER, T. R., WATKINS, J. G., & OSSEGE, J. (1990). Public health nursing research priorities. *South Carolina Nurse, 5*(1), 30-31.

MOONEY, K. H., FERRELL, B. R., NAIL, L. M., BENEDICT, S. C., & HABERMAN, M. R. (1991). 1991 Oncology Nursing Society research priorities survey. *Oncology Nursing Forum, 18*(8), 1381-1388.

NAPPIER, P., STANFIELD, J., SIMON, J. M., BENNETT, S., & COWAN, C. F. (1990). Identifying clinical nursing research priorities. *Nursing Connections, 3*(2), 45-50.

NAYLOR, M. D., MUNRO, B. H., & BROOTEN, D. A. (1991). Measuring the effectiveness of nursing practice. *Clinical Nurse Specialist, 5*(4), 210-215.

OBERST, M. (1978). Priorities in cancer nursing. *Cancer, 1,* 281-290.

RUTAN, R. L., CARROUGHER, G. J., MARVIN, J. A., BAYLEY, E. W., KNIGHTON, J., & WEBER, B. (1992). Research priorities for burn nursing: Report on physiologic issues. *Journal of Burn Care & Rehabilitation, 13*(3), 373-377.

TANNER, C. A., & LINDEMAN, D. A. (1987). Research in nursing education: Assumptions and priorities. *Journal of Nursing Education, 26*(2), 50-59.

THOMAS, B. S. (1984). Identifying priorities for prepared childbirth research. *Journal of Obstetrics and Gynecological Nursing, 13,* 400-408.

WALKER, C. L. (1992). Setting research priorities. *Journal of Pediatric Oncology Nursing, 9*(1), 29-30.

WORTHINGTON-ROBERTS, B. (1990). Directions for research on women and nutrition. *American Journal of Health Promotion, 5*(1), 63-69.

Appendix 4-2
RESOURCES FOR SELECTING TOOLS TO MEASURE NURSING VARIABLES

ANASTASI, A. (1985). *Psychological testing* (Ed. 6). New York: Macmillan.

ANDRULIS, R. (1977). *Adult assessment: A source book of tests and measurement of human behavior.* Springfield, Ill.: Charles C. Thomas.

BAUER, J. D., ACKERMAN, P. G., & TORO, G. (1982). *Clinical laboratory methods* (9th ed.). St. Louis: C.V. Mosby.

BEENE, C. A. (1979). *Women and women's issues: A handbook of tests and measurements.* San Francisco: Jossey-Bass.

BRONZINO, J. D. (1986). *Biomedical engineering and instrumentation: Basic concepts and applications.* Boston: PWS Publishers.

CATTELL, R. B., & JOHNSON, R. C. (1986). *Functional psychological testing: Principles and instruments.* New York: Brunner/Mazel.

CHUN, K., COBB, S., & FRENCH, J. R., JR. (1975). *Measures for psychological assessment: A guide to 3000 original sources and their application.* Ann Arbor, Mich.: Institute for Social Research, University of Michigan.

CIMINERO, A. R., CALHOUN, K. S., & ADAMS, H. E. (Eds.). (1986). *Handbook of behavioral assessment* (2nd ed.). New York: John Wiley & Sons.

COMREY, A. L., BACKER, T. E., & GLASER, E. M. (1973). *A sourcebook for mental health measures.* Los Angeles: Human Interaction Research Institute.

FERRIS, C. (1980). *A guide to medical laboratory instruments.* Boston: Little, Brown.

FRANK-STROMBERG, M. (1988). *Instruments for clinical nursing research.* Norwalk, Conn.: Appleton & Lange.

GEDDES, L. A., & BAKER, L. E. (1989). *Principles of applied biomedical instrumentation* (3rd ed.). New York: John Wiley & Sons.

GOLDMAN, B. A., & BUSCH, J. (1985). *Directory of unpublished experimental measures* (Vol. 4). New York: Human Science Press.

HART, S. E., & WALTZ, C. F. (1988). *Educational outcomes: Assessments of quality-state of the art and future directions.* New York: National League for Nursing. Pub. 18-2249.

KEYSER, D. J., & SWEETLAND, R. C. (1988). *Test critiques* (Vols. I-VI). Kansas City, Mo.: Westport Publishers, Test Corporation of America.

LYERLY, A. (1973). *Handbook of psychiatric rating scales* (2nd ed.). Rockville, Md.: National Institute of Mental Health.

JOHNSON, O. G. (1976). *Tests and measurements in child development: Handbook II* (Vols. 1 and 2). San Francisco: Jossey-Bass.

JOHNSON, O. G., & COMMARRITO, J. W. (1971). *Tests and measurements in child development: Handbook I.* San Francisco: Jossey-Bass.

MILLER, D. C. (1983). *Handbook of research design and social measurement* (4th ed.). New York: David McKay.

MITCHELL, J. V., JR. (1983) *Tests in print.* Lincoln, Neb.: Buros Institute of Mental Measurement.

MITCHELL, J. V. (Ed.). (1985). *The ninth mental measurements yearbook* (Vols. I and II). Lincoln, Neb: Buros Institute of Mental Measurement.

PFEIFFER, W. J., HESLEN, R., & JONES, J. E. (1976). *Instrumentation in human relations training* (2nd ed.). LaJolla, Calif.: University Associates.

PRICE, J. L., & MUELLER, C. W. (1986). *Handbook of organizational measurement.* Marshfield, Mass.: Sir Isaac Pitman & Sons.

REEDER, L. G., RAMACHER, L., & GORELNIK, S. (1976). *Handbook of scales and indices of health behavior.* Pacific Palisades, Calif.: Goodyear.

Robinson, J. P., & Shriver, P. R. (1973). *Measures of social psychological attitudes.* Ann Arbor, Mich.: University of Michigan.

Straus, M. A., & Brown, B. W. (1978). *Family measurement techniques: Abstracts of published instruments, 1935-1974* (Rev. ed.). Minneapolis: University of Minnesota Press.

Sweetland, R. C., & Keyser, D. J. (1986). *Tests* (2nd ed.). Kansas City, Mo.: Test Corporation of America.

Waltz, C. F., & Strickland, O. L. (1988). *Measurement of nursing outcomes (Vol. III: Measuring client outcomes).* New York: Springer Publishing.

Ward, M. J., & Felter, M. E. (1979). *Instruments for use in nursing education research.* Boulder Colo.: Western Interstate Commission for Higher Education.

Ward, M. J., & Lindeman, C. (Eds.). (1979). *Instruments for measuring nursing practice and other health care variables.* DHEW Pub No HRA 78-53, Vol. 1, and HRA 78-54, Vol 2. Hyattsville, Md.: Department of Health, Education, and Welfare.

Source: Waltz, C. F., Strickland, O. L., & Lenz, E. R. (1991). *Measurement in nursing research* (2nd ed.). Philadelphia: F.A. Davis.

CHAPTER 5

OVERVIEW OF QUANTITATIVE AND QUALITATIVE APPROACHES

JANET BLENNER

In the past nursing research has primarily focused on the use of quantitative methods. More recently nursing research has recognized the need for both qualitative and quantitative research in furthering the development of nursing science. Each method offers its own unique approach and purpose. For instance, quantitative research is useful in testing specific variables such as nursing interventions, whereas qualitative research seeks to grasp the essence of the holistic, subjective experience, such as an understanding of patients' experiences of their illness. In this way the two approaches are viewed as complementary. Both approaches are contrasted in Table 5-1.

QUANTITATIVE VERSUS QUALITATIVE NURSING RESEARCH

Commonly, the quantitative approach is referred to as "hard science" since it is perceived as rigorous, systematic, and objective, focusing on numerical data and using statistical analysis and controls in an attempt to eliminate bias. Quantitative research emerges from logical positivism, which contends that the researcher must be truly objective and that precise measurement is essential. Quantitative research seeks to establish relationships between variables and causal links when indicated.

While qualitative research is also systematic in its analysis, it is not interested in control and manipulation but in the preservation of the holistic, subjective experience of individuals. This approach is commonly referred to as an emic perspective since it is derived from the individual's experience rather than the researcher's perspective. Human behavior is predicated on human meanings. In the attempt to gain insight into the individual's perception, the researcher does not want to manipulate or control any aspect of the design but wants to capture the subject's holistic experience in a natural setting. Since the focus is holistic, the approach to the study remains broad in an effort to retain the experience of the whole.

Table 5-1

Contrasting Quantitative and Qualitative Research Designs

Quantitative	Qualitative
Specific focus on variables	Holistic broad focus
Objectivity	Subjectivity
Scientific rigor, manipulation, and control; often controlled setting	No manipulation or control; natural setting
Tests theoretical framework	Does not test theory; generates theory
Deductive	Primarily inductive
Hypothesis	Broad research questions
Uses psychosocial or physiological instruments	Uses flexible interview guide, observation, and other communicative methods
Subjects based on sampling procedures; subject numbers based on procedures	Key informants identified; number of informants based on concepts such as theoretical saturation
Statistical analysis of data	Coding of narrative data for patterns and themes; no statistical coding

GOALS AND PURPOSE OF THE STUDY

Typically, the goal of qualitative research is the synthesis or the generation of a theory. For instance, in a grounded theory study of infertility, patients' perceptions of their treatment yielded a stage theory of their passage through treatment (Blenner, 1990). In this way clinicians can gain a better understanding of how patients experience treatment in these various stages.

Quantitative research narrows and reduces its focus to study specific variables of interest. It tests a theoretical framework that consists of axioms and propositions that demonstrate the probable relationships of those variables based on prior related research. Based on previous studies, it uses evidence to predict the direction of the hypothesis. For example, in a study of hemodynamic and oxygen transport changes following endotracheal suctioning in trauma patients (Lookinland & Appel, 1991), the study provided a theoretical context for the proposed hypothesis.

Unlike quantitative research, which begins with a hypothesis, the qualitative approach does not test theory; thus it is inappropriate to include hypotheses. However, broad research questions are appropriate (Schatzman & Strauss, 1982). In fact, qualitative research questions are kept deliberately broad to gain in-depth understanding of some phenomenon. An example might read, "The purpose of this grounded theory study was to explore the perceptions that couples have during the several phases of their treatment" (Blenner, 1990, p. 153). Often these questions reflect general categories that can change as the study proceeds.

Although the qualitative approach does not test theory but seeks to generate it, a specific qualitative approach frequently operates out of its own theoretical orientation. For instance, a person using grounded theory method operates from a symbolic interactionist theory approach. This approach gives the researcher a perspective to the conceptual understanding of the phenomena under study.

APPROACH

Quantitative research uses a deductive approach, generating specific predictions in the form of research questions from more general principles. Qualitative research uses inductive reasoning to develop generalizations or theories from specific observations or interviews. The qualitative approach searches for patterns and themes rather than numerical analysis of the data collected.

LITERATURE REVIEW

The review of literature can be another source of difference between the two approaches. An exhaustive review of the literature is considered a necessity to the quantitative approach. By contrast, qualitative researchers are commonly cautioned to avoid an exhaustive review to reduce the risk of a biased perspective in the collection and analysis of data. Often in qualitative research, the literature review is treated as another source of data and is compared and contrasted to the evolving theory.

SAMPLE

A quantitative focus relies on random or nonrandom sampling procedures. The size of the sample needed for a particular study is based on sampling techniques and power analysis (Cohen, 1977). On the other hand, qualitative research does not rely on standard sampling procedures or power analysis for sample size but uses concepts like data saturation. Data saturation is reached when certain categories consistently emerge and less and less new information is discovered. Also, in qualitative research specific key informants rather than subjects are purposely selected for the type of information they can provide. Generally, the number of informants is much smaller than the sample size in quantitative research, and sampling procedures such as randomization are inappropriate. Glaser and Strauss (1967) and Lofland (1971) suggest that only 20 to 50 interviews are commonly needed for the qualitative interview due to the in-depth nature of the interviews.

DATA COLLECTION TOOLS

Quantitative research also relies on instruments, whether psychosocial or physiological, to collect data. These instruments need to exhibit significant reliability, validity, and sensitivity before they can be used as data collection tools. The qualitative approach does not use psychometrically developed instruments but uses an interview guide with broad themes and probes. This guide is meant to be flexible and may change or be redirected as the study proceeds.

RELIABILITY AND VALIDITY

Issues of reliability and validity also differ in the two approaches. In quantitative research the instruments used to collect the data need to have undergone rigorous psychometric testing before they can be used as data collection testing instruments. Interview guides do not undergo reliability and validity psychometric testing; such testing is perceived as irrelevant. However, qualitative research has become concerned with the credibility or relevance of the data (Glaser & Strauss, 1967). In recent years criteria have been developed for assessing credibility or trustworthiness of the qualitative findings (Lincoln & Guba, 1985; Leininger, 1990). Miles and Huberman (1984) have suggested a process of using two researchers to code the data. Agreements and disagreements are compared with a resulting coefficient. This approach is viewed as assisting in definitional clarity and reliability. Historical research, a form of qualitative research, is particularly concerned with the authentication of all its sources prior to its use in data analysis.

DATA ANALYSIS AND INTERPRETATION

Finally, quantitative study offers the analysis of data or numbers through the use of statistics. Qualitative analysis does not use statistics but analyzes narrations, searching for patterns and themes in the construction of a theory. However, there are systematic methods for coding, categorizing, and analyzing the data for each qualitative style.

Both quantitative and qualitative approaches are needed in nursing since they offer different perspectives, and both can work to enhance patient care. Often the approach is based on what is already known about the subject matter. If little is known or if the researcher's purpose is to get a more in-depth understanding of the subject, then a qualitative approach will help. The decision to use either approach largely depends on the researcher's purpose. For instance, a clinical intervention study would require scientific rigor, manipulation of variables, and statistical analysis that would indicate a quantitative approach. Essentially, the type of approach to be used depends on the knowledge to be obtained.

✎ QUANTITATIVE RESEARCH DESIGNS

As we have seen, quantitative research attempts to establish relationships between variables and tests the theoretical framework upon which hypotheses are derived. These designs are focused on the testing of relationships. Therefore, these designs require scientific rigor, appropriate sampling procedures, and statistical analysis. The degree of scientific rigor needed ranges from least, as in "exploratory research," which uncovers variables about which little is often known to the most rigorous scientific

manipulation of variables and controls, as seen in the "experimental design." The hypothesis for the experimental design is based on a theoretical framework composed of previous studies supporting the direction of the hypothesis. There is often concern over controlling the effects of extraneous variables. However, when there is little preexisting knowledge, quantitative designs such as exploratory and descriptive are used. The box gives an overview of quantitative designs.

NONEXPERIMENTAL RESEARCH
Exploratory Research
Exploratory research is commonly conducted when a review of the literature reveals that little is known about some phenomenon. This approach uses a more flexible rather than a more structured approach as in the other quantitative designs since it attempts to uncover relationships. This approach attempts to explore the dimensions of a phenomenon, the manner in which it is manifested, and any other factors that may be related to the area under investigation. In this approach the researcher gains a richer understanding of the phenomenon of interest. This fuller understanding often has the potential of generating hypotheses for future studies.

OVERVIEW OF QUANTITATIVE RESEARCH DESIGNS

Exploratory—Used to uncover relationships between variables
Descriptive—Examines relationships between variables
Correlational—Examines strength of the relationship between two or more variables
Quasi-experimental—Manipulation of the independent variable causing the depen-

dent variable (however, some element of control may be lacking)
Experimental—Manipulation of the independent variable causing the dependent variable (design exerts tremendous controls and rigor)

Descriptive Research

Although descriptive research may be similar to exploratory research, it is generally more structured. Descriptive research typically uses questionnaires or structured observations. Its main purpose is to examine the relationships among variables when enough information exists. At this point a descriptive rather than exploratory approach is used.

Correlational Research

Correlational research is used to examine the strength of the relationship between two or more variables. The correlation coefficient indicates the actual magnitude of that relationship's strength. A positive or negative sign indicates the direction of that relationship. However, causality cannot be inferred, and no manipulation of the independent variable takes place.

Quasi-experimental Research

Quasi-experimental studies are designed to study causal relationships between variables of interest. Manipulation of the independent variable is studied as the cause of an anticipated outcome or dependent variable. These designs are often limited in their ability to claim causality since they lack some element of control either in the form of a control group, randomization of subjects, or both. Clinical research poses particular problems since it is difficult to meet all the criteria of the true experimental model. However, these designs still offer some research controls over other quantitative designs when a true experimental design is not possible.

EXPERIMENTAL RESEARCH

Experimental research is also concerned with cause-and-effect relationships. However, this type of design is considered the most powerful since the investigator exerts tremendous controls and rigor in the study design. The characterizations of true experiments consist of manipulation of the independent variable, use of controls over the experimental condition, use of a control group, and random assignment of subjects to a control or experimental group. With these controls the researcher can infer that the manipulation of the independent (treatment) variable was the cause of change in the dependent (outcome) variable.

ISSUES AND PROBLEMS IN QUANTITATIVE RESEARCH

Quantitative research has been associated with some unique problems. A major problem with clinical intervention studies is the need for rigorous scientific methods. However, in clinical populations most of the subjects have preexisting pathologies and are undergoing a wide array of treatments. Hence, these studies require extensive identification of probable extraneous variables as patient exclusion criteria or analysis through statistical analysis to determine their influence. Another problem unique to clinical studies is the use of convenience rather than random sampling and assignment. Random sampling refers to the type of sampling procedure used to obtain subjects, whereas random assignment refers to the assigning of subjects to experimental or control groups in the study. This deficit has led to the use of more quasi-experimental rather than experimental methods in nursing research.

Ethical issues in quantitative research involve the protection of subjects from social, psychological, or physical harm during studies. With the increased use of physiological instrumentation and designs in nursing research, it is essential to carefully design protocols and anticipate potential risks to patients. As with any study, subject anonymity and privacy

EVALUATING QUANTITATIVE RESEARCH

1. Research Questions
   Hypotheses should be clear and directly stated. Variables should be clearly identified and operationally defined.
2. Theoretical Framework
   The theoretical framework should form a sound basis for the predicted relationship of the hypothesis. This framework is composed of theoretical suppositions and findings from related research that render a logical and sound basis for the hypothesis.
3. Method
   The researcher should give ample description of the overall method and protocol to be used in soliciting and testing subjects. Type of research design needs to be specified.
   Sampling—Type of probability or non-probability sampling technique should be stated. Size of the sample should also

be determined based on a form of power analysis.
   Procedure—Give a detailed description of the procedure that will take place (keep in mind that it should be clearly described and detailed).
   Instrument—Give specifics about each instrument to be used in the study. The type of instrument used should be congruent with what each variable intends to measure. Information regarding scoring, reliability, and validity should be given. Remember that even with physiological instrumentation data such as test-retest reliability, precision and sensitivity should be given.
4. Data Analysis
   Be detailed about how the data will be processed once collected. Specify type of software used and specific statistics.

---

must also be guarded. Guidelines for evaluating quantitative research are listed in the box.

QUALITATIVE RESEARCH DESIGNS

Qualitative research designs are often based on some theoretical or philosophical perspective. They attempt to preserve the wholeness of an individual's subjective experience rather than reduce it to distinct variables. Because it relies on inductive reasoning, qualitative research does not use numerical or statistical analysis but systematically engages in an interactive process

with narrative data. Such a holistic approach focuses on capturing the subjective experience of individuals, generating a theory rich in details of the overall experience. Data collection techniques include interviewing, observing, recording, collecting artifacts, and other related methods. Interviewing frequently uses process-oriented questions that are open ended, with probes to elicit further data when needed. Data collection often occurs in the natural setting and tends to describe the experiences of the individual. Data collection and analysis often are conducted simultaneously. Although qualitative research is relatively new to nursing research, it has long been used in the social and behavioral sci-

OVERVIEW OF QUALITATIVE DESIGNS

Phenomenological—Describes the "lived experience;" based on phenomenological philosophy

Grounded Theory—Develops a basic social process; based on sociological theory of symbolic interactionism

Ethnographic—Describes cultures and life-ways; based on an anthropological perspective

Historical—Describes patterns of past events to gain understanding of present; based on historical perspective

ences. The box gives an overview of the qualitative designs.

PHENOMENOLOGICAL RESEARCH

Phenomenological research originated from philosophers such as Husserl (1970), Heidegger (1962), and Merleau-Ponty (1962). The aim of phenomenological research is to examine the meaning of life through the interpretation of the lived experiences of individuals (Omery, 1983, 1987). Phenomenological research seeks to find differences among individuals. A major concern is capturing the totality of the human experience, which emphasizes the meaning that social behavior has for the individual. The data is examined through interpretive analysis or hermeneutics.

GROUNDED THEORY RESEARCH

The grounded theory approach was developed by sociologists Glaser and Strauss (1967) and is theoretically based on symbolic interactionism (Blumer, 1969). In grounded theory method, data collection and analysis occur simultaneously. The constant comparison method is used to develop and theoretically refine relevant categories. Through this process the investigator discovers fundamental patterns of social life or basic social processes, which leads to theory development.

ETHNOGRAPHIC RESEARCH

Ethnographic research originated from the anthropological perspective, with a focus on the study of cultures, subcultures, and life-ways within natural settings. The ethnographic researcher attempts to gain an understanding of the culture's world view as well as its rules, norms, and values. To be effective as an ethnographic researcher, it is essential to be accepted by the cultural group. Today the ethnographic approach is also used in health care research, not only to understand the health beliefs of certain cultural groups, but to understand institutions or groups of professionals or patients.

HISTORICAL RESEARCH

Historical research originated with historians, who searched for patterns to gain an understanding of history. Historical research rigorously collects and critically evaluates data to establish facts and relationships concerning past events. The historical researcher uses a systematic method to answer questions or test hypotheses by objectively evaluating and interpreting available historical evidence. The data are usually in the form of written records such as letters, diaries, artifacts, and audio or visual materials. Historical research is concerned with the authenticity of the source and its value. It is believed that through understanding past events, one can better understand human nature.

ISSUES AND PROBLEMS IN QUALITATIVE RESEARCH

Since increasingly more qualitative research is being conducted, concerns have arisen over how to critique qualitative research proposals and manuscripts for publication. Often criteria developed for critiquing quantitative research are used to judge qualitative research. This process of review can place the qualitative researcher at a distinct disadvantage. Hence, articles have been written that attempt to help qualitative researchers seek funding and give criteria for the judgment of qualitative proposals. Guidelines for evaluating qualitative research are listed in the box.

Another area of concern is the use of terminology in explaining the type of approach used in the methods section. For instance, it has been argued that the term *grounded theory method* cannot be used unless the researcher has actually developed a substantive theory (Morse, 1991). Yet the literature reflects a number of studies using the name grounded theory method when they simply describe the phenomenon and fail to develop a substantive theory.

A third area of concern is the mixing of different qualitative methods when each method is based on different philosophical assumptions (Morse, 1991). Such mixing can violate the assumptions of data collection techniques and methods of analysis of all the methods used. Attempts to quantify qualitative research are also perceived as an issue for debate.

Ethical considerations in qualitative research focus on ensuring the privacy of key informants. Informed consent needs to be obtained for interviews, recordings, and other data. It is also essential that taped recordings be erased immediately after transcription and that anonymity of informants be maintained.

EVALUATING QUALITATIVE RESEARCH

1. Research Questions
   The design should not address hypotheses since qualitative design does not test theory. However, broad research questions are appropriate.
2. Theoretical Framework
   Qualitative research does not test theory but generates it. Instead, the theoretical approach of the method should be explained. For instance, grounded theory method can explain the symbolic interactionist perspective.
3. Method
   The researcher should give sufficient description of the overall method.

Sampling—Concepts of *key informants* rather than *subjects* should be explained. Explain theoretical saturation with appropriate documentation.
Procedure—Give a detailed description of the procedure that will take place.
Instrument—Give a description of the interview guide with its broad themes and probes and include the guide in the appendix if writing a grant proposal.
4. Data Analysis
   Be detailed about your whole process of data analysis.
   Explain the criteria for assessing the credibility or trustworthiness of the findings.

Finally, another area of concern is the possibility of conflict between the roles of researcher and clinician. Munhall (1988) suggested that the clinical role of advocacy should always take precedence over the researcher's role. Continued discussion ensues regarding these concerns.

SELECTING QUANTITATIVE VERSUS QUALITATIVE RESEARCH

The decision to use quantitative rather than qualitative research largely depends on the type of research question asked, what was previously studied about the phenomenon, and what the overall purpose of the study is. For instance, if it was found that little was known about infertile patients' perceptions of their treatment, and the researcher wanted to get a more holistic sense of their experiences, it may be more logical to conduct a qualitative study. This type of study will enable a more complete understanding of the phenomenon and the overall patient experience of treatment. In this way the researcher gains an in-depth, holistic understanding of these experiences and builds a foundation for future research. Once this perspective is understood, more clearly defined research questions can be developed that are more congruent with individuals' experiences. If the investigator proceeds without the holistic perspective, he or she runs the risk of prematurely forcing research questions that do not truly reflect the population and phenomenon of interest.

A qualitative approach can also facilitate a more empathetic approach to the individual patient by making health professionals more aware of how patients perceive illness. This can also lead to better psychosocial therapeutic interventions in patient care. However, since qualitative research is not suited to establishing causal relationships and for rigorously testing research hypotheses, future quantitative studies can be designed that can test new interventions.

Quantitative approaches offer a systematic and objective way to test nursing interventions and other specific variable relationships. Controls, rigor, and attempts to remove any bias are essential components of the method and assure the researcher that the resulting outcome can be attributed to the manipulation of the treatment variable. Objectivity in the investigator and approach is essential. Nursing needs such rigorous research to test interventions used in everyday practice. Nursing also needs to continually develop new interventions, which also must undergo the same rigorous testing. Obviously both approaches contribute in their own way to the betterment of nursing practice. The box on p. 96 indicates steps to be taken in selecting a research design.

TRIANGULATION OF METHODS

Triangulation generally refers to the use of two or more research methods in the study of a particular phenomenon, although the term can refer to various combinations of research designs or instruments used in the same study. In nursing research it is more commonly used to refer to the use of both qualitative and quantitative approaches to data collection and analysis in a study (Duffy, 1987; Field & Morse, 1985; Mitchell, 1986; Morse, 1991). The two approaches are complementary and offer a more valid representation of reality due to their focus on different dimensions of the phenomenon. Triangulation also offers a more multidimensional understanding of the phenomenon of interest. The re-

STEPS IN SELECTING A RESEARCH DESIGN

1. Prior Documented Knowledge
   a. If very little is known about the subject matter, choose either a qualitative design or a quantitative exploratory design.
   b. If substantial knowledge exists, choose a quantitative design.
2. Purpose
   a. If little is known
      - Is your purpose to uncover relationships? Then use a quantitative exploratory design.
      - Is your purpose to gain in-depth understanding of the overall phenomenon? Then use a qualitative design. If you want to study culture and life-ways, use an ethnographic approach. If the purpose is to describe "the lived experience," use a phenomenological approach. To develop a substantive theory with a basic social process, use a grounded theory approach. If your purpose is to understand patterns of nursing's past, use a historical research approach.
   b. If preexisting knowledge exists, choose a quantitative design based on the purpose of the study.
      - If you simply wish to describe the relationship between specific variables, use a descriptive design.
      - If you wish to test an intervention (manipulating the independent variable), use an experimental design (if you can meet all the criteria for that design). If some element of control is missing, choose a quasi-experimental design.

searcher may use a combination of psychosocial instruments, interviews, and observations to capture a complex phenomenon. However, this requires substantial expertise on the part of the researcher.

Triangulation has also been used in the development of new instruments. The researcher may conduct a qualitative study and from the results of that study may form the theoretical basis for an instrument, based on the authentic verbalizations of the original study.

SUMMARY

- Quantitative research emerges from logical positivism and uses rigor, objectivity, and control. It seeks to establish relationships among variables and causality when appropriate.

- Qualitative research is interested in the emic perspective and in preserving the holistic, subjective experiences of individuals. It is not interested in control or manipulation but in the generation of theory.
- Quantitative research designs include exploratory, descriptive, correlational, quasi-experimental, and experimental designs. A true experimental design uses the most rigor of all, and therefore is considered the most powerful of the quantitative designs in inferring causality.
- Qualitative research designs include phenomenology, grounded theory, ethnography, and historical designs, with each approach based on its underlying philosophy.
- The decision to use quantitative rather

than qualitative research is based on the type of research question that needs to be asked and the extent of existing knowledge already available.

- Triangulation of methods usually refers to the use of two or more research methods to study a particular phenomenon. In nursing research it commonly refers to the use of both qualitative and quantitative approaches.

FACILITATING CRITICAL THINKING

1. As a researcher you want to study patients' perceptions of their hemodialysis treatment. You find that little has been studied in this area before.
   a. Would a qualitative or quantitative approach be more appropriate at this time? Give rationale.
   b. What type of specific research design would you choose? Give rationale.
2. You want to study a new nursing intervention that you developed. What type of research approach and design would be most appropriate for you to use? Explain why.

References

SUBSTANTIVE

BLENNER, J. L. (1990). Passage through infertility treatment: A stage theory. *IMAGE: Journal of Nursing Scholarship, 22,* 153-158.

LOOKINLAND, S., & APPEL, P. (1991). Hemodynamic and oxygen transport changes following endotracheal suctioning in trauma patients. *Nursing Research, 40,* 133-138.

CONCEPTUAL

BLUMER, H. (1969). *Symbolic interaction: Perspectives and methods.* Englewood Cliffs N.J.: Prentice Hall.

DILTHEY, W. (1961). *Pattern and meaning in history.* San Francisco: Harper Torchbooks.

GLASER, B., & STRAUSS, A. (1967). *The discovery of grounded theory.* Chicago: Aldine Publishing.

LEININGER, M. (1990). Ethnomethods: The philosophical and epistemic bases to explicate transcultural nursing knowledge. *Journal of Transcultural Nursing, 1,* 40-51.

LINCOLN, V., & GUBA, E. (1985). *Naturalistic inquiry.* Beverly Hills, Calif.: Sage Publications.

MUNHALL, P. (1988). Ethical considerations in qualitative research. *Western Journal of Nursing Research, 10,* 150-162.

STERN, F. (1956). *The varieties of history.* New York: Vintage Books.

WALSH, W. H. (1967). *Philosophy of history.* San Francisco: Harper Torchbooks.

METHODOLOGICAL

BLOCK, M. (1957) *The historian's craft.* New York: Vintage Books.

CHRISTY, T. E. (1975). The methodology of historical research. *Journal of Nursing Research, 24* (3), 189-192.

COHEN, J. (1977). *Statistical power analysis for the behavioral sciences.* New York: Academic Press.

DUFFY, M. E. (1987). Methodological triangulation: A vehicle for merging quantitative and qualitative research methods. *IMAGE: Journal of Nursing Scholarship, 19*(3), 130-133.

FIELD, P., & MORSE, J. M. (1985). *Nursing research: The application of qualitative approaches.* Rockville, Md.: Aspen.

GLASER, B. (1978). *Theoretical sensitivity: Advances in the methodology of grounded theory.* Mill Valley, Calif.: Sociology Press.

GUBA, E. (1981). Criteria for assessing the trustworthiness of naturalistic inquiries. *Educational Communication and Technology Journal, 29,* 75-92.

LOFLAND, J. (1971). *Analyzing social setting: a guide to qualitative observation and analysis.* Belmont, Calif.: Wadsworth.

MILES, M., & HUBERMAN, A. (1984). *Qualitative data analysis: A sourcebook of new methods.* Beverly Hills, Calif.: Sage Publications.

MITCHELL, E. S. (1986). Multiple triangulation: A methodology for nursing science. *Advances in Nursing Science, 8*(3), 18-26.

MORSE, J. M. (1991). Approaches to qualitative-quantitative methodological triangulation. *Nursing Research, 40*(1), 120-123.

Omery, A. (1983). Phenomenology: A method for nursing research. *Advances in Nursing Science, 5*(2), 49-63.

Saarman, L., & Freitas, L. (1990) Doing history. *Journal of Pediatric Nursing 7,* (1).

Schatzman, L., & Strauss, A. (1982). *Field research: Strategies for a natural sociology.* Englewood Cliffs, N.J.: Prentice Hall.

HISTORICAL

Heidegger, M. (1962). *Being and time.* New York: Harper & Row.

Husserl, E. (1970). *The crisis of the European sciences and transcendental phenomenology.* Evanston, Ill.: Northwestern University Press.

Merleau-Ponty, M. (1962). *Phenomenology of perception.* London: Routledge & Kegan Paul.

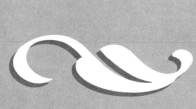

PART II

PRELIMINARY STEPS IN THE RESEARCH PROCESS

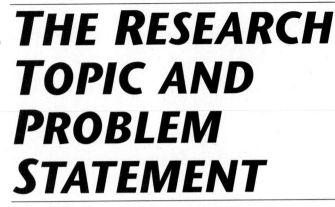

CHAPTER 6

THE RESEARCH TOPIC AND PROBLEM STATEMENT

LAURA A. TALBOT • PATRICIA A. DAVIS-LAGROW

Curiosity is an innate human quality. The ability to ask stimulating questions about the world provides a basis for identifying research topics and problems. *Research topics* are broad ideas or concepts from which many problems may be delineated. Nursing research topics may come from all areas governed by nursing. The topics investigated by nurses cover a wide variety of subjects, from thermoregulatory state in full-term infants (Bliss-Holtz, 1993) to activities used by healthy middle-aged women to promote well-being (Hartweg, 1993). Because a research topic can be very broad in scope, it must be narrowed to be researchable. The researcher must fine-tune the topic into a research problem.

This chapter differentiates between a research problem and purpose, examines criteria for the problem statement, and identifies sources for research problems. Criteria for determining the feasibility for the conduct of the study are also presented.

DIFFERENTIATING BETWEEN THE RESEARCH PROBLEM AND PURPOSE

A distinction must be made between the research problem and the research purpose. The research problem specifies the area of interest and describes, in general, the problem to be solved. The problem statement specifies *what* is being studied. The research purpose states specifically *why* the problem is being studied. The purpose is the aim of the study and provides clues as to how the results can be used. Although the research problem and purpose are related, they are not the same, and the terms should not be used interchangeably.

Identifying the research problem is the first step of the research process. The research problem provides direction for the rest of the study (see box on p. 102). The research purpose flows deductively from the problem statement. In writing the problem statement, the writer must con-

____ STEPS IN DEVELOPING A RESEARCH PROBLEM ____

1. Select a topic by identifying an area of interest.
2. Explore the phenomenon by examining the 10 related areas described by Rempushecki (1990) on page 108.
3. Narrow the topic to a specific problem.
4. Review the literature to determine the topic's present level of knowledge.
5. Evaluate the research problem for feasibility.
6. Write the statement of the problem.

vince the audience why it is important that the study be conducted. A written statement of the problem includes:

1. Information about the issue or concern that provoked the study or about which further knowledge is needed;
2. The scope of the problem area, for example, how many people are affected by it or how pervasive it is, the nature and scope of the problem to be studied;
3. Why it is important to study the problem;
4. How nursing science or practice would be influenced by the study; and
5. The overall goal of the proposed research or question to be answered (Woods & Catanzaro, 1988, p. 44).

The researcher first introduces the problem by providing background information about the issue or area of concern. The researcher wants to get the reader's attention in the introductory paragraph and to demonstrate the severity of the problem. The concluding statement usually indicates that further knowledge is needed through research.

The researcher then presents the scope or magnitude of the problem as well as why it is important to study the problem. The study population, major concepts or variables, and the present level of knowledge are introduced at this time. From the literature the researcher has determined the level of research and type of research design that are needed to solve the problem. Examples of different types of research designs and a corresponding problem statement may be found in the box on p. 103.

In research articles the research problem may be stated in the literature review or in the introductory paragraph. The following is an example of a problem statement with its corresponding purpose statement.

Problem statement: "Self-care is the most common and fundamental form of health care. Self-care is often of greater importance than professional health services and has been found to be an important determinant of health outcomes. Yet there is little research about older adults' management of symptoms and specific self-care practices." (Conn, 1991, p. 176)

Purpose statement: "The purpose of this study was to examine self-care behaviors that older adults use to manage cold and influenza episodes." (Conn, 1991, p. 176)

In this example the problem statement is very general and presents the need to research self-care practices of older adults. Self-care is a broad, encompassing concept.

A COMPARISON OF RESEARCH PROBLEM AND STUDY DESIGN

- *Exploratory:* "Little is known about the impact of the critical care experience on patients as they recall it. . . . A study of patient recollections during the early period after transfer would thus provide an essential knowledge base in which patients' perspectives of the experience are incorporated into nursing care of the critically ill." (Simpson, Armstrong, and Mitchell, 1989, p. 325)

- *Descriptive:* "Wife rape is the newest form of family violence to emerge as a significant problem; it is reported to be more traumatic for the victim and the marriage than battering alone. . . . Now prevalence studies are suggesting that rape by intimates is far more common than is a rape by strangers and that sexual assaults in marriage may be the most common kind of rape." (Weingourt, 1990, p. 144)

- *Correlational:* "Approximately 45% of those with chronic obstructive pulmonary disease (COPD) have a restriction in their activity. . . . As evidence is lacking to support a solely physiologic explanation for functional status, the exploration of the relationship between patients' perceptions of cause for their illness and the effect of the cause on affect, self-esteem, and functional status could provide insight into the psychological mechanisms operative in this population." (Weaver and Narsavage, 1992, p. 286)

- *Quasi-experimental:* "Unanesthetized circumcision has been found to cause severe abnormalities in the physiological indicators that imply that pain has occurred, including encephalographic (EEG) and rapid eye movement sleep patterns, respiratory rate, transcutaneous oxygen concentration, and heart rate. . . . Studies have not adequately evaluated and compared the effects of pacifiers, music, intrauterine sounds, and other nonpharmaceutical pain reduction methods for neonates undergoing painful procedures, used individually or in combination." (Marchette, Main, Redick, Bagg, & Leatherland, 1991, p. 241)

- *Experimental:* "Admission to the coronary unit (CCU) for patients with presumptive diagnosis of acute myocardial infarction (AMI) is a psychophysiologically stressful experience capable of adversely affecting the patient's prognosis and recovery. Although holistic techniques designed to reduce stress, such as relaxation and music therapy, are viewed within the realm of nursing practice, such techniques have been infrequently used and inadequately evaluated in critical care practice." (Guzzetta, 1989, p. 609)

- *Phenomenologic:* "The purpose of the study was to determine the essential structure of an experience from life through which or during which the elderly derived the sense life is meaningful." (Trice, 1990, p. 249)

- *Grounded theory:* "An understanding of the ways in which people manage difficult life events is crucial for nurses who care for individuals who face a variety of crises including changes in health, social network, finances and the ability to live independently. Older adults, in particular older women living alone, are the fastest growing population group and are projected to be the major recipients of health care in the future." (Wagnild & Young, 1990, p. 252)

- *Ethnographic:* "A central question was how hospice nurses met the varying needs of both terminally ill patients and those patients who were expected to recover." (Samarel, 1989, p. 132)

- *Historical:* "After weathering battles in the executive, legislative and judicial arenas, North Dakota became the first state to standardize educational requirements for two entry levels of practice. An analysis of that testimony can provide useful information related to the entry issue." (Warner, Ross, & Clark, 1988, p. 213)

Several purpose statements could come from this problem statement related to other self-care practices of older adults. For this study, the purpose statement focused on only one aspect of self-care behavior that was studied, the management of cold and influenza episodes by the older adult.

SOURCES OF RESEARCHABLE PROBLEMS

Ideas for research come from many sources. Some of these are listed in the box below. Moody, Vera, Blanks, and Visscher (1989) studied the origin of research ideas among established nurse researchers. Their findings indicated that 87% came from clinical practice, 57% from immersion into the literature, 46% from interactions with colleagues, 28% from interactions with students, and 9% from funding priorities. Researchers often use more than one source in identifying a research problem.

PRACTICE/EXPERIENCE

Research ideas can emerge from three broad areas: education, management/administration, and clinical practice. Education includes staff development and continuing education, as well as education in the college or university setting. Management/administration focuses on the organization and functioning of the health care institution, such as staffing and quality as-

surance. Clinical practice includes all areas related to patient care and its outcomes. All three of these areas are very broad, with numerous researchable problems.

The American Nurses' Association (ANA) has identified research priorities for the nursing profession (see Chapter 1). The priorities are broad and encompass all aspects of nursing practice. The ANA priorities may be utilized to stimulate interest in a particular research problem. However, many ideas for research come from everyday experiences. While at work, a nurse may notice a situation that occurs with a certain amount of regularity. For example, the more anxious a patient with chronic obstructive pulmonary disease (COPD) becomes, the more dyspneic he becomes. The nurse may want to validate or reaffirm the occurrence of that event through a systematic investigation to examine the event and factors that could influence its outcome or occurrence. The nurse might wonder, for example, if relaxation techniques, massages, or music would decrease the anxiety and dyspneic episodes of the COPD patients. Thus, from the clinical setting, an area of concern has been identified.

Nursing administration research is concerned with:

1. Establishing the costs of nursing care;
2. Examining the relationships between nursing services and quality patient care; and
3. Viewing problems of nursing service

SOURCES OF RESEARCH PROBLEMS

Practice/experience
Literature review
Previous research

Societal concerns
Special interest groups
Theory

NURSING ADMINISTRATION RESEARCH PRIORITIES

1. What are the cost-effective components of clinical nursing care that yield high patient satisfaction, decrease number of complications, and shorten hospital stay for identified groups of patients?
2. How can nursing research in the practice setting be used to decrease cost, improve the quality of care, and increase patient and nurse satisfaction?
3. What is the relationship of patient acuity to cost of care, to nursing resource needs, and to nursing judgment of acuity?
4. How is nursing productivity measured in units of service or nursing care hours, and how does it compare with the quality of care patients receive?
5. What are the actual direct and indirect costs of providing nursing services for patients in selected intensity classifications?

6. What are alternative approaches to measuring nursing intensity and patient need for nursing services?
7. How are the intensity of nursing care, selected patient characteristics, and the cost of nursing services related?
8. How can nursing costs be effectively and efficiently estimated?
9. What education and skill mix of nurses provides the highest quality care and is the most cost-effective in health care agencies of varying size, purpose, organization, and location?
10. What is the revenue-producing capability of nursing services?

Source: Henry, B., Moody, L. E., Pendergast, J. F., O'Donnell, J., Hutchinson, S. A., & Scully, G. (1987). Delineation of nursing administration research priorities. *Nursing Research, 36*(5), 312.

---

delivery within the broader context of policy analysis and delivery of health care services (Henry et al., 1987).

The top 10 priorities identified by Henry et al. (1987) for nursing administration research are presented in the box above.

Hermansdorfer, Henry, Moody, and Smyth (1990) examined the themes in nursing administration research studies published between 1976 and 1986 ($N = 220$) in *Nursing Research* and in the *Journal of Nursing Administration*. The top five recurring themes were:

1. Evaluation of care, programs;
2. Job satisfaction, recruitment, and retention;
3. Nursing productivity and accountability;
4. Interorganizational relations; and
5. Nursing intensity, patient acuity (p. 551).

Although all of these themes are still relevant, patient acuity is still a growing problem considering the changes in the health care industry.

LITERATURE REVIEW

Examining the nursing literature can generate ideas for possible areas of research. One can simply read nursing journals to search for ideas, or a computerized search can locate relevant articles if the researcher already has an idea or topic in mind. Commonly used computerized data bases for searching the literature include *CINAHL, Medline, ERIC, Psych Abstracts,* and *Soc Abstracts.* Three types of journals that can be explored are research journals, journals with a clinical focus, and specialty journals.

Examples of research journals include *Nursing Research, Western Journal of Nursing Research, Research in Nursing and Health, Advances in Nursing Science,* and *Applied Nursing Research.* Journals with a clinical focus present problems in the clinical sphere and imply areas of research. *Nursing '94, Nursing Outlook,* and *American Journal of Nursing* present current issues in nursing practice. Specialty journals focus on a specific area of nursing and are commonly published by a professional organization or association. These include *American Journal of Critical Care, Pediatric Nursing, Journal of Gerontological Nursing, Journal of Nursing Administration, Public Health Nursing, Journal of the American Association of Occupational Health Nursing,* and *Ostomy/Wound Management.* Most of these journals also include research studies. In general, refereed journals are preferred as sources of research topics. A refereed journal uses expert reviewers to determine whether an article is accepted for publication. In nonrefereed journals, the editor makes the decision regarding publication of manuscripts. Swanson, McCloskey, and Bodensteiner (1991) found that 94% of the 92 U.S. nursing journals examined were refereed.

Master's theses and doctoral dissertations are other sources of ideas. Whereas a research article is a brief write-up of the research findings, theses and dissertations contain a complete presentation of the research. The majority of theses and dissertations are not published. However, information can easily be accessed about them through abstracts such as *Dissertation Abstracts.* Complete copies of theses and dissertations may be purchased through University Microfilms. Toward the end of each thesis and dissertation (and some articles) is an area titled "Recommendations for Further Research." Here the researcher discusses modifications to the study and further areas to be investigated related to the topic. The researcher may wish to pursue these areas.

PREVIOUS RESEARCH

Repeating or replicating previous nursing research is another option for the nurse researcher. The purpose of replication is to validate and support earlier findings. Replication involves reproducing the study design and methods with a new group of subjects in order to determine whether similar findings will be obtained. The original methods and design must be held constant, but additional variables, new settings and populations, and procedural refinements are permitted. Similar results from both the original study and the replication study build confidence in the outcomes. Nursing science is concerned with the establishment of facts, theories, principles, and methods of nursing practice. Toward that end, replication studies should be given a higher priority for access to subjects in the clinical area than original studies when they are relevant to clinical problems and nursing care delivery (Taunton, 1989).

SOCIETAL CONCERNS

Societal concerns can generate research problems. Some issues presently in the news are health care reform, domestic violence, AIDS, drug abuse, and Medicare/Medicaid reimbursement.

SPECIAL INTEREST GROUPS

Special interest groups in nursing identify research priorities related to their specialty in nursing. Suzanne White (1990), president of the American Association of Critical-Care Nurses (AACN), wrote of the limited access to intensive care units and the future challenge of the 1990s. Numerous problems associated with limited access were identified, such as lack of intensive care beds, shortage of health care personnel, and increasing health care costs with decreasing reimbursement. Any one of these factors would make an excellent researchable problem. In addition, specific research priorities of the AACN for clinical practice and research on the context within which critical care nursing takes place may be found in the box on p. 19.

Gerontologic nursing research priorities have also been established and could provide ideas for research problems in the areas of patient welfare, nursing education, or nursing practice. Brower and Crist (1985) conducted a four-round Delphi survey to identify the impressions of practitioners as to research priorities for long-term care. The top five items identified as being extremely important for patient welfare were:

1. Prevention, formation, and treatment of decubiti;
2. Coping mechanisms needed by the family and patient after discharge;
3. Increased physician interest in geriatrics;
4. Age differences in response to medications; and
5. Improvement in gerontologic preparation of ancillary and nursing students and staff.

All of these topics, as well as those identified topics concerning gerontologic nursing education and practice, are still relevant areas for investigation today.

THEORY

Researchable problems can be derived from testing existing theories. When theory testing is the purpose of the research, only a portion and not the entire theory is tested. Generally, testing is limited to only a single propositional statement. A propositional statement is a relationship statement that indicates that one concept is associated with another concept. For example, Macnee (1991) used Lazarus's stress-coping theory to formulate a research problem related to smoking status and well-being. According to Lazarus and Folkman (1984), it is important to study antecedents, coping processes, and outcomes that are relevant to the stress phenomena.

Antecedents are the characteristics of the individual. Individuals differ in their sensitivity and vulnerability to certain events, as well as in their interpretations and reactions. External environmental demands or internal demands may impinge on or stress an individual. Stress is appraised when the relationship between the person and the environment is seen as taxing or exceeding a person's resources and endangering his or her well-being. The individual uses coping strategies or processes in an effort to manage the stressful demands that have been placed on him or her. Each individual has unique resources that he or she brings to every situation. Examples of resources are existential beliefs, beliefs about control, problem-solving skills, social skills, social support, and material resources.

Outcomes are the adaptational status of the individual (Lazarus & Folkman, 1984). The theoretical proposition of Macnee's study was that "quitting smoking may be stressful because it disrupts existing coping patterns, and because it introduces new demands which may exceed or tax a person's resources. . . . Stressors associated with quitting smoking have an effect on psychological and physical well-being similar to that of daily hassles" (p. 200). In that study Lazarus's whole theoretical model was tested, rather than only one propositional statement, which is generally the case in theory testing.

FORMULATING RESEARCHABLE PROBLEMS

Once a research problem has been identified, the researcher must then narrow down the research topic and develop a problem statement. The first two steps in this process are to systematically contemplate the idea and to examine the literature.

CONTEMPLATING THE IDEA

To organize one's thoughts into a researchable problem, time must be spent reflecting on and systematically examining the idea. The researcher can then refine the idea into a researchable topic. Rempushecki (1990) identifies 10 areas related to the idea to be explored:

1. Precipitating factors;
2. Situation as it was viewed by the nurse;
3. Responses of others involved in the situation, for example, patients, physicians, and other nursing and health care personnel;
4. Personal involvement in the situation;
5. Emotions felt;
6. Values and biases inherent in or related to the situation;
7. Economic of financial (cost) factors associated with the situation;
8. Care implications (positive, negative) of the situation as the nurse perceives them;
9. Care implications (positive, negative) as perceived by others; and
10. Dangerous or harmful (risk) factors associated with the situation. (p. 45)

EXAMINING THE LITERATURE

A review of pertinent articles may bring to light theoretical frameworks, methodologies, data-collection tools, and methods of data analysis that have been utilized to study the problem of interest. Exploring the literature will allow the researcher to identify what is and what is not known regarding the problem of interest. In new areas of study, a qualitative design may be used for the purpose of theory generation rather than theory testing.

DEVELOPING THE PROBLEM STATEMENT

The statement of the problem lays the foundation for the study. If the statement of the problem is incomplete or incorrect, the research findings could be irrelevant, causing a loss of time and money. Three criteria for a good problem statement are: (1) The problem should express a relation between two or more variables. (2) The problem should be stated clearly and unambiguously. (3) The problem should imply the possibility of empirical testing (Kerlinger, 1986). A problem statement may be stated in either the declarative or interrogative form. However, authors such as Kerlinger (1986) prefer the interrogative form of problem statement as it invites an answer and has the advantage of simplicity and directness.

Through the literature review, the researcher has determined, for example, that a correlational study would be appropriate. The next step would be to determine the population and major concepts of the study. A good idea would be to outline the research study before writing the research statement. Once specific areas are determined, the next step would be to write the statement of the problem. The box at the top of p. 109 presents criteria for evaluating the statement of the problem.

Although, the research topic may have scientific merit, it still may not be feasible to conduct the proposed study. Factors that the researcher needs to consider when eval-

_____ EVALUATING THE PROBLEM STATEMENT _____

1. Is background information provided on the research problem?
2. Does the reader get a feel for the magnitude of the problem?
3. Is the significance of the study stated?
4. Can the level of research be identified (descriptive, explanatory, correlational, or experimental)?
5. Do the population and variables stated relate to the level of research identified?
6. Does it provide the general significance of the investigation?
7. Is there a statement that clarifies how the research findings are significant to nursing?
8. Is the concluding problem statement clear and brief? Is it stated in declarative or interrogative form?
9. Does the study seem researchable based on the variables presented?
10. Does the study seem feasible with respect to time, money, and the availability of research participants, facilities, and equipment?
11. Are there any aspects of the research project in which the risks to the research participants outweigh the benefits?

DETERMINING THE FEASIBILITY OF A RESEARCH PROJECT

Time
Money
Availability of research participants
Ethical considerations

Facilities and equipment
Researchability
Experience and qualifications of the researcher

uating the feasibility for conducting the study are summarized in the box above.

TIME

The length of time needed for a research project is a major consideration in judging its feasibility. A timetable will help in estimating the length of time needed to complete the project. This is constructed by listing each phase of the research process and estimating the time needed to complete it. Factors to consider when developing the timetable include whether the study will utilize a cross-sectional or longitudinal study design. Availability of subjects influences the length of time necessary for collecting data. For example, a study that utilizes heart transplant recipients rather than the more commonly available myocardial infarction patient will require a longer time for data collection because of the proportiately small numbers of transplant recipients. The researcher must also take into account his or her own work schedule and other projects demanding time when constructing a timetable. Figure 4.1 (p. 65) provides a sample timetable for a descriptive correlational study.

MONEY

The cost of conducting the study must be considered. A budget is needed to estimate the overall costs of the study. The more extensive the study, the more detailed the budget should be. Some general areas a researcher would evaluate for costs are transportation/travel, consulting fees, cost of supplies, equipment, facilities, and payroll. Transportation and travel costs incurred during the research process are frequently overlooked. If a trip is required, hotel costs, food, and other expenses associated with it should be budgeted. Consulting fees come from various sources. The researcher may want to contract for the various services offered by experts. Some common uses of consultants are statistical analysis, data entry, editing of manuscripts, and typing. When lab assistants are utilized or when participants are paid, the research project will have a payroll. Administrative costs and tax considerations must also be included in the budget.

AVAILABILITY OF RESEARCH PARTICIPANTS

Good research studies have been abandoned because the researcher could not find enough subjects or because of excessive attrition from the study. Conducting a pilot study can help the researcher gauge subject availability, percentage of available subject enrollment, and subject attrition. A power analysis is quite helpful in determining sample size in quantitative studies. Difficulty in finding enough subjects may occur when specialty groups are used and a large sample is needed. An example of such is an experimental intervention that involves children going home on ventilators. These patients are more likely to be found in large medical centers than in small hospitals, but with what regularity? If a sample of 200 is needed, it may take the researcher several years to find subjects and collect the data.

ETHICAL CONSIDERATIONS

Risks are usually an inherent part of any study. Therefore, careful examination must be made to determine if the subjects' rights have been protected. If the study problem statement and purpose appear to infringe on the subjects' rights, they should be revised or abandoned. Refer to Chapter 3 for a more in-depth discussion of ethical considerations associated with the research process.

FACILITIES AND EQUIPMENT

The availability of facilities and equipment is part of the feasibility evaluation. An elaborate study may be planned, but if the facilities and equipment are not available to the researcher, the study cannot be conducted. For example, a study may require each participant to be extensively tested. This may include stress testing, magnetic resonance imaging, or other costly procedures. While planning the study, prospective costs must be estimated. Some institutions will donate costs and supplies, but funding may need to be secured prior to conducting studies that involve expensive protocols.

RESEARCHABILITY

The researcher must determine if the problem can be empirically tested. This is true for both quantitative and qualitative research. To be testable, the quantitative research problem must present concepts that can be formulated into research variables capable of being tested. If the variable(s) cannot be measured, the problem cannot be validated through empirical testing. In qualitative research little is known about the phenomenon. Thus the researcher seeks to get the emic perspective; that is, the participant's point of view. Researchability would be the logistics involved in getting to the participants perspective.

EXPERIENCE AND QUALIFICATIONS OF THE RESEARCHER

A research project must be within the researcher's scope of expertise. The ability to carry out the research process may require skills the researcher does not possess. An honest assessment of the researcher's ability to conduct the research is needed. Educational background and experience are factors to consider, as well as expertise in the research process and knowledge base of the topic of study. One means of overcoming this obstacle is to consult more experienced researchers in the area of concern. Many projects are comprised of groups of individuals with diverse backgrounds. These individuals may be either study investigators or consultants to the research project. Few individuals either possess all of the skills necessary for the conduct of the study or have the time required. A skilled methodologist or statistician may greatly enhance the scientific conduct of the study through the contribution of their knowledge to the development, conduct, and analysis of the project.

SUMMARY

- The research problem specifies the area of interest and describes, in general, the problem to be solved. The problem statement specifies what is being studied. The research purpose states specifically why the problem is being studied.
- Ideas for research come from many sources, including personal experience, the nursing literature, previous research, societal concerns, special interest groups, and nursing theory. Researchers often use more than one source in identifying a research problem.
- Possible ideas for research topics may come from examining the nursing literature. Three types of journals that can be explored are research journals, journals with a clinical focus, and specialty journals.
- The primary focus of the problem statement is to demonstrate why it is important to conduct the study. Background information, the scope of the problem, its significance to nursing, and the overall goal are discussed at this time. The final product should be evaluated for clarity and completeness as the statement of the problem provides direction for the entire study.
- The feasibility of conducting a research project is evaluated by examining time available, funds necessary for the conduct of the study, availability of subjects, ethical considerations, facilities and equipment necessary to conduct the study, the researchability of the problem, and the experience and qualifications of the researcher.

FACILITATING CRITICAL THINKING

1. After reading the following problem statements, decide which are researchable and which are not researchable. What are the reasons for your decision?
   a. Are men better administrators than women?
   b. Should Norplant devices or some other form of birth control be mandatory for mentally handicapped women of child-bearing age?
   c. What is the difference in the anxiety level of men and women prior to a course examination?
   d. Are nurse practitioners better health care providers than physicians?
   e. What is the relationship among stress, sense of humor, and social support for baccalaureate nursing students?
2. For each problem listed, state whether you think that a quantitative or qualitative design would be most appropriate and support your decision.

a. What factors have promoted a high level of wellness and longevity among people living to be over 100 years of age?

b. What is the relationship between self-esteem and grade point average of baccalaureate nursing students?

c. Is there a difference between the physical assessment skills of baccalaureate nurses and associate degree nurses?

d. What does spirituality mean?

e. Is there a relationship between the level of education and the practice of "safe sex" for women aged 15 to 25?

f. What is it like to be a woman, age 35 to 45, living with multiple sclerosis?

3. From the following list of independent variables, dependent variables, and populations, practice writing problem statements:

Independent variable	Dependent variable	Population
a. Positive reinforcement	Hours spent studying	Children between 8 and 10 years of age
b. Number of days of class attendance	Nursing grade point average	Baccalaureate nursing students
c. Sense of humor	Stress	Adult clients in the work force
d. Sense of well-being	Exercise	Women between the ages of 50 and 75

References

SUBSTANTIVE

BLISS-HOLT, J. (1993). Determination of thermoregulatory state in full-term infants. *Nursing Research, 42*(4), 204-207.

CONN, V. (1991). Self-care actions taken by older adults for influenza and colds. *Nursing Research, 40*(3), 176-181.

GUZZETTA, C., (1989). Effects of relaxation and music therapy on patients in a coronary care unit with presumptive acute myocardial infarction. *Heart & Lung, 18*(6), 609-616.

HARTWEG, D. L. (1993). Self-care actions of healthy middle-aged women to promote well-being. *Nursing Research, 42*(4), 221-227.

HENRY, B., MOODY, L. E., PENDERGAST, J. F., O'DONNELL, J., HUTCHINSON, S. A., & SCULLY, G. (1987). Delineation of nursing administration research priorities. *Nursing Research, 36*(5), 309-314.

HERMANSDORFER, P., HENRY, B., MOODY, L., & SMYTH, K. (1990). Analysis of nursing administration research, 1976-1986. *Western Journal of Nursing Research, 12*(4), 546-557.

MACNEE, C. (1991). Perceived well-being of persons quitting smoking. *Nursing Research, 40*(4), 200-203.

MARCHETTE, L., MAIN, R., REDICK, E., BAGG, A., & LEATHERLAND, J. (1991). Pain reduction interventions during neonatal circumcision. *Nursing Research, 40*(4), 241-244.

SAMAREL, N. (1989). Nursing in a hospital-based hospice unit. *IMAGE: Journal of Nursing Scholarship, 21*(3), 132-136.

SIMPSON, T., ARMSTRONG, S., & MITCHELL, P. (1989). American Association of Critical-Care Nurses Demonstration Project: Patients' recollections of critical care. *Heart & Lung, 19*(4), 325-331.

SWANSON, E. A., MCCLOSKEY, J. C., & BODENSTEINER, A. (1991). Publishing opportunities for nurses: A comparison of 92 U.S. journals. *IMAGE: Journal of Nursing Scholarship, 23*(1), 33-38.

TRICE, L. (1990). Meaningful life experience to the elderly. *IMAGE: Journal of Nursing Scholarship, 22*(4), 248-251.

WAGNILD, G., & YOUNG, J., 1990. Resilience among older women. *IMAGE: Journal of Nursing Scholarship, 22*(4), 252-255.

WARNER, S., ROSS, M., & CLARK, L. (1988). An analysis of entry into practice arguments. *IMAGE: Journal of Nursing Scholarship, 20*(4), 212-216.

WEAVER, T. E., & NARSAVAGE, G. L. (1992). Physiological and psychological variables related to functional status in chronic obstructive pulmonary disease. *Nursing Research, 41*(5), 286-291.

WEINGOURT, R. (1990). Wife rape in a sample of psychiatric patients. *IMAGE: Journal of Nursing Scholarship, 22*(3), 144-147.

WHITE, S. (1990). President's message: Access to care—The issue of the '90s. *Heart & Lung, 19*(1), 26A-30A.

WOODS, N., & CATANZARO, M. (1988). *Nursing research: Theory and practice.* St. Louis: The C.V. Mosby Company.

CONCEPTUAL

LAZARUS, R. S., & FOLKMAN, S. (1984). *Stress, appraisal, and coping.* New York: Springer.

METHODOLOGICAL

KERLINGER, F. N. (1986). *Foundations of behavioral research* (3rd ed.). Fort Worth, Tex: Holt, Rinehart & Winston.

MOODY, K., VERA, H., BLANDS, C., & VISSCHER, M. (1989). Developing questions of substance for nursing science. *Western Journal of Nursing Research, 11*(4), 393-404.

REMPUSHESKI, V. (1990). Ask an expert . . . formulating research questions. *Applied Nursing Research, 3*(1), 44-46.

TAUNTON, R. S. (1989). Replication: Key to research application. *Applied Research, 8*(3), 156-158.

HISTORICAL

BROWER, H. T., & CRIST, M. A. (1985). Research priorities in gerontologic nursing for long-term care. *IMAGE: The Journal of Nursing Scholarship, 17*(1), 22-27.

CHAPTER 7

THE LITERATURE REVIEW: SEARCH IN RESEARCH

SALLY DECKER • JANALOU BLECKE

Moving from a novice reviewer to a more competent reviewer includes realizing that to decide that "there is nothing out there" is probably a premature conclusion. Premature closure to a literature review can be a risk to the further development of research ideas, as well as to the credibility of the researcher. When the researcher is able to find the right number of quality resource articles to guide the study, a doorway is opened. This key group of articles may include research findings, theory articles, and published reviews of literature. The articles help with conceptualization of research problems and the determination of the specific methodology to be used for further exploration of the problems. When the group of articles has been synthesized, it allows the researcher to see the path of knowledge development that others in this area have followed and where it has taken them. It also suggests the limitations and biases that might be

contained as a result of this course of knowledge development.

A literature review is a compilation of resources that provides the groundwork for further study. It is frequently found as a subsection of a published research study. Reviews of literature are also published as freestanding explorations of a body of knowledge.

CONCEPTUALIZATION OF THE REVIEW

FORMS OF REVIEW

A literature review may be conducted as an end in itself or as part of a research study. Most of the emphasis in research texts has focused on the form of literature review that is part of, or embedded in, a research study. A closer examination of the freestanding form of research review is important however in view of the increased number of studies and nursing's new understanding of the conceptual and contextual nature of knowledge. Examination of this form

The authors gratefully acknowledge the assistance of Dr. Jean Houghton, Anita Dey, and Gayle Koehler.

114

of review can improve the substance for the embedded review.

This chapter will present the variety of ways in which a literature review can be conceptualized and the tasks that are both common and unique to the different forms of review. A pervasive theme will be that reviews of literature, whether embedded or freestanding in a study, can contribute to the body of nursing knowledge only if conducted in a valid, reliable manner. Attention will be drawn to considerations of concept, context, and content as the reviewer critically examines the literature and completes the literature review.

CLASSIFICATIONS OF REVIEW

In general, classifications of reviews provide the conceptual orientation to the review process. More specifically, they lead to the purposes of the review. Four major classifications of literature reviews were proposed by Jackson (1980). These classifications described the freestanding form of literature review. They included: (1) review of new substantive or methodologic developments in a field, (2) verification or development of a theory, (3) synthesis of knowledge from different disciplines, and (4) inferences and generalizations from a set of studies.

New Developments in Methodologic Issues

In nursing, articles representing the first classification, new developments in methodologic issues, are often seen in the "Methodology Corner" in *Nursing Research* and in *Western Journal of Nursing Research.* "State of the Science" articles in *IMAGE* summarize substantive developments, as do articles in specialty journals. Examples of these methodologic and substantive articles, respectively, include "Treating Ordinal Scales as Ordinal Scales" (Knapp, 1993) and "Nursing Blood Pressure Research, 1980-1990: A

Bio-Psycho-Social Perspective" (Thomas, Liehr, DeKeyser, & Friedmann, 1993).

Verification or Development of Theory

Verification or development of theory as a form of review of literature can be found in journals such as *Advances in Nursing Science* and *Nursing Science Quarterly,* as well as in general research journals. The use of this type of review of the literature in nursing has been described in theory texts. An example of this type of review is "Teetering on the Edge: A Substantive Theory of Postpartum Depression" by Beck (1993). Ganong (1987) noted that in the reviews published in nursing from 1978 to 1983, there was a notable absence of implications for theory development and suggestions for further research. These observations might be the result of the editorial traditions of the nursing discipline, as the four journals that served as sources for Ganong's study contained only one that published theoretical articles.

Synthesis of Knowledge from Other Disciplines

The third classification, synthesis of knowledge from other disciplines, has always been important to nursing. The idea of borrowed knowledge has received attention in the nursing literature. Although there has been a negative connotation to the word "borrowed," the emphasis in a synthesis is on the use of knowledge from a variety of viewpoints and paradigms to address an issue of importance in health care, rather than disciplinary ownership. The nature of nursing knowledge, as well as the current emphasis on interdisciplinary and multidisciplinary reviews, supports nursing's need to continue this type of review.

The word "synthesis" in the description of this type of review has been further clarified as "organize" and "put together" by Bangert-Drowns (1986). Viewing the category in this way implies more of a compilation, thus separating this classification from the fourth, which focuses on a new whole. This compilation reveals what is and is not known about a topic. An example of synthesis is "Physical and Psychosocial Effects of Antepartum Hospital Bedrest: A Review of the Literature" (Maloni & Kasper, 1991). The relatively small number of these synthesis articles may be the result of journals tending to be more discipline-specific; journals devoted to multidisciplinary subjects are not yet in strong evidence in nursing.

Inferences and Generalizations from a Set of Studies

The last classification, referred to by Jackson as "integrative," involves the creation of a new whole. This is new knowledge in that it forms a generalization that goes beyond a summary of existing data. This integrative step can be numerical and includes the various forms of metaanalysis. There has been an increasing number of meta-analyses conducted in nursing over the past 10 years. An example is "Nurses' Job Satisfaction: A Meta-Analysis of Related Variables" by Blegen (1993). The narrative integrative review has not been accepted to the same extent in the research publications in nursing. This may be because it is more likely to be seen within a conceptual analysis. An example of a narrative review within a conceptual analysis is "Empathy as an Ethical and Philosophical Basis for Nursing" (Olsen, 1991).

A fifth classification should be added to extend the scope of the four classifications so that they address both freestanding and embedded reviews. This classification is a focused, or directional, account that helps in the specific identification and refinement of study components. Examples of these reviews are seen at the beginning of quantitative studies and are incorporated into the conceptualization and analysis of qualitative studies. In "Physical and Psychosocial Side Effects of Antepartum Hospital Bed Rest," Maloni and others (1993) use the literature to document what is known about bedrest in this client group and to establish the need for their study. In contrast to this embedded review, a freestanding review of this same topic was written by Maloni and Kasper (1991). A comparison of these two articles illustrates the difference in synthesis and focused classifications, as well as the difference in the forms of review.

These classifications are not mutually exclusive. An integrative review, for example, will contain elements of the newest substantive ideas and may include articles from a variety of disciplines. The actual classification seems to reflect more specifically the emphasis of the review. Ganong (1987) has written about integrative reviews in nursing research and refers only to Jackson's (1980) integrative review category; yet this rubric seems to include the other classifications as well. Ganong suggests that integrative reviews should follow the tradition of primary research and should be reported in this fashion. It is probably not surprising that the only studies Ganong found to meet the criteria used quantitative analytic methods, as these can report the magnitude and direction of effect.

PURPOSES OF REVIEW

The corresponding purposes to the classifications for the review of literature described above are:

1. Summarization of new substantive or theoretical ideas
2. Formation or testing of theory
3. Organization of knowledge from different fields
4. Integration of knowledge into a new whole

5. Focused determination and explication of study components.

Additional purposes are suggested by the forms of review. Both freestanding and embedded reviews document the need for study. The embedded review does this as part of the justification for the respective study, whereas the freestanding review suggests a need for knowledge development related to a given topic. Another purpose that differentiates the two forms relates to sources of new knowledge. For the freestanding review, new knowledge is a direct outcome, whereas for the embedded review new knowledge is the study's findings supported by the literature. Finally, both forms serve as shorthand versions or methods of condensing information for readers. Although they differ in focus and scope, both provide updated information on a given topic, which is helpful to practitioners and educators.

Unique to the literature review embedded within a study is the purpose of refining certain parts of the study, specifically the problem statement, conceptual framework, design, and data analysis process. It also provides the comparative data for the interpretation of findings. Variations in the purpose of the embedded review differ for qualitative versus quantitative studies. In the quantitative study, the review of literature guides and refines the components of the research process. In the qualitative study, the review of literature serves to inform or support the study, especially in conjunction with the collection and analysis of data. It also orients the researcher before data collection.

PROCESS OF REVIEW

The process of review for the two forms shares common elements (see Figure 7-1). In both there is a time of focusing to determine the specific phenomenon or review

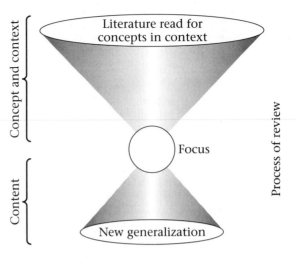

Figure 7-1. Process of review.

topic/question. During this time the conceptual and contextual analyses of the literature are important. Phillips (1992) accurately describes this part of the search as "the initial exploration pregnant with potential for research" (p. 50). Then, as the topic narrows and a more defined number of references become the focus, a content analysis approach can be used, taking into account the understanding of the conceptual and contextual issues. Having examined the narrowed topic, new generalizations can be formed that again widen the scope of thought.

Process in the two forms of review is differentiated by: (1) the amount of literature to include, (2) the kinds or types of literature, (3) the specificity or scope of the literature, and (4) the length of time covered by the review. Also, within reviews that are parts of research studies further differentiation in process is made by the specifications for quantitative or qualitative studies.

The amount of literature included in an article of a research journal may, for space reasons, reference only 25 sources and may not develop the ideas contained in more than a couple of studies. The review within a thesis or dissertation, however, would be more likely to contain over 100 references. A freestanding review article could contain either hundreds of articles or a much narrower subset for a review with strict inclusion criteria. Of course, the number actually referenced in the reviews is a subset of the entire number read and evaluated for inclusion.

The types of literature that might be reviewed include theory articles, methodological articles, empirical findings, and clinical reports or opinions found in books, journals, or pamphlets. Theoretical articles that explore the concepts, as well as the relationships between concepts, are important in both forms of review. In the embedded review of literature, however, less focus is placed on theory articles. Instead, methodological articles are more likely to be included as part of the review of literature in a study, as well as in a freestanding review focused on methodological developments. Empirical findings will comprise the largest number of cited articles in a study review of literature. Clinical reports and opinion articles may not appear in the reference list of either form of review, but will be helpful in the process of initial narrowing, and are more likely to be used in the freestanding review.

The process for the two forms of review will also vary along the dimensions of scope and length. The scope of the articles reviewed will be larger or more general in the freestanding review, and they are more likely to be from a variety of fields. Length of time covered is also broader in a freestanding review, as the historical background of knowledge development in the area is often important to understanding. Within each form, scope and length will also depend upon the nature of the research question.

In the embedded reviews, there is also a difference in the process involved in the literature review for quantitative and qualitative studies in relation to scope and timing. The use of the review of literature within the quantitative studies is generally agreed upon as to scope, length, and other dimensions. In qualitative study reports, however, the standard is less consistent and tends to differ by research tradition; for example, grounded theory versus ethnography versus phenomenology. Field and Morse (1985) best describe this difference with their three viewpoints about the use of literature in qualitative studies. These three include the extremes of no consultation of the literature prior to the fieldwork to a comprehensive review, like a quantitative study. The third view, and the one recommended by Field and Morse and supported by the authors of this chapter, includes a critical examination and selective review of the literature to inform researchers, but not influence their ability for analysis through a preconceived world view (p. 35).

Timing of the literature review differs in relation to the stage of the research process; specifically, in quantitative studies the review occurs early in the research process and is ongoing. In the qualitative study, generally only a cursory review occurs early, and the more expansive review is completed in conjunction with the data analysis and interpretation.

Although Figure 7-1 represents time along the X axis, suggesting that the conceptual review takes place prior to a more focused review, in reality individuals completing a literature review as part of a study may start with a focused idea and then backtrack to a larger conceptual review. Regardless of timing, it is important that this larger conceptual review explore the concepts in context in order to "disclose patterns that are manifest in the dances of the dynamic rhythmicities of the universe of knowledge" (Phillips, 1992, p. 50). By limiting the search to a very narrow topic from the beginning and bypassing this broader, conceptualizing step, the "patterns" may never be evident and the study may never develop its full potential as a contribution to knowledge. This review process is time-consuming and, it is hoped, can be done as a part of theoretical or substantive course work in graduate education as a preparation for the research study.

✍ TASKS IN THE REVIEW

A relatively predictable series of tasks needs to be completed in the literature review process. These will change with the form and purpose of the review, but the series of tasks is common. Each task is examined in light of specific procedures and issues related to concept, context, and content; methodological suggestions to address these issues are presented.

The five tasks presented were derived from a compilation of steps suggested by several authors (Cooper, 1982; Jackson, 1980; Light & Pillemer, 1984; Haller, 1988; Marchette, 1985; and Polit & Hungler, 1991). For each task a conceptualization of the ideas inherent in this task as understood in nursing is presented. The five tasks are summarized in the box. They include: (1) identify the focus question for your re-view (why you are doing the review); (2) identify and locate sources; (3) read and critique individual articles; (4) analyze, interpret, and critique the total group of articles; and (5) write the review.

The tasks do not occur in a rigid order. At each task the reviewer may identify reasons to repeat previous tasks such as identification and location of additional references. Figure 7-2 represents the relationships among the tasks. The issues at each task are important in determining the direction along the spiral. Also, the shape of the diagram suggests that the continual addition of references to the literature review makes the process of review potentially unending.

IDENTIFY THE FOCUS QUESTION

The focus question determines the form of review, the classification into which the review will likely fall, and the way in which the tasks will be completed. For example, if a nurse is updating a policy manual for the nursery and the focus question is, "What is the evidence for the use of 'hats' as a means of maintaining warmth in full-term infants?" this review is a freestanding one with a specific clinical focus—the main effect of "hats" on body temperature in the newborn. If the question relates to the importance of the use of "hats" when the newborn is placed into a warming device or the effect on preterm versus full-term infants, there occurs what Haller (1988) refers to as an interactive effect and a correspond-

---

TASKS IN THE LITERATURE REVIEW PROCESS

1) Identify the focus question
2) Identify and locate sources
3) Read and critique

4) Analyze and critique
5) Write the review

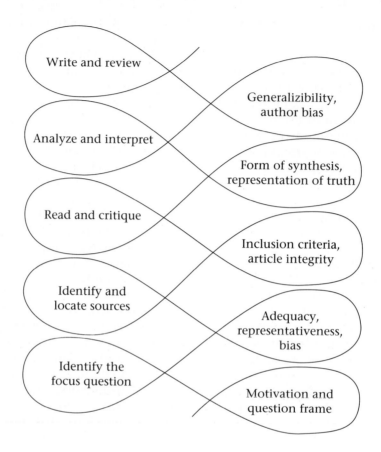

Figure 7-2. Interrelatedness of the review tasks with identification of issues for each.

ing change in the focus of the review. If a nurse is interested in conducting a study about the effectiveness of therapeutic touch in a psychiatric setting, the focus question for the embedded review might be, "What is known about the use of therapeutic touch and how has it been measured in specific settings?" The review is intended as a part of a study, and the purpose is to help further define the research problem and find potential methods for study.

Light and Pillemer (1984, p. 13) suggest

that the literature will be reviewed differently if the reviewer is asking the effect of a particular intervention on average, where and with whom an intervention is likely to be effective, or if the intervention will work in a specific setting. These authors further point out that if the purpose is to determine what is known about an intervention you "cast your net broadly" (p. 26). Using this wide angle for review will result in identification of a group of references with differing focus and methodology, and therefore statistical tests of analysis would not be appropriate for this group of study findings.

According to Smith, Smith, and Stullenbarger (1991, p. 51), the question serves as the conceptual foundation for the review. The decisions to be made at this stage are as follows: (1) Can the question be searched (studies identifiable and conceptually relevant); (2) Is the review needed (done by someone else already); (3) What approach will the review take (quantitative or qualitative); (4) What expertise is needed (librarian, statistician, research assistant); and (5) Is the review question feasibly answered within the constraints of time and availability of resources (Smith, Smith, & Stullenbarger, 1991). The answers to these questions may result in changes in the focus question for the review.

Focus questions for reviews of literature embedded within qualitative studies will look different from those embedded in quantitative studies. A focus question parallels the research question in both types of study. Research questions are addressed in Chapter 6. In a quantitative study the focus question will contain major variables and subject groupings, similar to those of the research question. This question may ask, for example, "What have been the findings of the relationships between locus of control and self breast exam?" or "What is the evidence for the effect of color therapy in surgical clients?" In contrast, the focus question of a qualitative study will be less structured. The question, for example, may be, "What is understood about responses to color?"

Issues
The issues in the question formation task relate to reviewer motivation for the review. The motivation might be to convince the faculty or funding agency that the reviewer knows enough about the project to proceed, or it might be to justify a change in clinical practice. The way in which the question has been framed is also an issue. The question itself will indicate the reviewer's conceptualization of the concept for study. Additionally, the scope of definitions included has been identified as an issue by Cooper (1982). Definitions that are either too narrow or too broad can limit generalization and understanding.

Methods
Methods to consider for this task are to explicate preconceived notions, state the assumptions, and try to reconceptualize the question from a different viewpoint to get a broader perspective. Clarity of rationale for decisions is important at this beginning point, as is the identification and recording of assumptions underlying the work. Development of a procedure manual similar to a data collection manual is suggested by Smith, Smith, and Stullenbarger (1991) as a very helpful method to record the coding and other procedural decisions regarding articles. This would also be a way of maintaining a record of the definitional decisions and assumptions.

Identify and Locate Sources
The next task involves the identification and location of sources. The library has been the traditional site for this. Through technology, however, any computer is now a potential site or link to a site. Additionally, identification of sources can occur through association with experts and colleagues, since success in this task often depends on mutual sharing of interests and resources. Success in this task also depends on knowledge of the way in which information can be retrieved from the literature.

Cooper (1982) identified the techniques of information retrieval as: (1) the "invisible college" (the informal network where resources are shared with peers), (2) ancestry (tracing a citation from one study to another), (3) descendancy approach (screening indexes using search terms), (4) abstracting, and (5) computer searching. Of these techniques, the ancestry approach has probably been used least in nursing. The idea in this approach is that when a seminal work is identified, references to that work are traced in work more recently published, using citation indexes. The *Nursing Citation Index* is found in the *International Nursing Index (INI)*. Other citation indexes that nurses might use are the *Science Citation Index* accessed as SCISEARCH and the *Social Science Index* accessed as SOCIALSCISEARCH.

Added to this list of ways to access the literature are the use of reference lists from articles previously obtained, a method labeled "network theory," and searching by names of authors known to have published in a particular area. Although potentially subjective, the network method avoids the disadvantages inherent in the use of search terms and helps to identify the most important works in the field early in the review process so that articles can be read in context. The use of the network method aids both in the identification of sources and in the analysis of the literature. Ryan, Scapens, and Theobald (1992) identified five steps in the network method, and O'Connor (1992) identified twelve steps. These authors acknowledge that they build on the work of Hesse. First, a small number of leading journals in the area are identified. As nursing has several journals that do not have a specific subject focus but contain important works about a variety of phenomena, the number may be closer to five than the two or three recommended by the authors. If the reviewer does not know which are the important journals, an expert in the area could be consulted or a

search of the last year's literature could be completed, using a broad key word related to the topic to identify where most of the literature related to this topic is published. In the next step in use of network theory, the reviewer looks through the current issues of these journals and identifies important articles related to the topic. For each of the articles (called source articles), the most important ideas are identified along with the work (previous publications referred to as primary articles) from which this study builds. Review articles are not used at this point. The primary articles are then charted with the X axis representing time; articles that build on each other are then connected by lines. In the Ryan, Scapens, and Theobald (1992) version of this process the literature is entered again at 3- to 5-year intervals, and the important source articles are again identified with the accompanying primary articles.

Figure 7-3 is an example of a network structure diagram.

Possible sources of information to be obtained through the search process selected include research and theoretical reports, editorials, and descriptive and explanatory works. These can be found in books, journals, and pamphlets. If the information sought is contained in historical records, these may not be published. Special libraries contain their own data bases (Miller, 1992). The number and types of sources to be identified and retrieved will depend upon the focus question that was asked. Decisions need to be made, based on the focus question, about use of primary and secondary sources, the currency of sources, the use of nonindexed sources, the range of sources, the use of human only or human and animal studies, and the use of foreign language studies. These decisions need to be documented with supporting rationale explaining how they were made.

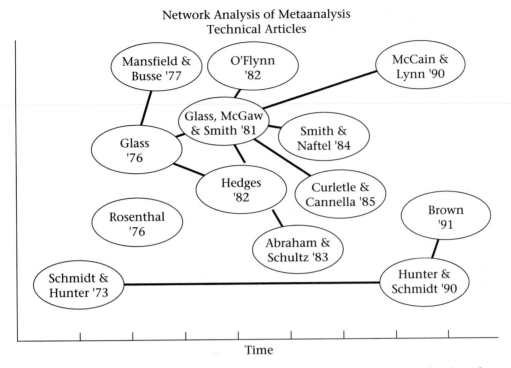

Figure 7-3. A network analysis of literature related to the technical application of metaanalysis.

Technology has provided the means to identify sources effectively and efficiently; however, some studies have questioned the accuracy of searches done by computer (Fox & Ventura, 1984; Bernstein, 1988; Heddle, Gagliardi, & Flemming, 1991). Although expanded indexing and increasingly sophisticated search mechanisms continue to improve accuracy of the search process, these studies are a reminder that not all of the relevant articles can be identified on the basis of one computer search. This is especially true if the topic is not well conceptualized in the literature. Fox and Ventura (1984) found that, compared with a criterion bibliography, only 22.5% of relevant articles were identified by a standard National Library of Medicine search, and 55% of the relevant articles were identified by a local search. Heddle, Gagliardi, and Flemming (1991) compared the number of relevant titles retrieved by MEDLINE, SCISEARCH, and EMBASE. The findings indicated little overlap among the three and represented 23 separate articles. Of particular importance was the finding that an additional 17 articles deemed to be relevant by criteria were obtained from the reference lists of the 23 articles.

A variety of ways exist in which the same data are accessed via technology. Figure 7-4 presents indexes, data bases, and end-user access used frequently in nursing. Note that the titles can be very similar for different levels in the figure. Understand-

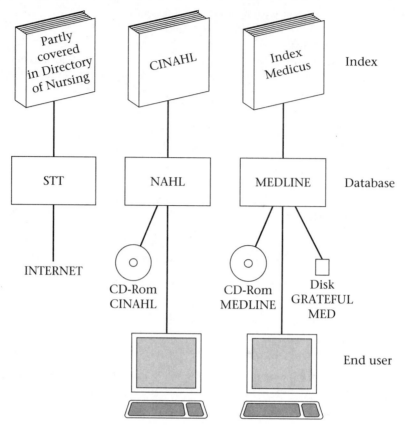

Figure 7-4. Relationships of selected data bases of concern to nursing to indexes and methods of access.

ing these is important, as access to the literature electronically can sometimes be confusing. In nursing, the most common indexes used are the *International Nursing Index* (INI), *Cumulative Index to Nursing and Allied Health Literature* (CINAHL), and *Index Medicus*. These can be searched manually or through data bases such as MEDLINE (MEDical Literature Analysis and Retrieval System onLINE) and NAHL (Nursing and Allied Health). Access to data bases can be from a personal computer with a modem and GRATEFUL MED software.

There is little difference in the journals

indexed by INI and CINAHL. Differences in the use of the indexes are due to the key words used for indexing. The INI uses the MeSH (U.S. National Library of Medicine's Medical Subject Headings) system, whereas CINAHL uses its own thesaurus, which is adapted from the MeSH system. As a result, the CINAHL key words are more nursing oriented. *Index Medicus* also uses the MeSH system, but the journals covered include a wide variety of medical literature and a more limited number of nursing journals. GRATEFUL MED includes all MeSH headings, and the EXPLODE command is an option that can be utilized. Sigma Theta Tau is creating a data base available to end users through INTERNET. Unpublished and current works of nursing researchers are available in this data base.

In addition, other indexes and data bases may reference the phenomena of concern to nursing. Examples include ERIC (Educational Resources Information Center), EMBASE, Health Planning and Administration (HLTH), AudioVisual catalog on LINE (AV-LINE), CANCERLIT (CANR), and DISS ABS EXCERPTA MEDICA (DISSertation ABStracts International @ EXCERPTA MEDICA).

One of the most common complaints from nursing students in their initial attempts to review the literature is that there is "nothing out there" that relates to their topic. This complaint is addressed by Delozier and Zingle (1992, p. 33), who suggest that symptoms indicating a problem with a search are either too much or too little information. Too much information is most likely to be obtained when a single search word is entered, similar to looking through a print index. These authors refer to this as "browsing." Too little information is likely to be obtained when the search is very specific, or the data base being searched is not a good match with the topic, or the search word is not correct. Delozier and Zingle note the importance of using qualifiers in the search so that the search is limited to those articles of interest to the question, e.g., to children only, to the last 5 years only, to research articles only. They also recommend using the EXPLODE command in MEDLINE searches, understanding that a search term may be found at two different locations in a MeSH tree structure. Finally, they recommend the searcher understand the types of journals available in different data bases.

Findley (1989) suggests that the reviewer needs a list of articles, of which at least 30% are relevant. Alternatively, there should be no more than 50 to 100 relevant articles. Findley further points out that the less time available to read, the smaller the final list, and that there is always a tradeoff between thoroughness (finding all the relevant and potentially relevant articles) and precision (percentage of articles retrieved that are relevant).

As an example of the identification process, "therapeutic touch" was searched using three data bases accessed using different methods. The searches were undertaken to answer the broad question: What is currently known about the practice of therapeutic touch? The results of the searches are presented in the box.

The steps in the identification portion of this identify and locate task are summarized in the box on p. 126. Use of network theory to locate references is presented in the boxed material.

In relation to the location portion of this task, based on the references provided by the search, the reviewer must decide which are relevant articles that need to be obtained. If there are abstracts that can be printed with the citation, these can be helpful in a retrieval decision. Frequently, however, titles are the only content information available. Using the system of classification by Findley (1989) (A = very relevant, B = questionably relevant, and C = irrelevant) and the specific criteria for decisions as to similar classifications as identified by Fox and Ventura (1984), most articles can be classified correctly by title. In the creation of relevance criteria, Fox and Ventura used a narrative summary of the content indicators in the titles of articles as well a list of key words that would likely identify each category of articles (p. 176). Additional considerations or heuristics for deciding which references to obtain relate

EXAMPLE OF SEARCH PROCEDURES

The Sigma Theta Tau (STT) data base is accessed through INTERNET. This data base contains a directory of nurse researchers, research conference proceedings (such as Midwest Nursing Research Society), an information resources data base, grant recipients from STT and projects, as well as *IMAGE.* The unique contributions of this data base allow the reviewer to identify current work in an area that may not have been published, or to identify a researcher's name under which to search for specific publications. The information about the studies is listed in such a way that the theoretical basis for each study, the data collection instruments, and the design are listed on lines of the printout. Information from the search is sent to the reviewer's E-Mail address. Although the data base is still growing (the library was established in 1989), this is a welcome addition to the other nursing data bases.

Searching "therapeutic touch" in this data base, an article in *IMAGE,* as well as the names of six nurse researchers, and the parameters of their studies were identified. In two cases detailed abstracts of the findings were included. As only one of the six identified their findings as published, this information was not available in either of the other two data bases.

MEDLINE can be searched as a paper index *(Index Medicus),* a CD-ROM, or an on-line data base and is available at many libraries. In addition, GRATEFUL MED is a software package compatible with IBM or Macintosh that allows users to search from their own computer, using a modem or direct INTERNET connection. Each method of access allows slightly different capabilities for searching; all use the MeSH categories for indexing the information. MEDLINE is accessed through the National Library of Medicine's MEDLARS or a commercial system such as DIALOG or BRS (Bibliographic Retrieval Service).

There is no MeSH term *therapeutic touch.* Using the index term *touch* to browse the data base, almost 5000 references were identified; this is obviously too many. When the search was limited to articles written in English, with *touch* as a major subject in the article, 840 references were identified. Using the document type of metaanalysis for *touch* there were no references identified; obviously not enough. Limiting the search references to 1992 and 1993, 138 were identified (as of August 1993); but the concept captured in these articles still included articles about the sensation of touch in victims of cerebral palsy. Using a text search of titles and abstracts where the word "therapeutic" appears with "touch," 52 articles were identified since 1985. These articles were more relevant based on their titles.

To search NAHL, the reviewer also has the possibility of using a paper index (CINAHL), CD-ROM (CINAHL), or on-line version. In contrast to MEDLINE, CINAHL includes virtually all English-language nursing journals. In CINAHL, *therapeutic touch* has been a search category since 1990. Searching *touch* before 1990 is by "touch!" Searching under *therapeutic touch* without qualifiers, 90 references were identified. Using the current thesaurus and identifying *touch* and then therapeutic touch, 60 references were identified. These are the same 60 that would be found without the thesaurus and using the search term *therapeutic touch* and the filter *in DE,* as only those articles using "therapeutic touch" as a major subheading were identified. Searches in CINAHL can filter results by methodology. One of the most commonly used heuristics for filtering results has been to use "research" as a document type. With therapeutic touch and document type research, 19 references were identified.

Comparisons of the findings of the three data bases suggest that different types of information can be identified in the three data bases. Even with all of this searching, the most current studies that have yet to be indexed would not have been identified or retrieved.

STEPS IN THE IDENTIFICATION OF SOURCES

1. Determine the search method.
   Network (see boxed material for steps)
   Data base search (continue with step 2)
2. Ensure the best match between the data base and the question being asked.
3. Know how the data base will be accessed.
   Paper index (e.g., INI)
   CD-ROM (e.g., CINAHL on silver platter)
   On-line (e.g., MEDLAR to search MEDLINE)
   End-user software (e.g., GRATEFUL MED)
4. Know the search mechanism and structure of the index.
   MeSH
   Other controlled vocabularies
5. Know how to limit the search by fields (e.g., document type, years, subject ages).
6. Decide if the parameters are too broad or too narrow based on the numbers of citations identified by the search; adjust if needed.
7. Identify a few of the most important current works in this area, or have an expert assist with this and make certain these are included in the printout. If not, find how these articles are referenced in the data set.
8. Use more than one data base.
9. Identify material for retrieval.
10. Retrieve the material.
11. Follow up with the reference lists of retrieved articles, and identify current references not yet indexed through journal search.

to the purpose for which the study was written and the reputation of the journal in which the article appears (Johnson, McKinin, & Sievert, 1992). Also, novelty can be a consideration if this is the only identified reference that seems to take a different approach to the topic.

The important factor is to assign criteria for inclusion into the categories of relevance based on the question to be addressed by the search. The desired sensitivity (proportion of relevant resources correctly identified) and specificity (proportion of irrelevant resources correctly identified) will differ with the research question and the number of references desired. With broader questions, for which a greater number of references are needed, false negatives (identified as irrelevant when relevant), create the biggest concern. Both qualitative and quantitative studies are used as sources of information for the review unless the review question is asked in a way that can be answered only quantitatively and by statistical analysis.

Although technology has facilitated the search for resources, manual searches are still important. There is a 3- to 4-month lag between the time an article is published and the time it is indexed. Additionally, the CD-ROM access is updated only at specific intervals, so an article might be published 6 months before it is available in a particular data base. Therefore, a manual search of the most current issues of the important journals in the search area needs to be completed on an ongoing basis.

One of the most common questions asked in relation to this task is, "How will I know when the literature review is adequate?" One method is to keep reading until the reference lists at the end of each article include only references that already have been read. Another way is to continue finding new articles until there are no new articles left to find. Of course, adequacy of the review will depend on whether it is an exhaustive or a representative review, an existing or a located review, and the cost benefit that might be gained from additional references (Jackson, 1980). The reviewer's experience with the literature will also be a major factor in determining when saturation or adequacy is reached. In network theory the pattern of the literature becomes visible, and adding additional articles is unlikely to change the picture. Both depth and breadth of review also need to be considered in determining adequacy of the review. While a review as part of a thesis or dissertation needs to be done in depth, the requirement for a Ph.D. degree also includes breadth as a criterion for review.

Findley (1989) recommends doing a last-year-only search of the literature based on the relevant subject headings and key words identified in two to four relevant articles. If fewer than 30 articles were identified in the past year, the author recommends going back until either a total of 30 articles is found or the 5-year point is reached. After this, print only the titles of the articles to determine relevance. If less than 30% are relevant, the reviewer should change the key words or search parameters. With the new parameters the reviewer should repeat the search. Next journals most likely to contain the relevant articles are identified, and the table of contents of each journal for the past 12 months is reviewed. The procedure is then repeated for the past 5 years, and articles are marked for relevance based on title. The final search is the basis for article retrieval.

Issues
During the search task, the issues include the adequacy of the search in terms of how the retrieved studies might differ from all studies and how the units contained in retrieved studies might differ from those of all studies (Cooper, 1982). This can be thought of as how the retrieved studies represent all studies on this topic. Other issues relate to the inherent biases contained in indexed and published sources. The published literature is more likely to contain statistically significant findings (Greenwald, 1975; Smith, 1980; Glass, McGaw, & Smith, 1981), and the indexed literature will not contain editorials. In addition to what is indexed, there is what is available to the reviewer due to language or interlibrary loan constraints. These concerns are summarized in Figure 7-5. The reviewer must decide if the group of retrieved articles is representative of all articles or if there are biases inherent in this final group.

Methods
To address the issues of this task, the reviewer should access as many information

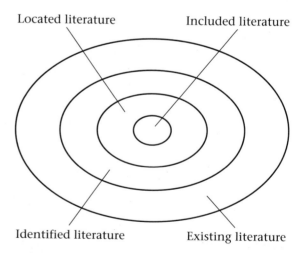

Figure 7-5. Relationships of existing sources of information and references selected for review.

sources as possible. Bias in one source can be partially overcome by use of other sources. Methods of searching need to be recorded carefully for reproducibility. Missing and/or overrepresented samples (of studies) should be documented for discussion in the written report. In addition, the reviewer should be present during the search when another person is conducting it in order to assist in the decisions as to limiters and descriptors used in the search process (it also helps to be friends with the librarian). The reviewer should remember that books as well as journals are potentially important sources of information, and books do not necessarily represent "older" information, due to the lag time for journal publication. It is also important to record the time lag between the most current literature and the last update of the indexed literature from the index being used. Gaining access to specialized data bases may require the assistance of an expert. A medical librarian is an invaluable resource for the identification of materials. These experts have advanced knowledge of the organization of data bases and methods of data retrieval.

In summary, the reviewer should use multiple sweeps of the literature, plus manual and computer searches as well as experts; and keep a code book of decisions and terms. The code book should contain a glossary that provides indicators and alternative terms to assist in decisions (Smith, Smith, & Stullenbarger, 1991); every term in the coding should be covered in the code book.

READ AND CRITIQUE

For the third task the articles retrieved are read and the process of screening and evaluating is completed. The trustworthiness of individual articles, as opposed to a group of articles, is determined in this task. Decisions about which articles are important to consider and which articles are methodologically sound are important here. Retrieval of articles can be accomplished using LONESOME DOC if a medical library is not available ("Using Loansome Doc," 1991). GRATEFUL MED users retrieve citations and the DOCLINE library fills the order, photocopying articles, and sending them to the user.

Critique for the two types of research tradition is addressed in detail in Chapter 23 on critique. Briefly, the critique of a qualitative study concentrates more on the procedure and analysis, noting especially adherence to the research tradition. In quantitative studies more emphasis is placed on the sample size and the limitations of the design. Critique of the individual articles is important to evaluate article integrity.

Findley (1989) suggests that articles should be read in an integrated fashion, using a framework of important concepts so that the reviewer does not get lost in the mass of published material and lose the main focus (p. 89). Findley also recommends not automatically rejecting methodologically flawed studies. Although the results of these studies should not be immediately incorporated, Findley feels that in the context of other studies, these papers can be supportive of more general concepts. Furthermore, the reviewer should look for overall trends as well as detail. The combination of literature search and construction of conceptual framework may require several attempts. This conceptualization process begins to take place as the reviewer reads. In this method, after determination of the major categorizations in the literature, a table needs to be constructed, listing the author and year of each relevant article under the conceptual category. This is another way to track the literature search by determining if an adequate number of studies correspond to each category.

The order in which the articles are read may also be important. The network approach to the identification of literature previously described (see Figure 7-3) can be an important way to determine the order of articles. Using this method, the seminal works in an area should be read first to identify the overall conceptualizations and create a picture of the development of knowledge over time. This is similar to Findley's (1989) idea of conceptualization and may be a reasonable starting place for individuals new to a field of knowledge.

Information about the individual article needs to be recorded in a summary form to allow for decisions about inclusion and later synthesis. Decisions about information to be included differ somewhat depending on whether the study is quantitative or qualitative. The sample needs to be described in both studies. In a qualitative study, the characteristics of the sample are as important as its size. Procedures should be briefly described in records for both study types. The research and study questions need to be recorded for qualitative studies and the research question and instrument for quantitative studies. Notations regarding reliability and validity, theoretical framework, design/tradition, data analysis, and findings need to be identified for both.

Notes can be taken on a standard bibliography card or can be entered into a computer, using bibliographic management software such as Pro-Cite. This software allows the user to collect, store, retrieve, sort, and print. It permits the downloading of data from other sources and allows output of bibliographic references into standard word processing programs (Aronson, 1993). As the notes are taken, it is imperative that any quotes or close paraphrases be set in quotation marks or identified as closely paraphrased to avoid plagiarism at the later stage of writing the review. A complete bibliography reference with page numbers on the notes will save a great deal of time later. It is also possible, and sometimes preferable, to use photocopies of articles as an alternative or addition to bibliographic notes. The copies need to be labeled with attached cards, color coding, or some other form of identification as belonging to a theme in the data.

Issues

Issues related to this task include the critical analysis of individual articles, with special attention to the results in the context of the other study components. Decisions about inclusion criteria based on quality of articles are also an issue. If only the studies using experimental design are included in the review, for example, what types of data are excluded? If other forms of criteria are used, such as sample size or definition of variable, again, how does this further influence the representativeness of the study findings? Incomplete reporting by the primary reviewers is a potential source of error in the critical analysis of the individual articles, but this is not under the control of the reviewer (Cooper, 1982).

Methods

Methods to be considered to address the issues at this task include documentation of inclusion criteria, interrater reliability in relation to the criteria, and documentation of study concepts for later synthesis. Inclusion criteria should be developed before the search and written clearly in the code book to maintain clarity and consistency in decision making about inclusion in the final review. Light and Pillemer (1984, p. 32) have identified possible criteria to be used at this juncture. These criteria include use of every available study without regard to "flaws," a subset of the studies that have the same characteristics (stratified sampling), only published studies, and selected studies as identified by a panel of experts.

As the articles are read, some condensation and coding of the information for later retrieval in the writing of the review are needed. While the first reading will decide inclusion or noninclusion, it is still important to keep track of all articles reviewed and why they were or were not included. The extensiveness of the notes will depend on the inclusion criteria decision and the number of concepts identified for coding. The coding will help the reviewer keep the results in the context of other study components and evaluate the integrity of the individual studies.

Examples of coding of study characteristics might include form, design, sample size, and other substantive characteristics (Smith, Smith, & Stullenbarger, 1991). Coding for context over time is an important criterion in some searches. If the reviewer were investigating length of hospitalization, coding for institution of DRG policy might be an important consideration when comparing data. If the analysis were a cost analysis, the inflation rates during the data collection or since the data were collected (versus article published) may be an important coding characteristic. Jackson (1980) stresses the importance of representing relevant characteristics of studies. Two of these characteristics may be time (in relation to period in history) and environment (in relation to relevant events, paradigms, or conditions). Of course, both supporting and nonsupporting articles need to be included in the review. A chart may be used to log the articles and record selected criteria.

ANALYZE AND INTERPRET

In the task of analysis and interpretation, the differences within the data set (group of references) are explored, and another critique is completed. In this critique, differences across and not within studies are considered. Looking for the "holes in the whole" is another way of conceptualizing this task. At this stage the rules of inference must be considered; some may be inappropriate. In nonquantitative review approaches, the rules frequently are not stated, making it more difficult to judge appropriateness. According to Light and Pillemer (1984, p. 74), there are several methods of evaluating the group of articles and combining the findings. The first is to sort the articles by findings—all of those with significantly positive findings, all of those with significantly negative findings, and all of those with a finding of no significant difference. Other methods are to combine significance tests and develop an average effect size or other common metric. The final method is to choose a subgroup of studies based on criteria from this task (analyze and interpret) or the previous task (read and critique). Any subgroup of studies has the potential to be nonrepresentative.

Combining data from qualitative and quantitative traditions can be a challenge. In qualitative studies, results are presented in descriptive terms that create a picture in which relationships and differences may be evident. This picture may be enhanced and further focused by differences and/or relationships identified from quantitative studies. Conversely, the qualitative study can also provide a deeper understanding of relationships identified within quantitative studies. Lack of congruence between study findings from these two different traditions again provides the potential for exploitation of differences. Here the differences may be the result of the questions asked, the research tradition, the sample choice and context, and the conceptualization of the phenomenon being studied.

Important in this task is the consideration of reliability or reproducibility of the synthesis. Frequently, scholars have taken a body of knowledge and interpreted it to mean different things. An example of this is the research on calcium intake and human disease. This literature contains studies on individuals with different amounts of bone mass and other outcomes and uses calcium as a potential contributor across groups. Using these findings, two panels of experts identified the recommended daily allowance (RDA) for calcium, the amount of intake that is recommended to prevent disease. In this country, the RDA for adult females was set at 800 to 1200 mg per day, depending on age; in England, using the same body of literature, the RNI was set at 550 mg per day—two different generalizations from the same literature ("Food & Nutrition," 1989; "Proposed Nutrients," 1993).

Examples of these conflicts in reliability are found in many fields and are one of the reasons that metaanalysis has become more popular in the recent past. Metaanalysis is a quantitative review of the quantitative literature. The unique aspects of the metaanalysis are the objective basis for comparing findings from different studies and the reproducibility of analysis (Graney & Engle, 1990). Literature reviews that develop from the traditional and research model approaches are compared in Figure 7-6. The traditional review uses study conclusions to form new generalizations, whereas the research model review uses the original study data as the basis for new generalizations. Characteristically, the traditional review has been used for freestand-

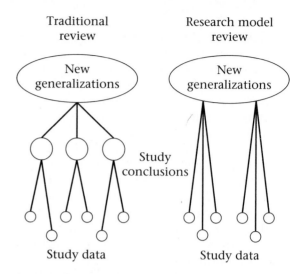

Figure 7-6. Comparison of traditional review and research model review approaches.

ing reviews or reviews of qualitative studies. In the latter case this is appropriate, because the original data sets are not available. The metaanalysis approach is a type of research model review. Individual aspects of each study are data points for this synthesis. Metaanalysis closely follows the steps of quantitative research methodology, and data collection here is the identification of studies.

Five separate approaches to metaanalysis have been identified by Bangert-Drowns (1986), but the nursing literature has used the Glassian metaanalysis approach most extensively. Using this approach, the sample articles are determined based on inclusion and exclusion criteria, and the variables for the groups of studies are defined. Then the study outcomes are transformed to a common metric and an average outcome of a group of studies and its variance is reported. While Glass used effect size as the common metric, there are four commonly used metrics for synthesis of data using metaanalysis including: r (the square root of variance shared), vote counting, pooled probability, and effect size (Graney & Engle, 1990).

Limitations of metaanalysis have been addressed by several authors (Curlette & Cannella, 1985; Smith & Naftel, 1984; McCain & Lynn, 1990; and Lederman, 1992) and include the combination of studies in which the concept of interest was conceptualized and/or operationalized in different ways, making it difficult, if not impossible, to compare the results. Other limitations arise from the need to treat nonindependent findings independently in analysis and the exclusion in the original article of data needed for the metaanalysis. Lederman (1992) suggests several ways to minimize the limitations of metaanalysis, including combining qualitative review with quantitative review. Probably the biggest limitation in metaanalysis as a form of synthesis is the omission of qualitative references from the review necessitated by using the metaanalytic approach.

While metaanalysis has a number of limitations, the sheer number of studies in the literature has made it important that methods be developed to deal with this increasingly complex data set of references. The established review tradition has used the narrative conclusions reached by the authors as a data source (Figure 7-6); but there is a great deal of promise in a synthesis method that uses the specific results in the synthesis. By relating outcomes to study characteristics, those characteristics that explain the differences across studies may be identified (Curlette & Cannella, 1985). In both narrative and quantitative methods of review, the selection of the set of studies for review as well as the decisions about the integrity or quality for individual studies are important issues.

McCain and Lynn (1990) compared the conclusions regarding the effectiveness of patient teaching reached in a narrative review with those of a metaanalysis of the same group of studies. These authors noted the difficulty in determining the "quality of study" score in the metaanalysis and obtained an interrater reliability of $r = 0.66$ in the quality ratings between two reviewers. McCain and Lynn also noted that only 15 of the 29 studies used in the narrative review reported sufficient data to enable the calculation of effect size, therefore eliminating about half of the studies from the metaanalysis. Based on the metaanalysis of the remaining studies, McCain and Lynn reported that there was a statistically significant mean effect for patient teaching. Although the general finding of the importance of patient teaching agreed with that of the previously written narrative summary, the findings within the specific categories of teaching goals (improved knowledge, compliance, physical well-being, psychological well-being, and self-care) varied with the synthesis method.

Issues

Issues for this task relate to the way in which synthesis is conceptualized, the necessity of synthesis in all cases, and the larger issues of the completeness of the data set in terms of representing the "truth" about the phenomenon. For example, the studies completed on heart disease using males as subjects so far outweigh those using women as subjects that it would be difficult to say that the body of knowledge holds the "truth" about this phenomenon. Discussion of conflicting findings needs to focus on differences in the sample (e.g., gender, age, education, setting; methods used for data collection; and the phenomenon studied). Even though the phenomenon being studied may be labeled the same way in both studies, it may be conceptualized in such a way that a different phenomenon is captured. The original researcher's choice of variables at this point may be very confused with the reconceptualization.

Methods

Methods to address the issues concerning the need for synthesis or representation of "truth" focus on the reviewer's sense of awareness and scrutiny. The reviewer needs to identify the method of synthesis and its limitations. The issue of reproducibility within this task is addressed within meta-analysis with identification of specific inclusion and scoring criteria and interrater reliability using these criteria. The inclusion criteria can also be identified for narrative reviews. The process of synthesis needs to be identified in narrative reviews to promote reproducibility of results.

Both forms of synthesis must address the representativeness of the studies included. Light and Pillemer (1984, p. 52) suggest assessing the representation of "truth" from a group of published studies by examining the spread of study findings. The question is, are differences in outcomes just random sampling variations or evidence of clusters that respond differently? Light and Pillemer (p. 65) suggest that a funnel diagram can help to locate publication bias. If the true effect is 0, the diagram should look like a funnel; if there is publication bias, the middle of the funnel diagram will be hollow, as illustrated in Figure 7-7. These authors also suggest this type of pictorial representation of articles to display historical trends in the data.

The extent to which the phenomenon of concern has been captured with the designs, samples, and procedures of the completed studies also needs to be evaluated. An examination of the categories from the note cards or data base may be helpful in this process.

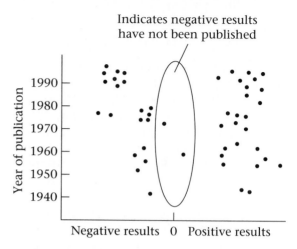

Figure 7-7. Funnel diagram of fictitious data.

WRITE THE REVIEW

For the written report the target audience needs to be considered. This affects the generalizations that are drawn from the synthesis and their limits. A useful review may emphasize differences as opposed to similarities and point out the clusters in which the differences were found. Although this would not be appropriate if the original question was a "main effect" question, there are many types of questions that would be addressed by an exploration of differences. Also of concern in writing the report is plagiarism; the rules for quoting and paraphrasing must be followed.

Writing the review of literature as part of a qualitative study differs from the quantitative. The written review at the beginning of the qualitative study is sufficient only to introduce or "inform"; the more extensive review is found in conjunction with the analysis of data and discussion of findings. In contrast, the review written for the quantitative study includes a complete section on review of literature at the beginning and refers only briefly to this in the discussion to generalize further the study results.

For either type of review, the reviewer should write the outline or tree structure of the major content ideas first and then write the major sections of the review, watching for a flow of ideas from one section to the next. At this point it is important to return to the focus question and see if it is addressed by the review.

Issues

Issues from previous tasks have included differences in the studies at the level of the participant (subject), but potential differences at the compilation of studies level also need to be considered. The administrative and contextual differences should be addressed, as well as potential differences based on characteristics of the authors. If all of the study authors for a phenomenon were female, or white, or from one educational institution, for example, bias may be introduced into the body of knowledge. The degree to which the combined studies' results can be generalized becomes important to the reviewer. Also, the biases of the reviewer are an issue in this task.

Methods

Haller (1988) points out that the review is not a chronological or a serial listing of study findings and that the conclusions of the review contain specific suggestions (generalizations) for policy and/or research and practice, depending upon the original question. The decision may be that, based upon the data to date, policy changes are not warranted.

The style in which the review is written uses tentative language and past tense. The style will depend on the style manual or publication guidelines the reviewer has been given to follow. The key is to guard against distortion of the data and to give appropriate credit for ideas. As Findley (1989) notes, similar to the tasks of analysis and synthesis, this task requires large blocks of time. Although a review of individual articles can be accomplished in shorter time blocks, the work of synthesis and writing is best done in 4-hour blocks to allow for assimilation of information and to maintain consistency in context.

The generalizability of the compiled data can be partially assessed by attention to the characteristics of the authors, institutions, funding sources, or other potential sources of bias. The reviewer bias can be addressed with a statement in the review of assumptions, experiences, and opinions about the phenomenon that the reviewer held prior to the review process.

CRITICAL THINKING: REFLECTIONS ON THE REVIEW

In the process of literature review, the value of the literature to the reviewer and to others must be identified. The use of critical thinking provides a means to examine these values. The key issue is to decide if "true knowledge" has been captured by the accumulated literature and what that knowledge conveys. The critical analysis of the literature is the bridge to further knowledge development as it is "one area which most distinctively links methodology with method . . ." (Ryan, Scapens, & Theobald, 1992, p. 147).

A framework that can be used to guide the critical analysis of the literature is provided by Brookfield (1987). Brookfield's four components of critical thinking include: (1) assumption analysis, (2) contextual awareness, (3) exploration of alternatives, and (4) reflective skepticism (pp. 7-9). These four components will be used to suggest issues and methods for critical review of the consistency and integrity of a literature review.

ASSUMPTION ANALYSIS

Assumptions are closely tied to and reflected in the language used to convey meanings. The changes in the meanings of the words that make up a body of literature, and the conceptualizations that were described with words, are determined by social and ideological standards. Language, therefore, is an important issue to consider in the critical analysis of the literature. Some idea of language use and meaning will have emerged from the search process. For example, since *therapeutic touch* was not an index term until 1990 in the NAHL data base and still is not an index term in the MEDLINE data base, it seems reasonable to consider this concept "new" to the scholarly community. The fact that references relating to therapeutic touch are frequently indexed under "alternative medicine" in MEDLINE also gives an indication of how therapeutic touch is conceptualized and implies some assumptions about the concept. Another, more formal, approach to the analysis of language is to create a network of core terms designed to represent the theoretical development of terms within a particular research center. Papineau (1979) used an ordering of terms from those shared by all researchers to those within subdivisions of disciplines, to schools of thought within a subdivision, to a group of researchers. Tracing the use of core terms in the language of the literature provides an understanding of the derivation of words used to describe phenomena. Ryan, Scapens, and Theobald (1992) note that this network tree can be further extended to attach assumptions to each branching of the terms.

CONTEXTUAL ANALYSIS

The network process used to identify articles for review can also be helpful to aid in critical analysis of a body of knowledge. This method helps to identify the context of the body of knowledge, why certain articles appear when they do, and how they are interconnected. Ryan, Scapens, and Theobald (1992, p. 154) suggest selecting a small number of high-quality, representative journals and, in turn, identifying antecedent articles. The primary articles and the antecedent articles in the network are then positioned on a time axis with the interconnections among them. The process continues, reentering the literature for a small number of representative articles and their antecedents at 3- to 5-year intervals. Similar assumptions among groups of articles can also be identified. The literary antecedents of an article and the methodologic rationale that bind the articles can be examined in the network. The interconnections and the historical, empirical, and theoretical changes in the school of thought and conceptualization of knowledge through a body of literature can then be traced. If review articles exist in this subject area, they can be compared to the network for corroboration. This process may be difficult, however, in a poorly organized body of literature with many methodologic disputes (Ryan, Scapens, & Theobald, p. 155). O'Connor (1992) suggests that a simplification of the network can reveal several patterns that need to be considered in the critical analysis. These patterns include seminal articles, updated theme or concept articles, and fashionable trends in the literature. Finally and most important, any pattern of ideas in conflict may be identified. When two theories with competing ideas evolve over time, there will be two pattern lines that appear on the graph as opposed to one.

EXPLORATION OF ALTERNATIVES

Exploration of alternatives can occur through examination of competing explanations generated by analyzing both the assumptions and the context, as well as by comparing previous reviews and the generalizations that others have drawn from the literature. These generalization may be in the form of consensus forum reports, review articles, or state-of-the-art types of papers. The language of the arguments is examined for another way to interpret the body of knowledge or interpret the "truth" of a body of evidence. This process can occur more formally through identification of conclusion indicators (terms such as *therefore, thus, infers, so, it follows that . . .*) and reason indicators (terms such as *assuming, because, since, it follows from the fact . . .*). Studying these indicators allows analysis of the conclusions reached and the reasons provided as justification (Ryan, Scapens, & Theobald, 1991, p. 161). Another approach to providing alternative explanations is to find other generalizations that fit the findings in addition to the ones offered by the authors. This requires looking at the compiled literature with a different set of assumptions or from the viewpoint of another field, or in some way providing another approach.

REFLECTIVE SKEPTICISM

An attitude of reflective skepticism helps the reviewer to be wary of overgeneralizations, embedded social structures within knowledge bases, and potentially falsified results in the literature. This attitude of reflective skepticism helps in self-reflection. Biases can be found not only in individual or collective knowledge, but also in the reviewer. The generalizations drawn may reflect the world view or values the reviewer is unconsciously trying to maintain. Bracketing the assumptions embedded in one's understanding of the phenomenon under study may help to provide the review reader an understanding of potential bias and help the reviewer to guard against some forms of this bias.

In summary, critical thought is important throughout the review process. The reviewer must consider concept, context, and content of the resources that comprise the review and the new generalizations drawn in the integration of these. The standards of review identified in the box below, based on Ganong's (1987) work, can be related to these considerations. Attention to the concept will help to ensure that theory, as well as results, methods, and subjects are considered in the review. Attention to the context will provide the reader with information about the studies that goes beyond mere results to enrich the interpretation and meaning. Attention to the content will help ensure that methods are identified that relate to the accuracy and thoroughness of the review. Additionally, this will help ensure a

---

EVALUATING THE REVIEW OF THE LITERATURE

1. Were the methods used to identify references appropriate?
2. How many existing references were retrieved?
3. Is the information retrieved accurate?
4. Is the review readable? Does it synthesize the available information?
5. Are assumptions and potential biases addressed? Are discrepancies in findings among studies discussed?
6. Are both conceptual and theoretical issues addressed?

review that includes content that informs instead of overwhelms the reader.

CRITICAL EVALUATION

Critical thought leads to evaluation of written reviews. The boxed criteria for review will help to focus the attention of the reviewer. Evaluation for inclusiveness and accuracy refers to how many existing references have been retrieved and the methods that were used to identify and retrieve them. In addition, the accuracy of the information is evaluated. Individual findings reported out of context would be identified at this point. The readability criteria indicates that the review should tell a story and not be a series of paraphrased or quoted material, but a synthesis that leads the reader to an understanding of the current state of the art about the topic. The review should not overwhelm the reader with isolated pieces of information but should keep the reader focused on the issues in the literature. The evaluation of the total study indicates that the authors have addressed the assumption and potential biases when considering the results. These are especially important as a way of addressing any discrepancies in the group of findings. Within a review, both conceptual and theoretical issues need to be addressed. The individual concept, as well as the relationship of concepts within explanatory theories, can provide insights, and both need to be included.

SUMMARY

- Reviews can be freestanding or embedded.
- There are different classifications of reviews and evidence of each classification can be found in the nursing literature.
- The five purposes for the review are:
  1. Summarization of new ideas

2. Formation or testing of theory
3. Organization of knowledge
4. Integration of knowledge
5. Focused determination of study components

- The process of review includes an initial focusing with attention to the concept and context followed by creation of a new generalization with accompanying concern for content.
- The five tasks of the review (with accompanying issues for each task) are:
  1. Identify the focus question (motivation and question frame)
  2. Identify and locate sources (adequacy, representativeness, bias)
  3. Read and critique (inclusion criteria, article integrity)
  4. Analyze and critique (form of synthesis, representation of truth)
  5. Write and review (generalizability, author bias)
- Critical thinking is important for the integrity of the review process. The components of critical analysis can be used as a framework to guide in the review.

FACILITATING CRITICAL THINKING

1. If you have decided to complete a freestanding review, what choices will you make that are different from those that would be made for an embedded form of literature review?
2. In the second task of identifying and locating resources, what are the problems associated with doing a search of one data base using one index term or phrase?
3. If all of the studies completed on the health of home caregivers is completed on females, what are the potential problems of understanding the "truth" about the influence of caregiving on health outcomes?
4. Trace the ordering of terms in the phe-

nomena of self-care as these words are used:
  a. in the large group of researchers attending to this topic;
  b. within nursing;
  c. within community health nursing;
  d. and then within a group of researchers you can identify.
5. Evaluate the freestanding review by Ingham, "A review of the literature relating to touch and its use in intensive care," using the evaluation criteria.
6. References relating to bonding can be classified to include the following: sample (size, sex of infant), design type, and instruments. What important classification criteria could potentially be missed?

References

SUBSTANTIVE

BECK, C. T. (1993). Teetering on the edge: A substantive theory of postpartum depression. *Nursing Research, 42*(1), 42-48.

BLEGEN, M. A. (1993). Nurse's job satisfaction: A meta-analysis of related variables. *Nursing Research, 42*(1), 36-40.

FOOD AND NUTRITION BOARDS. (1989). *Recommended dietary allowances* (10th ed.).Washington, D.C.: National Academy of Science.

INGHAM, A. (1989). A review of the literature relating to touch and its use in intensive care. *Intensive Care Nursing, 5,* 65-75.

KNAPP, T. A. (1993). Treating ordinal scales as ordinal scales. *Nursing Research, 42*(3), 184-186.

MALONI, J. A., CHANCE, B., ZHANG, C., COHEN, A. W., BETTS, D., & GANGE, S. (1993). Physical and psychosocial side effects of antepartum hospital bedrest: A review of the literature. *IMAGE 23*(3), 187-191.

MALONI, J. A., & KASPER, C. E. (1991). Physical and psychosocial effects of antepartum hospital bedrest: A review of the literature. *IMAGE 23*(3), 187-192.

OLSEN, D. P. (1991). Empathy as an ethical and philosophical basis for nursing. *Advances in Nursing Science, 14*(1), 62-75.

PROPOSED NUTRITION AND ENERGY INTAKE FOR THE EUROPEAN COMMUNITY. (1993). Report of the Scientific Community for Food of the European Community. *Nutrition Reviews, 51*(7), 209.

THOMAS, S. A., LIEHR, P., DEKEYSER, F., & FRIEDMANN, E. (1993). Nursing blood pressure research, 1980-1990: A bio-psycho-social perspective. *IMAGE, 25*(2), 157-164.

CONCEPTUAL

BANGER-DROWNS, R. L. (1986). Review of developments in meta-analytic methods. *Psychological Bulletin, 99*(3), 388-399.

BERNSTEIN, F. (1988). The retrieval of randomized clinical trials in liver diseases from the medical literature. *Controlled Clinical Trials, 9,* 23-31.

BROOKFIELD, S. D. (1987). *Developing critical thinking.* San Francisco: Jossey-Bass.

COOPER, H. M. (1982). Scientific guidelines for conducting integrative research reviews. *Review of Educational Research, 52*(2), 291-302.

CURLETTE, W. L., & CANNELLA, K. S. (1985). Going beyond the narrative summarization of research findings: The meta-analysis approach. *Research in Nursing and Health, 8*(3), 293-301.

DELOZIER, E. P., & LINGLE, V. A. (1992). MEDLINE and MeSH: Challenges for end users. *Medical Reference Services Quarterly, 11*(3), 29-45.

FIELD, P. A., & MORSE, J. M. (1985). *Nursing research: The application of qualitative approaches.* Rockville, Md: Aspen.

FINDLEY, T. W. (1989). Research in physical medicine and rehabilitation: The conceptual review of the literature or how to read more articles than you ever want to see in your entire life. *American Journal of Physical Medicine and Rehabilitation, 68*(2), 97-102.

FOX, R. N., & VENTURA, M. R. (1984). Efficiency of automated literature search mechanisms. *Nursing Research, 33*(3), 174-177.

GANONG, L. H. (1987). Integrative reviews of nursing research. *Research in Nursing and Health, 10,* 1-11.

GLASS, G. V., McGAW, B., & SMITH, M. L. (1981). *Meta-analysis in social research.* Beverly Hills, Calif: Sage.

GRANEY, M. J., & ENGLE, V. F. (1990). Meta-analysis techniques. *Journal of Gerontological Nursing, 16*(9), 16-19.

GREENWALD, A. G. (1975). Consequences of prejudice against the null hypothesis. *Psychological Bulletin, 82,* 1-20.

HALLER, K. B. (1988). Conducting a literature review. *American Journal of Maternal Child Nursing, 13,* 148.

HEDDLE, N. M., GAGLIARDI, K., & FLEMMING, T. (1991). Searching the scientific literature. *Canadian Journal of Medical Technology, 53,* 210-213.

JOHNSON, D. E., MCKININ, E. J., & SIEVERT, M. (1992). The application of quality filters in searching the clinical literature: Some possible heuristics. *Medical Reference Services Quarterly, 11*(4), 39-59.

LIGHT, R. J., & PILLEMER, D. B. (1984). *Summing up.* Cambridge, Mass: Harvard University Press.

MARCHETTE, L. (1985). Research: The literature review process. *Perioperative Nursing Quarterly, 1*(4), 69-75.

MCCAIN, N. L., & LYNN, M. R. (1990). Meta-analysis of a narrative review: Studies evaluating teaching. *Western Journal of Nursing Research, 12*(3), 347-358.

MILLER H. S. (1992). Registering the history of nursing. *IMAGE, 24*(3), 241-245.

PAPINEAU, D. (1979). *Theory and meaning.* Oxford: Clarendon Press.

PHILLIPS, J. R. (1992). Search in research. *Nursing Science Quarterly, 5*(2), 50-51.

SMITH, M. C., & NAFTEL, D. C. (1984). Meta-analysis: A perspective of research synthesis. *IMAGE, 16*(1), 9-13.

SMITH, M. L. (1980). Publication bias and meta-analysis. *Evaluation in Education, 4,* 22-24.

METHODOLOGICAL

ARONSON, A. R. (1993). Bibliography manager. *JAMA, 270*(14), 1751.

LEDERMAN, R. (1992). Guidelines for using meta-analysis. *American Journal of Maternal Child Nursing, 17,* 265.

O'CONNOR, S. E. (1992). Network theory—a systematic method of literature review. *Nurse Education Today, 12,* 44-50.

O'FLYNN, A. I. (1982), Meta-analysis. *Nursing Research, 31*(5), 314-316.

RYAN, B., SCAPENS, R. W., & THEOBALD, M. (1992). *Research method and methodology in finance and accounting.* San Diego: Academic Press.

SMITH, J. T., SMITH, M. C., & STULLENBARGER, E. (1991). Decision points in the integrative review process: A flow-chart approach. *Medical Reference Services Quarterly, 10*(2), 47-72.

HISTORICAL

GLASS, G. (1977). Integrating findings: The meta-analysis of research. *Review of Research in Education, 5,* 351-379.

GLASS, G. (1976). Primary, secondary, and meta-analysis of research. *The Educational Researcher, 5,* 3-8.

JACKSON, G. B. (1980). Methods for integrative reviews. *Review of Educational Research, 50,*(3), 438-460.

USING LOANSOME DOC (1991). *Gratefully yours: From the National Library of Medicine.* March/April. U.S. Department of Health and Human Services.

CHAPTER 8

THE THEORETICAL FRAMEWORK

SUZANNE H. BROUSE

Janice, a community health nurse working for the local Visiting Nurses Association, has been increasingly concerned that new mothers she visited often did not continue the positive life-style changes they had made during pregnancy. Many returned to smoking, eating fewer vegetables and fruit and more junk food, and stopped doing their regular exercise program. In her literature search she found the Pender Health Promotion Model (1987), which identifies cognitive-perceptual and modifying factors that may explain the occurrence of health-promoting behaviors. According to Pender, the model is derived from social learning theory and is structurally related to the Health Belief Model. Janice was using the Betty Neuman (1989) conceptual model to guide her practice and believed that the Pender Health Promotion Model was consistent with the Neuman model. Further review of the literature disclosed partial support of the Pender model components but also indicated conflicting results among studies that examined the same variables. Janice found that few studies examined

new mothers in relation to their health habits, so she decided to design and conduct a research study. Given the lack of current research, she chose a descriptive study approach. The cognitive-perceptual factors of the Pender model that she decided to add to the study included the importance of health, perceived control of health, and perceived benefits of and barriers to health-promoting behaviors. The modifying factors she selected were the interpersonal demographic factors of education, age, employment status, and income. Janice needed to delineate a theoretical framework for her study that would be congruent with the Neuman systems model (1989), which guided her overall approach to nursing.

❧ THE IMPORTANCE OF A THEORETICAL FRAMEWORK

The importance of a theoretical framework for any research study has long been recognized in the nursing literature. Fawcett

(1978) uses the image of the DNA double-helix molecule to describe the research-theory relationship (Figure 8-1). The theory helix is described as spiraling from the idea stage, through transformations, to eventual support or refutation. The research helix is described as spiraling from the formation of research questions, through collection and analysis of data, to interpretation and recommendations for future study. The core of the helix is the critical pairing of research and theory. Fawcett believes that only when theory directs research and research shapes theory development the potential triviality of each is avoided and science is advanced.

Schlotfeldt (1975) proposes that to be meaningful, systematic inquiry must be guided by a conceptual framework that influences all phases of the research process, from problem selection to data analysis. Brown (1964) focuses on the role of research in theory testing. She suggests that for nurse scientists to meet the challenge of developing the body of knowledge to guide practice and education, new criteria must be used to evaluate research effort. We need to ask how a particular study and its theoretical framework are linked to nursing theory and what it contributes to the scientific body of nursing knowledge. Batey (1971) has described the research process as having three phases: (1) the conceptual, (2) the empirical, and (3) the interpretive. The investigator's organizing image (i.e., the theoretical framework) determines what questions will be addressed by the research and how other aspects of the research process will be used to answer these questions.

Moody (1990) notes that the theoretical perspective allows the investigator to "weave together the facts into a meaningful pattern" (p. 74). Fawcett and Downs (1992) propose that research is the vehicle for theory development and that theory gives data their meaning. This concept applies whether the intent of the research is theory development or theory testing.

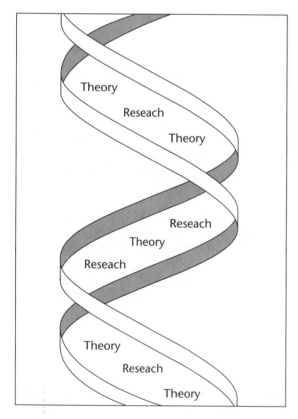

Figure 8-1. The theory-research spiral of knowledge. (From Chinn, P. L. and Kramer, M. K. (1991). *Theory and nursing: A systematic approach* (3rd ed.). St. Louis: Mosby-Year Book.)

✎ METAPARADIGMS, CONCEPTUAL FRAMEWORKS, THEORY, AND STUDY THEORETICAL FRAMEWORKS

Before discussing the development of a theoretical framework for a research study, it is necessary to differentiate among a metaparadigm, conceptual framework, theory, and study theoretical framework.

METAPARADIGMS

Metaparadigms are the constructs and relationship statements that single out the concerns that are unique to a discipline. In a discipline a metaparadigm is the most abstract level of knowledge. According to Fawcett (1989), there is a general agreement that the concepts central to nursing are: person, environment, health, and nursing. As early as 1971, Walker proposed that nursing encompassed four distinct aspects: persons with health problems receiving care; persons providing care; the environment in which this care is provided; and well-being, the end-state of care. In 1975 Yura and Torres identified person, health, society, and nursing as the four central concepts in the conceptual frameworks guiding baccalaureate curricula in nursing. Neuman (1989) concurred that the central concepts of nursing were health, client, environment, and nursing. In all these variations, "person" may refer to an individual, family, group, or community (Schultz, 1987). Donaldson and Crowley's (1978) review of nursing literature led them to propose three themes that interrelate the metaparadigm concepts:

1. The principles and laws that govern the life process, well-being, and optimum function of human beings, sick or well;
2. The patterning of human behavior in interaction with the environment in normal life events and critical life situations; and
3. The processes by which positive changes in health status are effected. (p. 119)

For Meleis (1991) the concepts central to the discipline of nursing are interactions; the nursing client; environment; actual or anticipated transitions; nursing process; nursing therapeutics; and health:

> It is proposed that the nurse interacts (interaction) with a human being in a health/illness situation (nursing client) which is an integral part of his sociocultural context (environment) and who is in some sort of transition or is anticipating a transition (transition); the nurse-patient interactions are organized around some purpose (nursing process, problem solving, or holistic assessment), and the nurse uses some actions (nursing therapeutics) to enhance, bring about, or facilitate health (health). (p. 101)

Kim (1987) also varies slightly from the four more generally accepted concepts of the metaparadigm, identifying domains of nursing knowledge as: client, client-nurse, environment, and practice. The client domain focuses on health care experiences and development. The client-nurse domain comprises the interactions that occur between client and nurse during the provision of care. The quality, time, and space attributes of the client's environment constitute the environment domain. Finally, the practice domain focuses on the social, behavioral, and cognitive aspects of the nurse's professional activities.

CONCEPTUAL FRAMEWORKS

As other disciplines, nursing has several conceptual frameworks derived from the metaparadigm, as outlined in the works by Johnson (1959, 1980), King (1981, 1992), Levine (1967, 1989), Neuman (1991), Newman (1979, 1986), Nightingale (1859/ 1969), Orem (1991), Orlando (1961), Parse (1981, 1992), Rogers (1970, 1990), Roy and Andrews (1991), and Watson (1979, 1985, 1989). Each represents the theorist's somewhat unique view of nursing and offers differing definitions of health, person, environment, and nursing, as well as additional, more specific concepts. As Fawcett (1989) points out, conceptual models are not new to nursing. However, the first models, such as those of Nightingale (1859/1969), Peplau (1952), and Johnson (1980), were not formalized as such with explicit definitions of the four metaparadigm concepts. The concepts and propositions of conceptual frameworks are slightly less abstract than those at the metaparadigm level of knowledge.

THEORY

The definition of a theory may vary widely among authors. Following Kerlinger (1986), "A *theory* is a set of interrelated constructs (concepts), definitions, and propositions that present a systematic view of phenomena by specifying relations among variables, with the purpose of explaining and predicting the phenomena" (p. 9). We also define a *concept* as "an idea or complex mental image of a phenomenon (object, property event). Concepts are the major components of theories" (Powers & Knapp, 1990, p. 22). Third, a *proposition* is a general statement about the relationship among concepts in the theory. Theories contain concepts and relationships that are more concrete than those of conceptual models.

Several nurse theorists have developed theories from their conceptual frameworks. Orem (1991) has developed the theory of self-care, the theory of self-care deficit, and the theory of nursing systems. Roy (Roy & Andrew, 1991) has developed the theory of persons as adaptive systems. Rogers (1992) has developed the theory of accelerating evolution and the theory of paranormal phenomena. Neuman (1989) is now developing the theory of optimum client stability. Because of the complexity of human experiences, multiple theorists are necessary to provide structure or explanation for these experiences. Many theories are also

necessary to address the phenomena of interest to a discipline. Nursing uses teaching-learning, systems, adaptation, coping, social support, social learning, and many other theories from other disciplines in addition to nursing theories. They permit us to provide order in a disorganized world and to interpret events, situations, and behaviors in practice and research.

Classification of Theories

Theories may be classified as descriptive, explanatory, or predictive, *Descriptive* theories describe or classify specific dimensions or characteristics of individuals, groups, situations, or events by summarizing the commonalities found in discrete observations. These are needed when very little is known about particular phenomena. *Explanatory* theories delineate relationships among the dimensions or characteristics of individuals, groups, situations, or events. *Predictive* theories, sometimes referred to as *practice* theories, express precise relationships among the dimensions or characteristics of a phenomenon or differences between groups.

Theories may also be categorized according to their scope. Grand theories are those broadest in scope. The concepts are very abstract and not easily empirically tested. Some authors have designated nursing conceptual frameworks as grand theories (Kim, 1983; Stevens, 1984). Fawcett (1989) advocates separating the two for clarity and because grand theories derived from nursing conceptual models are appearing in the literature (Newman, 1979, 1986). Theories with fewer concepts and that purport to explain a smaller part of the universe are labeled *middle-range theories*. Merton (1957) recommends that efforts in theory development concentrate on middle-range theory, which can be directly tested and thus be most useful. Some authors support this view, but others propose that middle-range theories be derived from one of the nursing conceptual frameworks in order to build a knowledge base rooted in the nursing perspective.

THEORETICAL FRAMEWORKS FOR STUDIES

The theoretical framework for a particular research study is made up of the concepts and the relational statements between the concepts to be examined or tested.

The theoretical framework for a specific study may be a nursing middle-range theory or one derived from another discipline. It may be a unique synthesis of more than one theory to describe the phenomenon under study. Depending on the scope of the study, the framework may be composed of only some of the concepts from a particular theory or synthesis of theories, or it can comprise only some of the relationships among concepts.

RELEVANCE TO RESEARCH STUDIES

The relationships between metaparadigm concepts, conceptual frameworks, theories, and theoretical frameworks for research studies are illustrated in Figure 8-2. Each discipline focuses on specific phenomena,

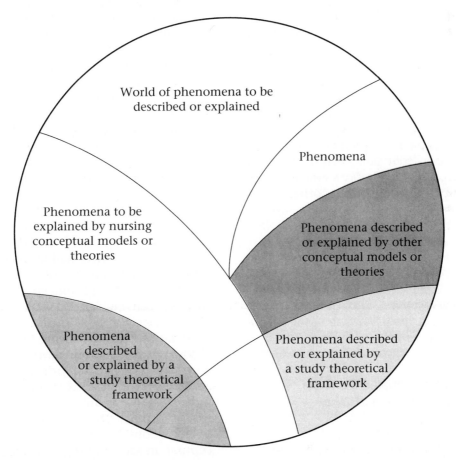

Figure 8-2. Relationship of metaparadigm concepts, conceptual frameworks, theories, and study conceptual frameworks.

described at a highly abstract level in the metaparadigm of the discipline. The metaparadigm provides the perspective of the discipline and direction for knowledge development. As we have seen, for nursing the metaparadigm concepts generally accepted are person, environment, nursing, and health. Each discipline also has several communities of scholars who support a particular focus or vision of the metaparadigm, embodied in a particular conceptual framework. The conceptual framework is made up of concepts and relationship statements (propositions) that are less abstract than metaparadigmatic concepts but that may still not be directly testable. A conceptual framework may not have sufficient scope to explain all aspects of the metaparadigm in the early stages of development. Theories, particularly middle-range theories, are derived from conceptual frameworks and are characterized by less abstract, more testable concepts and relationship statements. Each theory attempts to describe, explain, or predict a portion of a phenomenon that falls within the more limited scope of that theory's concepts and relationships. Theories from other disciplines may be integrated into a nursing theory or theoretical framework to explain the phenomenon of interest better. Because nursing's perspective is different from that of other disciplines, a borrowed theory will change to become congruent with the nursing perspective. Walker and Avant (1988) describe this process as *theory derivation*.

⚬ DEVELOPING CONCEPTUAL FRAMEWORKS FOR STUDIES

QUANTITATIVE STUDIES

How does Janice, the nurse described at the beginning of the chapter, or any other researcher develop a theoretical framework, the organizing framework for a research study? How does the researcher select from the body of knowledge available what will provide direction for a particular study?

A given field's metaparadigm determines what a discipline's activities focus on. As discussed, the consensus is that nursing is concerned with the four metaparadigmatic concepts of person, environment, health, and nursing in relation to the three themes described by Donaldson and Crowley (1978): (1) principles and laws that govern life processes and well-being in health and illness; (2) patterning of human behavior in interaction with the environment; and (3) the processes by which positive changes in health occur. The body of knowledge about these real-world events is composed of conceptual frameworks, theories and empirical generalizations, and facts not organized into theories developed by nursing and other disciplines (Batey, 1971).

Janice selected the nursing conceptual framework of Betty Neuman to guide her professional activities. Selecting a nursing conceptual framework helps the researcher identify problems that are of significance to the discipline of nursing. It provides theoretical definitions of the four metaparadigm concepts as well as other concepts specific to the conceptual framework. Nursing conceptual frameworks also specify relationships between concepts from which theories can be derived at a less abstract level. Janice noticed from her own clinical observations while using the Neuman (1989) model that new mothers did not incorporate postpartum primary prevention activities that had strengthened flexible lines of defense during pregnancy. Janice first described the problem she is concerned about in terms of the nursing conceptual model guiding her practice. This problem would be consistent with the

Donaldson and Crowley (1978) theme of patterning of behavior in interaction with the environment (health-promotion activities) in critical life situations (pregnancy and postpartum).

The state of the existing knowledge base influences how the researcher proceeds to develop the study framework (Batey, 1971). When the accumulated knowledge base about the phenomenon of interest is not well developed or systematized, the researcher uses generalized theories that may be relevant, as well as knowledge from direct observation and insight from creative reflection. Initially, the accumulated body of knowledge may be acquired through a review of existing literature. Computerized literature reviews may be combined with direct review of journals and other written materials that are judged likely to contain material relevant to the phenomenon under study. Batey (1971) points out that the framework guiding a research study is not merely a review of the literature but also a creative product of the researcher's appraisal of the literature. The researcher may also gain current knowledge by direct contact and discussion with colleagues in nursing and other disciplines to obtain unpublished data and creative ideas or thoughts applicable to the study. At this point, the researcher may again review and further systematize those clinical observations that first led to identifying a problem. With such new information about current knowledge and perhaps some new insights from clinical data, the problem can be further defined.

If the accumulated body of knowledge immediately related to the phenomenon of interest is not well developed, the literature should be further explored for theories that are more general or explain similar phenomena. Then, the researcher can begin to actually choose the concepts (potential variables for the study) and relationships (potential hypotheses) and organize them into a study framework. It is helpful to draw a visual picture or model of the concepts and known or proposed relationships between concepts in the framework. Omissions or inconsistencies may be become more evident as the model is visualized. As these occur the researcher can select those concepts (variables) and relationships (hypotheses) that will actually be included in the study. As Batey (1971) notes, it is through this process of developing and refining the theoretical framework that the interaction between the real world of events and the systematized body of knowledge is discovered. These steps are summarized in the box.

QUALITATIVE STUDIES

When developing a qualitative study, the researcher does not start with a completely blank slate. The tension that motivated the researcher to want to learn more about a phenomenon comes from "somewhere"— perhaps from clinical, teaching, or personal experiences, discussions with colleagues, or reading the literature. However, the qualitative researcher approaches the research endeavor with a different philosophical stance regarding knowledge development, the role of the participant, and the role of the researcher.

Some qualitative methodologies require the researcher to put aside, or "bracket," any biases or presuppositions about the phenomenon under study (Lincoln & Guba, 1985; Oiler, 1986). The intent is to learn about the phenomenon from the viewpoint of those participating in the study, to frame it as they would rather than as the researcher would. The concepts and relationships, and thus the theoretical framework, will emerge from the data as the study progresses. Theory develops from

STEPS IN DEVELOPING A STUDY THEORETICAL FRAMEWORK

1. State the problem as clearly as possible.
2. Select a nursing conceptual framework, or review relevant components of the nursing conceptual framework already used to guide professional activities.
3. Try to systematize your clinical observations and creative insights about the problem.
4. Review the literature for theories, theoretical generalizations, empirical generalizations, and systematized facts related to the phenomenon of interest (problem).
5. If the accumulated knowledge immediately related to the phenomenon of interest is not well developed, review the literature for general theories or theories about similar phenomena that may be relevant.
6. Contact researchers and theorists who may have recently developed knowledge about the problem that has not yet been published.
7. Restate and redefine the problem as needed.
8. Identify the important concepts and relational statements, and organize these into a study framework.
9. Draw a visual model of concepts and known or proposed relationships.
10. Select those concepts (variables) and relationships (hypotheses) that will be the focus of this particular study; if not all concepts and relationships of the framework will be tested.

the study rather than guiding it from the beginning.

Other qualitative studies may be guided by a theory that is to be tested by the researcher and validated from the data provided by participants. The researcher is still continually open to the possibility that data will dictate revision of the model or theory, new questions, and a new way of looking at real events. Hutti's (1992) study of parents' perceptions of the miscarriage experience using Dougherty's (1984) cognitive representation framework is an example.

CRITERIA FOR EVALUATING A STUDY'S THEORETICAL FRAMEWORK

A variety of criteria have been developed to evaluate nursing conceptual frameworks (Chinn & Kramer, 1991; Fawcett, 1994; Fawcett & Downs, 1992) and theories (Barnum, 1990; Ellis, 1968; Johnson, 1974; Meleis, 1991). Meleis (1991) maintains that the ultimate purpose of a theory is to systematize data and to provide a unique insight into the study phenomena. A set of criteria for judging a theoretical framework for research studies is also needed to determine whether it makes a contribution to guiding the knowledge base of the discipline. The box on p. 149 lists questions that can be used to evaluate the theoretical framework a researcher has developed to guide the methodology and data analysis of a particular research study.

Not all study theoretical models will meet every criterion listed. The quality and usefulness of the study theoretical model must be determined by the researcher when developing the research study further and when analyzing results by others evaluating the model. The practitioner must also determine its practical usefulness in di-

EVALUATING A RESEARCH STUDY'S THEORETICAL FRAMEWORK

1. Is the theoretical framework derived from a nursing conceptual framework?
2. Does the theoretical framework address a phenomenon of importance and of interest to the discipline?
3. Does the theoretical framework provide direction for planning and methodology and for data analysis?
4. Does the theoretical framework improve the precision with which the phenomenon can be described and predicted?
5. Is the theoretical framework congruent with professional values?
6. Is the theoretical framework congruent with society's view of nursing?
7. Is the theoretical framework testable?
8. Does the theoretical framework render practice more efficient and effective?
9. Is the theoretical framework internally consistent?
10. Is the theoretical framework as simple as possible yet still contains all essential concepts and relationships?

rect client care, in education, or in administration.

✎ EXAMPLES OF NURSING CONCEPTUAL FRAMEWORKS IN RESEARCH

Examining several nursing conceptual frameworks that have been useful in guiding research studies may be helpful. The original works of nursing theorists should be consulted for more detailed descriptions of the conceptual models. Several secondary sources that describe and evaluate the conceptual frameworks are also available (Barnum, 1990; Fawcett, 1994; Fitzpatrick & Whall, 1989; Marriner-Tomey, 1993; Meleis, 1991; Parse, 1987). Examples of specific studies will be used to illustrate how concepts from a nursing conceptual framework are related to study variables. For more complete listings of research studies guided by Orem's, Roy's, Roger's, Johnson's, Levine's, and Neuman's models, the reader is referred to Fawcett (1994). An updated list of Neuman-guided studies has been published in the *Neuman News*

(March, 1992). Parse model-directed studies are frequently published in *Nursing Science Quarterly, IMAGE,* and other journals.

OREM'S GENERAL SELF-CARE THEORY

Dorothea Orem (1980) has described her model as a general theory of nursing composed of three interrelated theories: theory of self-care, theory of self-care deficits, and theory of nursing systems. The six central concepts of Orem's overall conceptual framework are self-care, self-care agency, therapeutic self-care demand, self-care deficit, nursing agency, and nursing systems. The peripheral concept is basic conditioning factors (Orem & Taylor, 1986).

Theory of Self-Care
The theory of self-care focuses on self-care as learned behavior that is performed purposely in response to three types of self-care requisites: universal, developmental, and health-deviation requisites. *Universal self-care* requisites are related to life processes and to the maintenance of human structure and function. *Developmental self-care* requisites are related to human

development in all stages of the life cycle and to events that may adversely affect development. Health-deviation self-care requisites are due to structural and functional deviations, genetic or not, and their effects, as well as medical diagnostic and treatment measures (Orem, 1985, 1991).

Two other dimensions of the theory of self-care are self-care agency and dependent-care agency. *Self-care agency* is the ability to perform care of self. *Dependent-care agency* is the capability to care for infants, children, and dependent adults. Self-care or dependent-care agency is affected by the basic conditioning factors of age, gender, developmental stage, sociocultural orientation, health state, family system factors, health care system factors, patterns of living, environmental factors, and resource availability and adequacy (Orem, 1991).

Theory of Self-Care Deficits

The central idea of the theory of self-care deficit is that at times self-care agency may not be sufficient for the therapeutic self-care demand (i.e., the sum of those actions required to maintain life, health, and well-being over time) (Orem, 1991). When a self-care deficit occurs, nursing interaction is appropriate.

Theory of Nursing Systems

The theory of nursing systems describes three types of systems: wholly compensatory nursing system, partially compensatory nursing system, and supportive-educative nursing system. A nursing system is defined as "all the actions and interactions of nurses and patients in nursing practice situation" (Orem, 1985, p. 148). When a patient is unable to perform self-care actions, the *wholly compensatory nursing* system is appropriate. The nurse performs all necessary actions. In the *partially compensatory* nursing system, the nurse performs some self-care measures for the patient, compensates for self-care limitations of the patient, and assists the patient as needed. With the third type of nursing system, the supportive-educative, the patient is able to perform self-care measures, but the nurse still needs to provide teaching, support, a developmental environment, and guidance for a period of time. Orem describes the ability to nurse as nursing agency, "the complex property or attribute of nurses developed through specialized education and training in the theoretical and practical nursing sciences and through their development of the art of nursing in reality situations (Orem & Taylor, 1986, p. 53). Those same conditioning factors that influence self-care agency, education, and experience affect nursing agency.

Person

The metaparadigm concept of person in the Orem (1991) framework is the recipient of care who functions biologically, symbolically, and socially. Human beings differ from other living things in their capacity for self-reflection, symbolization of experience, use of symbols in thinking, communication, and making objects that are beneficial for themselves and others.

Environment

Environment as a concept is not defined, although the term *developmental environment* is described in detail. A positive developmental environment includes opportunities to pursue individual decisions with provisions for assistance when needed, respect, trust, recognition and encouragement of potential, and opportunities for both solitude and companionship. The person and environment are described as an integrated system (Orem, 1985). One aspect of the role of the nurse is to assist individuals or groups to maintain or change conditions in their environments.

EXAMPLE OF RESEARCH GUIDED BY THE OREM MODEL

Research guided by the Orem model is extensive (Fawcett, 1994). A study by Frey and Denyes (1989) illustrates how Orem's (1991) theory of self-care served as the theoretical framework for a study examining the relationship of basic conditioning factors to self-care activities of adolescents with insulin-dependent diabetes mellitus (IDDM). (See Figure 8-3.)

According to Orem (1991), basic conditioning factors influence an individual's universal self-care and health deviation self-care. Universal self-care in response to universal self-care requisites is directed to the maintenance of structure functioning (i.e., health). Health deviation self-care in response to health deviation self-care requisites is related to structural and functional deviations such as diabetes mellitus.

Study variables included basic conditioning factors, universal and health deviation self-care, health, and a physiologic control marker of adolescents with IDDM.

Conditioning factors were age, gender, birth order, socioeconomic status (SES), religious participation, health symptoms, and mother's employment outside the home. Universal self-care for this study was the Denyes Self-Care Practice Instrument (DSCPI) (Denyes, 1980, 1988). Health deviation self-care followed the Diabetic Self-Care Practice Instrument (DiSCPI). Health was operationalized by a combination of scores on the Self-Perception Profile for Children (SPPC) (Harter, 1985) and the Denyes Health Status Instrument (DHSI) (Denyes, 1980). The value of the adolescent's glycosylated hemoglobin was used as an index of pathology.

Health

Orem (1985) defines health as a "state of the person that is characterized by soundness or wholeness of developed human structures and of bodily and mental functioning" (p. 179). Health includes the achievement of innate potential and the ability to live within one's physical, biological, and social environments. Health and well-being are seen as related but differing human states. Well-being is "a state characterized by experiences of contentment, pleasure, and kinds of happiness, by spiritual experiences, by movement toward fulfillment of one's self ideal; and by continuing personalization" (Orem, 1991, p. 184).

Nursing

Nursing, according to Orem (1985), is a field of knowledge and a practice discipline. The practice discipline is a helping service originating from a societal mandate distinguished from other human services by the way in which it focuses on its proper object, human beings. The special concern of nursing is the individual's ability for self-care. The nurse may provide assistance to another by teaching, acting or doing for, guiding, supporting another person, or by providing for a developmental environment. The nursing process guides the activities of the nurse in consciously selecting actions that meet nursing goals.

THE ROY ADAPTATION MODEL

Sister Callista Roy identifies the general systems model of vonBertalanffy (1968), the adaptation-level theory of Helson (1964), humanism, and veritivity as influential in the formation of her conceptual model

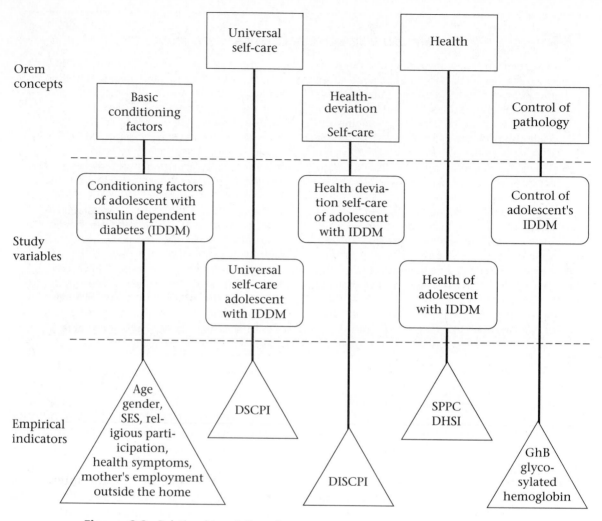

Figure 8-3. Relationship of Orem's concepts to study variables of Frey and Denyes (1989).

(Roy, 1988). In line with the widely accepted concepts of nursing's metaparadigm, Roy (Roy & Andrews, 1991) considers the broad concepts of the Roy adaptation model to be *person, environment, health,* and *nursing.* The major concepts of the theory of person as an adaptive system (developed from the Roy adaptation model) include the coping mechanisms of

the cognator and regulator; the four adaptive modes (interdependence, physiological, self-concept, and role function); three types of stimuli (focal, residual, and contextual); and adaptation level.

Person

Person in Roy's model is the recipient of care. In a holistic adaptive system the per-

---

EXAMPLE OF RESEARCH GUIDED BY THE ROY ADAPTATION MODEL

Fawcett (1994) and a review of nursing periodicals document numerous doctoral dissertations and research studies guided by the Roy Adaptation Model. A program of research by Fawcett (1990) is directed at developing and testing a nursing educational intervention derived from the Roy Adaptation Model to prepare expectant parents for unplanned caesarean birth. The fourth study of Fawcett's program of research was designed to test the educational intervention with 81 pregnant women and their husbands.

Concepts of the Roy Adaptation Model serving as the basis for the study theoretical framework included focal and contextual stimuli and adaptation in the four modes: physiologic, role function, interdependence, and self-concept. (See Figure 8-4.) Childbirth was the focal stimulus for this study; the experimental and control childbirth education interventions were the contextual stimuli being tested.

Physiologic mode adaptation was defined as the mother's pain and distress. Functional status postpartum constituted adaptation in the role function mode. The study variables of feelings for the baby and marital relations indicate adaptation in the interdependent mode, and mother's self-esteem indicated adaptation in the self-concept adaptation mode.

Childbirth was classified as a vaginal delivery, an unplanned caesarean section, or a planned caesarean section. The control intervention was operationalized as the standard childbirth preparation classes; the experimental intervention included pamphlets and focused discussion of caesarean sections.

Physiologic mode adaptation was operationalized as the mother's scores on the Pain Intensity Scale and the Distress Scale. The mother's score on the Inventory of Functional Status operationalized the variable of functional status postpartum. Feelings for the baby were evaluated as the mother's score on the Feeling about Baby Scale, and marital relation by Relationship Change Scale scores. Mother's self-esteem scores were measured by the Rosenberg Self-Esteem Scale.

---

son is more than a sum of parts and functions adjusting to and affecting the environment. The person is seen an adaptive system that receives either *internal stimuli* from the self or *external stimuli* from the environment. The *focal stimulus* is "the internal or external stimulus most immediately confronting the person" (Roy & Andrews, 1991, p. 8). *Contextual stimuli* are other stimuli present which may influence the focal stimulus. *Residual stimuli* are "environmental factors within or without the person whose effects in the current situation are unclear" (Roy & Andrews, 1991, p. 9). When residual stimuli are identified, they become contextual stimuli.

The three types of stimuli interact to make up the changing point indicative of the person's ability to respond positively to the situation. Roy and Andrews (1991) have labeled this point the *adaptation level*. Adaptive responses are those behaviors that promote the integrity of the person; ineffective responses do not contribute to the goals of adaptation and may threaten survival, growth, reproduction, or mastery (Roy, 1988). According to the Roy model the two major internal control processes of the adaptive system are the regulator and the cognator subsystems (Roy, 1984). The *regulator* deals primarily with physiologic stimuli. The *cognator* deals with perception/in-

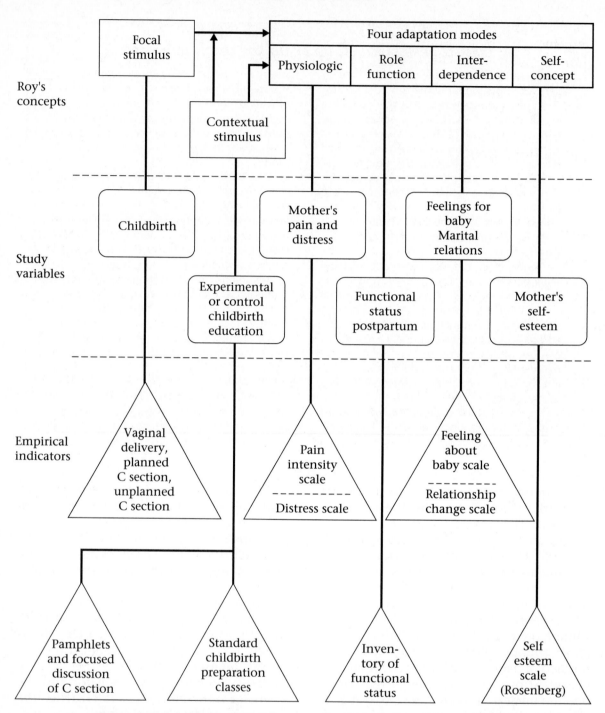

Figure 8-4. Relationship of Roy's concepts to study variables of Fawcett (1990).

formation processing, learning, judgment, and emotion. These two subsystems are intimately interrelated as the person responds holistically (Roy & Roberts, 1981).

Regulator and cognator activities are observed in the four adaptive modes identified by Roy: (1) The behaviors in the *physiologic mode* are related to oxygenation, nutrition, elimination, activity and rest, and protection. (2) The *self-concept mode* focuses on the psychologic and spiritual factors of the person. This mode has two components, physical self and person self. (3) The *role function mode* focuses on the individual's societal roles. (4) Interdependence is based on affectional adequacy. Roy and Andrews (1991) emphasize that although the modes may be studied independently for convenience, they are interrelated.

Environment

In the Roy Adaptation Model, environment is defined as "all of the internal and external conditions, circumstances, and influences surrounding or affecting the development and behavior of persons or groups" (Roy, 1984, p. 39). All stimuli are part of the environment. As the environment changes, new adaptive responses are required, providing opportunities for growth, development, and enhancement of life (Roy & Andrews, 1991).

Health

Roy considers health as a reflection of adaptation, but the definition is not yet fully developed. Health needs to be viewed in light of individual goals and of the fulfillment of one's purpose in life as reflected in becoming an integrated and whole person. Thus health is a state and process of being and becoming an integrated person; lack of integration is lack of health (Roy & Andrews, 1991). As a state, health reflects

the adaptation process in the interrelated four modes; as a process it is observed in the behaviors of individuals as they strive to achieve their full potential.

Nursing

Nursing is a practice-oriented scientific discipline. It is distinguished from other disciplines by the activities of the nursing process. The Roy nursing process consists of six steps: (1) assessment of behavior, (2) assessment of stimuli, (3) nursing diagnosis, (4) goal setting, (5) intervention, and (6) evaluation. Collaboration at each step of the process with the person or group is emphasized as essential (Roy & Andrews, 1991). A nursing diagnosis is a statement of behaviors in one or more of the four modes and may include relevant influencing stimuli. Goal setting includes development of short-term and long-term behavioral outcomes that are thought to promote adaptation. The goal of nursing intervention is the promotion of adaptation in each of the four modes. Interventions may include altering, increasing, decreasing, removing, or maintaining relevant stimuli to achieve the stated goals. The final step of evaluation includes judging whether the person exhibits adaptive behavior after the nursing intervention was performed—was the desired goal attained?

NEUMAN SYSTEMS MODEL

Betty Neuman believes that the systems view from which her model is derived presents an opportunity for developing new ways of thinking and methods for disciplined inquiry into complex phenomena (Neuman, 1989). Concepts unique to the Neuman conceptual framework include the flexible line of defense, normal line of defense, lines of resistance, and central core in describing person.

EXAMPLE OF RESEARCH GUIDED BY THE NEUMAN SYSTEMS MODEL

Fawcett (1989), Neuman (1989), and other authors cite multiple applications of the Neuman model to clinical, educational, and administrative situations. However, examples of research studies guided by the Neuman framework are not as evident in the literature. Zeimer (1983) examines the use of different types of preoperative data as primary prevention tools in promoting coping strategies (see Figure 8-5). The concepts of the Neuman Systems model guiding this study are stressors, primary prevention, lines of defense, and impact of stressors.

Surgery is the stressor, and a nursing education intervention is primary prevention. The lines of defense were defined as physiologic and psychophysiologic coping behaviors. The impact of stressors would be symptoms experienced by the surgical patients postoperatively, such as pain, nausea and vomiting, and urinary retention.

Surgery for this study was operationalized as gynecologic or gastrointestinal surgery. The primary prevention nursing intervention was one of three types of surgery-related information provided preoperatively: description of the procedure only; procedural information plus descriptions of sensations that accompany the procedure; and procedural and sensory information plus physiologic and psychophysiologic coping measures including cognitive reappraisal relaxation techniques. Coping behaviors are scores on the Physical Coping Behavior Scale and the Psychophysiologic Coping Behavior Scale. Reactions to stressor are scores on the Pain Intensity Scale and patient reports of nausea, vomiting, and difficulty voiding.

Person

Neuman uses the term client-client system for person, based on the new collaborative relationship between client and caregiver. The person is viewed as a system composed of five variables. The physiologic variable refers to body structure and function, the psychologic to mental processes and relationships, the sociocultural to combined social and cultural functions, the developmental to life development processes, and the newest, spiritual, to spiritual belief influence (Neuman, 1989).

The client-client system is seen as a series of concentric rings about a basic or core structure. The outermost ring, the *flexible line of defense,* acts as a buffer system for the person's usual state to prevent reactions to stressors. The five variables described by Neuman interact within this buffer system and, as with other defensive mechanisms, are in differing states of development. The flexible line of defense is visualized as an accordionlike mechanism that can react rather quickly to alterations in the client-client system.

The next ring is the *normal line of defense.* This is the usual wellness state that the individual has developed over time. The integrity and stability of the normal line of defense are influenced by the five system variables, as well as by life-style, coping patterns, cultural and spiritual influences, and developmental state. This line is considered dynamic in that it can expand or contract over time. When the normal line of defense has been penetrated by one or more stressors, instability or symptoms of illness occur.

The innermost protective mechanisms for the central core, which contains the basic factors common to all organisms, are

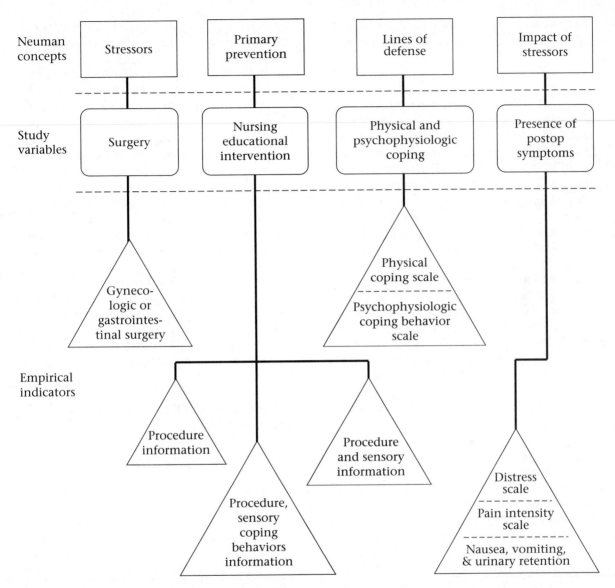

Figure 8-5. Relationship of Neuman's concepts to study variables of Ziemer (1983).

the *concentric lines of resistance.* These lines of resistance are activated when the normal line of defense has been ineffective in response to stressors in an attempt to move the client-client system back in the direction of stability and health. The abil-

ity of each protective mechanism to protect against stressors depends on the interaction of the five system variables at each level, as well as the timing, number, and strength of the stressors. Reconstitution can begin at any level of reaction to stressors, with the result extending beyond the previous normal line of defense in some instances.

Environment

Neuman (1989) defines environment as all the influences, whether they be internal or external, that affect the client-client system. The *internal environment* is composed of all forces within the client-client system itself and is related to intrapersonal stressors. The *external environment* is all the forces external to the defined client-client system and corresponds to the interpersonal and extrapersonal stressors. The third type of environment is the *created environment,* which is developed unconsciously by the client and acts as a reservoir or protector for the maintenance of system integrity. The created environment changes the response or possible response of the system to stressors; it may be expressed consciously, unconsciously, or at both levels at the same time. The created environment is intra-, extra-, and interpersonal in nature (Neuman, 1989).

Health

In the Neuman Systems Model health and wellness are interchangeable concepts, dichotomous with illness on a continuum. The best possible wellness state is optimal system stability, but it may vary within a normal range throughout the life cycle. To determine the level of wellness, the effect of stressors on the energy level of the client-client system is assessed. Neuman (1989) refers to a theory of optimal client system stability she and a colleague developed from the model but does not provide details of this theory.

Nursing

The major concern for nursing is "keeping the client system stable through accuracy both in the assessment of effects and possible effects of environmental stressors and in assisting client adjustments required for an optimal wellness level" (Neuman, 1989, p. 34). To implement the Neuman System Model a specific nursing process format has been developed. It is organized into three sections: nursing diagnosis, nursing goals, and nursing outcomes. Interventions to keep the system stable are primary, secondary, or tertiary. The intent of primary intervention is to strengthen the flexible line of defense in order to protect the normal line of defense through stress prevention or risk reduction. The intent of secondary prevention is to strengthen the internal lines of resistance to protect the basic core. Reconstitution can begin at any point following the initiation of treatment. Should secondary prevention interventions not be effective, death occurs. Tertiary prevention is directed at protecting client system reconstitution.

ROGERS'S SCIENCE OF UNITARY HUMAN BEINGS

Although Martha Rogers's ideas have often been controversial and have generated heated debate, she is acknowledged as one of the most influential scholars in the discipline (Garon, 1992; Meehan, 1990; Meleis, 1985; Sarter, 1988). Rogers (1989) includes the concepts or "building blocks" of energy fields, a universe of open systems, pattern, and four-dimensionality as unique to nursing science. More recently (Lutjens, 1991), the term *pandimensional* has replaced the term *four-dimensionality.*

Person

Person, or "unitary human being," is defined as "an irreducible, indivisible pandimensional energy field identified by pattern and manifesting characteristics that are specific to the whole and which cannot

---

EXAMPLE OF RESEARCH GUIDED BY ROGERS'S SCIENCE OF UNITARY HUMAN BEINGS

The use of Rogers's conceptual model as a guide for many research studies is documented in Barrett (1990), Fawcett (1989), Ference (1986), Malinski (1986), and in nursing journals. Fawcett notes that Rogers's focus on the unity of the person-environment interaction dictates that both be taken into account when designing a study and choosing statistical analysis techniques. Meehan (1993) tested the hypothesis that therapeutic touch would decrease postoperative pain in 108 patients undergoing major elective surgery. (See Figure 8-6.) Meehan used Rogers's (1980, 1989) theory of paranormal phenomena derived from the theorists science of unitary human beings. This derived theory states that in a pandimensional unitary world there is no separation between the human and environmental field. Action-at-a-distance phenomena, such as therapeutic touch, are congruent with this new reality (Meehan, 1990).

The two major Rogerian concepts guiding this study are nursing practice as knowledgeable purposive patterning of the patient-environmental field process and a patient's experience of health or illness as a manifestation of the mutual person-environmental energy field patterning process.

Nursing practice for this study is the intervention of therapeutic touch. Postoperative pain is the selected energy field patterning process.

Therapeutic touch is a standardized 5-minute procedure using focused intent and hand movements. Pain is the patient's subjective report as measured by the Pain Visual Analogue Scale (VAS, Huskisson, 1974).

---

be predicted from knowledge of the parts" (Lutjens, 1991, p. 22). Pattern is the distinguishing characteristic of a field. The concept of "universe of open systems" underscores the focus on the continual openness and evolving diversity of the human and environmental energy fields. These energy fields are infinite and the unifying concept for the model. Pandimensionality is considered by Rogers (1989) as "a nonlinear domain without spatial or temporal attributes" and "characteristic of all reality" (p. 185).

Environment
Environment is seen as an irreducible energy field perceived as a single wave and integral with the human field. Rogers (1986) proposed three principles of homeodynamics to summarize her conceptualization of the human and environmental field patterning.

> *Principle of resonancy.* Continuous change from lower to higher frequency wave patterns in human and environmental fields.
> *Principle of helicy.* Continuous innovative, unpredictable, and increasing diversity of human and environmental field patterns.
> *Principle of integrality.* Continuous mutual human field and environment a field process (p. 8).

Health
Health and illness are viewed by Rogers (1970) as expressions of the life process. Each society infuses these concepts with unique cultural meanings. Those manifes-

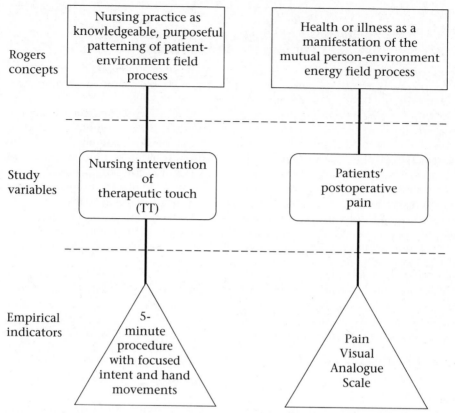

Figure 8-6. Relationship of Rogers's concepts to study variables of Meehan (1993).

tations of the life process with high value are termed *health,* and those with low value are termed *illness.* Health and wellness exist on the same continuum but are not dichotomous.

Nursing
Rogers considers nursing to be a learned profession and therefore a science and an art. The art of nursing is the creative use of the organized abstract body of knowledge to assist people to achieve maximum wellness within their potential (Rogers, 1989). Nursing science is defined as "the study of

unitary, irreducible, indivisible human and environmental fields: people and their world" (Rogers, 1989, p. 6). Rogers believes that a science has many theories, and she has derived three from her conceptual model: the theory of accelerating evolution, the theory of paranormal phenomena, and the theory of rhythmical correlations of change (Rogers, 1980). Fawcett (1989) notes that other nurse theorists have drawn from Rogers: Newman's theory of health (1979, 1986), Parse's unified person theory (1981, 1992), and Fitzpatrick's life perspective rhythm model (1983, 1989).

PARSE'S HUMAN BECOMING THEORY

Parse's human becoming theory of nursing was originally labeled man-living-health: theory of nursing. Recently, it has been retitled, and the language of the assumptions and principles have been revised because of changes in the dictionary definition of the term *man*. Currently, the term usually refers to the male gender rather than to mankind as the author originally intended. No other aspects of the theory were changed. The new name, human becoming, is intended to maintain the unitary man-living-health focus of the theory (Parse, 1992). Assumptions for this model were derived from Rogers's (1970, 1990) concepts of energy field, pattern and organization, openness, and four-dimensionality (now pandimensionality) and principles of helicy, integrality, and resonancy (now integrality). The existential-phenomenologic influences of Heidegger (1962), Sartre (1963), and Merleau-Ponty (1963) are also noted by Parse (1987). The concepts of coconstitution, coexistence and situated freedom and the tenets of intentionality and human subjectivity are integral to her model (Parse, 1981).

Coconstitution is the active participation of the person in creating meaning with others and the world. *Coexistence* involves living with one's predecessors, contemporaries, and successors all at once. *Situated freedom* involves the freedom to choose from various options in situations (Parse, 1981). Each of the nine assumptions connects three of the theory concepts. For example, one assumption states: "The human is coexisting while coconstituting rhythmical patterns with the universe" (Parse, 1992, p. 38). Parse's theory is a human science theory focusing on participation of the human being with the universe in the cocreation of health.

The underlying assumption of the interrelatedness of person, environment, and health in Parse's model makes it difficult to discuss these concepts separately. Parse places her model in the simultaneity paradigm, distinguishing it from the totality paradigm of most nursing models. The totality paradigm according to Parse (1992) describes the human-environment relationship as cause-effect, and the language of the theories tends to promote separation of mind, body, and spirit. The simultaneity paradigm is based on a mutual process view of the person-environment interaction. Human beings are recognized through patterns, and practice focuses on pattern recognition (Parse, 1992). Parse also differentiates her human becoming theory from Rogers's life process theory within the simultaneity paradigm (Parse, 1992). The central phenomenon of concern is human becoming, in contrast to Rogers's unitary human beings or the focus on self-care, adaptation, goal attainment, or caring of other nurse theorists.

Person-Environment

The human being in the human becoming theory is an open being who is cocreating with the universe rather than simply interacting with the environment. Coconstituted patterns are illuminated through body movements, positions, speech, touch, and gaze (Parse, 1987). The individual is defined by interrelationships rather than the field pattern of Rogers or physiological, psychological, sociological, and spiritual attributes found in the totality theories. The person freely chooses in each situation encountered. As new actual events illuminate other possibilities, the person becomes more complex. The human-environment mutual energy occurs at many universe levels, and space and time are interconnected.

EXAMPLE OF RESEARCH GUIDED BY PARSE'S MODEL

An increasing number of research studies using the Parse Human Becoming Theory of Nursing and research method are appearing in the literature (Cody, 1991; Heine, 1991; Jonas, 1992; Kelley, 1991; Mitchell, 1990; Parse, 1990; and Smith, 1990). Pilkington (1984) used the Parse theory and methodology to learn about the lived experience of grieving for an important other of five mothers who had lost their babies at birth. Three of Parse's nine principles were supported from the data with extraction-synthesis and heuristic interpretation (Parse, 1987); cocreation of meaning (valuing), paradoxical unity of rhythmical patterns of relating (connecting-separating), and moving beyond the now moment to greater unfolding (transforming). The relationship of the three core concepts uncovered in the study to Parse's three principles is illustrated in Figure 8-7.

Health

Health is a continuous process experienced by the person rather than the well-being defined by norms in totality theories. It is described by Parse (1981) as nonlinear and cannot be described as *good* or *bad* or *more than* or *less than*. Rather, as the person simultaneously connects with and separates from the environment and other persons in the environment, changes occur and values are experienced. Parse (1981) describes this as health.

Nursing

Nursing is a human scientific discipline; its practice is a performing art (Parse, 1992). The goal of nursing for Parse's human becoming theory is the individual's personally defined quality of life, not well-being and optimal health as defined by the individual in Rogers's theory or the prevention of disease and promotion of health found in other nursing models. Parse's (1987) practice methodology consists of the following:

1. Illuminating meaning is shedding light through uncovering the what was, is, and will be, as it is appearing now. It happens in explicating what is. Explicating is a process of making clear what is appearing now through languaging.
2. Synchronizing rhythms happen in dwelling with the pitch, yaw, and roll of the interhuman cadence. Dwelling with is giving self over to the flow of the struggle in connecting-separating.
3. Mobilizing transcendence happens in moving beyond the meaning moment to what is not yet. Moving beyond is propelling toward the possibles in transforming. (p. 167)

The nurse's attentive presence is what inspires the individual or family to illuminate meaning, synchronize rhythms, and move beyond the here and now.

Research Methodology

Based on a belief that a mature discipline has its own research methodologies consistent with its ontologic base, Parse (1992) developed a research methodology unique to the human becoming theory. The focus for study is universal human health experiences, and the purpose is to uncover the structure of lived experience of individuals or groups who are able to articulate the

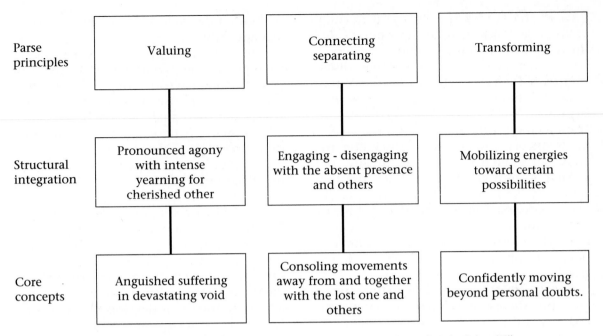

Figure 8-7. Relationship of uncovered core concepts to Parse's principles (Pilkington, 1984).

meanings. Findings, that is, descriptions of the lived experience, are woven into theory, the language of science, through extraction-synthesis and heuristic interpretation. These processes move from the language of the participants to a more abstract level of theory and beyond. Parse (1992) differentiates her research methodology from other qualitative methods. She describes the primary differences as the way in which processes are lived. Description of the lived experience is not elicited from the participant in the usual interview, but in a unique way of "becoming with." In addition, the way in which findings are taken to the more abstract theory level and interwoven with other concepts of the human becoming theory through extraction-synthesis and heuristic interpretation is unique to this method.

THEORY DEVELOPMENT METHODS

Many authors emphasize the importance of developing middle-range theories with more specific concepts and propositions to guide practice and research to provide the basis for the more specific study theoretical framework used to guide a particular research project (Dickoff & James, 1968; Ellis, 1968; Jacobs & Huether, 1978; Meleis, 1991).

Whall (1986) suggests four approaches to knowledge development for the practice of nursing based on assumptions that each discipline is responsible for developing its distinct body of knowledge within its unique perspective and that knowledge can be developed in a variety of ways. One method for knowledge development is to deduce a theory from one of the major nursing conceptual models.

A second approach is to use a nursing conceptual framework to reformulate deductively an existing theory developed within the perspective of another discipline. For example, Whall (1986) reformulates Madanes's (1981) strategic family theory using Roy's (1984) nursing model. A third method is the reformulation of an existing theory from another discipline by using an inductively derived nursing approach. Corbin and Strauss (1991) use the trajectory framework of Strauss and associates to develop a nursing model of chronic illness for use in practice and education. The fourth approach is the inductive development of a nursing theory in practice.

Meleis (1991) suggests four major strategies for theory development based on analysis of the theory literature in nursing. The first is the theory-practice-theory strategy. The clinical theorist selects an established theory from another discipline, uses it in practice, and refines and adapts the theory to the nursing situation. Examples cited include Johnson's (1980) adaptation of Parson's concept of behavioral systems to develop her seven behavioral subsystems and Roy's (1984) use of adaptation, systems, and interactionist models to develop her nursing adaptation model.

The second strategy for theory development is the practice-theory strategy. Impetus for this strategy comes from questions in the practice situation for which no theory is available to explain the phenomenon. Observation of phenomena, description and labeling of concepts, and linking of concepts to form relational statements are the major activities. The grounded theory techniques of Glaser and Strauss (1967) have provided guidance for theorists using this strategy. An example cited by Meleis (1991) is Reed and Leonard's (1989) devel-

opment of the concept of self-neglect using grounded theory.

The third strategy, the research-theory strategy, is the traditional inductive approach. Characteristics of a selected phenomenon are measured in a variety of situations and then analyzed for the existence of significant patterns that are formalized into theoretical propositions.

The fourth strategy for theory development proposed by Meleis (1991) is the theory-research-theory strategy. The theorist selects a theory for use in developing research variables and questions or hypotheses for testing and goes further to modify the original theory. This approach differs from the research-theory strategy in that the theorists start with an intent to test and refine the theory or develop a new theory. The findings are specific to selected phenomena (Meleis, 1991).

A fifth "ought-to-be" strategy is also recommended, practice-theory-research-theory strategy. This strategy is based on acknowledging the integral relationship among research, practice, and theory. The theorist or researcher brings to any situation previous experience as well as theoretical and empirical knowledge that provides a unique nursing perspective. According to Meleis (1991) this approach assumes that a patterned and orderly reality exists that can be comprehended and explained. However, the uniqueness of individuals and situations reminds the theorists to consider patterns of diversity that add to the complexity of theory. The essential starting point for this strategy for theory development is often difficult to isolate.

Walker and Avant (1988) have described nine strategies for theory development synthesized from the three elements of concepts, statements, and theories and the three approaches of analysis, synthesis, and derivation (see Table 8-1). Con-

Table 8-1
Walker and Avant's (1988) Methods of Theory Construction

Concepts	Statement	Theory
ANALYSIS	ANALYSIS	ANALYSIS
Examines the attributes and defines the characteristics of a concept as a formal linguistic exercise	Examines relational statements for the relationship of each part to each other and to the whole	Systematically examines a theory's parts and whole to determine the strengths and weakness of the theory
SYNTHESIS	SYNTHESIS	SYNTHESIS
Develops concept on the basis of observation or other forms of empirical evidence	Specifies relationships between two or more concepts based on evidence	Pulling together available information about a phenomenon and organizes concepts and statements into a network or whole
DERIVATION	DERIVATION	DERIVATION
Transposes a concept from one field to another and redefines the concept as a new concept that fits the second field of study	Develops a set of statements about a phenomenon in a second field analagous to those in the first field by using statements from the first field	Transposes a theory from one field to another and restates the theory as a new theory that fits the second field of study

cepts provide the basis for classifying elements of experiences into some kind of meaningful whole and are the building blocks for theories. Statements specifying the relationships between concepts and providing definitions are also essential theory components. In the *analysis* approach the whole is divided into its component parts, and these parts and their relationships to one another and to the whole are examined. In contrast, *synthesis* uses information from a variety of sources to construct a new whole, a concept. *Derivation* as an approach uses the techniques of metaphor or analogy to modify or refine a concept from one context for use in another.

ETHICAL ASPECTS OF THEORY DEVELOPMENT

The ethical implications of any nursing conceptual framework, theory, or study theoretical framework are considerable. The purpose of theorizing is to determine what is essential knowledge for the discipline. Yeo (1989) maintains that the key concepts of nursing theories are value-laden, making the theories themselves examples of value or normative statements. Gadow (1979) has described the definition of nursing as the most pressing ethical problem of nursing. In determining what is essential, decisions are made as to what to include and what not to include. Decisions are made as to what is the focus of the discipline. By defining theories, the values, beliefs, and assumptions of the theorist affects what is deemed essential knowledge for nursing. In discussing nursing conceptual framework, a growing consensus is that the concepts for nursing are person, environment, health, and nursing. Most of the nursing conceptual frameworks propose that the goal for nursing is health or well-being. However, the nursing conceptual frameworks vary in their definitions of the metaparadigm concepts, or worldview (Fawcett, 1989). The nurse theorist's values, beliefs, and assumptions are ultimately translated into nursing knowledge that guides nurses' actions in research, practice, education, and administration (Reed, 1989).

RESEARCH

The nursing conceptual framework and theories from nursing and other disciplines that form the basis for a research study's theoretical framework influences decisions about what phenomena are worthy of study, methods of data collection, the role of participants, risks deemed appropriate for participants, what is termed valid and reliable, and what are considered significant findings.

PRACTICE

The clinician's practice framework's underlying values reflected in the definition of person will help determine the individual's role in attaining, maintaining, or promoting health supported by the nurse, and in the degree of mutuality in goal setting be-

tween client and nurse. The definition of health will determine when this has been reached, as well as what is promoted as the "good" and when this too has been reached. The definition of nursing will determine the role of the nurse, what is assessed, what are appropriate interventions, and methods for evaluation.

EDUCATION

The nursing conceptual framework and other theories chosen by educators to guide curriculum development are expressions of values and beliefs of the faculty and theorists. Such values and beliefs will be reflected in the philosophy, program objectives, course objectives and content, type of clinical experiences offered, teaching methodologies, roles of the teacher and student as active, passive, or mutual, and the degree to which the environment promotes health for all.

ADMINISTRATION

Similarly, for administrators in health care facilities, values and beliefs underlying the conceptual framework and theories chosen guide administrative activities. They will in large part determine what are considered legitimate nursing activities, authority, and responsibility; the role of the clients and other health care providers; the goals of the institution; the preferred ways to achieve goals; and the role of the institution in research and the development of knowledge relevant to health care.

Reed (1989) also points out that as the values, beliefs, and assumptions of theorists are translated into the essential knowledge of the discipline there are fundamental implications for what "ought to be." Standards for the discipline are implicitly or explicitly provided as nursing conceptual frameworks, and theories are developed and used to guide practice and research. The ethical implications of nursing theory development and use need to be recognized and examined more fully because of the critical consequences of knowledge development. This knowledge is ultimately translated into actions for the good of society.

SUMMARY

- The study theoretical framework guides all phases of the research process and contributes to the development of the discipline's body of knowledge.
- A nursing conceptual framework provides the theorist's perspective of nursing and direction for knowledge development.
- The state of existing knowledge about the phenomenon to be studied influences how the researcher proceeds to develop the study theoretical framework.
- The relationship of a study theoretical framework to the qualitative research process usually differs from the relationship of the framework to the quantitative research process.
- A study theoretical framework is evaluated on its contribution of knowledge building in nursing, its contribution to development of the study from question to methodology, congruence with professional and societal values, its internal consistency, and contribution to practice.
- The ethical implications of nursing theory development and use need to be more fully examined for their critical consequences as they influence nurses' actions.

FACILITATING CRITICAL THINKING

1. Select a research article from the literature that describes a study guided by a nursing conceptual framework. From the researcher's description of the theorist's model and the study hypotheses, draw a diagram of the relationship of study variables to the conceptual framework concepts. State whether you believe that the study variables as described are congruent with the model and provide supporting rationale.

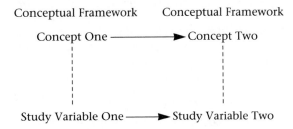

2. Wha t would you say to try to convince a fellow researcher that it is advisable to develop a study theoretical framework before proceeding further in the research project?
3. Select a research study with a well-developed study theoretical framework. Analyze how the framework influenced the steps in the research process.
4. Describe how the hypotheses or research questions would have been different for a research study guided by one nursing conceptual framework if the study had been guided by a different nursing conceptual model.
5. Using the criteria for evaluation of a study theoretical framework, evaluate a study framework based on a nursing conceptual model and one not based on a nursing conceptual model.

References

SUBSTANTIVE
CODY, W. K. (1991). Grieving a personal loss. *Nursing Science Quarterly, 4,* 78-82
DENYES, M. (1980). Development of an instrument to measure self-care in adolescents. (Abstract) *Nursing Research, 31,* 63.

DENYES, M. (1988). Using Orem's theory for health promotion: Directions for research. *Advances in Nursing Science, 11*(1), 13-21.

FAWCETT, J. (1990). Preparation for caesarean childbirth: Derivation of a nursing intervention from the Roy Adaptation Model. *Journal of Advanced Nursing, 15,* 1418-1425.

FREY, M. A., & DENYES, M. J. (1989). Health and illness self-care in adolescents with IDDM: A test of Orem's theory. *Advances in Nursing Science, 129*(1), 67-75.

HEINE, C. (1991). Development of gerontological nursing theory: Applying the man-living-health theory of nursing. *Research in Nursing and Health Care, 12*(4), 184-188.

HUSKISSON, E. C. (1974). Measurement of pain. *Lancet, 9,* 1127-1131.

JONAS, C. M. (1992). The meaning of being an elder in Nepal. *Nursing Science Quarterly, 5*(4), 171-175.

KELLEY, L. S. (1991). Struggling with going along when you do not believe. *Nursing Science Quarterly, 4,* 123-129.

MEEHAN, T. C. (1990). Theory development. In E. A. Barrett (Ed.), *A vision of Rogers' science-based nursing.* New York: National League of Nursing.

MEEHAN, T. C. (1993). Therapeutic touch and postoperative pain: A Rogerian research study. *Nursing Science Quarterly, 6*(2), 69-78.

MITCHELL, (1990). The lived experience of taking life day by day in later life: Research guided by Parse's emergent method. *Nursing Science Quarterly, 3,* 29-36.

PARSE, R. R. (1990). Parse's research methodology with an illustration of the lived experience of hope. *Nursing Science Quarterly, 3,* 9-17.

PILKINGTON, F. B. (1984). The lived experience of grieving the loss of an important other. *Nursing Science Quarterly, 6*(3), 130-139.

POWERS, B. A., & KNAPP, T. R. (1990). *A dictionary of nursing theory and research.* Newbury, CA: Sage.

SMITH, M. J. (1990). Struggling through a difficult time for unemployed persons. *Nursing Science Quarterly, 3,* 18-28.

ZEIMER, M. M. (1983). Effects of information on postsurgical coping. *Nursing Research, 32*(5), 282-287.

CONCEPTUAL

CORBIN, J. M., & Strauss, A. (1991). A nursing model for chronic illness management based upon the trajectory framework. *Scholarly Inquiry for Nursing Practice, 5*(3), 155-174.

DOUGHERTY, E. (1984). Cognitive models of face-to-face interaction: A semiotic approach. Published doctoral dissertation, State University of New York at Buffalo.

FERENCE, H. M. (1986). Foundations of a nursing science and its evolution: A perspective. In V. M. Malinski (Ed.), *Explorations on Martha Rogers' science of unitary human beings.* Norwalk, CT: Appleton-Century-Crofts.

FITZPATRICK, J. J. (1983). A life perspective rhythm model. In J. J. Fitzpatrick & A. L. Whall (Eds.), *Conceptual models of nursing: Analysis and applications.* Bowie, MD: Brady.

FITZPATRICK, J. J. (1989). A life perspective rhythm model. In J. J. Fitzpatrick & A. L. Whall, *Conceptual models of nursing: Analysis and application* (2nd ed.). Norwalk, CT: Appleton & Lange.

GADOW, S. (1979). ANS open forum. *Advances in Nursing Science, 1*(3), 92-95.

GARON, M. (1992). Contributions of Martha Rogers to the development of nursing knowledge. *Nursing Outlook, 40*(2), 67-72.

HEIDEGGER, M. (1962). *Being and time.* New York: Harper & Row.

HELSON, H. (1964). *Adaptation-level theory.* New York: Harper & Row.

JOHNSON, D. E. (1980). The behavioral system model for nursing. In J. P. Riehl & C. Roy (Eds.), *Conceptual models for nursing practice* (2nd ed.). New York: Appleton-Century-Crofts.

KIM, H. S. (1983). *The nature of theoretical thinking in nursing.* New York: Appleton-Century-Crofts.

KIM, H. S. (1987). Response to "Structuring the nursing knowledge system: A typology of four domains." *Scholarly Inquiry for Nursing Practice, 1*(2), 111-114.

KING, I. M. (1981). *A theory for nursing: Systems, concepts, process.* New York: Wiley.

KING, I. M. (1992). King's theory of goal attainment. *Nursing Science Quarterly, 5*(1), 19-26.

LEVINE, M. E. (1967). The four conservation principles of nursing. *Nursing Forum, 6,* 45-49.

LEVINE, M. E. (1989). The four conversation principles: Twenty years later. In J. P. Riehl-Sisca (Ed.), *Conceptual models for nursing practice* (3rd ed.). Norwalk, CT: Appleton & Lange.

LUTJENS, L. R. (1991). *Martha Rogers: The science of unitary human beings.* Newbury Park, CA: Sage.

MADANES, C. (1981). *Strategic family theory.* San Francisco: Jossey-Bass.

MALINSKI, V. M. (1986). *Explorations on Martha Rogers' "Science of unitary human beings."* Norwalk, CT: Appleton-Century-Crofts.

MERLEAU-PONTY, M. (1963). *The structure of behavior.* Boston: Beacon Press.

MERTON, R. (1957). *On theoretical sociology: Five essays, old and new.* New York: The Free Press.

NEUMAN, B. (1989). *The Neuman systems model: Application to nursing education and practice.* Norwalk, CT: Appleton & Lange.

NEUMAN, B. (1991). *The Neuman Systems model* (2nd ed). Norwalk, CT: Appleton & Lange.

NEWMAN, M. A. (1979). *Theory development in nursing.* Philadelphia: Davis.

NEWMAN, M. A. (1986). *Health as expanding consciousness.* St. Louis: Mosby.

NIGHTINGALE, F. (1859/1969). *Notes on nursing: What it is and what it is not.* New York: Dover.

OREM, D. (1980). *Nursing: Concepts of practice* (2nd ed.). New York: McGraw-Hill.

OREM, D. (1985). *Nursing: Concepts of practice* (3rd ed.). New York: McGraw-Hill.

OREM, D. (1991). *Nursing: Concepts of practice* (4th ed.). New York: McGraw-Hill.

OREM, D., & TAYLOR, S. G. (1986). Orem's general theory of nursing. In P. Winstead-Fry (Ed.), *Case studies in nursing theory.* New York: National League for Nursing.

ORLANDO, I. (1961). *The dynamic nurse-patient relationship.* New York: G. P. Putnam's Sons.

PARSE, R. R. (1981). *Man-living-health: A theory of nursing.* New York: Wiley.

PARSE, R. R. (1992). Human becoming: Parse's theory of nursing. *Nursing Science Quarterly, 5*(1), 35-42.

PENDER, N. J. (1987). *Health promotion in nursing practice* (2nd ed). Norwalk, CT: Appleton & Lange.

PEPLAU, H. (1952). *Interpersonal relations in nursing.* New York: G. P. Putnam's Sons.

REED, P. G. (1989). Nurse theorizing as an ethical endeavor. *Advances in Nursing Science, 11*(3), 1-9.

ROGERS, M. E. (1970). *An introduction to the theoretical basis of nursing.* Philadelphia: Davis.

ROGERS, M. E. (1980). Nursing: A science of unitary man. In J. P. Riehl & C. Roy (Eds.), *Conceptual models for nursing practice* (2nd ed.). New York: McGraw-Hill.

ROGERS, M. E. (1986). Science of unitary human beings. In V. M. Malinski (Ed.), *Exploration on Martha Rogers' "science of unitary human beings."* Norwalk, CT: Appleton-Century-Crofts.

ROGERS, M. E. (1989). Nursing: A science of unitary human beings. In J. Riehl-Sisca (Ed.), *Conceptual models for nursing practice* (3rd ed.). Norwalk, CT: Appleton & Lange.

ROGERS, M. E. (1990). Nursing: Science of unitary, irreducible, human beings: Update 1990. In E. A. Barrett (Ed.), *Visions of Rogers' science based nursing.* New York: National League for Nursing.

ROGERS, M. E. (1992). Nursing science and the space age. *Nursing Science Quarterly, 5*(1), 27-34.

ROY, C. (1984). *Introduction to nursing: An adaptation model* (2nd ed). Englewood Cliffs, NJ: Prentice-Hall.

ROY, C. (1988). An explication of the philosophical assumptions of the Roy adaptation model. *Nursing Science Quarterly, 1*(1), 26-34.

ROY, C., & ANDREWS, H. A. (1991). *The Roy adaptation model: The definitive statement.* Norwalk, CT: Appleton & Lange.

ROY, C., & ROBERTS, S. L. (1981). Theory construction in nursing: *An adaptation model.* Englewood Cliffs, NJ: Prentice-Hall.

SARTER, B. (1988). *The stream of becoming: A study of Martha Rogers' theory.* New York: National League for Nursing.

SARTRE, J. P. (1963). *Search for a method.* New York: Braziller.

SCHULTZ, P. R. (1987). When client means more than one: Extending the foundational concept of person. *Advances in Nursing Science, 10*(1), 71-86.

VONBERTALANFFY, L. (1968). *General systems theory.* New York: Braziller.

WALKER, L. O. (1971). Toward a clearer understanding of the concept of nursing theory. *Nursing Research, 20*(5), 428-435.

WATSON, J. (1979). *Nursing: The philosophy and theory of human caring.* Boston: Little Brown.

WATSON, J. (1985). *Nursing: Human science and human care.* Norwalk, CT: Appleton-Century-Crofts.

WATSON, J. (1989). Watson's philosophy and theory of human caring. In J. Riehl-Siska (Ed.), *Conceptual models for nursing practice* (3rd ed.). Norwalk, CT: Appleton & Lange.

WHALL, A. H. (1986). *Family therapy theory for nursing: Four approaches.* Norwalk, CT: Appleton-Century-Lange.

YEO, M. (1989). Integration of nursing theory and nursing ethics. *Advances in Nursing Science, 11*(3), 33-42.

METHODOLOGICAL

BARNUM, B. J. (1990). *Nursing theory: Analysis, application, and evaluation* (3rd ed.). Boston: Little, Brown.

BARRETT, E. A. (1990). *Visions of Rogers' science-based nursing.* New York: National League of Nursing.

CHINN, P. L., & KRAMER, M. K. (1991). *Theory and nursing: A systematic approach* (3rd ed.). St. Louis: Mosby.

FAWCETT, J. (1989). *Analysis and evaluation of conceptual models of nursing* (2nd ed.). Philadelphia: Davis.

FAWCETT, J. (1994). *Analysis and evaluation of conceptual models of nursing* (3rd ed.). Philadelphia: Davis.

FAWCETT, J., & DOWNS, F. (1992). *The relationship of theory and research* (2nd ed.). Philadelphia: Davis.

FITZPATRICK, J. J., & WHALL, A. (1989). *Conceptual models of nursing: Analysis and application,* (2nd ed.). Norwalk, CT: Appleton & Lange.

GLASER, B. G., & STRAUSS, A. (1967). *The discovery of grounded theory: Strategies for qualitative research.* Chicago: Aldine.

HARTER, S. (1985). *Manual for the Self-Perception Profile for Children.* Denver: University of Denver Press.

HUTTI, M. H. (1992). Parents' perceptions of the miscarriage experience. *Death Studies, 16,* 401-415.

KERLINGER, F. N. (1986). *Foundations of behavioral research* (3rd ed.). New York: Holt, Rinehart & Winston.

LINCOLN, Y. S., & GUBA, E. G. (1985). *Naturalistic inquiry.* Beverly Hills, CA: Sage.

MARRINER-TOMEY, A. (1989). *Nursing theorists and their work* (2nd ed.). St. Louis: Mosby.

MELEIS, A. I. (1985). *Theoretical nursing: Development and progress.* Philadelphia: Lippincott.

MELEIS, A. I. (1991). *Theoretical nursing: Development and progress* (2nd ed.). Philadelphia: Lippincott.

MOODY, L. E. (1990). *Advancing nursing science through research.* Newbury Park, CA: Sage.

OILER, C. J. (1986). Qualitative methods: Phenomenology. In P. Moccia (Ed.), *New approaches to theory development.* New York: National League of Nursing.

PARSE, R. R. (1987). *Nursing science.* Philadelphia: Saunders.

REED, P. G., & LEONARD, V. E. (1989). An analysis of the concept of self-neglect. *Advances in Nursing Science, 12*(1), 39-53.

STEVENS, B. J. (1984). *Nursing theory: Analysis, application, evaluation* (2nd ed.). Boston: Little, Brown.

WALKER, L. O., & AVANT, K. C. (1988). *Strategies for theory construction in nursing* (2nd ed.). Norwalk, CT: Appleton & Lange.

HISTORICAL

BATEY, M. V. (1971). Conceptualizing the research process. *Nursing Research, 20*(4), 296-301.

BROWN, M. I. (1964). Research in the development of nursing theory. The importance of a theoretical framework in nursing research. *Nursing Research, 13*(2), 109-112.

DICKOFF, J., & JAMES, P. (1968). A theory of theories: A position paper. *Nursing Research, 17*(3), 197-203.

DONALDSON, S. K., & CROWLEY, D. M. (1978). The discipline of nursing. *Nursing Outlook, 26*(2), 113-120.

ELLIS, R. (1968). Characteristics of significant theories. *Nursing Research, 17*(3), 217-222.

FAWCETT, J. (1978). The relationship between theory and research: A double helix. *Advances in Nursing Science, 1*(1), 49-62.

JACOBS, M. K., & HUETHER, S. E. (1978). Nursing science: The theory-practice linkage. *Advances in Nursing Science, 1*(1), 63-73.

JOHNSON, D. E. (1959). Theory in nursing: Borrowed and unique. *Nursing Research, 17*(3), 206-209.

JOHNSON, D. E. (1974). Development of theory: A requisite for nursing as a primary health profession. *Nursing Research, 23*(5), 372-377.

SCHLOTFELDT, R. M. (1975). The conceptual framework of nursing research: The need for a conceptual framework. In P. J. Verhonick (Ed.), *Nursing research.* Boston: Little, Brown.

YURA, H., & TORRES, G. (1975). *Today's conceptual frameworks with the baccalaureate nursing programs.* New York: National League for Nursing.

CHAPTER 9

THE PURPOSE AND PROPOSITIONS OF THE STUDY

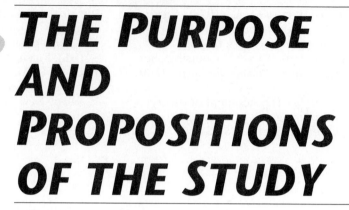

LAURA A. TALBOT

Administering a tube feeding to a patient in nutritional need is a common nursing task. Part of the care associated with this task is checking tube placement. Traditionally, tube placement has been checked by aspirating gastric contents and/or attaching a syringe to the distal end of the nasogastric tube, injecting 10 to 20 cc of air into the tube, and simultaneously listening over the stomach.

Another promising method of verifying tube placement was recently studied by Metheny et al. (1993). From clinical experience the team had noted the potential for small-bore soft tubes to become dislodged and enter the respiratory tract. This life-threatening event can go undetected because few respiratory symptoms may surface, especially if the patient has a neurologic deficit. At present radiographic placement verification is the method of choice, especially with initial placement.

This team of researchers tested the pH of aspirated body fluid to differentiate gastric, intestinal, and respiratory placement. The authors' review of the literature revealed

the following pH values for various body fluids: gastric fluid ranged from 1.0 to 3.5, intestinal fluid ranged from 6.0 to 8.0, and pleural fluid was 7.5. However, intervening factors could affect the pH readings. For example, malignancy in the lung lowered the pH to 7.00, whereas that of an empyema was 5.5. Medications such as cimetidine and ranitidine elevated the pH. The researchers then voiced a need for a nonradiological, bedside method for verification of tube feeding position and proposed the use of pH testing.

The above scenario provides a framework for developing the purpose of a research study. The study's purpose is derived from the theoretical framework, clinical experience, and review of the literature. The theory states that tube placement can be determined based on the pH of body fluids. Clinical experience validates the difficulty in determining accidental respiratory placement based on symptoms. The review of the literature provides guidelines for the range of the pH for various body fluids, although various factors change the pH.

Based on this information, the researchers identified an alternative, nonradiological, bedside method for verifying tube placement: pH testing.

The research purpose, established in response to the theory, clinical practice, and the review of the literature, states specifically why and how the research is being conducted. For this research study the purpose was "to provide more definitive information on the ability of pH to differentiate gastric and intestinal placement and gastric and respiratory placement of feeding tubes" (Metheny, 1993, p. 326).

STATEMENT OF THE PURPOSE

The purpose statement should include (1) the aim of the research, (2) the target population, (3) the setting, and (4) the research variables. The researcher specifies the aim of the research and type of research category by using phrases such as "to identify," "to describe," "to explore," or "to explain." If the phrase states "the purpose of this study is *to identify . . .*" or *"to describe . . . ,"* it is understood that little is known about the phenomenon, and the purpose of the study will be to identify and/or describe the phenomenon as it exists in nature (exploratory or descriptive study). "The purpose of this study is *to explore the relationships* among . . ." suggests that variables have been identified and the study is examining the relationship between these variables (correlational study). If a cause-and-effect relationship is the focus of the study, the statement may read: "The purpose of this study is *to determine . . .*" The research category will be experimental or quasi-experimental. Table 9-1 shows examples of research aims as used in the literature and their corresponding statements of the purpose.

Mitchell et al. (1994), in a study describing the three patterns of symptoms associated with the menstrual cycle, stated the following: "The purpose of this study was to differentiate women with three perimenstrual symptom severity patterns: premenstrual syndrome (PMS), premenstrual magnification (PMM), and low symptom (LS)" (p. 25). The reader can tell that the aim of the research is descriptive in nature because the statement specifies that the researcher is going to describe the differences between perimenstrual symptom severity patterns.

The target population is stated in the purpose. This is the population to which the researcher wants to generalize the findings of the research study. The setting is the location where the study will be conducted. Crosby et al. (1990) identified the target population, variables, and implied the setting in this statement: "The primary purpose of this study was to evaluate backrest position, nursing activities, patient activities, and diurnal variations as factors that may contribute to the onset of supraventricular tachyarrhythmias (SVT) after coronary artery bypass surgery (CABG)" (p. 667). The target population consists of patients who have undergone CABG. The research variables are back-rest position, nursing activities, patient activities, and diurnal variations, and the dependent variable is onset of supraventricular tachyarrhythmias (SVT). The implied setting is a hospital in which CABGs are performed.

The variables of the study are stated in the purpose. The aim of the research can also be determined based on how the variables are presented. If a single variable is being described, the aim of the research will be to describe (descriptive study). If more than one variable (multivariate) is examined, the use of independent (cause) and dependent (effect) variables will assist

Table 9-1
Comparison of Research Aim and Research Purpose

Research Aim	Research Purpose	Source
To describe	Because little is known about positive as well as negative patient recollections within the immediate posttransfer period, the purpose of the current study is to identify patient recollections of the critical care experience within 24 to 48 hours after transfer from the unit using an open-ended series of questions.	Simpson et al., 1989, p. 325
To explore	The reactions to wife rape reported in clinical samples are strikingly similar to the clinical picture of psychiatric patients diagnosed with major affective or anxiety disorders . . . to determine the extent to which wife rape is a precipitating or complicating factor in these disorders.	Weingourt, 1990, p. 144
To explain	The purpose of this descriptive correlational study was to examine the relationships among the measures of (1) observed sleep, (2) patient perception of sleep, and (3) polysomnograph sleep data on the sleep traits of SL, MSA, and WASO in one common group of critical care patients, those with multisystem trauma.	Fontaine, 1989, p. 402
To predict	The purpose of this research was to determine during unanesthetized circumcision the effects of pain reduction interventions (music, intrauterine sounds, pacifiers, music plus pacifiers, and intrauterine sounds plus pacifiers) versus no pain reduction intervention on neonatal pain.	Marchette et al., 1991, p. 241

in focusing the study. If the purpose states the study will explore the relationship between the independent and dependent variables, the aim of research will be to explain (correlational study). If the purpose states the study is to determine the relationship between the independent and dependent variables, the aim of the research will be to predict (experimental study).

Whitney et al. (1993) in a study examining the effects of activity and bed rest stated, "The purpose of this preliminary study in normal subjects was to investigate the influence of activity on physiologic responses related to wound healing. Specifically, the effects of bed rest and activity at 50% of maximum capacity on subcutaneous oxygen tension, subcutaneous perfusion, and plasma volume were examined"

(p. 349). The reader can infer from the phrase "to investigate the influence" and the use of independent and dependent variables that the aim of the research is to predict. This implies that a cause-and-effect relationship between the variables will be examined. The target population is normal subjects experiencing wound healing; the setting is a research center. The variables are activity and bed rest as the independent variables and subcutaneous oxygen tension, subcutaneous perfusion, and plasma volume as the dependent variables.

REFINING THE PURPOSE INTO A RESEARCH PROPOSITION

The research purpose is now refined into a research proposition. A research proposition is a premise from which conclusions about the research variable(s) will be drawn. The proposition will be put in the form of a research question or hypothesis. The manner in which the research purpose is stated reflects the aim of the research, as well as the research category. Table 9-2 summarizes the types of research propositions commonly used with various research categories.

When the aim of the research is to describe, the proposition used is a research question. Descriptive research is used when little is known about a phenomenon. It is often difficult and premature to use a hypothesis that states a relationship between the variables. The research categories are phenomenological, grounded theory, ethnographic, historical or exploratory. The research method will be qualitative or quantitative, and the research proposition should be a statement of the variable(s) of a population to be identified or described.

When the aim of the research is to explore, the proposition may be either a research question or a hypothesis. The research category is either exploratory, descriptive, or descriptive-correlational. The research method will be quantitative, and the research proposition should be a statement of the variable(s) of the population to be explored.

When the aim of the research is to explain, the proposition used is either a research question or a hypothesis with a correlational study. Through the quantitative method, the researcher investigates a proposition that states the relationship between two or more variables.

When the aim of the research is to predict, the proposition used is a hypothesis with either quasi-experimental or experimental quantitative research used. A hypothesis states an effect on the dependent variable(s) when the independent variable is manipulated.

Another factor affecting the type of research proposition to be used is whether the focus of the study is to *develop* theory or to *test* theory. If the purpose of the study is to develop theory, a research statement is used. Data analysis is used to identify and analyze concepts and their relationships. The researcher starts with a research question about a phenomenon. Through the

Table 9-2

Comparison of Research Method, Aim, and Approach with the Types of Research Propositions

Research Method	Research Aim	Research Levels	Research Proposition
Qualitative	To describe	Phenomenological Grounded Theory Ethnographic Historical	Research Question
Quantitative	To explore	Exploratory Descriptive Comparative (descriptive-correlational)	Research Question or Hypothesis
Quantitative	To explain	Correlational	Research Question or Hypothesis
Quantitative	To predict	Quasi-experimental Experimental	Hypothesis

verification of concepts and linkages, theory evolves.

If the purpose of the study is to test theory, a hypothesis would be used. The purpose of a theory testing study is to reject an invalid hypothesis. Research findings never confirm or prove a theory; rather a portion of the theory is tested to determine its validity or applicability. As more hypotheses are supported (i.e., not rejected), the validity of the theory gains strength.

℘ THE RESEARCH QUESTION

A research question is the premise on which the final research conclusions are based. It is used when prior knowledge of the phenomenon is limited and research is descriptive in nature. The research question can also be used when an associative relationship can be identified in the review of literature, and research is at the descriptive, exploratory, correlational category of quantitative research. Methodological studies also use a research question when the development of a research instrument is being conducted.

The research question may be written in one of two forms, interrogative or declarative. When the research question is written in the interrogative form, it seeks an answer. All research variables and the population to be studied are included in this interrogative statement. When contrasted to the problem statement, research questions are more precise and specific. It naturally flows from the research purpose, narrowing the focus of the study.

Aber and Hawkins's (1992) study is an example of how the research purpose is refined into a research question using the interrogative form. The purpose of the Aber and Hawkins's (1992) study was to examine "the content of advertisements in med-ical and nursing journals to determine if the images of nurses reflect the roles nurses play in health care" (p. 289). From this purpose, the reader can ascertain that the target population is medical and nursing journals. The research variables are the image of nurses and their reflective roles. The research aim is descriptive; thus a descriptive study is used to address the following research questions:

1. What are the images of nurses in picture advertisements in nursing and medical journals?
2. Are there differences between the images of nurses and those of physicians when both appear in the same advertisements?
3. Do the images of the roles of nurses presented differ from the actual roles nurses play in the health care system?
4. Is the portrayal of nurses stereotyped in characteristics such as uniforms and caps? (p. 290)

When the research question is written in the declarative form, the research variables and the target population are also included in the statement. Blenner (1992) demonstrates a logical flow of the research question from the purpose of the study using the declarative form.

The purpose of this qualitative study was to describe infertility treatment from the patient's perspective. Specifically, the following issues were explored:

1. The aspects of infertility assessment and treatment that are hardships, and how they are managed;
2. The aspects of the health care system that facilitate or inhibit tolerance of treatment; and
3. Patient's perceptions of health providers' management of their infertility

treatment and the psychosocial issues surrounding infertility. (p. 92)

STATING A HYPOTHESIS

A hypothesis is the researcher's prediction of the outcome of the research study based on the research variable(s). It provides direction for the type of research design and statistical analysis to be used in the study. Because it suggests the direction of the study outcomes, it must be stated clearly, concisely, and in measurable terms.

For hypotheses to be stated clearly, concisely, and measurably, three criteria should be considered. First, only one variable, condition, or relationship and only one statistical analysis should be addressed in each hypothesis. A single study may have one hypothesis statement or several. When a single hypothesis states several variable relationships, it is often difficult to decipher what the researcher is examining. This is why using several hypotheses with each stating a single variable, condition, or relationship adds to clarity and brevity of the hypothesis.

Second, the variable, condition, or relationship must be testable. Clear implications for testing should be indicated in the stated hypothesis.

Third, the aim of the research guides what is included in the hypotheses. When the research aim is to explore, the hypotheses include the target population and variables being described in the study. When the research aim is to explain, the research hypotheses make predictions about the population and the relationship among the variables. Finally, when the research aim is to predict, the hypotheses center on the population and a cause-and-effect relationship between the independent and dependent variables.

While the purpose of the study states why there is a need for the research, the hypotheses seeks to provide the solution by predicting the outcome. Stated in the present tense, hypotheses are deduced from theoretical propositions taken from the theoretical framework. Theoretical concepts are converted into measurable variables. Hypotheses are used to test the theoretical concepts and propositions in the real world. Hypotheses foster the expansion of scientific knowledge by either providing support for the theory or failing to support the theory. Hypotheses are the operational tools of a theory connecting abstractions to the real world.

TYPES OF HYPOTHESES

Hypotheses can be categorized several different ways, including (1) simple versus complex hypotheses, (2) null versus alternative hypotheses, (3) directional versus nondirectional hypotheses, (4) causal versus associative hypotheses, and (5) statistical versus research hypotheses. These categories are not mutually exclusive. For example, you can have a complex null hypothesis that may or may not be directional.

Simple versus Complex Hypotheses

A simple hypothesis predicts the relationship between one independent variable and one dependent variable. You may recall the independent variable is the predicted cause of some effect on the dependent variable. It is common to see several simple hypotheses listed in one study. Hollerbach and Sneed (1990) use a simple hypothesis in their study on radial pulse assessment: "The accuracy of radial pulse rate assessments per minute taken by nursing personnel will differ on the basis of number of years of experience" (p. 259). In this example the number of years of experience is the independent variable and the accuracy of radial pulse rate assessment is the dependent variable.

A complex hypothesis predicts the relationships among two or more independent variables and two or more dependent variables. O'Malley et al. (1991) used a complex hypothesis in their study of "Critical care nurse perceptions of family needs": "There will be differences in responses to three categories of family needs (psychologic, cognitive, and physical or person comfort) from nurses in differing ICUs and with differing lengths of employment in the units" (p. 192). In this example, the dependent variables are the three categories of family needs: (1) psychological, (2) cognitive, and (3) physical or personal comfort. The independent variables are (1) nurses in differing ICUs and (2) differing lengths of employment.

While advanced statistics allow for testing of complex hypotheses, if only one part of the hypothesis is rejected, it may be difficult to determine which parts should be accepted and which rejected. Using several simple hypotheses makes interpretation simpler.

Null versus Alternative Hypotheses

The null hypothesis, sometimes designated as H_0, is a statement that there will be no difference, no change, or no effect on the dependent variable for the population under study. It predicts that a proposed treatment will have no effect. The null hypothesis is used when statistical testing procedures are applied to the data.

Williamson (1992) stated the following null hypothesis in her study of "the effects of ocean sounds on sleep after coronary artery bypass graft surgery": "The null hypotheses for this study stated that there were no differences in (1) sleep depth scores, (2) falling asleep scores, (3) awakening scores, (4) return to sleep scores, (5) quality of sleep scores, or (6) total sleep scores between postoperative CABG patients exposed to white noise/ocean sounds and those exposed to usual ambient sounds after transfer from an intensive care unit" (p. 94).

The alternative hypothesis (H_1) is the opposite of the null hypothesis. It predicts that the independent variable will make a difference, have an effect, or make a change on the dependent variable for the population under study. Spees (1991) used an alternative hypothesis in her study of "knowledge of medical terminology among clients and families." The hypothesis proposed: "There is a significant difference between nurses' perceptions of clients' and families' knowledge of medical terms and their actual knowledge of medical terms" (p. 226).

When testing a hypothesis, statistical procedures are applied to sample data to draw inferences about the target population. First the researcher proposes a hypothesis about the target population. A sample drawn from the target population is used to collect data. It is then determined, through the sample data, if the information collected is consistent with the hypothesis. The sample data provides evidence the researcher uses to support a position for or against a hypothesis. Sometimes the evidence is overwhelming and conclusions can be made confidently. Often the evidence is inconclusive, however, and conclusions cannot be made confidently, which leaves the possibility for error to occur.

When testing a hypothesis the alternative hypothesis is supported when the null hypothesis is rejected. The rationale for this method is that it is often easier to prove that a hypothesis is false than it is to prove it is true. For example, a conjecture is made that "all girls have blond hair." To test this conjecture a sample of one girl is selected. If that girl has blond hair, is the conjecture proven? On the other hand, if the girl chosen has brown hair, the conjecture has definitely been proven false. This also applies with the null hypothesis. Support is sought for the alternative hypothesis by disproving the null hypothesis. When the null hypothesis states that a treatment has no effect, the researcher tries to prove it false to demonstrate there is an effect.

Directional versus Nondirectional Hypotheses
A directional hypothesis predicts the type of relationship between the variables, which in turn specifies the expected direction of the treatment effect. The conceptual framework or theory is used as the basis for the determination of the direction of the relationship between the variables.

Directional hypotheses allow for the use of a one-tailed statistical test. The one-tailed statistical test is a directional hypothesis test in which the critical region is located in only one tail of the theoretical sampling distribution (either the right or left tail). The advantage for using a one-tailed statistical test is that it is more sensitive in detecting a treatment effect and statistical significance is more easily achieved. The disadvantage is that it is easier to commit a type I error. That is, the null hypothesis is actually true and the researcher decides to reject it. By rejecting the null hypothesis the researcher is saying the treatment had an effect on the dependent variable, when in reality the treatment had no effect.

Gaydos and Farnham (1988) used a directional hypothesis to predict the effects of stroking on heart rate and blood pressure. Their hypothesis stated: "Persons petting a dog with whom they have a companion bond will experience a greater reduction in heart rate and blood pressure than when petting an unknown dog or reading quietly" (p. 75).

With nondirectional hypotheses the researcher predicts only that a relationship exists. It does not specify the direction of the relationship. Nondirectional hypothe-

ses are used when the research is not theory based, if past research provides conflicting results, or if the direction of the relationship is not known.

The two-tailed statistical test is a nondirectional hypothesis test in which the critical region is located in both tails of the theoretical sampling distribution. With the two-tailed test, a large statistical difference is needed to show significance, but a type I error is less likely to be committed.

Aber (1992) used a nondirectional hypothesis in her study of spousal death: "The independent variables of work history and work attitude are statistically significant predictors of the dependent variable of health during bereavement, as measured by the Widowhood Questionnaire, an instrument specifically developed for use in this study" (p. 96).

Statistical versus Research Hypotheses
The statistical hypothesis is the null and alternative hypothesis written in statistical terms. It states the research hypothesis in quantifiable terms by making a statement about the values of the mean of the population under study. An example of a null and alternative hypothesis is as follows:

$$H_0: u_1 = u_2 \quad \text{(Null hypothesis)}$$
$$H_1: u_1 > u_2 \quad \text{(Alternative hypothesis)}$$

In this example, the null hypothesis (H_0) states in statistical terms that the population mean 1 (u_1) is equal to population mean 2 (u_2). This means that there is no difference between the two means.

It also states that for the alternative hypothesis (H_1) the population mean 1 (u_1) is greater that the population mean 2 (u_2). This indicates that there is a difference between the two means and that the effect will be greater for the population mean 1.

A research hypothesis makes a prediction about the outcome of the study and about the relationship between the variables. It is written in a narrative format versus using statistical symbols.

COMPONENTS OF THE HYPOTHESIS STATEMENT

A hypothesis statement should communicate the intent of the study as outlined by the study problem statement and purpose by including the target population, the research variables, and a predictable outcome. In addition, the hypothesis statement should be in the form of a declarative statement and be theory based (see box).

Problem Statement and Purpose

The hypothesis must have the same population, variables, and predicted outcome as stated in the problem statement and purpose. To assure congruency, the researcher should write the hypothesis using the same terminology expressed in the problem statement and purpose.

Target Population

The target population is stated in the hypothesis. This is the group of subjects or objects to which the findings will be generalized. The target population should not be confused with the subjects in the research sample. The sample is a subset of the target population. The sample is selected from the target population to represent it.

Research Variables

The variables in the hypothesis must be measurable. Variables are characteristics or attributes that differ among research subjects. As their name implies, they *vary* or have different values. There needs to be some means of measuring this variance. The term measurable implies a means in which changes to the variables can be measured. Since the hypothesis states the predicted effect the independent variable has on the dependent variable, there needs to be a means of measuring this effect.

Predicted Outcome

The hypothesis predicts the exact relationship anticipated between the variables. A directional hypothesis states the direction the dependent variable is expected to take as a result of the independent variable.

Rentschler (1991) predicted the outcome in her study of correlates of successful breastfeeding. Her hypothesis was, "There would be a positive relationship between pregnant women's level of information about breastfeeding and success in breastfeeding" (p. 152). In this example level of information is the independent variable

---

STEPS IN STATING THE HYPOTHESIS

1. Review the research problem statement and purpose to be sure the stated hypothesis is reflective of the statement.
2. Identify the target population.
3. Review the theoretical propositions of the theory, and state the hypothesis using the propositions as a theoretical base.
4. Determine if a directional or nondirectional hypothesis is appropriate.
5. Write the hypothesis using a declarative statement with a single relationship between variables.
6. State the research variables in measurable terms, being clear and concise in the hypothesis statement.

EVALUATING THE RESEARCH HYPOTHESIS

1. Is the target population stated in the hypothesis?
2. Are the variables identifiable and measurable in the hypothesis?
3. Is there one relationship or condition stated in each hypothesis?
4. Do the hypotheses flow from the research problem and purpose?
5. Is the hypothesis stated in declarative form?
6. Is the hypothesis stated clearly, concisely, and limited to two sentences?
7. Is the hypothesis theoretically based?
8. Does the hypothesis express a predictable outcome?

and success in breastfeeding is the dependent variable. The predicted outcome was that as the level of information on breastfeeding increases, success in breastfeeding also increases.

Declarative Statement

The hypothesis should be a declarative statement written in the present tense, although it is not unusual to see it written in the future tense in the literature. It should be stated clearly and concisely with a maximum length of two sentences. A single statement is preferred, using only one relationship between variables per hypothesis.

Theory Based

A hypothesis is a prediction based on a theory or a specific portion of a theory (proposition). The purpose of a study is to test the theory or theoretical propositions. For example, Meininger et al. (1991) wanted to investigate theoretical explanations for the developmental origin of type A behavior. One component or proposition of this theory is that "anger and hostility components of type A behavior may stem from a profound sense of insecurity" (p. 222). The sample used was composed of two sets of twins aged 6 to 11 years old. From this theoretical proposition, the hypothesis read: "Teachers' ratings of social competence and behavioral conduct will be negatively correlated with the impatience-aggression subscale score of the MYTH" (Matthews Youth Test for Health) (p. 222).

EVALUATING THE PROBLEM STATEMENT AND HYPOTHESIS

Since the problem statement and hypothesis provide the foundation for a research study, it is important that they state clearly how and why the research will be conducted. Guidelines for evaluating hypotheses are summarized in the box.

SUMMARY

- The research purpose is derived from the review of the literature, the conceptual framework, and the clinical practice.
- The purpose statement includes the aim of the research, the target population, the setting, and the research variables.
- The purpose statement is then refined into a research proposition. It can be in the form of a research question or hypothesis.
- The research question is used when the aim of the research is to describe, explore, or explain.
- The research question may be written in

declarative or interrogative form with the research variables and target population included in the statement.

- The research hypothesis is used when the aim of the research is to explore, explain, or predict.
- Hypotheses may be classified into several ways: (1) simple versus complex hypotheses, (2) null versus alternative hypotheses, (3) directional versus nondirectional hypotheses, and (4) statistical or research hypotheses.
- Components to be included in the hypothesis are the target population, the research variables, and a theory based on a predictable outcome.

FACILITATING CRITICAL THINKING

1. Select a current nursing research article. Identify in the article the following components of the research process:
   a. The theoretical framework
   b. The problem statement
   c. The purpose of the study
   d. The research question or hypothesis
   Write each of the components in the table below.
2. Is there a logical interrelationship between each of the components of the research study? If not, where are the inconsistencies? How would you correct them?

Theoretical Framework	Problem Statement	Purpose	Research Question or Hypothesis

References

SUBSTANTIVE

ABER, C., & HAWKINS, J. (1992). Portrayal of nurses in advertisements in medical and nursing journals. *IMAGE: Journal of Nursing Scholarship, 24*(4), 289-293.

ABER, C. S. (1992). Spousal death, a threat to women's health: Paid work as a "resistance resource." *IMAGE: Journal of Nursing Scholarship, 24*(2), 95-99.

BLENNER, J. (1992). Stress and mediators: Patients' perceptions of infertility treatment. *IMAGE: Journal of Nursing Scholarship, 41*(2), 92-97.

CLIFTON, G., BRANSON, P., KELLY, H., DOTSON, L., RECORD, K., & PHILLIPS, B. (1991). Comparison of normal saline and heparin solutions for maintenance of arterial catheter patency. *Heart & Lung, 20*(2), 115-118.

CROSBY, L., WOLL, K., WOOD, K., & PIFALO, W. (1990). Effect of activity on supraventricular tachyarrhythmias after coronary artery bypass surgery. *Heart & Lung, 19*(6), 666-670.

FONTAINE, D. (1989). Measurement of nocturnal sleep patterns in trauma patients. *Heart & Lung, 18*(4), 402-410.

GAYDOS, L. S., & FARNHAM, R. (1988). Human-animal relationships within the context of Rogers' principle of integrality. *Advances in Nursing Science, 10*(4) 72-80.

GUZZETTA, C. (1989). Effects of relaxation and music therapy on patients in a coronary care unit with presumptive acute myocardial infarction. *Heart & Lung, 18*(6), 609-616.

HOLLERBACH, A., & SNEED, N. (1990). Accuracy of radial pulse assessment by length of counting interval. *Heart & Lung, 19*(3), 258-264.

KOLANOWSKI, A. (1990). Restlessness in the elderly: The effect of artificial lighting. *Nursing Research, 39*(3), 181-183.

MARCHETTE, L., MAIN, R., REDICK, E., BAGG, A., & LEATHERLAND, J. (1991). Pain reduction interventions during neonatal circumcision. *Nursing Research, 40*(4), 241-244.

MEININGER, J., STASHINKO, E., & HAYMAN, L. (1991). Type A behavior in Children. Psychometric properties of the Matthews Youth Test for Health. *Nursing Research, 40*(4), 221-227.

METHENY, N., REED, L., WIERSEMA, L., McSWEENEY, M., WEHRLE, M., & CLARK, J. (1993). Effectiveness of pH measurements in predicting feeding tube placement: An update. *Nursing Research, 42*(6), 324-331.

MITCHELL, E., WOODS, N., & LENTZ, M. (1994). Differentiation of women with three perimenstrual symptom patterns. *Nursing Research, 43*(1), 25-30.

OSGUTHORPE, S., TIDWELL, S., RYAN, W., PAULL, D., & SMITH, T. (1990). Evaluation of the patient having cardiac surgery in the postoperative rewarming period. *Heart & Lung, 19*(5), 570-573.

RENTSCHLER, D. (1991). Correlates of successful breastfeeding. *IMAGE: Journal of Nursing Scholarship, 23*(3), 151-154.

SAMAREL, N. (1989). Nursing in a hospital-based hospice unit. *IMAGE: Journal of Nursing Scholarship, 21*(3), 132-136.

SIMPSON, T., ARMSTRONG, S., & MITCHELL, P. (1989). American Association of Critical-Care Nurses Demonstration Project: Patients' recollections of critical care. *Heart & Lung, 19*(4), 325-331.

SPEES, C. (1991). Knowledge of medical terminology among clients and families. *IMAGE: Journal of Nursing Scholarship, 23*(4), 225-229.

TRICE, L. (1990). Meaningful life experience to the elderly. *IMAGE: Journal of Nursing Scholarship, 22*(4), 248-251.

TROUMBLEY, P. F., & LENZ, E. R. (1992). Application of Cox's interaction model of client health behavior in a weight control program for military personnel: A preintervention baseline. *Advances in Nursing Science, 14*(4), 65-78.

WAGNILD, G., & YOUNG, H. (1990). Resilience among older women. *IMAGE: Journal of Nursing Scholarship, 22*(4), 252-255.

WARNER, S., ROSS, M., & CLARK, L. (1988). An analysis of entry into practice arguments. *IMAGE: Journal of Nursing Scholarship, 20*(4), 212-216.

WEINGOURT, R. (1990). Wife rape in a sample of psychiatric patients. *IMAGE: Journal of Nursing Scholarship, 22*(3), 144-147.

WHITNEY, J., STOTTS, N., GOODSON, E., & JANSON-BJERKLIE, S. (1993). The effects of activity and bed rest on tissue oxygen tension, perfusion, and plasma volume. *Nursing Research, 42*(6), 349-355.

WILLIAMSON, J. W. (1992). The effects of ocean sounds on sleep after coronary artery bypass graft surgery. *American Journal of Critical Care, 1*(1), 91-97.

CHAPTER 10

VARIABLES, ASSUMPTIONS, AND LIMITATIONS

LAURA A. TALBOT

Heparin locks are a common sight in acute care facilities. They are used to administer intermittent doses of medications intravenously. How long can a heparin lock be left in place before complications occur? This question was posed by Smith, Hathaway, Goldman, Ng, Brunton, Simor, and Low (1990). To answer this question, they designed a study to focus on the complications associated with the use of a heparin lock over a 7-day period without changing the site. However, before taking even the first step, the researchers needed to specify how they were going to measure the concept of such complications; in other words, they had to identify the specific complications associated with continuous intravenous therapy. These included blocking, leaking, interstitial edema, phlebitis, purulence at the insertion site, and cannula-related septicemia. Now the concept of "complications" had been expressed in terms that could be measured by objective observation and by laboratory cultures of the heparin lock cannulas. When an ab-

stract concept is defined in terms that can be measured, it is called a variable.

VARIABLES

A concept is an abstract idea conjuring a mental image of a phenomenon. Concepts constitute the vocabulary of the theoretical framework, putting us in touch with the properties of the phenomenon under study. The concept is not the phenomenon itself, only the image thought of when the word is mentioned. For example, consider the concept "kiss." One individual might think of the union of two individuals' lips while another may think of a chocolate candy. These are two diverse images of the same concept.

Concepts enable the phenomenon to be described, categorized, interpreted, and structured. When conducting a quantitative research study, the researcher is attempting to describe a phenomenon or find a predictable relationship between two

184

concepts. A predictable relationship exists when changes occur interdependently between the two concepts. For example when X changes, Y also changes in a predictable manner based on the change in X. This predictable change is usually expressed as a value. As we have just seen, a concept is abstract and therefore not measurable in its initial form. Once a concept has been operationalized through its expression in measurable terms, it is called a variable. The nature of a variable is that it can vary in form or measurement. A concept that does not change and has only a single value is called a constant. If the variable has an infinite number of possible values from positive to infinity to negative to infinity, it is called a continuous variable. A discrete variable has a finite number of possible values, which is usually a factor of the instrument used to measure the concept. For example, if you were measuring a patient's temperature, the thermometer is marked in specific increments of degrees. Temperature is a continuous variable, for it has an infinite number of possible values, but when using the thermometer as a measuring device, the degrees on the thermometer provide discrete (degrees) units.

CATEGORIES OF VARIABLES

Since a variable is a quantifiable concept that changes or varies, a researcher may need to manage and assess several different categories of variables. The following discussion will focus on potential categories of research variables in a research study, and an example from the literature will be used as an illustration of each.

Independent and Dependent Variables

When a researcher is looking at a proposed relationship, at least two variables are identified: the independent variable and the dependent variable. In experimental research the independent variable is the presumed "cause" for some "effect" on the dependent variable. The value of examining cause-and-effect relationships is that if the researcher knows the probable cause, the effect can be predicted and controlled.

The independent variable is manipulated by the researcher: it is the intervention or treatment that the researcher performs to see the resulting change in the dependent variable. Conversely, the dependent variable is the outcome variable. The independent variable is the presumed cause for the resulting effect on the dependent variable. This is why a change in the dependent variable's measured value is presumed to be the result of the manipulation of the independent variable.

An example of an independent variable and dependent variable are presented in a randomized trial study by O'Sullivan and Jacobsen (1992). The researchers wanted to evaluate the effectiveness of a health care program focused on first-time adolescent mothers and their infants. A quasi-experimental design was used. "The purpose of the study was to test the effectiveness of a special health care program for adolescent mothers and their infants in preventing second pregnancies, maintaining attendance at clinic so that the infant would have up-to-date immunizations, having adolescent mothers resume their schooling, and reducing the use of the emergency room for routine infant care" (p. 210). In this study the independent variable is the type of health care program, in this case a constant or unchanging variable. The dependent variables are subsequent pregnancies, attendance at the clinic, infant immunizations, return to school, and a reduction in the use of the emergency room. These variables may vary in frequency and occurrence and have readily observable outcomes.

Independent and dependent variables are used in some nonexperimental designs. In nonexperimental research, there is no manipulation of variables. Variables are observed as they occur. If changes in one variable occur when changes in another variable occur, it is presumed that the independent variable had some effect on the dependent variable.

The same is true for correlational studies. If changes in one variable occur when changes in another variable occur, the two variables are considered correlated.

Research Variables

Research variables are the operationalized concepts being examined in the research study. They are the logical groupings of attributes, characteristics, or traits of the phenomenon. These variables should be clearly identified in the research problems and propositions that are to be examined in the study.

In qualitative research, variables are qualified by the terms *qualitative* or *categorical*. These are groupings of common characteristics, qualities, or categories of a phenomenon. Again, they must be quantifiable or qualifiable to be a variable. These variables are clearly delineated in the research question.

In a historical study Olson (1990) wanted "to explore the relationship between the minutes of the alumnae association of a training school for nurses, from 1895 to 1916, and the occupational evolution of nursing" (p. 53). The research question was, "Which set of ideas most accurately describes the occupational evolution of nursing as portrayed in the alumnae minutes of a midwestern training school for nurses?" (p. 54). The research variable under investigation in this study was the "set of ideas." The author defined this variable as professionalization and the work group paradigms. Those associating with the professionalization paradigm "view the apprenticeship system of early nursing education as an unfortunate and repressive part of nursing's past . . ." (p. 54). Historians who operate under the "work group" paradigm "see ordinary nurses as active participants in the 'apprenticeship culture' rather than victims of an unfortunate system of training and work" (p. 54).

In quantitative research, questions are used to guide the research and identify the variables. Research variables are seen in exploratory, descriptive, and some correlational research designs. Miller and Holditch-Davis (1992) studied high-risk preterm infants and their interactions with their parents and with the nurses who cared for them during hospitalization. One research question asked, "How do nurses and parents differ in the level of caregiving involvement and in the amount of interactive behaviors?" (p. 188). The research variables were the level of caregiving involvement and the amount of interactive behaviors. The researcher defined the following levels of caregiving involvement: "contact—touching, holding, or carrying without direct caregiving; routine care—feeding by bottle or gavage, or changing and bathing; low-level nursing care—noninvasive examination such as taking vital signs; and high-level nursing care—respiratory care, needle stick, or procedures that involve more manipulation than a simple examination" (p. 190). Three interactive behaviors of the caregiver were positive "touch, talk, and move" (p. 190). Six behaviors of the infant were "large movement, jitter, startle, hiccup, spit-up or gag, yawn, and negative facial expression" (p. 190).

Extraneous and Intervening Variables

Extraneous variables are uncontrolled variables that influence the findings of the research study. These variables are specific to the type of study design and the data-gathering process used by the researcher. Knowing the type of extraneous variable associated with a particular research design helps the researcher estimate the effects of the independent variable on the dependent variable.

In experimental and quasi-experimental research, extraneous variables are referred to as threats to internal and external validity (Campbell & Stanley, 1963; Cook & Campbell, 1979). For example, in a test-retest research design, the researcher first tests the participants, administers an intervention, then retests the participants. If the same test is used, the participants become familiar with the test and may score higher in subsequent tests even if no intervention is used. In such a case the reseacher must control for test familiarity or wait a designated length of time so the participants will not remember the items in the first testing.

Intervening variables (sometimes called confounding variables) are a type of extraneous variable that cannot be controlled but are innate to the participant in the study and whose effect on the study cannot be measured. Examples of intervening variables are maturation, intelligence, perception, stress, personality, or anxiety. For example, if a researcher does a teaching intervention during the elapsed time between the pretest and the administration of the posttest, the participant will experience increasing maturation. Because of that ongoing developmental process, the participant will become more experienced and possibly wiser. This life experience is an intervening variable. The score on the posttest is representative of both the teaching (independent variable) and the developmental experience (intervening variable). The phenomenon of maturation would be particularly noticeable for re-

search using children as subjects and longitudinal studies.

Another example is in Brown's (1992) metaanalysis of diabetic patient education literature. In reviewing the literature on diabetic patient education research, she found that many researchers did not perform a comparison of learning outcomes between the type I and type II diabetic. Nevertheless, conclusions were drawn concerning diabetics treated with insulin versus those treated with other methods of medical management; those treated with insulin learned more and showed greater metabolic control. The influencing factor may not have been the method of diabetic teaching (independent variable) but the improved metabolic control (intervening variable), which resulted in higher learning scores. Another factor could have been that more type I's were young persons who were more attentive and motivated, whereas interventions for elders (type II's) mandated more difficult behavioral changes such as weight reduction.

Attribute Variables

Attribute variables are variables that cannot be manipulated (Kerlinger, 1986) or influenced by the researcher, yet they may be present or vary in the population under study. Examples are characteristics of the research participants in a study such as gender, age, ethnicity, or height. The participants come to the study with these existing attribute variables. Attribute variables can also be employed in the study design and provide fuel for alternative hypotheses.

Cimprich (1992) used a descriptive study to examine attentional fatigue in women following breast cancer surgery. One of the research questions was focused on the attribute variables of the sample. The research question asked, "What is the relationship between selected variables such as age, educational level, narcotic pain medication, proximity of testing to surgery, and attentional performance following breast cancer surgery?" (p. 200). The attribute variables were age, educational level, narcotic pain medication, and interval (number of days) between research testing and surgery. Age and educational level were clearly attribute variables, but narcotic pain medication and interval between research testing and surgery need more clarification. The type of narcotic pain medication is also an attribute variable because the participants were prescribed either acetominophen/codeine or acetaminophen/oxycodone prior to entry into the study. The medication was not manipulated in the study. The interval between research testing and surgery is also an attribute variable. The participants were recruited into the study the day before their scheduled discharge. The interval was examined retrospectively and not manipulated by the researcher.

OPERATIONALIZING THE CONCEPTS
When operationalizing the concepts several variables may be identified. To start, the researcher reviews the literature to identify uses of the concept in previous research studies and notes how the previous researchers have operationalized the concept(s).

Next the researcher ascertains what the concepts mean in relation to the purpose of the study and its theoretical framework. This process involves examining the abstract theoretical definition of the concept(s) and identifying instances where it exists in concrete settings.

The overall research plan is then examined. This includes taking into consideration the research design, the degree of precision wanted, the level of measurement, and the type of data to be collected.

Variables can be in any type of research study, with various degrees of precision, and at any level of measurement. The researcher needs to determine what type of research design will best answer the overall research question, that is, explanatory, descriptive, correlational, or predictive. Next the degree of precision needed to quantify and qualify the variables of interest is determined.

Using the theoretical definition as a basis, the method of measurement, which can demonstrate the occurrence or presence of the concept, is chosen. To assist in the selection process, the researcher asks, "What means can I use to measure this concept or determine its existence in the real world?" Levels of measurement are discussed in Chapter 14.

Theoretical Definitions
A theoretical definition defines the concepts under study in terms of the theoretical framework; that is, the concepts are defined in abstract terms using other concepts from the theory. To assist the researcher in exploring the concepts, a concept analysis is frequently used to discern the essence of the concept or concepts under study. Concept analysis is the process of extracting the critical attributes of the concept under study to state a precise theory-based definition.

Lauver (1992) explored the influence of "affect," "utility," "norm," and "habit" on seeking medical care for breast cancer symptoms. The researcher theoretically defined the variables under investigation based on the theory of care-seeking behavior. With reference to the care-seeking behavior theory, "*affect* refers to feelings about care seeking, *utility* to beliefs about worth of care seeking, *social norm* to others' beliefs, and *habit* to how one usually acts regarding this behavior. *Facilitating* condi-

STEPS IN OPERATIONALIZING THE CONCEPTS

1. Review the literature to identify uses of the concept in previous research studies. Note how the previous researcher has operationalized the concept(s).
2. Write out what the variables mean in relation to the purpose of the study and theoretical framework.
3. Determine what type of research design will best answer the overall research question, that is, explanatory, descriptive, correlational, or predictive.
4. Ascertain the degree of precision needed to quantify and qualify the variables of interest.
5. Write the operational definition. Be sure to operationally define all of the major variables in the propositions (research question or hypothesis).

tions are objective conditions, such as insurance coverage, that make it easier to seek care" (pp. 236-237).

Operational Definitions

In contrast, operational definitions specify how the concepts will be measured in terms of the research protocol or measurement instrument to be used. Although a theoretical definition is an abstract statement, operational definitions are stated in specific, measurable terms. The definition should be so specific that another researcher replicating the study could reconstruct the measurement techniques in the exact same way, based on the operational definition of the earlier study.

When evaluating research for use in practice, the practitioner needs to examine how the researcher operationalized the concept (see box). A vital question to ask is, "Does the operational definition of the concept fit the way in which I plan to utilize this concept in practice?" The researcher may have been measuring a different facet of the concept, contrary to the way the practitioner is trying to adapt the research.

Miller, Wikoff, and Hiatt (1992) studied the compliance of hypertensive patients with their prescribed medical treatment programs. Five variables were operationalized based on the Fishbein theory of reasoned action: attitudes, perceived beliefs of others, motivation to comply, intentions, and compliance behavior. Attitudes were measured using the Miller Attitude Scale. The perceived beliefs of other significant individuals were measured by the responses given on the Perceived Beliefs of Others Scale. Each patient's intentions, compliance behavior, and motivation to follow prescribed treatment were measured by responses on the Motivation to Comply Scale and the Health Intention Scale.

ASSUMPTIONS

Assumptions are overt and/or innate beliefs held by the researcher about phenomena that are accepted as truths without proof or empirical evidence. They often concern relations between phenomena. There are several types of assumptions: universal, theoretically based, empirically based, and research assumptions.

Universal assumptions are beliefs accepted as universal truths by a majority of the population. These assumptions help us to explain the world around us. One universal assumption is that man is a biopsychosocial, cultural, spiritual being. Many theories build on this universal belief of holistic man, yet this phenomenon is not measurable per se.

Theoretically based assumptions are beliefs associated with a specific theory. To accept the theory, one must accept the underlying assumptions associated with that theory. An example is Dorothea Orem's (1971; 1980) nursing theory of self-care. A vital assumption of her theory asserts that self-care is a necessity for every individual and is a basic human need. Her entire theory builds on this assumption. This assumption is assumed to be true, although it has not been empirically tested. If an individual espouses her theory, this assumption must be accepted as true. If a theory is used as the basis for a research study, the assumptions of the theory also become the assumptions of the research study.

Empirically based assumptions are those derived from previous research studies; they are therefore also considered the most reliable. Lindsay et al. (1991) acknowledged a previously researched assumption based on B. F. Skinner's linear program technique. Skinner's assumption was that linear programmed techniques increase knowledge because they are self-paced and accommodate to individual learning differences. The assumption of increased knowledge with the use of programmed instruction had been tested on patients having warfarin therapy, postthoracic surgery, ischemic heart disease, precoronary artery bypass graft surgery, and prenatal lessons on the care of the newborn. The Lindsay et al. (1991) study focused on using programmed instruction for cardiac rehabilitation in patients following an MI.

Research assumptions are beliefs about the research design itself. For research studies, assumptions are embedded in the theoretical framework, the research methodology, the statistical analysis, and the interpretation of the findings. One assumption related to the research methodology is that the researcher assumes all the participants are going to respond truthfully whether in an interview or on a questionnaire. Another assumption is that the participants will read the questionnaire correctly and answer appropriately. A participant could be unable to read a scale properly. For example, when a response scale interprets a score of 1 to mean "strongly disagree" and 4 to mean "strongly agree," a respondent may interpret the scale incorrectly and reverse the meaning of the responses.

Further, all research studies have assumptions that form the basis of the investigation. These assumptions may simply be implied or explicitly stated in the text of the study. In research journals, assumptions are frequently unstated because of space constraints yet are implied throughout the article. In theses and dissertations, assumptions are expected to be explicitly stated by the researcher. The identification of the assumptions, whether implied or explicit, strengthens the research study. It allows for more rigorous study and objective examination of the phenomenon under study.

LIMITATIONS

When a researcher is investigating a problem, it is impossible to examine every aspect of the phenomenon or to control for every intervening or extraneous variable. Limitations are factors over which the researcher has no control or purposely chooses to disregard because of cost or time involved to modify the limitation. These factors are called extraneous variables. As previously discussed, extraneous variables are threats to internal and external validity.

The researcher thus delineates the limitations of the study, which may subsequently influence the study results, by identifying variables that cannot be modified or controlled.

Hannemann (1994) studied predictors of successful or unsuccessful weaning from short-term mechanical ventilation after cardiac surgery. The researcher discussed one limitation of the study as "the use of clinical instrumentation for research purposes. The lack of assurance that these instruments were operating according to manufacturers' specifications was countered by the desire to study routine bedside measures for clinical decision making" (p. 9). This limitation could potentially influence the study results, yet the researcher felt that using the clinical setting for the study far outweighed the exactness of conducting the study in a controlled laboratory setting.

Limitations restrict the generalizability of the findings and should be considered when the conclusions of a study are dis-cussed and recommendations made for further research. Lindsay et al. (1991) discussed generalizability when a programmed instruction booklet was used to educate post-MI patients on basic information related to cardiac rehabilitation. Limitations were discussed: "Generalization of the study findings are limited because of the demographic characteristics of the study subjects. The sample generally was an affluent and well-educated group who scored relatively high even on the pretest. Consequently, the study results might differ with a more heterogeneous sample" (p. 652).

✎ EVALUATING THE VARIABLES, ASSUMPTIONS, AND LIMITATIONS

When evaluating a research study, key areas to examine are how the researcher operationalizes the variables, states the study's assumptions, and acknowledges the limitations (see box). The reader considers whether the variables are relevant to the re-

EVALUATING THE VARIABLES, ASSUMPTIONS, AND LIMITATIONS

1. Are all research variables identified that are relevant to the research question(s)?
2. Are the research variables consistent with the theoretical/conceptual framework and the review of the literature?
3. Can you identify any/all intervening variables?
4. Are the attribute variables identified as such?
5. Are the variables operationally defined?
6. Are the intervening and extraneous variables defined and controlled for as well as possible within the research design/plan?
7. Which assumptions are implied and which are explicit in the study?
8. Does the researcher sufficiently outline the assumptions associated with the theoretical framework?
9. Are there other implied assumptions associated with the research methodology?
10. What assumptions about the properties of data are also associated with the statistical analysis to be used in the study?
11. Are the assumptions used to temper the interpretation of the findings?
12. Are the limitations fully discussed in the study?
13. Have other limitations that can weaken generalizability not been considered?

search question and if they reflect the study's theoretical/conceptual framework. The review of the literature shows the transition from theoretical concepts to measurable variables operationally defined. In addition, intervening and extraneous variables need to be identified and controlled for within the study's design.

With respect to research assumptions, the evaluator identifies all assumptions, both those that are explicitly stated and those that are implied. The evaluator must then determine which assumptions should be stated in the report and which should be omitted. If an assumption is a basic belief on which the research project is built, it should be stated. In addition, assumptions that are theoretically based, associated with the research methodology, needed for data interpretation, and instrumental to the study's findings, conclusions, and utilization should be explicitly stated. For example, a common assumption in research relating to abuse is that neglect is a form of child abuse. This assumption would affect all of these areas.

Limitations should be fully discussed, especially where they limit the generalizability of the results to other situations and populations. The evaluator should also consider other limitations not discussed in the report that would affect generalizability. For example, the researcher should not generalize results to women if the sample consisted only of men.

SUMMARY

- A concept is an abstract notion based on the theoretical framework of the research study. A variable is a measurable expression of the value of the concept. There are different types of variables in a research study.
  - Independent and dependent variables

are used in research studies that focus on cause-and-effect relationships. The independent variable is the variable manipulated by the researcher. The dependent variable is the outcome variable whose changed value is purported to represent the result of the researcher's manipulation.
  - Research variables are operationalized concepts in research studies in which a single phenomenon is being examined. They are the logical groupings of attributes, characteristics, or traits of the phenomenon.
  - Extraneous variables are uncontrolled variables specific to the phenomena under study, the research design, and the data-gathering process. Intervening variables are innate to the participant and come into play after the intervention, but before the response.
  - Attribute variables are descriptive characteristics of the phenomena under study that cannot be manipulated.
- The researcher operationalizes the variables by examining previous research, the research design, the highest level of measurement attainable, the degree of measurement precision, and the type of data to be collected.
  - The theoretical definition is an abstract description of concepts based on the research theory.
  - The operational definition is the concrete definition of variables that specifies the procedure or instrument to be used to measure the variables.
- The researcher states all assumptions. Assumptions are beliefs accepted as truth without proof. There are several types of assumptions: universal, theoretically based, empirically based, and research assumptions.
- The research limitations are acknowl-

edged. These are factors over which the researcher has no control or chooses to disregard.

FACILITATING CRITICAL THINKING

1. Select a research article from any research journal. Critically evaluate the research, answering the following questions:
   a. Does the research article have an independent and dependent variable?
   b. Does the researcher discuss attribute variables?
   c. What type of research design was used?
   d. Do the variables fit the type of research design?
   e. Are the variables theoretically defined?
   f. How are the variables operationally defined?
2. Identify the extraneous variables in the article. Suggest possible ways to control for these variables.
3. Examine the selected research article for assumptions and limitations. Be sure to answer the following questions.
   a. Does the author discuss assumptions?
   b. Are limitations presented?
   c. Can you identify other implicit or explicit assumptions or limitations to the study?

References

SUBSTANTIVE

BROWN, S. (1992). Meta-analysis of diabetes patient education research: Variations in intervention effects across studies. *Research in Nursing & Health, 15*(6), 409-419.

CIMPRICH, B. (1992). Attentional fatigue following breast cancer surgery. *Research in Nursing & Health, 15*(3), 199-207.

HANNEMAN, S. K. (1994). Multidimensional predictors of success or failure with early weaning from mechanical ventilation after cardiac surgery. *Nursing Research, 43*(1), 4-10.

LAUVER, D. (1992). Psychosocial variables, race, and intention to seek care for breast cancer symptoms. *Nursing Research, 41*(4), 236-241.

LINDSAY, C., JENNRICH, J., & BIEMOLT, M. (1991). Programmed instruction booklet for cardiac rehabilitation teaching. *Heart & Lung, 20*(6), 648-653.

MILLER, D., & HOLDITCH-DAVIS, D. (1992). Interactions of parents and nurses with high-risk preterm infants. *Research in Nursing & Health, 15*(3), 187-197.

MILLER, P., WIKOFF, R., & HIATT, A. (1992). Fishbein's model of reasoned action and compliance behavior of hypertensive patients. *Nursing Research, 41*(2), 104-109.

OLSON, T. (1990). Competing paradigms and the St. Luke's Alumnae Association minutes, 1895-1916. *Advances in Nursing Science, 12*(4), 53-62.

O'SULLIVAN, A., & JACOBSEN, B. (1992). A randomized trial of a health care program for first-time adolescent mothers and their infants. *Nursing Research, 41*(4), 210-215.

SMITH, I., HATHAWAY, M., GOLDMAN, C., NG, J., BRUNTON, J., & SIMOR, A. (1990). A randomized study to determine complications associated with duration of insertion of heparin locks. *Research in Nursing & Health, 13*, 367-373.

CONCEPTUAL

KERLINGER, F. (1986). *Foundations of behavioral research.* New York: Holt, Rinehart & Winston.

HISTORICAL

CAMPBELL, D., & STANLEY, J. (1963). *Experimental and quasi-experimental designs for research.* Chicago: Rand McNally.

COOK, T., & CAMPBELL, D. (1979). *Quasi-experimentation: Design & analysis issues for field settings.* Boston: Houghton Mifflin.

OREM, D. (1971; 1980). *Nursing: Concepts of practice.* New York: McGraw-Hill.

PART III

THE QUANTITATIVE RESEARCH PROCESS

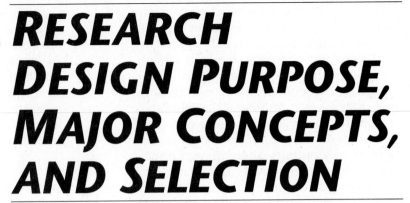

CHAPTER 11

RESEARCH DESIGN PURPOSE, MAJOR CONCEPTS, AND SELECTION

LYNN I. WASSERBAUER • IVO L. ABRAHAM

The research process can be thought of as a circular process that begins and ends with a conceptual issue, or one that evolves from a research question to its empirical answer. Within this circular process, the research design shifts from expressing and reflecting the stated research aims to providing the structure in which to conduct the study. At this point of transition the researcher faces the dual tasks of rationally selecting a research design, often from many options and variants, and subsequently technically implementing this design.

This chapter provides an orientation to the purpose and major concepts of quantitative research available to nurse researchers and offers guidelines for the selection of designs. It is organized in three major parts. First, the purpose of the research design in the research process is described in detail. Second, major concepts that may vary from one research design to

Preparation of this chapter was supported in part by grants from the W. K. Kellogg Foundation, the Pew Charitable Trusts, the National Institute of Mental Health, the DHHS Division of Nursing, and the National Center for Nursing Research.

another are reviewed. The third and final part discusses the issue of validity of research designs, differentiating between four types and levels of validity and describing threats to each of them.

PURPOSE OF THE RESEARCH DESIGN

Within the circular process of research, the research design is established at the point of transition from asking the question to attempting to find an answer to that question. When selecting a research design, the researcher crystallizes what is known to date about a certain phenomenon or set of phenomena, explanations and counterexplanations, as well as possible causes and potential confounds. Yet, at the same time, the research design is the platform from which the researcher explores new knowledge in an effort to better describe and understand phenomena, clarify plausible explanations, and (sometimes) identify potential causative factors.

Thinking of the research design as the transition point from old knowledge to new knowledge implies that the researcher must carefully choose a research design, argue and defend its choice rationally, and recognize the consequences of choosing one design over another. Unfortunately perhaps for the beginning researcher, there are no rules of thumb for selecting research designs, only options, alternatives, implications, and consequences. Fortunately for the advanced researcher, the multitude of research designs available, with their various advantages and disadvantages, offers scientific opportunities to tailor the methodology of a study to the conceptual issues at hand. Indeed, the great variety of research designs permits researchers to conduct studies in which the research questions, not the methods used to find answers to the research questions, are the focal point of attention.

The choice of an appropriate research design, then, is a matter of examining how it will optimize exploration, discovery, and explanation. Certainly, selecting a research design is not a matter of choosing the more sophisticated over the less complex ones, or the more fashionable over the less common ones—errors often made by researchers who believe that the credibility of their research is determined by complexity and sophistication of methodology, not by the conceptual issues it attempts to address.

The research design provides the backbone structure of a study. It determines how the study will be organized, when data will be collected, and when interventions, if any, are to be implemented. The research design is also a statement of commitment by the researcher to:

- Organize a study in a certain way, defending the advantages of doing so while being aware of and cautious about the potential disadvantages;
- Maximize objectivity in study protocol implementation and data collection; and
- Use generally accepted methods of inquiry that safeguard researchers from drawing incorrect inferences and conclusions from their investigations.

✍ MAJOR CONCEPTS

To fully appreciate the principles of research design, several concepts must first be understood. These are summarized in the box on p. 199 and discussed below.

MANIPULATION

Manipulation means that, within the specification of a given research design, the researcher actively initiates, implements, and terminates procedures. In most instances manipulation is linked to the independent variable(s) under consideration. Essential to manipulation is that the researcher has complete control over the process. The researcher decides what is to be manipulated (e.g., selected nursing intervention protocols), to whom the manipulation applies (e.g., samples and subsamples of subjects), when the manipulation is to occur according to the specification of the research design, and how the manipulation is to be implemented.

For instance, Abraham, Neundorfer, and Currie (1992) reported a quasi-experimental study in which nursing home residents with mild to moderate cognitive impairment participated in one of three cognitively oriented group interventions of 24-weeks' duration: cognitive-behavioral group therapy, focused visual imagery group therapy, and educational discussion groups (a comparison group). In this study,

---

CONCEPTS TO CONSIDER WHEN DESIGNING A RESEARCH STUDY

Manipulation. What is actively directed or managed by the researcher.

Control. The extent to which the researcher can manage extraneous sources that might affect a study and lead to incorrect scientific conclusions.

Random selection. Randomly drawing research subjects from the target population.

Random assignment. Allocating subjects to treatment and control conditions in a non-systematic way, using a method that is known to be random.

Probability. The likelihood that research findings are low in uncertainty and error or are trustworthy and believable.

Bias. The difference between the true and the observed.

Causality. Determining the cause-and-effect relationship(s) that exist between variables.

---

manipulation was expressed in many forms. The fact that three different interventions were developed and applied to three different subject groups implies manipulation. The protocols of the interventions were clearly specified, both in terms of content, adaptation of generic therapeutic principles to a frail and impaired nursing home population, and timing within the 24 weeks of intervention (Abraham, Niles, Thiel, Siarkowski, & Cowling, 1991). The decision to have the interventions last 24 weeks (as opposed to the usual 8 to 12 weeks) was an active decision based on clinical considerations about group work with the elderly.

CONTROL

Manipulation implies—*and* is impossible without—researcher control over extraneous sources that might affect a study, sometimes positively but most often negatively, and might lead to incorrect scientific conclusions. Control aims "to rule our threats to valid inference." It also adds precision, the "ability to detect true effects of smaller magnitude" (Cook & Campbell, 1979, p. 8). Unlike laboratory studies, where total control is often possible, control is a relative matter in clinical research. The researcher is responsible for ensuring as much control over extraneous forces as possible. For instance, in the Abraham, Neundorfer, and Currie (1992) study, group sessions were conducted in quiet locations in each nursing home, in an attempt to exert control over possible distracting sounds. Subjects also had to meet specific sampling criteria about minimal levels of vision, hearing, and comprehension to participate in group activities, to avoid the possibility that some subjects might not benefit because of severe sensory or comprehension impairment.

Control also pertains to "the ability to determine which units receive a particular treatment at a particular time" (Cook and Campbell, 1979, p. 8). This can be interpreted incorrectly as the researcher having control over the *decisions* about which subjects receive a given treatment at a specified time. The correct interpretation has to do with the researcher having control over the *processes* that determine who gets what at what time. Two processes can be identified. The first process refers to the researcher's use of random methods to assign subjects to treatments. As we will see, this is one of the most preferred methods of exerting control over subjects and their treatment as, theoretically, it ensures that known *and* unkown extraneous forces inherent to subjects are dispersed equally across the different treatment options. This may not always be possible, in which case the second process comes into play—that of structuring the assignment process in such a way that major, known extraneous forces are controlled. For example, a researcher studying various protocols of discharge planning and follow-up of low-birthweight infants may choose to randomly assign infants to various protocols. However, if the researcher is concerned that such factors as socioeconomic status or the availability of additional caretakers beyond the mother (e.g., father, grandparent) may affect infants' health and well-being, the researcher may want to control for such factors. One approach might be to ensure that, within each treatment group, there is approximately even representation of these variables in each of the treatment groups (this is achieved by using a method called *blocking,* which is discussed in Chapter 12 as *block design).*

Another example of ensuring active control over known extraneous forces is *matching,* a weaker but very common method of control. In matching, the researcher identifies one or more (usually up to three) extraneous variables to be controlled. As soon as a subject is recuited for one of the treatment groups, the researcher tries to find a subject for the other group(s) identical to the first subject on the specific matching variables. For instance, if age and gender are the matching variables of interest in a two-group study, and a 75-year-old male is recruited for the first group, the researcher would try to find another 75-year-old male to be included in the second group.

The use of *counterbalancing* is another way to exert active control over extraneous forces. Counterbalancing is used in studies in which the researcher is concerned that the order in which treatments are administered influences the results. With counterbalancing, all subjects receive all treatments; however, the order of administration of treatment is varied. Varying the order of treatments allows the researcher to determine more effectively the way in which differential responses are influenced by the order of treatment administration. For example, counterbalancing can be used to study the effects of several different relaxation techniques by varying the order in which they are administered to subjects. Subject 1 might receive guided imagery, listening to a relaxation tape, and then self-hypnosis, while subject 2 received self-hypnosis, relaxation tape, then guided imagery. Note that these approaches to controlling the influence of extraneous sources are all integral parts of the design. The researcher can also exert control statistically and independently of the design. Various statistical methods for controlling the influence of one or more variables have been proposed. The beginning researcher in particular might benefit from appropriate statistical consultation.

RANDOMIZATION

A major concept, randomization entails two separate processes: random selection of subjects from the population and random assignment of subjects to treatment and control conditions. In both processes, randomization provides a way to ensure that characteristics of subjects are dispersed across sample and/or subsamples in a non-systematic fashion. This way, if any of these characteristics has extraneous or confounding effects, the likelihood of such effect occurring is dispersed in a probabilistically equal way. As Cook and Campbell (1979) point out, "formally speaking, the most representative samples will be those that are randomly chosen from the population, and it is possible for these randomly selected units to be randomly assigned to various . . . groups" (p. 75). Random selection is virtually nonexistent in nursing research; moreover, a large proportion, 55.3%, of nursing intervention studies do not use random assignment methods (Abraham, Chalifoux, & Evers, 1992).

Random Selection

Random selection refers to the process of randomly drawing research subjects from the target population, about which the researcher wants to gain knowledge and to which the researcher hopes to generalize the findings of a study. Unless the population is defined very narrowly and all its members are known and potentially recruitable, *or* one has quasi-unlimited funds and time for implementing large and complex sampling schemes, random selection of a sample from a population is seldom possible in nursing and health research. Instead, the researchers has to forgo the relative objectivity of probabilistic sampling methods in favor of the potential shortcomings of nonprobabilistic methods of recruiting subjects.

At issue, truly, is the representativeness of the sample relative to the characteristics of the population it is intended to exemplify. If random methods of drawing a sample from its reference population cannot be implemented, the researcher has to defend the representativeness of the sample. An effective way of doing this is to demonstrate statistically how the sample compares favorably to known, critical parameters of the reference population. For instance, with reasonable margins of cost and feasibility, it was impossible for Abraham, Neundorfer, and Currie (1992) to draw their study sample from all nursing home residents in the United States or all nursing homes in a smaller geographic area. In addition, not every nursing home is necessarily interested in participating in a complex, longitudinal intervention study. As there is a specific pattern of gender distribution in nursing homes in the United States, these researchers had to demonstrate that the gender mix of their study sample corresponded to the gender mix typical in American long-term care (Abraham, Neundorfer, Cowling, & Sutorius, 1990).

Sometimes critical parameters might not be known, or are known with less certainty than, for instance, the mix of men and women in nursing homes. In these situations, the argument of representativeness has to be a logical, conceptual one, in which a cogent case is made that the sample may indeed be similar to, and representative of, the target population. In recent years, for instance, increasing attention has been given to the health needs of rural populations (Midwest, South, Northeast, Northwest), especially the rural elderly. Initially, there was a tendency to consider all rural elderly the same, without attention to regional differences in demography, epidemiology, topography, economic infrastructure, and health and human services infrastructure (Abraham & Neese, 1993; Abraham, Buckwalter, Snustad, Smullen, Thompson-Heisterman, Neese, & Smith, 1993; Buckwalter, Abraham, Smith, & Smullen, 1993). In addition, it has become increasingly evident that race (white, black, Latino, native, Asian) determines health needs and health care utilization and that within certain races, important subgroups of rural elderly populations can be identified: coastal versus plateau versus Appalachian blacks; white Appalachians of Scottish-English descent, to name a few (Abraham, Buckwalter, Neese, & Fox, 1994). Thus findings from studies in one region or with subpopulations will not be generalizable to rural elderly at large. This example also shows that effectively arguing the representativeness of a sample is determined by the clarity with which the researcher defines the population—a narrow definition may be more helpful than a broader one.

Random Assignment
Random assignment entails allocating sampling units (e.g., patients) to treatment and control conditions in a nonsystematic way, using a decision method that is known to be random (e.g., coin toss, random drawing, use of random tables, computer-generated random sequences of options). Theoretically, random assignment is intended to ensure that, on the average, subjects in one condition are similar to those in other conditions—and that thus the influence of potential extraneous and confounding sources of variability is dispersed across subsamples. In a randomized trial to test the effectiveness of a health care program, O'Sullivan and Jacobsen (1992) utilized random assignment to allocate 243 subjects to a treatment group and a control group. The treatment group received well-baby care and extra care, while the control group received routine well-baby care.

Random assignment of subjects themselves may not always be possible. Abraham, Neundorfer, and Currie (1992), for instance, had to use seven nursing homes to attain a sample size that was sufficiently powerful. The numbers of subjects generated by each nursing home were not

enough to implement each of the three interventions in each nursing home (Abraham et al., 1990). To achieve some random assignment, nursing homes were randomly assigned to the interventions. Although this method was suboptimal, it allowed at least some degree of random assignment.

PROBABILITY
Because research is most often conducted under suboptimal conditions, there is a degree of uncertainty and thus error about any findings that may come from it. In research and statistics, this uncertainty and error are translated into likelihoods or probabilities: the likelihood that findings are unjustified and incorrect, expressed as a probability between 1.00 (completely erroneous finding) and 0.00 (completely exact finding). Uncertainty and error also reflect the "trustworthiness" and "believability" of research findings. We want findings that are low in uncertainty and error and thus are trustworthy and believable. In turn, it will also be easier to convince others that findings can be generalized beyond the study sample, even if random selection of the sample from the population did not occur.

Probability is the language of certainty and uncertainty, accuracy and error, trust and distrust, belief and disbelief in research data. In research, the aim is to pursue findings with a high probability of certainty, accuracy, trust, and belief. This can take either one of two forms. For instance, in studies testing the effectiveness of nursing interventions, we want to be able to conclude with high certainty that a given intervention indeed generates the hypothesized changes in health status among patients. Or, likewise, we want to be sure that, if the interventions prove to be ineffective, we can be reasonably assured of this as well. In other words, whether the interventions are effective or not, we want to be certain.

Researchers use probability to convey their confidence in findings. The most common form is to use an error margin that is deemed acceptable. The allowable margin of error is determined by the nature of the phenomenon under investigation. Nursing research has tended to follow the behavioral, social, and biomedical sciences and has taken a 5% error margin (usually expressed as an α of 0.05) as the maximum error margin. However, often a 1% ($\alpha = 0.01$) or 0.1% ($\alpha = 0.001$) margin might be more appropriate. To put the issue of margin of error in perspective, values such as the ones discussed here would be unacceptable in certain fields of engineering. A bridge engineer cannot accept a 5% construction error. The bridge engineer, then, works with margin errors that are infinitely small.

One may wonder why research findings should be expressed probabilistically at all. Why can we not express findings as they present themselves, in absolute values (e.g., two postoperative complications; a depression score of 23) without the constraints of a probabilistic context? Why can't we believe the statistics as they are, just as much as we believe the statistics of a baseball player ("He's hitting only 0.221 this season")? In fact, the baseball situation not only underscores the need for a margin of error, but also it is an incorrect application of probability. First, is 0.221 really 0.221, or might it not be 0.219 or 0.223, or an even wider deviation from the known 0.221? Second, hitting statistics are a performance ratio of a numerator (base hits) to a denominator (at bats) and are expressed as a value from 0.000 to 1.000. Implicitly, it assumes that every baseball player is perfect and will

only hit the ball and make it to base because of his technical ability, regardless of how the pitch is thrown, of atmospheric conditions such as a strong side wind, of distraction noise from the audience, and so on. However, these and many other known and unknown factors create an environment of uncertainty and do not make all things equal at any point. In addition, there is also a perhaps small but nonetheless real likelihood that, just by mere chance, the trajectory of the bat will intersect with the trajectory of the ball. Or, to put the example in reverse, if the second author of this chapter—who, growing up in Europe, never played baseball and whose experience is limited to playing with his small son in the backyard—would step up to home plate at a major league stadium, there would be a finite (but admittedly extremely small) chance that, after many pitches and many relief pitchers, it would so happen that his bat is swung in a (random) way that just happens to intersect, at the right time and place, with an oncoming ball. For every professional baseball player of whatever ability, then, there is theoretically always a probability that some of his base hits are due (mostly) to chance and not to skill.

Now that we understand the concepts of uncertainty, error, and probability, we can make the link to randomness. With randomness is understood the likelihood that an event occurs without understanding of factors and determinants. This randomness, again, is expressed probabilistically, and a process that has a random component to it—full or part—is called a probabilistic process. Specific to this type of process is that there are unknown factors that we have not been able to clarify, describe, and causally link to antecedents and consequences. Scientific studies are about probabilistic processes: no matter how well our study is designed, there are always additional, unknown factors that affect the independent and dependent variables. These factors, which may be related to individual differences among subjects as well as factors in the environment, create variability among our study subjects—and thus uncertainty in the results.

Probabilistic processes stand in contrast to *deterministic* processes. The latter are processes about which all determinants and their relative impacts are known. Take gravity, for instance. Newton's proverbial apple has been studied so extensively that the course, speed, and impact of its fall can be described faultlessly, and we can predict the same for other apples, given, of course, that we know the weight, height, biological composition of the apple, relevant atmospheric conditions, and soil and surface characteristics, among others. Deterministic processes are devoid of randomness: everything has been discovered, identified, and quantified.

An implication of this difference between probabilistic and deterministic processes is that, through extensive study, a phenomenon might progress from the former to the latter. We can even extend this to so-called random processes, which are probabilistic processes about which we believe we do not know anything. We use random processes, for instance, to make random assignments to treatment conditions. A common method is the coin toss with an evenly weighted and unbiased coin. Persi Diaconis, one of the greatest contemporary statisticians but also one of the greatest magicians, has combined his dual skills to demonstrate that randomness is only a matter of not having fully discovered, identified, and quanitified many of the processes involved in the presumably random act of tossing a coin and obtaining

either heads or tails. Asking his audience what result they would like, he is able to toss an unbiased coin time after time and obtain the same result over and over—just because he knows exactly the correct angle of the launch position of the coin from his hand, force to be applied, rotations to be allowed, and so on.

It is unlikely that scientific knowledge in nursing will move from the probabilistic to the deterministic. However, as investigations build on one another and studies grow from tentative explorations to tightly controlled and empirical knowledge within which the discipline progresses, we might see a gradual narrowing of the error margin associated with nursing knowledge.

BIAS

Bias refers to the difference between what we observe about a phenomenon and the phenomenon itself as it exists. Unfortunately, the true is never known; research can only give us observations. There are many potential scores of bias that researchers must be aware of and that will be discussed more fully later in this chapter as threats to validity. It is important to remember that all bias cannot be eliminated, but it can be minimized. The task is to design studies in such a way that observations are as accurate as possible and thus minimize bias. Strategies include adequately conceptualizing constructs of interest and appropriately turning them into variables; selecting designs with minimal threats to validity; using valid, reliable, and sensitive measurement methods; and applying statistical methods that maximize quantitative yield and conceptual relevance.

Many techniques are used to minimize bias. However, the use of blinding warrants more discussion. *Blinding* is one common technique that, if used correctly, can minimize many potential sources of bias. In blinding, subjects are unaware of the study hypotheses or the specific details of the treatment they receive until the completion of the study. For example, elderly adults may be enrolled in a research study designed to test the hypotheses that participation in an exercise program will increase socialization and decrease isolation and depression. Prior knowledge of these hypotheses could influence the behavior and responses of participants. Therefore, to reduce the threat of bias, subjects remain blind to the hypotheses until the data are collected.

In some situations it may not be possible to blind subjects to a study's hypotheses, but it may be possible to blind subjects to the specific intervention or treatment they receive. Drug trials frequently use this kind of blinding when participants with a specific illness seek treatment and know the type of study they are enrolled in. In a blinded drug trial all subjects receive a treatment; however some participants receive the drug under investigation and others receive a placebo. When both the subjects as well as the person(s) collecting and/or analyzing the data are blind to the study hypotheses or treatments, *double-blinding* is used.

CAUSALITY

It is beyond the scope of this chapter to review the major philosophical perspectives on causality, nor is this necessary to underscore the importance of causal thinking in nursing research. (We refer the interested reader to such sources as Cook and Campbell, 1979; Kourany, 1987; Polkinghorne, 1983; and Reynolds, 1971.) Rather, we choose to adopt the perspective of Cook and Campbell (1979), who are less interested in finding out what causes a certain result all of the time and are more interested in determining what things lead to a

certain result most of the time. In this perspective, we recognize some of the major concepts discussed: manipulation and control; uncertainty, error, and probability; and bias. This perspective distances itself from the traditional approach to causality, in which one attempts to unambiguously pinpoint cause, effect, and causal process. Pinpointing these three elements imposes on the researcher three separate scientific tasks of proof:

- Proving that one or more hypothesized causes are indeed unquestionably and verifiably the cause(s) of something else, and that there are no other possible causes (again, unquestionably and verifiably).
- Proving that one or more observable effects indeed occur in association with the hypothesized cause(s).
- Proving that there is an identifiable process that causally links the hypothesized cause(s) with the observed effect(s).

To do this for any phenomenon of interest to nursing would be a monumental task. In much of nursing research, rather than attempting to empirically prove cause, effect, and empirical processes it may be more prudent to focus on the conceptualization and operationalization of both hypothesized causes and effects. Studies in which causes and effects are conceptualized and operationalized well, and in which both are argued convincingly, do not need empirical proof of the adequacy and appropriateness of causes and effects. Rather, the emphasis should be on repeatedly underscoring the causal link between cause and effect across the same and similar situations. Thus the issue of causality is one of repeated observation in which conceptually defensible (yet still hypothesized) causes, through manipulation, produce conceptually defensible outcomes consistently in the same situation (and perhaps in similar situations). They produce these outcomes perhaps not always and perhaps with some error—but certainly most of the time with minimal variability.

The causal perspective of Cook and Campbell (1979) adopted here certainly does not provide the researcher with "tight and unyielding" conclusions. Then, again, we already discussed that all scientific knowledge is probabilistic and tentative by nature. The goal of nursing research, and with it the goal of selecting and implementing research designs, should be focused, therefore, on demonstrating that manipulation of putative causes consistently, but not necessarily always, produces certain results, whether anticipated or not. This is a dual call to reject a traditionalist perspective on causality for a pragmatic approach to conceptualization, manipulation, observation, and interpretation; and to adopt a probabilistic view of change as something that, across replications, will withstand alternative explanations.

❧ SELECTION FACTORS

In this section, we review four types of validity of research designs and potential threats to each (see also Cook & Campbell, 1979). *Statistical conclusion validity* addresses the extent to which, at the mathematical/statistical level, covariation is present between the independent and dependent variables; that is, the extent to which a relationship exists between the independent and dependent variables. *Internal validity* refers to whether an observed relationship between variables is indeed causal; or in the absence of a relationship whether there is no real causal link. *Construct validity of putative causes and effects* asks whether the causal relationship between two variables is indeed *"the one"* and tries to refute the possibility that a confounding variable may explain the presumed causal relationship. *External validity* refers to the generalizability of an observed causal relationship "across alternate measures of the cause and effect and across different types of persons, settings, and times" (Cook & Campbell, 1979, p. 37). Validity of any type is not a yes/no issue of whether or not it is present. Rather, it is a matter of degree, determined by the extent to which the researcher has tried to cope with the various potential threats to each type of validity. The four types of validity are summarized in Table 11-1.

There is a clear hierarchy among these four levels of validity, with no level of validity except the first being possible without first reasonably ensuring that the previous level has been sufficiently attained. Statistical conclusion validity is necessary for internal validity to be considered. If, by means of appropriately selected measurement and analysis procedures, we cannot show within a reasonable margin of statistical error that covariation between variables does or does not exist, there is neither ground for, nor use in, exploring the nature of the relationship and whether extraneous influences may have influenced the emergence (or nonemergence) of the association. In turn, without sufficient internal validity, we cannot examine whether the presumed independent and dependent variables are indeed representations of the higher theoretical constructs of interest. Finally, only after sufficiently ensuring statistical conclusion, internal, and construct validity of a given design, are we in a position to examine the generalizability or external

Table 11-1
Threats to Validity of Research Designs

Statistical Conclusion Validity	Internal Validity	Construct Validity	External Validity
Low statistical power	History	Inadequate preoperational explication of constructs	Hawthorne effect
Violated assumptions of statistical tests	Maturation	Mono-operational bias	Rosenthal effect
Fishing and the error rate problem	Testing	Mono-method bias	Testing
Low reliability of measures	Instrumentation	Hypothesis-guessing within experimental conditions	Novelty
Low reliability of treatment implementation	Statistical regression	Evaluation apprehension	Selection
Random irrelevancies in the experimental setting	Selection	Experimenter expectancies	Setting
Random heterogeneity of respondents	Mortality	Confounding constructs and levels of constructs	History
	Interactions with selection	Interaction of different treatments	
	Lack of clarity in direction of causality	Interaction of testing and treatment	
	Diffusion of experimental conditions	Restricted generalizability across constructs	
	Compensating equalization of treatments		
	Compensatory rivalry		
	Demoralization of controls		

Based on Cook, T. C., & Campbell, D. T. (1979). *Quasi-experimentation: Design & analysis issues for field settings.* Boston: Houghton Mifflin.

validity of a research design and the findings generated by it.

THREATS TO STATISTICAL CONCLUSION VALIDITY

This first level of validity seeks to establish three indications of credibility for a study; statistical power available to detect covariation, adequacy of the empirical evidence to infer covariation, and the strength of this covariation. Several threats to statistical conclusion validity have been identified (Cook & Campbell, 1979).

Low Statistical Power
This threat occurs when either sample sizes are too small, the allowable margin of error

too high, and/or the statistical test chosen too weak and inadequate.

Violated Assumptions of Statistical Tests
Statistical tests are governed by assumptions that must be met for the test to be appropriately applied and adequately executed. Violating assumptions may lead to inaccurate statistical results and consequently to incorrect inferences about the presence or absence of covariation.

Fishing and the Error Rate Problem
When we adopt a certain error level (say, an α of 0.05), this only applies to the execution of *one* statistical test. It has been shown that conducting multiple tests

within the same study inflates the α error beyond its original limits according to the following equation:

$$\alpha_{inflated} = 1 - [\Pi(1 - \alpha_i)]$$

where $\alpha_{inflated}$ refers to the α error rate due to multiple statistical testing, to serial multiplication of the elements defined in the argument, and α_i to the chosen α error rate. Application of this equation to, for instance, a study involving five statistical tests at an original α error rate of 0.05 reveals that the true error rate for this study would be:

$$\alpha_{inflated} = 1 - (0.95 \times 0.95 \times 0.95 \times 0.95 \times 0.95) = 1 - 0.774 = 0.226.$$

Reducing the original error rate to 0.01 would bring the α error rate down to:

$$\alpha_{inflated} = 1 - (0.99 \times 0.99 \times 0.99 \times 0.99 \times 0.99) = 1 - 0.951 = 0.49.$$

Low Reliability of Measures
This threat occurs when the researcher uses measurement instruments with low reliability and thus poor accuracy and consistency. Unreliable measures cannot be expected to detect covariation when there is covariation. They may lead us to conclude there is no covariation, which in turn leaves two questions unanswered: Is covariation present? Or, on the other hand, may covariation perhaps be absent? Neither question can be answered without reliable measures, and in both situations statistical conclusion validity is compromised.

Low Reliability of Treatment Implementation
When treatments are not implemented according to tightly standardized protocols, the variability in treatments will cause variability in subjects' responses. In turn, this

will make it difficult to detect change if it is present and to determine that there is no change if it is not present.

Random Irrelevancies in the Experimental Setting
This refers to extraneous factors in the experimental setting that co-occur with the implementation of treatment protocols. As with the previous threat, these factors may cause variability and impair statistical conclusion validity. If it is impossible to control the extraneous factors the researcher should try to determine which variables affect all subjects and incorporate them as factors in the data analysis.

Random Heterogeneity of Respondents
It may happen that participants in a study may differ from one another on variables that, known of unknown, affect their responses to treatments. This, in turn, may cause variability and thus affect the accuracy of statistical inferences drawn from the sample.

THREATS TO INTERNAL VALIDITY
The second type of validity that must be considered is internal validity. Internal validity is the degree to which the outcome can be attributed to the experimental treatment, not to extraneous factors. In essence it involves making a determination about how credibly the researcher can claim that the experimental treatment caused the observed effect. Cook and Campbell (1979) provide a comprehensive discussion of the threats to internal validity. Several of these threats will be described in greater detail.

History
History refers not to what subjects bring to the treatment setting but to what may occur between a pretest and posttest that

may affect the outcome of the treatment. Extraneous events are not as problematic in settings in which the researcher has greater control over the experimental environment, such as in a laboratory. However, in most instances social scientists, including nurse researchers, must be aware that events during the time of the experimental treatment can alter results.

Maturation

When research is conducted over time, it is possible that subjects themselves can change, and these changes can affect treatment results. Maturation may be a threat when subjects manifest changes that are not related to the experimental treatment. These changes may include physical growth, mastering new developmental skills, intellectual maturity, and normal healing following an injury or illness. In general, the longer the treatment, the harder it will be to rule out the effects of maturation.

Testing

One of the difficulties inherent in research that utilizes a pretest-posttest design is the effect of testing. If the same or similar test is given at both intervals, posttest results may be influenced by subjects being familiar with the format of the test. The more frequently a test is administered, the greater will be the influence of testing.

Instrumentation

Threats to internal validity as the result of instrumentation occur when the instrument used to record measurements changes over time. These changes can occur when humans are the instrument, when physical equipment is used, or when measuring scales are utilized. Human observers can gain experience and become more proficient in their observations or interviewing skills. Equipment can record inaccurate readings, and with repeated use equipment may need to be recalibrated to maintain accuracy of measurement. Measuring scales that change sensitivity along the instrument is another way instrumentation may affect validity.

Statistical Regression

Statistical regression toward the mean occurs as the result of testing. At any given test administration some individuals may do better than expected, and others may do much worse than expected. Research subjects, like the rest of the population, can have good or bad days, and this may affect their test scores. If subjects are retested, those who initially did very well will tend to do worse, and those who did poorly will tend to improve their scores. Thus scores will move toward the mean or average score.

Selection

Selection becomes a problem when differences exist in the way subjects are recruited for a study and assigned to groups. Unless subjects in each group can be shown to be similar before the treatment, the researcher will have difficulty attributing causality to the experimental treatment. As much as possible the researcher should take steps to ensure that the subjects in all treatment groups are as similar as possible. Random selection and assignment will decrease the potential for selection to be a threat to validity.

Mortality

In almost any research involving human subjects it is expected that some individuals will drop prematurely. When this occurs the researcher must attempt to determine why subjects have withdrawn from the study and if subjects from one group have dropped out at a disproportionate rate. If one group loses more subjects than another, the treatment groups may no longer be equivalent and a selection bias may then exist.

Interactions with Selection
Selection can interact with history, maturation, and instrumentation to produce additional threats to internal validity. Selection history, like the effect of history, occurs when events happen between the pretest and the posttest that influence the outcomes. However, in selection history the events are local, and not all treatment groups are affected. This is most problematic when groups are geographically separated or when a treatment is administered to groups after a significant time. In selection maturation, subjects within treatment groups mature at different rates, making it difficult to determine the extent to which the treatment effect is observed. Selection instrumentation results when treatment groups score differently on a measuring scale that changes sensitivity along the instrument.

Lack of Clarity in Direction of Causality
When the researcher is attempting to establish causality, situations may arise in which it is impossible to determine the direction of the causal relationship. For instance, consider this question: Does a diet rich in beta carotene lower the risk of heart disease, or do people with a low risk of heart disease eat foods rich in beta carotene? Correlational studies where one event does not clearly precede the other in time are most susceptible to this threat. Correlation studies are generally not used in isolation to establish the direction of causality because in most instances a correlation study only indicates that an association exists between two variables.

Diffusion of Experimental Conditions
Diffusion of experimental conditions becomes a threat to validity when the control group gains knowledge of the experimental intervention. This can occur when groups have contact with one another and when the control group gains access to information that was intended for the treatment group. This may occur if the treatment and control groups are in close proximity. Contact between subjects in different groups may occur if they share a waiting area or a hospital unit or are part of a common social group. When the control group becomes aware of the treatment and inadvertently receives it, it will be impossible to determine what effect the experimental treatment had. Whenever possible, the researcher should prevent contact between the treatment and control groups.

Compensation Equalization of Treatments
This threat also produces a situation in which the control and treatment groups receive essentially the same experimental treatment. However, compensating equalization of treatments occurs when the researcher is unable to restrict the access the control groups have to components of the experimental intervention. This may happen in situations where the researcher provides a beneficial treatment and thus is unable, for ethical or political reasons, to limit this intervention to the treatment group.

Compensatory Rivalry
There are times when both the treatment and control groups are aware of the experimental treatment. Compensatory rivalry is frequently a problem in studies that involve groups of people (hospital unit staff, hospital divisions) who perceive (accurately

or erroneously) that the outcome of the study will affect them negatively. In these instances compensatory rivalry may result if the control group thinks that what they receive is inferior to the treatment other groups receive. A rivalry is established between the groups and the control group may actually begin to compete with subjects in the treatment groups and do better than expected. This may mask the effects of the experimental treatment.

Demoralization of Controls

Demoralization of controls is the opposite reaction of compensatory rivalry. As with compensatory rivalry, both treatment and control groups are aware of the experimental treatment and the control group perceives that what they receive is inferior to what the treatment groups receive. However, with demoralization of controls members of the control group become less motivated and do worse than anticipated. When this happens, the differences between the treatment and control groups will be inflated, and the treatment may appear more effective than it actually is. Demoralization also frequently involves groups of subjects on different hospital units. For example, units of hospitalized psychiatric patients in which the control unit receives only group therapy while the treatment groups receive individual and/or family therapy in addition to group therapy. The control group may respond to these differences by sabotaging their treatment or by acting out against the staff.

THREATS TO CONSTRUCT VALIDITY OF PUTATIVE CAUSES AND EFFECTS

This type of validity of research designs is concerned with the "confounding" of the presumed causal relationship between two variables. Specifically, it examines whether the effects noted on the dependent variable(s) are indeed due to the proposed independent variable(s); or whether known or unknown confounding, independent variables may be held responsible, in total or in part, for the observed effects. Conceptually, evaluating the construct validity of causes and effects involves assessing whether the independent and dependent variables, respectively, are appropriate representations of the theoretical constructs of interest. Operationally, it entails examining whether different versions of the same manipulations and measures *converge* (i.e., are they manipulating and measuring the same thing), as well as whether different versions of different manipulations and measures *diverge* (i.e., are they manipulating and measuring discrete things).

Inadequate Preoperational Explication of Constructs

If we think through and define the constructs of interest poorly, the ensuing process of conceptualization and operationalization is irrevocably compromised. This situation can be likened to doing a study when you do not know what you are really studying.

Mono-Operation Bias

Many studies include only one operationalization of the independent variable(s) and/or only one measure for each dependent variable. This may lead to an underrepresentation of the constructs of interest.

Mono-Method Bias

Similarly, many studies include only one possible treatment protocol for each level of the independent variable and/or only one method or strategy of measurement for each dependent variable. Again, the constructs of interest may end up being underrepresented and inadequately captured.

Hypothesis Guessing within Experimental Conditions

Hypothesis guessing pertains to the situation in which participants are able to figure out the hypothesis under investigation and thus the effects the investigators hope to achieve. Subjects may attempt to respond or alter their behavior to reflect what they think the research wants or expects to hear or see. This introduces bias and can alter the results of the study.

Evaluation Apprehension

Some people just do not like to be evaluated or only want to be evaluated in a positive manner. Evaluation apprehension may cause them to "clam up," which may hinder data collection, or they may withhold or underreport information thought to be negative or controversial, such as a history of drug or alcohol abuse. Subjects may also exaggerate or overreport information that is thought to be positive or socially acceptable, such as compliance with medications or adherence to treatments.

Experimenter Expectancies

It may happen that the expectations of the experimenter bias the researcher and interfere with data collection. In other words, researchers can find exactly what they are looking for. This threat can be especially problematic in studies in which the person collecting the data is aware of the study hypotheses. Researchers can inadvertently influence subjects, and willingly or unwillingly, subjects act and respond according to what hypotheses the researcher wants to prove or disprove. The use of double-blinding will help to reduce the effect of this threat.

Confounding Constructs and Levels of Constructs

Some studies are focused on independent variables that are continuous but have been operationalized into several discrete levels. For instance, a topical anesthetic may have a continuous range of application dosages (e.g., by gram or fraction thereof), yet it may be impossible or clinically irrelevant to study the effectiveness of each possible level of the continuum. Selecting target dosage levels may entail the danger of unrepresentative dosages. This is particularly problematic if the dosages sampled fall below the threshold level of therapeutic efficacy. This would lead the researcher to conclude that the drug is ineffective when, in fact, at higher dosages it might very well be effective.

Interraction of Different Treatments

Interaction of different treatments refers to the situation in which more than one treatment affects subjects. Unless this occurs within the context of a carefully designed factorial experiment (see Chapter 12), in which all possible treatments and treatment levels are administered in every singular and combined form, it will be difficult to ascertain which treatment produced which effects, if any at all.

Interraction of Testing and Treatment

This threat occurs when the schedule and timing of testing or of data collection interferes with the treatment; for instance, testing may intentionally or unintentionally influence subjects' receptivity to the stimuli embedded in the treatment. In these situations, we cannot speak anymore of the treatment producing an effect but, rather, of the interaction of testing and treatment bringing about change. Likewise, the interaction of both may extinguish any effects, leading us to infer that no effect occurred, when in fact change was achieved.

Restricted Generalizability Across Constructs

Interventions may produce effects on many possible outcome variables. In the conceptualization stage of a study it is important to think broadly and comprehensively and to examine the full range of outcomes that might be achieved by one or more treatments. If the range is restricted, researchers will be limited to generalizations about only those outcomes that were included. They may be able to speculate about the effects on related outcomes and, by extension, constructs, but this will be limited to speculation. Careful and thoughtful planning might lead to a broadened spectrum of outcome variables and constructs and thus avoid the problem of restricted generalizability.

THREATS TO EXTERNAL VALIDITY

External validity refers to the degree to which the results of a study can be generalized. Nursing research often seeks to demonstrate that an intervention has been successful with a particular problem. If the research has external validity, the researcher may argue that the intervention is applicable to other populations and in other settings. There are several threats to external validity that must be considered.

Hawthorne Effect

The Hawthorne effect derives its name from the Hawthorne experiment conducted by Elton Mayo at the Hawthorne works of the Western Electric Company in Chicago. From 1927 to 1932, using a control and an experimental group, Mayo studied the effect of lighting conditions on workers. Conditions were held constant for the control group, and the light for the experimental groups was first made brighter, then more dim. Mayo anticipated that there would be some difference in the rate of production between subjects in the control and experimental groups. What he found was that both groups had increased production. From this and other studies on human behavior, Mayo concluded that informal organizations develop within groups, and because all subjects knew they were being watched, both the treatment and control groups increased production (Pugh, Hickson, & Hinings, 1985).

It is important for researchers to be aware of the potential impact that the Hawthorne effect can have. In light of the need to obtain informed consent, it is often difficult to conduct research without participant awareness. The burden is on the researcher to show that the effect was caused by the intervention, not simply by participation in the study.

Rosenthal Effect

Research subjects may be influenced when they know they are participating in a study. Likewise, because of their awareness of study participation, researcher's may influence subjects. They may unwittingly influence participants by verbal or nonverbal cues. Researchers may also exert bias in recording observations in a way that produces more favorable results. One useful way to control for this effect is for the researcher to remain blind to group assignment.

Testing

In addition to being a threat to internal validity, testing may also be a threat to external validity. When a pretest is utilized or subjects are asked extensive background information, this may create a situation in which they are then different from other populations who do not participate in these measurement procedures.

Novelty

There is a first time for everything, and this can pose a threat to the validity of research. Subjects may react to a treatment because it is new. This reaction, either positive or negative, can produce an effect that can skew

EVALUATING THE SELECTION OF A RESEARCH DESIGN

1. In what way are the independent variables manipulated by the researcher?
2. How are extraneous forces controlled?
3. How is randomization used in the study?
4. What is the maximum error margin that the researcher has established?
5. What are the potential sources of bias in the study?
6. Does the researcher try to infer causality?
7. What threats to validity exist in the study?

results. As the experimental situation or treatment becomes more familiar, different results may be obtained.

Selection

How participants are selected for a study has implications for the generalizability of findings. Typical methods of recruitment include soliciting volunteers or using a convenience sample. However, there may be inherent differences between people who volunteer for research and those who do not or between clinic and nonclinic populations. Although ultimately subjects must agree to participate, and in that sense are volunteers, it may be possible to utilize selection procedures that provide for a broader representation of participants rather than including only those who participate as volunteers or only those who are available in convenient settings.

Setting

It is essential for the researcher to consider the setting in which the experimental treatment is conducted. There may be a significant difference between the treatment setting and other settings to which the researcher may want to apply the results. The experimental setting may pose a threat to validity when it is artificial and controlled, such as in a laboratory. The setting may also influence generalizability when the preferred site is not available and a substi-

tution must be made. In these instances the results obtained may not be applicable in other settings.

History

History is another factor that can pose a threat to external validity. Events occur in the world that the researcher has no control over. If a significant world or personal event occurs during an experimental treatment, it may be difficult to rule out the effect this event had on the results. When the treatment is repeated, different results may be obtained because history changes and new events or no significant event may occur during treatment.

✑ EVALUATING THE RESEARCH DESIGN'S MAJOR CONCEPTS AND SELECTION

Understanding the major concepts and the rationale for the selection of a specific research design is important for the nurse researcher or for those who want to benefit fully from reading research reports in the literature. Several questions can be used to evaluate the selection of a specific research design (see box above).

SUMMARY

- The purpose of the research design is to provide the backbone structure of a study. It determines how the study will be organized, when data will be collected, and when interventions, if any, are to be implemented.

- When designing a research study it is necessary to consider the concepts of *manipulation, control, random selection, random assignment, probability, bias,* and *causality.*
- The major types of validity of a research design that are vulnerable to potential threat are:
  - *Statistical conclusion validity.* Determining the statistical power available to detect covariation, the adequacy of the empirical evidence to infer covariation, and the strength of this covariation. Threats to *statistical conclusion validity* include: low statistical power; violated assumptions of statistical tests; fishing and the error rate problem; low reliability of measures; low reliability of treatment implementation; random irrelevancies in the experimental setting; and random heterogeneity of respondents.
  - *Internal validity.* The degree to which the outcome can be attributed to the experimental treatment and not to extraneous factors. Threats to *internal validity* include: effects of history (extraneous events); maturation; testing; instrumention; statistical regression; selection; mortality; interactions with selection; lack of clarity in direction of causality; diffusion of experimental conditions; compensating equalization of treatments; compensatory rivalry; and demoralization of controls.
  - *Construct validity of putative causes and effects.* Whether the effects noted on the dependent variable(s) are indeed due to the proposed independent variable(s), or whether confounding independent variables may be responsible for the observed effects. Threats in-

clude: inadequate preoperational explication of constructs; mono-operation bias; mono-method bias; hypothesis guessing within experimental conditions; evaluation apprehension; experimenter expectancies; confounding constructs and levels of constructs; interaction of different treatments; interaction of testing and treatment; and restricted generalizability.
  - *External validity.* The degree to which the results of the study can be generalized to other populations. Threats include: Hawthorne effect; Rosenthal effect; testing; novelty; selection; setting; and history.

FACILITATING CRITICAL THINKING

1. You are designing a study to test the effectiveness of three different types of preoperational teaching. The three interventions are an informational pamphlet, one-to-one teaching, or small group teaching. Answer the following questions.
   a. What variables are manipulated in the study?
   b. List ways in which you can increase control and decrease the effect of extraneous forces.
   c. How would you select subjects for the study?
   d. How would you assign subjects to treatment groups?
   e. What are the potential sources of bias in this study?
2. In your study of preoperative teaching you decide to administer a questionnaire to subjects at two time intervals; before teaching and after surgery. Answer the following questions.
   a. What are the potential threats to statistical conclusion validity?
   b. What are the potential threats to internal validity?

c. What are the potential threats to construct validity of putative causes and effects?

d. What are the potential threats to external validity?

References

Substantive

Abraham, I. L., Buckwalter, K. C., Neese, J. B., Fox, J. C. (1994). Mental health of rural elderly: A research agenda. *Nursing Issues in Mental Health Nursing, 15*(3), 203-213.

Abraham, I. L., Buckwalter, K. C., Snustad, D. G., Smullen, D. E., Thompson-Heisterman, A. A., Nesse, J. B., & Smith, M. A. (1993). Psychogeriatric outreach to rural families: The Iowa and Virginia models. *International Psychogeriatrics, 5*(2), 203-210.

Abraham, I. L, Chalifoux, Z., & Evers, G. C. M. (1992). Conditions, interventions, and outcomes: A quantitative analysis of nursing research (1981-1990). In P. Moritz (Ed.), *Patient outcomes research: Examining the effectiveness of nursing practice* (pp. 70-87). Bethesda, MD: National Institutes of Health (NIH Publication No. 93-3411).

Abraham, I. L., & Neese, J. B. (1993). Outreach to elderly and their families: Focus on the rural south. *Aging, 365,* 26-31.

Abraham, I. L., Neundorfer, M. M., Cowling, W. R., & Sutorius, S. D. (1990). Changes in resident mix in nursing homes: Cognitive and sensory data from a (redesigned) sampling plan. *Psychological Reports, 66,* 547-550.

Abraham, I. L., Neundorfer, M. M., & Currie, L. (1992). Effects of group interventions on cognition and depression in nursing home residents. *Nursing Research, 41,* 196-202.

Abraham, I. L., Niles, S. A., Thiel, B. P., Siarkowski, K. I., & Cowling, W. R. (1991). Therapeutic group work with depressed elderly. *Nursing Clients of North America, 26,* 635-650.

Buckwalter, K. C., Abraham, I. L., Smith, M. A., & Smullen, D. E. (1993). Nursing outreach to rural elderly people who are mentally ill. *Hospital and Community Psychiatry, 44,* 821-823.

O'Sullivan, A. L., & Jacobsen, B. E. (1992). A randomized trial of a health care program for first-time adolescent mothers and their infants. *Nursing Research, 41,* 210-215.

Conceptual

Kourany, J. A. (1987). *Scientific knowledge: Basic issues in the philosophy of science.* Belmont, CA: Wadsworth.

Polkinghorne, D. (1983). *Methodology for the human sciences: Systems of Inquiry.* Albany: State University of New York Press.

Pugh, D. S., Hickson, D. J., & Hinings, C. R. (1985). *Writers on organizations.* Beverly Hills, CA: Sage.

Reynolds, P. D. (1971). *A primer in theory construction.* New York: Macmillan.

Methodological

Brink, P. J., & Wood, M. J. (Eds.). (1989). *Advanced design in nursing research.* Newbury Park, CA: Sage.

McLaughlin, F. E., & Marascuilo, L. A. (1990). *Advanced nursing and health care research: Quantification approaches.* Philadelphia: Saunders.

Oyster, C. K., Hanten, W. P., & Llorens, L. A. (1987). *Introduction to research: A guide for the health science professional.* Philadelphia: Lippincott.

Polit, D. F., & Hungler, B. P. (1991). *Nursing research: Principles and methods* (4th ed.). Philadelphia: Lippincott.

Waltz, C., & Bausell, R. B. (1981). *Nursing research: Design, statistics and computer analysis.* Philadelphia: Davis.

Woods, N. F., & Catanzaro, M. (1988). *Nursing research: Theory and practice.* St. Louis, Mosby.

Historical

Cook, T. C., & Campbell, D. T. (1979). *Quasi-experimentation: Design and analysis issues for field settings.* Boston: Houghton Mifflin.

CHAPTER 12

QUANTITATIVE DESIGNS

LYNN I. WASSERBAUER • IVO L. ABRAHAM

Within the research process, the research design or methodology can be considered the backbone or structure of the study. The structure of the research design then becomes the framework that supports the study and holds it together. Having a knowledge of many different research designs provides the researcher with flexibility and the tools needed to choose the most appropriate design for each particular question and to adapt designs to fit the situation at hand. It is important to remember that in most instances the research questions or hypotheses dictate the type of research design that can be used. Theoretically, with every research question there is one research design that may be considered the most appropriate; however, researchers should not lose sight of the fact that the theoretically best design might prove to be impractical or impossible in any given situation. With experience researchers can

adapt and tailor designs to provide the most effective framework for each study.

The focus of this chapter is a review of the many quantitative research designs. Experimental, quasi-experimental, nonexperimental, and nontraditional designs are described in terms of structure, advantages, and disadvantages. Examples of several designs are also provided. The chapter concludes with guidelines for evaluating research designs.

In conducting any study careful consideration must be given to the type of research design that is chosen. The choice of design is dependent on the question(s) to be answered, the resources available to the researcher (such as time, money), and the personal preferences of the researcher. The three main categories of research are experimental, quasi-experimental, and nonexperimental. While much of nursing research falls within these three categories, a fourth category of importance is nontraditional research. Each design will be described briefly, followed by its advantages and disadvantages.

Preparation of this chapter was supported in part by grants from the W. K. Kellogg Foundation, the Pew Charitable Trusts, the National Institute of Mental Health, the DHHS Division of Nursing, and the National Center for Nursing Research.

217

In the descriptions that follow standard notation will be used to illustrate each research design. R represents randomization, O represents observation, and X represents treatment. Numerical subscripts will represent the order of implementing treatments or the order of recording observations.

EXPERIMENTAL DESIGN

True experimental design is considered to be the classic form of research, and experiments have the potential to provide the most evidence for the strength of the association between variables. Experiments are concerned with testing hypotheses and establishing causality. Experiments achieve this strength because they are characterized by manipulation, control, and randomization. (Manipulation, control, and randomization were defined in Chapter 11. A thorough grasp of these concepts is necessary to understand experimental research designs. The reader is encouraged to review these concepts, if necessary, before proceeding further.) In general, these factors contribute to increasing the internal validity of a study. To achieve a high degree of control, experimental studies are usually conducted in laboratories under very artificial conditions; however, the amount of control required makes experimental design an inappropriate choice for many research problems. Moreover, while a well-controlled study allows the researcher to more easily determine the impact that the experimental intervention had, the results of such a study can only be generalized to similar settings and populations. This limits the external validity of the findings. To gain external validity, many trials must be conducted with different populations and under different conditions. Several of the most widely used experimental designs will be described, and the advantages and disadvantages of each type will be discussed. Although each design will be illustrated with a treatment group and a control group, more than two groups can be incorporated in each design. The first three experimental designs are summarized in Table 12-1.

PRETEST-POSTTEST CONTROL GROUP DESIGN

In the pretest-posttest control group design subjects are randomly assigned to either the control or the experimental group. Each group is observed (the pretest); one group receives a treatment, while the other does not. The researcher then observes the groups again (the posttest) to determine what effect, if any, the treatment had. The pretest-posttest control group design is illustrated in Figure 12-1. In this design each group should receive the same pretest and the same posttest. Based on the hypotheses to be tested, the researcher can make a prediction as to the way in which the treatment will affect the treatment group.

Advantages and Disadvantages

The pretest-posttest control group design has several advantages; however, as with most of the designs that will be described, the amount of control achieved is significantly dependent on the ability of the researcher to structure the research environment. By using a control group, several threats to internal validity can be minimized. These include history, maturation, testing, statistical regression, selection, and interactions with selection. In a well-designed experiment the only differences between the control and experimental groups should be the treatment; whatever extraneous events that happen between one observation and the next should hap-

Table 12-1
Experimental Designs

Name of Design	Notation*				Advantages	Disadvantages
Pretest-posttest control group	R O_1 X O_2 R O_1 O_2				Decreases threats to internal validity: history, maturation, testing, statistical regression, selection, and interactions with selection	Differential influence of mortality, limited generalizability of results
Posttest-only control group	R X O R O				Controls for threats to internal validity as listed above, eliminates effect of testing	Lack of randomization decreases ability to determine strength and direction of response
Solomon four-group	Treatment group 1 R O_1 X O_2 Control group 1 R O_1 O_2 Treatment group 2 R X O_2 Control group 2 R O_2				Strong design, increased internal validity, controls for the effects of history, testing, and maturation	Increased resources needed, may require multiple researchers, potential for increased observational bias

*R, Randomization; O, observation; X, treatment.

$$R \quad O_1 \quad X \quad O_2$$

$$R \quad O_1 \quad \quad O_2$$

Figure 12-1. Pretest-posttest control group design.

pen to both the control and treatment groups. Therefore, the threat of history can be reduced significantly. Depending on the length of the intervention there may be some maturation in the group over time; however, with randomization and the use of a control group, it is possible to determine the changes in both samples that can be attributed to maturation over time and not to the treatment. The effects of testing are minimized when each group receives the pretest. If the pretest does in some way influence the posttest, each group will be similarly affected, which diminishes the effect. The threat of statistical regression is minimized because extremes in testing would not generally occur in only one group. The use of random selection and random assignment can control for the bias of selection and strengthen the internal and external validity of the study. The use of a control group does not automatically control for the effects of testing and instrumentation. These biases can still exist, but may not be manifest in between-group comparisons.

One disadvantage of the pretest-posttest control group design is the possibility that mortality may affect one group more than the other. This attrition may be unavoidable and may skew the study results. The other major disadvantage of this design is that results can only be generalized to similar groups and settings.

POSTTEST-ONLY CONTROL GROUP DESIGN

This design is quite similar to the pretest-posttest control group design; however, it is considered a weaker experimental design. In the posttest-only control group design there is no pretest (Figure 12-2). This design is particularly useful in situations in which it is not possible to obtain a pretest measure.

Advantages and Disadvantages
With randomization the posttest-only control group controls for many of the same threats to internal validity as the pretest-posttest control group design. Another advantage is that the effect of testing would be eliminated because of the lack of a pretest. Although this design does allow a researcher to undertake studies that are not amenable to other designs, there are several disadvantages that limit its usefulness. Randomization to groups does provide some control, but without pretest measures the

$$R \quad X \quad O$$
$$R \quad \quad O$$

Figure 12-2. Posttest-only control group design.

researcher is less able to determine the strength and direction of the response. Given these weaknesses, the pretest-posttest design is preferred.

SOLOMON FOUR-GROUP DESIGN

The Solomon four-group design is particularly complex and is a combination of the pretest-posttest control group design (treatment group 1 and control group 1 in Figure 12-3). In the Solomon four-group design there are two control groups and two experimental groups. Subjects are randomly assigned to one of the groups. With randomization of a large enough number of subjects the groups can be considered equivalent at the onset of the study. The experiment is conducted concurrently on all groups in an effort to reduce the threat of history on the external validity. Analysis of the posttest scores gives an indication of the degree to which the treatment influenced outcome.

Advantages and Disadvantages
The Solomon four-group design is a very strong study design and greatly increases the level of internal validity that can be achieved. The effects of history and maturation are controlled for by the pretested groups. Groups without the pretest control for the effect of testing. Moreover, the non-pretested control group allows the researcher to assess the impact of maturation

Treatment group 1	R	O_1	X	O_2
Control group 1	R	O_1		O_2
Treatment group 2	R		X	O_2
Control group 2	R			O_2

Figure 12-3. Solomon four-group design.

without treatment. In spite of the strength of this design, the Solomon four-group design does have some disadvantages. The main disadvantage of this design is the amount of resources required to conduct the study correctly. The design requires a large number of subjects who are available at the same time. Many nurse researchers do not have access to the number of subjects required; therefore it may be necessary to collaborate with researchers from other disciplines. Moreover, when more than one researcher is involved in data collection, observational bias may be introduced. Thus it is necessary to develop a system to ensure interrater reliability, and great care must be taken to ensure that there is consistency between researchers in recording observations.

FACTORIAL DESIGN

The designs discussed so far have involved the manipulation of one independent variable. At times a researcher may want to study the effect of one or more independent variables. A factorial design is particularly useful when there are multiple independent variables, which are called factors, to be tested. Typical factorial designs incorporate a 2×2 factorial or a 2×3 factorial, but any combination is possible. The first number refers to the independent variables and the second number to the levels of treatment. For example, types of therapy (individual or group) can be factors (independent variables), and lengths of treatment (brief, intermediate, or long-term) can be levels of treatment. This would yield a 2×3 factorial design, and subjects would be randomly assigned to one of the six treatment combinations (cells) that would results from this design.

A factorial design permits the analysis of both main effects and interaction effects. A main effect is the effect of one variable alone; that is, the effect of individual or group therapy. In studying the main effects a researcher could determine if long-term individual therapy was more effective than short-term individual therapy or which level of group therapy was most effective. However, at times it is also useful to be able to determine the way in which factors interact to produce an effect. Interaction effect is the effect produced by a combination of variables and helps to determine if a combination of group and individual therapy is more effective than either treatment alone.

Advantages and Disadvantages

The primary advantage of the factorial design is the ability to test multiple independent factors. This is particularly useful when levels of interventions and specific combinations of interventions are being assessed. The disadvantage of a factorial design is the increased number of subjects required to obtain statistical significance.

RANDOMIZED BLOCK DESIGN

A specific type of factorial design is the randomized block design. A traditional factorial design is used when the researcher can randomly assign subjects to each of the cells created. At times there may be factors the researcher is interested in studying that cannot be manipulated or that the researcher suspects may be confounding variables. Variables such as the age, race, sex, geographic location, or hospital unit of the subject cannot be changed, and the researcher may suspect that they may be confounding variables. To control for this problem the researcher can design a study in which the potentially confounding variable is incorporated into the study design as an independent variable; this is known as blocking. Subjects are then randomly assigned within each block. For instance, a researcher could block by age to test the effectiveness of a geriatric rehabilitation program if it was suspected that younger subjects would show a much more significant improvement than older subjects. Specific age categories are developed, and subjects within each age category are randomly assigned to each treatment group.

Advantages and Disadvantages

The randomized block design has essentially the same advantages as the factorial design. However, because confounding can be controlled for, the randomized block design extends the usefulness of the factorial design. As with factorial designs, the randomized block design requires a large number of subjects. It is also necessary to have equal numbers of subjects with the blocking variable.

CLINICAL TRIALS

Clinical trials or intervention studies are considered to be one of the most rigorous study designs. The focus of clinical trials is on clinical outcomes. Clinical trials can be either experimental or quasi-experimental based on the degree to which randomization is used to select subjects and assign them to treatment groups. The two major types of clinical trials are preventive and therapeutic. Preventive trials are designed to determine if a specific treatment reduces the risk associated with developing a specific disease. In therapeutic trials the aim is to determine how effective a treatment is in reducing symptoms, preventing relapse, or reducing risk of death associated with a specific illness. Drug studies are one of the most common types of clinical trials and are designed to test the efficacy of new types of medications.

Advantages and Disadvantages

Randomized clinical trails have several advantages over other study designs. In a well-designed randomized clinical trial the temporal relationship between treatment and outcome is more clearly established; this can provide strong evidence for inferring causation. When randomization is used in a clinical trial, the threats to internal and external validity are reduced and both known and unknown confounders are controlled. The major disadvantages of clinical trials is that they are usually quite expensive, there may be ethical consideration in administering treatments for which the risks and benefits are not completely understood, and when they are experimental studies, the study may lack generalizability because of the structured and contrived research setting.

༄ QUASI-EXPERIMENTAL DESIGN

True experimental design is considered to provide the strongest evidence for assessing causality between the independent and dependent variables. However, when conducting research in field settings, it is not always possible to implement a design that meets the three criteria of an experimental study: manipulation, control, and randomization. Quasi-experimental research is similar to experimental research in that there is manipulation of an independent variable. It differs from experimental research because either there is no control group or random assignment is not used to assign subjects to groups. Quasi-experimental research is a useful way to test causality in settings when it is impossible or unethical to randomly assign subjects to treatment and control groups or to withhold treatment from some subjects. The main disadvantage of quasi-experimental research is the increased threat to internal validity as a result of utilizing a design in which randomization and/or a control group is lacking.

The first three quasi-experimental de-

Table 12-2
Preexperimental Designs

Name of Design	Notation*	Advantages	Disadvantages
One-group posttest-only	X O	Simple and quick, minimizes threat of testing, possible increased cooperation of subjects	Cannot assess causality, without a control group decreased internal validity of results
Static-group comparison	X O ------ O	Useful when pretest measures are impossible to obtain, control group decreases the threat of history and maturation	Lack of pretest limits ability to determine if groups were similar before treatment
One-group pretest-posttest	O_1 X O_2	Control group improves one-group posttest-only design; however, few real advantages	Multiple threats to internal validity, impossible to rule out effect of history, maturation, instrumentation, and statistical regression

*O, Observation; X, treatment.

signs that will be described are also known in the literature as preexperimental designs. These designs are summarized in Table 12-2. In general they are considered the weakest quasi-experimental designs, which greatly limits the usefulness of the results obtained in research utilizing these approaches. The other quasi-experimental designs that will be discussed are non-equivalent control group designs and time series designs.

ONE-GROUP POSTTEST-ONLY DESIGN
As the name implies, the one-group posttest-only design utilizes one treatment group and only a posttest. There is no control group or pretest (Figure 12-4). The one-group posttest-only design can be used to study the effects of natural or man-made catastrophes, such as hurricanes, floods, or plane crashes. In these unplanned situations it is highly unlikely that pretest data will be available; however, some demographic data may be available from other sources that could be used instead of a

$$X \qquad O$$

Figure 12-4. One-group posttest-only design.

pretest to strengthen the study design. Cook and Campbell (1979) point out that the one-group posttest-only design is not the same as the one-shot case study. The one-group posttest-only design provides relatively little data, while a well-done case study quite often assesses many variables that provide detailed descriptions for further analysis.

Advantages and Disadvantages
The main advantage of the one-group posttest-only design is that it is simple and quick. Subjects may be more cooperative when only a posttest is given, and without a pretest testing is not a threat to internal validity. The study can be used to provide information on the impact of a treatment and the experiences individuals have with it. One disadvantage of this design is that it

cannot be used to assess causality. Without the use of a pretest and with only one group, the researcher cannot be sure that the outcome observed had any relationship to the treatment. The lack of a control group significantly reduces the internal validity of the results, because there is no evidence that the results obtained would not have occurred in the absence of the treatment.

STATIC-GROUP COMPARISON

A second relatively weak design is the static-group comparison. The static-group comparison is also known as the posttest-only design with nonequivalent groups (Figure 12-5). This design is quite similar to the posttest-only experimental design. However, the static-group comparison does not use randomization to assign subjects to groups. As Cook and Campbell (1979) point out, the researcher may use existing information to obtain some pretreatment data. It is possible for the researcher to gather some information such as demographic data from other sources (e.g., the medical record) rather than administering a pretest.

Advantages and Disadvantages

The static-group comparison can be used in situations in which it is not possible to obtain pretreatment information. This may be an appropriate design for unanticipated events that cannot be repeated. The information gathered from such a study may help to stimulate further research as well as

generate questions that can be tested in the future. The static-group comparison is an improvement on the one-group posttest-only design because the use of a control group decreases the impact of history and maturation as threats to internal validity. Yet the static-group comparison does have disadvantages. Without pretest data it is impossible to conclude that the results obtained were related to the treatment and not to pretreatment differences in the groups. The use of archival data for pretest measures is another disadvantage that may threaten the validity of the findings.

ONE-GROUP PRETEST-POSTTEST DESIGN

This is a relatively straightforward research design in which there is a treatment group without a control group (Figure 12-6). All subjects are given a pretest, receive the treatment, and are given a posttest. In the absence of a control group, subjects act as their own controls and pretreatment and posttreatment data are analyzed for differences.

Advantages and Disadvantages

The use of a pretest does improve on the one-group posttest-only design and allows further analysis, yet the one-group pretest-posttest design has few real advantages. With this design there are multiple threats to internal validity, and it is impossible to rule out the effects of history, maturation, instrumentation, and statistical regression. Causality cannot be determined using this design, but it may provide some information that may be useful in generating further research.

$$X \qquad O$$
$$\text{-------}$$
$$O$$

Figure 12-5. Static-group comparison. Dashed line indicates non-random assignment to group.

$$O_1 \qquad X \qquad O_2$$

Figure 12-6. One-group pretest-posttest design.

NONEQUIVALENT CONTROL GROUP DESIGNS

The nonequivalent control group design is one of the standards of quasi-experimental research. A nonequivalent design is often used when there are naturally occurring groups of subjects or when it is impossible or unethical to withhold treatment from one group. Subjects may be selected on the basis of hospital or specific units within the hospital, or patients may self-select into various treatment groups. In situations where it is impossible or unethical to withhold treatment, the control group may also receive a treatment.

One of the most frequently used nonequivalent control group designs, the untreated control group with pretest and postest, is the same as the experimental pretest-posttest control group design, except that in the nonequivalent control group design subjects are not randomly assigned to groups. There are several other variations of the nonequivalent control group design that are used by nurse researchers. These designs include the untreated control group design with proxy pretest measures, the untreated control group design with separate pretest and posttest samples, the untreated control group design with pretest measures at more than one time interval, the removed-treatment design with pretest and posttest, the repeated-treatment design, and the reversed-treatment nonequivalent control group design with pretest and posttest (counterbalanced design). Nonequivalent control group designs are summarized in Table 12-3.

Advantages and Disadvantages

Use of a nonequivalent control group design does have several advantages. In spite of the absence of randomization, nonequivalent control group designs can be considered relatively strong designs. The use of a control group and a pretest significantly increases the strength of nonequivalent control group designs. Good pretest data will enable the researcher to improve the level of analysis of results. In nonequivalent control group designs the researcher is interested in analyzing the differences between group scores on pretest and posttest measures and not simply the differences within group scores on these measures. When subjects from different settings are used, a nonequivalent control group design may control some threats to internal validity, such as compensatory rivalry and demoralization of controls. When subjects in each group are naturally kept separate, it is less likely that they will have contact with each other, and it is often useful to minimize contact between treatment and control groups.

The disadvantages in using a nonequivalent control group design are the threats to internal and external validity. Selection is a threat because subjects are not randomly selected for the study. Another threat is interactions with selection, including selection-history and selection-maturation. These are especially problematic in studies in which subjects come from two different settings such as two hospitals. It is impossible to ensure that events between the pretest and the posttest are identical for the two settings. Therefore, there are limits to the extent that one can infer causality. Whenever a pretest is used, testing is potentially a threat to validity. The main threats to external validity are selection and setting. When subjects self-select for a study or for a specific treatment group, the generalizability of the findings is limited. Setting can be a threat when the researcher attempts to generalize the results to individuals from multiple settings. While the results of any one study cannot be ex-

Table 12-3
Nonequivalent Control Group Designs

Name of Design	Notation*	Advantages	Disadvantages
Untreated control group with pretest and posttest	O_1 X O_2 ------------------ O_1 X O_2	Provides very interpretable results, useful in situations where other designs are not possible, controls for most threats to internal validity	Does not control for selection-maturation, instrumentation, statistical regression, and interaction of selection and history.
Untreated control group with proxy pretest measures	O_{A1} X O_{B2} ------------------ O_{A1} X O_{B2}	Useful when it is impossible to use the same instrument as the pretest and posttest	Pretest instrument may not correlate well with posttest instrument
Untreated control group with separate pretest and posttest samples	O ┊ X O -------┊-------- O ┊ X O	Eliminates the effect of testing as a threat to internal validity	Relatively weak design, does not control other threats to internal validity, difficult to achieve homogeneous samples
Untreated control group with pretest measures at more than one time interval	O_1 O_2 X O_3 ------------------------------------ O_1 O_2 O_3	Can look at trends in the data, findings more interpretable, controls for selection-maturation	More time-consuming and expensive to obtain multiple pretest measures, may not be possible
Removed treatment with pretest and posttest	O_1 X O_2 O_3 x O_4	Useful when an appropriate control group is not available, same subjects used for all measures	Impossible to use in some situations, may be unethical to remove a treatment, observations must be made at equal time intervals, difficult to use in situations in which the effects of the treatment last over time
Repeated treatment	O_1 X O_2 x O_3 X O_4	Subjects act as their own control group, fewer subjects required	Does not eliminate threats of maturation and resentment when treatment is removed, construct validity a threat
Reversed treatment nonequivalent control group with pretest and posttest	O_1 X+ O_2 ------------------ O_1 X− O_2	Reduces threat of selection-maturation, potential increase in construct validity	Complex design, construct validity dependent on treatment producing effect in opposite directions, does not eliminate threat of maturation or statistical conclusion validity

*O, Observation; X, treatment; x, treatment removed; vertical line indicates separate samples; *subscripts A and B*, different measures; $X+$, treatment that produces an effect in one direction, $X−$, treatment that produces an effect in the opposite direction.

tended to all individuals, nonequivalent control group designs can assist the researcher in gaining knowledge and inferring causality.

INTERRUPTED TIME SERIES DESIGNS

The second standard type of quasi-experimental design is the interrupted time series design. In time series designs the researcher does not always use a control group and does not use randomization. An interrupted time series study uses several observations of subjects over time with a treatment given at a specified point. A time series study can be designed to study the same individuals at specified intervals or to study different individuals at some common point in time such as admission to the hospital or birth. When the researcher studies one group of subjects, the subjects act as their own controls, which provides the researcher with equivalent control groups. Time series designs are used when a control group population is not available. When only one group is available to the researcher, the time series design significantly increases the strength of the research.

The simple interrupted time series is the most straightforward and involves the use of one group of subjects. Several pretest observations are made, the treatment is administered, and several posttest observations are made. Other variations of the interrupted time series design are the interrupted time series with a nonequivalent no-treatment control group time series, interrupted time series with nonequivalent dependent variables, interrupted time series with removed treatment, interrupted time series with multiple replications, and interrupted time series with switching replications. The interrupted time series designs are summarized in Table 12-4.

Advantages and Disadvantages

One of the advantages of the interrupted time series is that repeated pretreatment observations help to control for maturation. If there is any trend, it should be apparent as a result of the pretreatment observations. Another advantage of time series designs is that repeated posttreatment measures allow the researcher to determine if posttreatment change is maintained over time. There are also several disadvantages to the interrupted time series design. History may be a threat to internal validity. However, according to Cook and Campbell (1979), there are several ways to control for this threat. Increasing the frequency of observations and recording any significant events during the study period will help to determine the effect outside events may have had on the outcome. The use of a control group with an interrupted time series design will also decrease the threat of history. Threats that are more difficult to control for are instrumentation and selection. With repeated observations instrumentation is a threat to validity. This is especially problematic when the pretreatment data is obtained from archival records in which uniformity is not always possible. Selection becomes a threat when some subjects drop out of treatment at the time the treatment is administered.

❧ NONEXPERIMENTAL DESIGNS

Nonexperimental designs are those that do not involve manipulation of an independent variable, control, or randomization. Frequently the focus of nonexperimental designs is to describe and to measure the independent and dependent variables. Nonexperimental research is important because there are situations in which an experimental or quasi-experimental design is

Table 12-4
Interrupted Time Series Designs

Name of Design	Notation*	Advantages	Disadvantages
Simple interrupted time series	O_1 O_2 O_3 O_4 X O_6 O_7 O_8 O_9	Uses only one group of subjects, maturational and seasonal trends more apparent, reduces threat of statistical regression	Does not eliminate the threat of history, instrumentation, and selection
Interrupted time series with a nonequivalent no-treatment control group time series	O_1 O_2 O_3 O_4 X O_6 O_7 O_8 O_9 O_1 O_2 O_3 O_4 O_6 O_7 O_8 O_9	Controls for threats listed above and decreases the threat of history and statistical regression	Does not eliminate threat of the interaction of selection and history, more expensive and time-consuming
Interrupted time series with nonequivalent dependent variables	O_{A1} O_{A2} X O_{A4} O_{A5} O_{B1} O_{B2} X O_{B4} O_{B5}	Useful to control the threat of history, increased statistical conclusion validity, able to test the effect of multiple independent variables	Dependent variables used must be conceptually related, more complex design
Interrupted time series with removed treatment	O_1 O_2 O_3 X O_4 O_5 O_6 x O_8 O_9	Reduces threat of history, selection, and instrumentation	Difficult to determine that removal of treatment caused the observed effect, may be resentful demoralization of subjects, or selection-maturation, ethical issues in removing a treatment
Interrupted time series with multiple replications	O_1 O_2XO_3 O_4xO_5 O_6XO_7 O_8xO_9 O_{10}	Strong design, able to infer causality, reduces threats of maturation and seasonal trends	Scheduling of treatments should be random, cannot be used in situations where the effects of treatment persist over time, requires greater experimental control
Interrupted time series with switching replications	O_1 O_2 O_3 O_4 O_5 O_6 O_7 X O_8 O_9 O_1 O_2 O_3 X O_4 O_5 O_6 O_7 O_8 O_9	Control for many threats to internal validity, increased external and construct validity	Requires two very similar populations, history remains a threat if the two populations differ

*O, Observation; X, treatment; x, treatment removed; *subscripts A and B, different dependent variables.*

TYPES OF NONEXPERIMENTAL DESIGNS

DESCRIPTIVE DESIGN: SURVEY RESEARCH
    Simple descriptive survey
    Comparative descriptive survey
    Developmental survey

EX POST FACTO DESIGNS
    Descriptive correlational design
    Retrospective design
    Prospective design
    Path analysis design
    Predictive design

inappropriate for a particular research question. Manipulation of variables is not always possible, especially for variables like sex, age, or diagnostic category. Randomization is not always ethical, because with human subjects it may be impossible to randomly assign subjects to groups. Randomization is especially problematic in situations in which the experimental treatment is known to provide some benefit. To withhold treatment and assign some subjects to a control group would be unethical.

Nonexperimental research is designed to overcome these limitations. The goal of nonexperimental research is not to prove causality, but rather to describe phenomena, and explore and explain the relationships between variables. The two main categories of nonexperimental research are descriptive, and ex post facto (see box).

DESCRIPTIVE DESIGN

As the name implies, the goal of descriptive research is to describe phenomena. Although descriptive research is a comparatively weak design, it is frequently used when very little is known about a topic or to initially explore a research question. Descriptive research encompasses a wide variety of different designs that utilize both quantitative and qualitative methods. The present discussion will be limited to quantitative survey research.

Survey Research

Survey designs are concerned with gathering information from a segment of the population. It is impossible to collect data from every individual, because most researchers do not have unlimited time and resources. Therefore a sample is selected from the population, and information is obtained from this sample. There are specific research techniques that are frequently utilized with any survey design. Two of the most common are interviews and questionnaires, and each type has advantages and disadvantages.

Interviews can be conducted in person or over the telephone, and questionnaires can be mailed or administered in person. The technique chosen is dependent on the amount of time, money, and personnel available to the researcher. Interviews conducted in person generally provide the most complete information; however, they are also the most expensive and time-consuming for the researcher. Although telephone interviews are usually not as effective as personal interviews, they are much cheaper and less time intensive. However, subjects are limited to individuals who have telephones. This may decrease the sample size and act as a form of selection bias because individuals who have telephones may be different from those who do not have telephones. Another source of bias during interviews is the interviewer. It is important for interviewers to ask questions in a standard format using predetermined criteria for recording answers. If more than one interviewer is used, steps must be taken to ensure that there is interrater reliability between the interviewers.

Questionnaires are self-administered interviews; however, they are not as sensitive as interviews. Questionnaires may acquire less information from subjects because there is less contact between the person administering the questionnaire and the subject. Mailed questionnaires are very cost-effective, but may pose some additional problems for the researcher. The return rate may be low, questionnaire development may be complex, and the researcher may encounter subjects who are illiterate. Administering questionnaires in person may increase response rate, and allow the researcher to assist those who cannot read; however, this would increase both the time and cost required.

Simple Descriptive Survey Design.
Simple descriptive survey design involves describing and documenting the world as it currently exists. The goal of this type of research is to provide as complete a description as possible. The researcher does not manipulate any variables, and there is no effort to determine the relationship between variables. In simple descriptive survey research, the researcher identifies the variables of interest and ascertains the frequency of occurrence of these variables. The census is one example of a simple descriptive survey.

ADVANTAGES AND DISADVANTAGES. A simple descriptive survey design is used for preliminary research on a topic. Variables can be identified, and further research questions can be generated. In comparison to experimental and quasi-experimental research, survey research is faster and much less expensive. A disadvantage of this design is that the information obtained is necessarily limited. Simple descriptive survey research cannot be used to infer causality or the extent of the relationship between variables.

Comparative Descriptive Survey Design. A comparative descriptive survey is designed to be a comparison between two or more groups. Information is obtained on each group, and using statistical analysis, the researcher tries to identify what differences exist between the groups. When conducting a comparative survey, it is important for the study samples to be as similar as possible in all variables except the variables under study. To achieve this, random sampling procedures and, when appropriate, stratified random sampling should be used.

ADVANTAGES AND DISADVANTAGES. Comparative descriptive surveys can provide detailed descriptive information about several groups. This type of research design can be used to determine if the groups are the same or different on specific variables. This design can also be used to stimulate further research on a topic. The disadvantages of comparative descriptive designs include the relative weakness of the design and the inability to determine the degree of association between variables.

Developmental Survey Design. Developmental surveys are conducted when the researcher wants to examine the way variables change over time. Two main types of developmental surveys are longitudinal surveys and cross-sectional surveys. Longitudinal surveys allow the researcher to collect data at several points in time. Three of the more commonly used longitudinal survey designs are trend studies, cohort studies, and panel studies. In trend studies the researcher selects samples from the general population at specified time intervals, and at each interval new subjects are chosen. In cohort studies different subjects are also selected at specified time intervals; however, these subjects are drawn from previously identified groups within the population. Panel studies involve the repeated measurement of the same subjects at specified time intervals.

Cross-sectional surveys involve obtaining data from a cross section of the population. In cross-sectional surveys data can be obtained on all individuals at one point in time, or data can be obtained on individuals at a fixed event during life such as birth or death.

ADVANTAGES AND DISADVANTAGES. Each type of developmental survey has specific advantages. Trend studies are used to provide data about the amount of change that has occurred over a specific period of time. The advantage of cohort studies is that they allow the researcher to study segments of the population for changes over time. Panel studies can provide detailed information on specific individuals and the changes that occur with these individuals over time. An advantage of cross-sectional studies is that they are fast, easy to do, and cost-effective. Cross-sectional studies can also provide valuable information for administrators who plan health care services.

There are also several disadvantages to using developmental surveys. Depending on the variables of interest, longitudinal studies may be very lengthy and expensive. With a long study there is an increased chance there will be a loss of subjects for follow-up as a result of subjects dropping out, dying, or moving. The main disadvantage of cross-sectional studies is difficulty in determining what contributed to any observed differences in the data. Another disadvantage is that when a section of the population is surveyed at the same time, differences may be attributed to generational differences between groups rather than changes that occur over time.

EX POST FACTO DESIGN

The second type of nonexperimental research is ex post facto or "after the fact." Ex post facto designs are frequently referred to as correlational studies. In ex post facto research there is no manipulation of the independent variable, because the event of interest (the dependent variable) has already occurred. This type of research is conducted to describe existing relationships between variables and to determine if there is a correlation between variables. When a correlation exists, a change in one variable corresponds to a change in other variables. However, it must be kept in mind that a correlation does not indicate causation. Ex post facto research may confirm the existence of a correlation, but it is generally insufficient to prove that a causal relationship exists. The ex post facto designs that will be described in more detail are descriptive correlational, retrospective, prospective, path analysis, and predictive.

Descriptive Correlational Design. In a descriptive correlational design the researcher attempts to determine and describe what relationships exist between variables. Subjects are not randomly assigned to treatment and control groups, and there is no manipulation of the independent variable. The researcher identifies the variables of interest and then determines the most appropriate way to measure them. Data are usually collected by using a questionnaire or through interviews.

ADVANTAGES AND DISADVANTAGES. The advantages of descriptive correlational research are that it is straightforward, it is usually inexpensive, and it can be done quickly. It may also be important preliminary research for further studies that do attempt to determine causation between variables. The disadvantage of this research is that it determines correlation and not causation.

Retrospective Design. When using a retrospective design the researcher starts with an effect and works back to determine what in the past is associated with this effect. Epidemiological studies frequently use a retrospective design. In retrospective studies subjects are chosen based on having the effect of interest; information is then obtained from subjects or from archival records to determine what variables in the past may have contributed to the development of the effect. For example, in a retrospective epidemiologic study subjects are chosen based on disease status (whether they have the disease), and information about past history is then obtained to determine what may have contributed to the development of a specific disease.

ADVANTAGES AND DISADVANTAGES. Retrospective studies are particularly useful when investigating rare occurrences. When using other sampling methods it may not be possible to obtain a large enough sample that contains the variable of interest. Retrospective studies can also utilize existing data and therefore may be faster and less expensive. One of the disadvantages of retrospective studies is that subjects may have recall bias in which they are more aware of their personal histories and overreport events. Overreporting may lead the researcher to conclude that a stronger association exists than actually does exist. Underreporting may also be a problem in retrospective studies. Subjects may have difficulty recalling an event as the result of memory problems, or the event may be un-

derreported because of a socially undesirable outcome, for example, research on the prevalence of falls. Another disadvantage of retrospective studies is that causation cannot be inferred. The presence of temporal antecedence, that is, when one event precedes another in time, does not automatically indicate that one event caused the other.

Prospective Design. In a prospective study the researcher selects a population and follows it over time to determine outcomes. Subjects are usually selected because they have the potential to develop a specific disease or effect of interest. Prospective studies are frequently used in epidemiologic research to determine what effect exposure to certain risk factors has on the development of disease. Subjects are chosen based on exposure status and followed over time to determine the incidence of disease.

ADVANTAGES AND DISADVANTAGES. One advantage of prospective studies is that they are a stronger research design than retrospective studies and can provide more convincing evidence of the nature of the relationship between variables. The results obtained from prospective studies may provide essential preliminary research to generate hypotheses that can be tested with other experimental or quasi-experimental methods. In prospective research it is easier to determine the sequencing of events over time, which makes prospective studies more useful in determining temporal antecedence. Disadvantages of prospective studies is that they are time-consuming and expensive and may require large samples. Although prospective studies are a stronger design than retrospectve studies, they still cannot be used to infer causality.

Path Analysis Design. Path analysis is a complex research design that uses statistical analysis to test hypothesized causal relationships. Path analysis is a nonexperimental design; therefore there is no manipulation of variables. The hypothesis to be tested is often a theory or model that has been developed. Using path analysis the model can be tested to determine if it is supported or rejected by the data. If data supports the model, the model is not proven to be correct, but only shown to be plausible. In path analysis the structural model that is developed can be used to determine the impact that one variable has on other variables. This is important if the results are to be used to project future trends or the future demand for services. Path analysis also allows the researcher to determine both main effects and interaction effects. Main effects are the effects of one variable on another variable. Interaction effects are the effects of the interaction of two or more variables on other variables.

ADVANTAGES AND DISADVANTAGES. The advantage of path analysis is that it is a means to test theories and conceptual frameworks. Path analysis is particularly useful for problems that have several aspects and multiple variables. Another advantage of path analysis is that it provides stronger evidence for causality than other types of ex post facto research. However, the disadvantage of path analysis is that it is weaker than experimental or quasi-experimental designs.

Predictive Design. In a predictive design the researcher analyzes data on one group of subjects to predict how another group of subjects will respond. Predictive research can be retrospective and can study the relationships among variables for which the outcome is known, or it can be prospective in which an attempt is made to determine how one group will do based on data previously obtained from another group. For instance, in studying the health service utilization patterns of the rural elderly based on functional and physical impairments, it is possible to use a retrospective or a prospective design. Data on physical impairments, functional impairments, and health service utilization can be collected. From this information the researcher can determine what physical and functional impairments are predictive of increased health service utilization. Once these predictor variables are known, it is possible to apply them to other populations to prospectively predict, based on physical or functional impairments, who is at high risk for increased utilization of health care services. When using a predictive design, data are analyzed, and a regression equation is developed. This equation serves as a model to predict how groups that are similar to the sample population will respond in the future.

ADVANTAGES AND DISADVANTAGES. One of the advantages of predictive research is that it can serve as a tool in the decision-making process regarding specific programs or treatments. The disadvantage of predictive research is that the behavior of one group will never correspond exactly to that of another group. Predictions are always subject to error.

♋ NONTRADITIONAL DESIGN

The final type of research that will be described is nontraditional research. There is some discrepancy in the literature about the categorization of nontraditional research, and several authors classify nontraditional designs as experimental, quasi-experimental, or descriptive. This is because categories overlap and several nontraditional designs do use methods from other

---

NONTRADITIONAL DESIGNS

Case studies   Secondary analysis
Historical research   Evaluation research
Methodological research   Needs assessment
Metaanalysis

---

major categories of research designs. Non-traditional research is considered separately here because many of the designs do not fit easily in one of the other categories. The nontraditional designs that will be described are listed in the box.

CASE STUDIES

Case studies are often considered a detailed analysis of one individual. However, case studies can also be used to study specific groups or organizations. A case study is frequently used when there is a new phenomenon about which not much is known or for very rare events in which few subjects can be found. An example is the case studies of the first HIV+ individuals that were conducted before much was known about the disease. Case studies provide significant amounts of descriptive information, and they can also provide some explanatory information about *why*, as well as *what*.

Advantages and Disadvantages

One of the advantages of case studies is the detailed level of analysis that results when research is confined to a small number of subjects. Another advantage of case studies is that a complete analysis can provide evidence for the relationships among variables. This may stimulate additional research questions in an area of study. A disadvantage is that when research is limited to a small number of subjects, the results are not readily generalized to other populations. Case studies are also difficult

to replicate because future researchers may not have access to the same subjects, and if another subject is used, results may differ.

HISTORICAL RESEARCH

Historical research does study past events; however, historical research should never be confused with ex post facto research in which a retrospective design is used. Historical research is a type of nonexperimental research, because there can be no randomization or manipulation of past events and a retrospective design is used. However, the focus of historical research is usually quite different than the focus of ex post facto research. Historical research involves a detailed study of individuals, events, institutions, or specific time periods. Often historical researchers are able to use the data they have obtained to more accurately explain current trends in society or health care. Historical research involves more than just describing past events; good historical research is guided by research questions and hypotheses. The major data sources for historical research are divided into primary and secondary sources. Primary sources are original documents such as letters, books, written records of proceedings, and other first-hand accounts. Primary sources can also include nonprint media such as oral histories, photographs, or movies. Secondary sources are those that are not written or obtained directly from the subjects. These include books and articles about a subject, such as biographies.

Advantages and Disadvantages

One advantage of historical research is that it can provide insights into the past. This information is valuable in its own right, but it is also valuable because it can enlighten the present. A present-day situation may be more clearly understood when it is viewed in the context of history. The disadvantage of historical research is that the researcher must rely on available data sources. This may pose some difficulties if documents have been destroyed and subjects of interest are no longer alive. Frequently, available sources dictate the type of questions that can be asked. For example, in a study of a significant leader in nursing history, the following two questions could only directly be asked of an individual who was still living: (1) What factors contributed to your decision to become a nurse? (2) What factors contributed to your development as a leader within the nursing profession? When studying a person who is no longer alive the researcher could use a personal journal, if available, to answer the preceding questions, but information could not be obtained directly from the subject. Moreover, if a personal journal was not available, an attempt could be made to obtain the data from secondary sources. These secondary sources may or may not provide accurate data. Another disadvantage of historical research is that the researcher must determine the validity of sources and must contend with the possibility that sources and data are not reliable.

METHODOLOGICAL RESEARCH

Methodological research is conducted to improve the methods used in other research investigations. Frequently methodological research centers on the development of specific data collection tools such as instruments and `questionnaires. The goal of methodological research is to improve the reliability and validity of data collection tools, which increases the control and reduces the threats to internal and external validity that can result from using instruments and questionnaires. Using this design the researcher also attempts to improve the construct validity of data collection tools. Although methodological research may appear tedious, it is extremely important to other research endeavors. In the absence of methodological research it would be impossible to conduct many quantitative studies, and every study would have to develop a new research instrument.

Advantages and Disadvantages

The advantage of methodological research is that when good instruments are developed, they may be used across studies and across disciplines. A disadvantage is that instrument development can be very difficult and time-consuming. Some individuals would also argue that it is not possible to develop an instrument that is completely reliable and valid and that the use of instruments always creates problems in interpreting the data. While there are some limitations inherent in using instruments, essential research could not be conducted without them.

METAANALYSIS

In a metaanalysis the results from a large number of previously conducted studies are used as data for statistical analysis. A metaanalysis is usually done on a topic such as a specific aspect of pain (i.e., pain management or assessment of pain). The researcher consults the published pain literature for relevant studies, and the results of each of these studies become one piece of data. Metaanalysis is becoming a more popular design for nurse researchers as the amount of well-conducted nursing research has increased.

Advantages and Disadvantages

One of the advantages of a metaanalysis is that because it uses previously conducted research, it may be faster than several other methods. Another advantage is that when results from several studies are combined, the results of a metaanalysis may point to relationships that were not apparent in the analysis of each individual study. A disadvantage is that the researcher may combine studies that measure conceptually different things. In these instances a metaanalysis may combine data that should not be combined. Another disadvantage is that because a metaanalysis makes use of data from published studies, selection of those published studies may be biased toward those that showed a result rather than no result. In using metaanalysis the researcher must also rely on the validity of the findings as reported by the authors of the selected studies.

SECONDARY ANALYSIS

Secondary analysis, like metaanalysis, uses data that has previously been collected. It differs from metaanalysis in that secondary analysis uses data from one specific data base. The data can come from large data bases that have been collected through large surveys or from smaller research projects. In conducting a secondary analysis the researcher formulates hypotheses and then uses existing data for the statistical analysis. When using a large data base for a secondary analysis, the researcher frequently analyzes only a portion of the data rather than the entire data base.

Advantages and Disadvantages

One of the main advantages of a secondary analysis is that it is much less expensive and time-consuming than research that involves data collection. The disadvantage of secondary analysis is that the data available may not be exactly what the researcher would like. Some important information may be missing, which may make it impossible to answer all the questions of interest to the researcher. Another disadvantage is that the data may not be in the exact form the researcher would like. This may limit the type of statistical tests that can be used to analyze the data.

EVALUATION RESEARCH

When a specific program is instituted, it becomes necessary at some point to evaluate its effectiveness. Evaluation research is conducted to determine how well a program was implemented and how well it accomplished its purpose. There are two broad categories of evaluation research: formative and summative. Formative evaluation of an existing program determines if it was implemented as planned, if it is working as planned, and if it can be improved. A summative evaluation is conducted on an ongoing or completed program to determine whether the program met the stated objectives.

Advantages and Disadvantages

The advantages of evaluation research is that it can provide important and useful results. Evaluation research is helpful in combination with policy analysis to determine which programs should be continued and which should be terminated. Evaluation research also provides a mechanism for quantifying the results of a program, which can be useful in obtaining ongoing funding or to demonstrate program effectiveness. One disadvantage of evaluation research is that it can be difficult to obtain unbiased and accurate information from individuals connected with a program who have a financial or emotional investment in the continuation of the program. Another disadvantage is that a program may be diffi-

EVALUATING THE RESEARCH DESIGN

1. What specific type of research design is used?
2. Is the research design appropriate for the study question(s)?
3. What other research designs could have been used for this study?
4. Are the research methods clearly described?
5. How well does the research design control threats to statistical conclusion validity, internal validity, construct validity of putative causes and effects, and external validity?
6. What threats to validity are not controlled by the research design? How does this affect usefulness of the results?
7. How well does the research design determine causality between the independent and dependent variables?

cult to evaluate because it does not have clearly defined goals. It is also possible that while some of the goals of the program may have been met, other goals may not have been met. In these instances it may be difficult to evaluate the effectiveness of the total program.

NEEDS ASSESSMENT

A needs assessment is used to determine what would be most beneficial to a specific group of individuals. Needs assessments have many different applications. They can be used by organizations to determine what is needed by their employees or by agencies to determine what is needed by those they serve. A needs assessment is conducted by obtaining input from agency insiders, by getting a broader perspective through a survey of needs, or by addressing problems as they present themselves.

Advantages and Disadvantages

One of the advantages of conducting a needs assessment is that it is then possible to make changes that more clearly reflect perceived need. Another advantage is that with a well-conducted needs assessment, the researcher is in a position to make rec-

ommendations for interventions or programs. The disadvantage of needs assessment is that a decision must be made as to who will have input into the process. For example, in an effort to improve patient care, hospital administrators may have a specific idea about what is needed. However, a survey of general hospital employees may produce conflicting data. Another disadvantage is that while the results of a needs assessment may indicate that a specific problem must be addressed, it may not be politically feasible to do so.

EVALUATING THE RESEARCH DESIGN

An analysis of any research study or research article should include an evaluation of the research design utilized. There are several specific criteria that can be used when evaluating a research design. These criteria are summarized in the box above.

SUMMARY

- The type of research design used for a particular study is dependent on the research question(s), resources available to the researcher, and the personal preferences of the researcher.

- The four types of research design described in this chapter are the following:
  - *Experimental.* Provides the strongest evidence for causality and is characterized by manipulation, control, and randomization. *Experimental designs* include pretest-posttest control group design, posttest-only control group design, Solomon four-group design, factorial design, randomized block design, and clinical trials.
  - *Quasi-experimental.* Useful design to test causality in field settings when complete control or randomization is not possible. *Quasi-experimental designs* include one-group posttest-only design, static-group comparison, one-group pretest-only design, nonequivalent control group designs, and interrupted time series designs.
  - *Nonexperimental.* Designs that do not involve manipulation, control, or randomization, but are useful to describe and measure the independent and dependent variables. *Nonexperimental designs* include descriptive designs and ex post facto designs. Descriptive designs include survey research (simple descriptive survey design, comparative descriptive survey design, and developmental survey design). Ex post facto design includes descriptive correlational design, retrospective design, prospective design, path analysis design, and predictive design.
  - *Nontraditional.* Designs that do not fit easily into one of the other categories. Designs categorized as *nontraditional* include case studies, historical research, methodological research, metaanalysis, secondary analysis, evaluation research, and needs assessment.

FACILITATING CRITICAL THINKING

1. Answer the following questions based on your knowledge of the four types of research design presented in the chapter (experimental, quasi-experimental, nonexperimental, and nontraditional).
   a. What features characterize each type?
   b. In what ways do the major research types differ from one another?
   c. What are the strengths and limitations of each type of research design?
   d. List specific research questions that could be explored with each type of design.
2. You would like to study the relationship between level of care provider in a community mental health center (clinical nurse specialist, psychiatrist, psychologist, social worker), diagnosis, and psychological and physical health and functioning.
   a. What research design is appropriate to explore the research question?
   b. Is it possible to allocate subjects to control and treatment groups?
   c. What are the potential threats to validity in using the chosen research design?
   d. How could the researcher reduce bias in this study?

References
CONCEPTUAL

HENNEKENS, C. H., & BURING, J. E. (1987). *Epidemiology in medicine.* Boston: Little, Brown.

METHODOLOGICAL

BRINK, P. J., & WOOD, M. J. (Eds.). (1989). *Advanced design in nursing research.* Newbury Park, CA: Sage.

HOLM, K., & LLEWELLYN, J. G. (1986). *Nursing research for nursing practice.* Philadelphia: W. B. Saunders.

HULLEY, S. B., & CUMMINGS, S. R. (1988). *Designing clinical research: An epidemiological approach.* Baltimore: Williams & Wilkins.

Leedy, P. D. (1989). *Practical research: Planning and design* (4th ed.). New York: Macmillan.

McLaughlin, F. E., & Marascuilo, L. A. (1990). *Advanced nursing and health care research: Quantification approaches.* Philadelphia: W. B. Saunders.

Oyster, C. K., Hanten, W. P., & Llorens, L. A. (1987). *Introduction to research: A guide for the health science professional.* Philadelphia: J. B. Lippincott.

Polit, D. F., & Hungler, B. P. (1991). *Nursing research: Principles and methods* (4th ed.). Philadelphia: J. B. Lippincott.

Waltz, C., & Bausell, R. B. (1981). *Nursing research: Design, statistics and computer analysis.* Philadelphia: F. A. Davis.

Woods, N. F., & Catanzaro, M. (1988). *Nursing research: Theory and practice.* St. Louis: Mosby-Year Book.

HISTORICAL

Cook, T. C., & Campbell, D. T. (1979). *Quasi-experimentation: Design & analysis issues for field settings.* Boston: Houghton Mifflin.

CHAPTER 13

POPULATIONS AND SAMPLES

LAURA A. TALBOT

There is a generalization that all women who develop gallstones have three major characteristics (often called the three Fs): fair, fat, and forty. This generalization was made from observations that women with fair skin and excess weight and who were approximately 40 years of age were more likely to develop gallstones. These observations were based on a select group or sample of patients with gallstones requiring surgical intervention; they were then generalized to the entire population of patients with gallstones. The description may or may not apply in every case, but because the "three Fs" are common characteristics, all women with gallstones are grouped in this category.

Sampling is a complex process. To avoid inappropriate generalizations, the researcher needs to take appropriate steps to ensure that the sample is a true representation of the population. In the above example a reviewer of research would question the sampling approach used by the researcher. Was this a sample of convenience or a simple random sample? Are the conclusions generalizable to the total population? Was there a large enough sample size?

In 1972 the Nurses' Health Study did conduct a 4-year study to explore the risk factors associated with gallstone formation. The sample consisted of 88,837 women who were registered nurses. They ranged in age from 34 to 59 years. Factors examined included diet, alcoholic intake, weight, and height. The findings supported previous beliefs about gallstone formation. Moderately overweight women were two times more likely to develop gallstones than lean women. Obese women were six times more likely to develop gallstones than lean women. An unexpected finding was that women who drank two to three servings of alcoholic beverages per week were less likely to develop gallstones than nondrinkers (Maclure et al, 1989).

This chapter discusses the steps in making decisions about the type of sample needed for a research project. Sampling theory is reviewed, sampling terms defined, and a step-by-step sampling plan is detailed.

240

SAMPLING THEORY

Sampling theory is a mathematical method of decision making for determining the most efficient means of selecting a sample that represents the population under study. Theorems backed by proof enable the researcher to estimate the precision or accuracy of a sampling procedure and thus ensure greater accuracy in the resulting generalization to the larger population. This refers to the ability of the sampling method to generalize the results to the general population.

Sampling theory is the foundation for current sampling methods used in research. To understand the rationale behind the sampling process, critical concepts need to be defined and discussed as they relate to sampling theory.

SAMPLING TERMS

Sampling is the process of selecting a portion of the population to obtain data regarding a problem. Terms specific to the process of sampling include *population, sample, parameter, statistic, randomization, sampling error,* and *sampling bias.*

POPULATION

A population is a group whose members possess specific attributes that a researcher is interested in studying. The population may consist of events, places, objects, animals, or individuals. In research two populations are described: the target population and the accessible population. The target population is the population under study, the population to which the researcher wants to generalize the research findings. An example of a target population is all institutionalized older adults with dementia in the United States. Institutions would in-clude nursing homes, hospitals, retirement centers, and board-and-care facilities. The researcher would have to contact all the institutions in the United States who care for older adults with dementia. Then a list of all residents with the diagnosis of dementia would have to be generated by the institution and sent back to the researcher. It would be very expensive and time consuming to list all the people in this target population.

A more realistic approach would be to use an accessible population. An accessible population is that part of the target population that is available to the researcher. An example of an accessible population would be all hospitalized older adults with dementia in Parkland Hospital.

Lynn, McCain, and Boss (1989) in their study of the "Socialization of R.N. to B.S.N." identify their target population as all registered nurse students pursuing bachelor degrees. The accessible population for their study was registered nurses and generic students enrolled in "a moderately sized, upper-division baccalaureate degree program in a state university in the southeastern United States" (p. 233). By accessing only a portion of the target population, the researchers saved time and money.

SAMPLE

A sample is a portion of the population that has been selected to represent the population of interest. A sampling unit is the overall entity used for sample selection. The sampling unit can be a specific site or setting. For example, if a researcher was studying diet changes of first trimester women, the sampling unit for the study could be the office of an obstetrician. In the Lynn, McCain, and Boss (1989) study, the sample was 30 registered nurses and 193 generic students who participated in the study based on a population of 359 students enrolled in the baccalaureate program. The sampling unit for the study was the baccalaureate program located in the state university.

ELEMENT

The element is a single member of the population under study. It is from the sampling elements that data are collected. Other common terms used interchangeably for sampling element are *subject* or *participant*. The sampling element can be an animal, person, object, event, or group.

SAMPLING FRAME

The sampling frame is a comprehensive list of all the sampling elements in the target population. The study sample is drawn from the sampling frame. The sample is only as accurate as the sampling frame from which it is selected. Every element in the population must be included in the sampling frame. If an element is listed more than once, the chances for selection into the study are increased. Conversely, if an element is omitted, then every element in the population does not have an equal chance of being selected.

An example of a sampling frame is used by the Nurses' Health Study. "In 1976, 121,700 female registered nurses 30 to 50 years of age who were living in 11 large U.S. states completed a mailed questionnaire on known and suspected risk factors for cancer and coronary heart disease" (Willett et al, 1990, p. 1665). The sampling frame for this study was a list of all the registered nurses in these 11 states provided by each state's Board of Nurse Examiners; all were sent a questionnaire. The study sample was drawn from the sampling frame. This sample consisted of the 121,700 female registered nurses who completed the questionnaire and mailed it back

to the researchers. If the state board had omitted a name from the list, then the list would not be representative of all registered nurses in that state.

PARAMETER AND STATISTIC

Data are information collected from a source. It is important to identify the source from which the information is obtained. Information (data) collected from a sample is called a statistic. Information (data) collected from a population is called a parameter. An even more important difference is that we estimate parameters, and statistics represent parameters.

RANDOM SELECTION AND REPRESENTATIVENESS

Random selection is a process of selecting a representative sample of the target population. Its purpose is to ensure that every element in the target population has an equal, independent, and nonzero chance of being selected for inclusion in the study.

Representativeness is how well the sample represents the variables of interest in the target population, as well as other demographic information. The sample should replicate the population in approximately the same proportions as it occurs in the target population. Demographic information commonly looked at includes educational level, gender, ethnicity, age, and income level. One method of achieving representativeness is by using random selection techniques when selecting the sample from the sampling frame. These techniques ensure, to a degree of confidence, that the data collected from the sample represent the characteristics of the target population.

SAMPLING ERROR

The advantage of using a sample instead of the entire population is that it saves time, money, and resources. The disadvantage is that a sample is not identical to the population. When sample data are collected and statistically analyzed, the statistics calculated for the sample will differ from the population parameters. Even if two samples are drawn from the same population, both samples will vary to some degree. Sampling error is the difference or error between the sample statistic and the population parameter. When random selection is used to obtain a sample, sampling error can be estimated statistically by the researcher by calculating the standard error.

STANDARD ERROR

Standard error is the measurement of the standard distance (deviation) between a sample measure and the population measure. This measure can be the mean or the correlation coefficient. For example, if a researcher were looking at a specific characteristic of older adults with diagnosed glaucoma, it would be impossible to measure every diagnosed older adult in the universe. Using a random selection technique to select 100 older adults with diagnosed glaucoma in the Oklahoma City area would be more feasible. If the mean were calculated for that characteristic, it would be important to know how close the sample mean was to the population mean. Unfortunately we cannot calculate the population mean; we can only estimate its value based on the sample mean. The standard error tests to see if the sample mean is an accurate estimate of the population mean.

The sampling error estimates the amount of error the researcher can anticipate if the sample measure (e.g., mean, standard deviation) is used to estimate the population measure. Sampling error is based on chance variations in the data resulting from selecting a sample with few subjects as compared to the population's many possible subjects. Sampling error can

be decreased by increasing the sample size. In general, the larger the sample size, the smaller the sampling error and the more closely the sample will represent the population. Unfortunately, error is inherent and even a large sample is not always a panacea to correct it (Slakter et al, 1991).

SAMPLING BIAS

Sampling bias occurs when the researcher shows a preference in selecting one participant over another. This could be conscious or subconscious on the part of the researcher. Whereas sampling error is the result of chance, sampling bias is based on nonchance occurrence. When using any sampling method, there is always the chance that sampling bias will occur. The probability of sampling bias occurring increases when random selection is not used.

SAMPLING APPROACHES

There are two basic approaches to sampling: probability and nonprobability sampling. The randomness of probability sampling offers the advantage of being the most representative, allowing more accurate generalization to the target population. The advantage of nonprobability sampling is that it is less expensive and more time efficient. Both approaches are examined in more detail on the following pages.

PROBABILITY SAMPLING

Probability sampling is a randomized method of selecting participants in a research study who are the most representative of the target population. In probability sampling, each element or participant has an independent chance (or probability greater than zero) of being included in the study. By using this method, the researcher can estimate the probability each population element has of being represented in the sample.

Probability sampling also allows for appropriate use of inferential statistics. The basic assumption of inferential statistics is that random sample selection was used. The researcher then applies inferential statistics to the sample data and generalizes the results to the target population. When the sample is an accurate representation of the population, the sample statistics will approximate the population more precisely.

Probability sampling designs are plans to obtain a probability sample. Four types of probability sampling designs are simple random sampling, stratified random sampling, cluster sampling, and systematic sampling. Examples of all four types of probability sampling designs as seen in the literature are presented in Table 13-1.

Simple Random Sampling
The characteristics of simple random sampling include (1) an independent chance for each element to be selected into the study, (2) a complete list of the accessible population, and (3) a one-stage selection process.

To start, the researcher identifies the target population. A sampling frame, or list of all the elements of the target population, is created. In the McCabe (1989) study, a sample of 318 registered nurses was drawn at random from a sampling frame of RNs with current licensure and residency in a midwestern state (Table 13-1).

After the sampling frame is created, the next task is to randomly select participants. Each element in the sampling frame is assigned a consecutive identification number, and a method of randomizing the sample selection is then chosen. Three means of randomizing are (1) placing the numbers in a bowl and drawing out the numbers one at a time, (2) using a table of random numbers, or (3) using a computer-generated selection of random numbers.

When a bowl is used, the numbers are drawn out of the bowl one at a time and placed back in the bowl after each drawing. This is to ensure that each participant has an equal and independent chance of being selected. Using this approach, each 100 names would have a 1/100 chance of being selected each time. This is called random sampling with replacement. By returning the numbers to the bowl, there is also a chance that the same number would be selected twice.

If the researcher does not return the number to the bowl, each participant does not have an equal and independent chance of being selected. For example, if the sample frame has 100 names, each participant will initially have a 1/100 chance of being selected. After 20 names have been selected, there would be a 1/80 chance of being selected in the sample. This is called random sampling without replacement. The bowl method of random sampling has largely been replaced by the two other methods: a table of random numbers and computer-generated selection.

A table of random numbers can be used to randomize identification numbers for participant selection. Such a table can be found in most statistical books, or the researcher can generate a set of random numbers with the use of a computer. A table of random numbers is presented in Figure 13-1.

To use this method, select a starting point on the table by pointing to a number on the table without looking. This number is the first sample element. You may then move in any direction on the page (e.g., horizontally, vertically, diagonally, backward) as long as a consistent approach is

Table 13-1
Probability Sampling

Sampling Procedure	Research Article Example	Description of Method
Simple random sample	McCabe, B. (1989). Ego defensiveness and its relationship to attitudes of registered nurses toward older people. *Research in Nursing & Health, 12,* 85-91.	A sample of 318 registered nurses was drawn at random from a listing of RNs with current licensure and residency in a midwestern state.
Stratified random sample	Franks, F., & Faux, S. (1990). Depression, stress mastery, and social resources in four ethnocultural women's groups. *Research in Nursing & Health, 13,* 283-292.	From a community ethnic master list, a stratified random sample of 212 subjects were chosen to make up four strata of Chinese, Vietnamese, Portuguese, and Latin American immigrant women.
Cluster sample	Jackson, B., Taylor, J., Pyngolil, M. (1991). How age conditions the relationship between climacteric status and health symptoms in African-American women, *Research in Nursing & Health, 14,* 1-9.	From 27 predominantly black neighborhoods, 9 neighborhoods were randomly selected. From those 9 neighborhoods, 1500 households were randomly selected. The final sample consisted of 522 African-American women.
Systematic random sample	Gross, D., Rocissano, L., Roncoli, M. (1989). Maternal confidence during toddlerhood: Comparing preterm and full-term groups. *Research in Nursing & Health, 12,* 1-9.	A systematic random sample of 146 mothers of toddlers was selected from a population of 4000 mothers who delivered full-term babies at a northeastern metropolitan hospital. Hospital chart codes were used to select the sample. A comparative sample of 116 mothers of preterm infants was also selected.

used. Circle each element on the sampling frame whose number coincides with the one on the table of random numbers. When the same number is selected twice, simply ignore it. If there is a number higher than the numbers in the sampling frame, ignore it also. Continue selecting numbers until the desired sample size is attained.

Many existing tables are large enough to accommodate five-digit numbers. if the sample is to consist of 150 subjects, the researcher uses three columns of random numbers. It could be the first three or the last three columns. As long as the approach is consistent, the choice of columns does not matter.

A computer-generated selection of ran-

	00-04	05-09	10-14	15-19	20-24	25-29	30-34	35-39	40-44	45-49
00	54463	22662	63905	70639	79265	67382	29085	69831	47058	08186
01	15389	85205	18850	39226	42249	90669	96325	23248	60933	26927
02	85941	40756	82414	02015	13858	78030	16269	65978	01385	15345
03	61149	69440	11286	88218	58925	03638	52862	62733	33451	77455
04	05219	81619	10651	67079	92511	39888	84502	72095	83463	75577
05	41417	98326	87719	92294	46614	50948	64886	20002	97365	30976
06	28357	94070	20652	35714	16249	75019	21145	05217	47286	76305
07	17783	00015	10806	83091	91530	36466	39981	63481	49177	75779
08	40950	84820	29881	85966	62800	70326	84740	62660	77379	90279
09	82995	64157	66164	41180	10089	41757	78258	96488	88629	37231
10	96754	17676	55639	44105	47361	34833	86679	23930	53249	27083
11	34357	88040	53364	71726	45690	66334	60332	22554	90600	71113
12	06318	37403	49927	57715	50423	67372	63116	48888	21505	80182
13	62111	52820	07243	79931	89292	84767	85693	73947	22278	11551
14	47534	09243	67879	00544	23410	12740	02540	54440	32949	13491
15	98614	75993	84460	62846	59844	14922	48730	73443	48167	34770
16	24856	03648	44898	09351	98795	18644	39765	71058	90368	44104
17	96887	12479	80621	66223	86085	78285	02432	53342	42846	94771
18	90801	21472	42815	77408	37390	76766	52615	32141	30268	18106
19	55165	77312	83666	36028	28420	70219	81369	41943	47366	41067
20	75884	12952	84318	95108	72305	64620	91318	89872	45375	85436
21	16777	37116	58550	42938	21460	43910	01175	87894	81378	10620
22	46230	43877	80207	88877	89380	32992	91380	03164	98656	59337
23	42902	66892	46134	01432	94710	23474	20423	60137	60609	13119
24	81007	00333	39693	28039	10154	95425	39230	19774	31782	49037
25	68089	01122	51111	72373	06902	74373	96199	97017	41273	21546
26	20411	67081	89950	16944	93054	87687	96693	87236	77054	33848
27	58212	13160	06468	15718	82627	76999	05999	58680	96739	63700
28	70577	42866	24969	61210	76046	67699	42054	12696	93758	03283
29	94522	74358	71659	62038	79643	79169	44741	05437	39038	13163
30	42626	86819	85651	88678	17401	03252	99547	32404	17918	62880
31	16051	33763	57194	16752	54450	19031	58580	47629	54132	60631
32	08244	27647	33851	44705	94211	46716	11738	55784	95374	72655
33	58497	04392	09419	89964	51211	04894	72882	17805	21896	83864
34	97155	13428	40293	09985	58434	01412	69124	82171	59058	82859
35	98409	66162	95763	47420	20792	61527	20441	39435	11859	41567
36	45476	84882	65109	96597	25930	66790	65706	61203	53634	22557
37	89300	69700	50741	30329	11658	23166	05400	66669	48708	03887
38	50051	95137	91631	66315	91428	12275	24816	68081	71710	33258
39	31753	85178	31310	89642	98364	02306	24617	09609	83942	22716
40	79152	53829	77250	20190	56535	18760	69942	77448	33278	48805
41	44560	38750	83635	56540	64900	42912	13953	79149	18710	68618
42	68328	83378	63369	71381	39564	05615	42451	64559	97501	65747
43	46939	38689	58625	08342	30459	85863	20781	09284	26333	91777
44	83544	86141	15707	96256	23068	13782	08467	89469	93842	55349
45	91621	00881	04900	54224	46177	55309	17852	27491	89415	23466
46	91896	67126	04151	03795	59077	11848	12630	98375	52068	60142
47	55751	62515	21108	80830	02263	29303	37204	96926	30506	09808
48	85156	87689	95493	88842	00664	55017	55539	17771	69448	87530
49	07521	56898	12236	60277	39102	62315	12239	07105	11844	01117

Figure 13-1. Table of random numbers. From *Statistical Methods* (6th ed.), G. W. Coebran. Copyright © by Iowa State University Press, Ames, Iowa. Reprinted by permission.

dom numbers is a must for large samples and large sampling frames. When compared to the bowl or table of random numbers methods, computer-generated selection will save the researcher a great deal of time. The actual steps in obtaining the random numbers will depend on the software package used by the researcher.

The advantages of using simple random sampling are that it eliminates researcher bias, requires limited knowledge about the population, and provides a means for estimating sampling error. The disadvantage is that a complete list of the accessible population is needed. In addition, for large samples and large sampling frames, simple random sampling can be very time consuming unless a computer is used to assist in the process. Also random sampling is still no guarantee that the sample is representative; this increases with sample size.

Stratified Random Sampling
Stratified random sampling is used to ensure representativeness of different groups within the population. Strata are determined by mutually exclusive variables such as ethnicity, gender, age, or educational level. The term *mutually exclusive* means that each sample element belongs to only one group or stratum. After the population is divided, a simple random sample is taken within each stratum.

Herth (1990) used simple stratified random sampling in her study of the relationship of hope, coping styles, concurrent losses, and setting to the resolution of grief in the elderly widow(er). A list of bereaved spouses was identified through the records of two hospices, two hospitals, and two skilled nursing homes in a midsize southwestern United States city. "Simple stratified random sampling with replacement was used to ensure that an equal number of subjects (25 each) was obtained according

to setting (hospital, hospice, nursing home)" (p. 111).

Proportional stratified sampling is a method of increasing the representativeness of the variable in the sample. The number of participants taken from each stratum would be proportional to the number in the population. If the strata were to be gender-based and the target population consisted of 3000 men and 7000 women, the sample size would be calculated proportionally: 30% men and 70% women. So for a sample of 100, the stratum of men would consist of 30 and the stratum of women would consist of 70.

Disproportional stratified sampling occurs when the number of elements in each stratum is not proportional to the number in the population. So in the above example, instead of using 30 men and 70 women, the researcher may choose to use 50 men and 50 women to get responses from both sexes that are more representative of the general population versus the target population. When using disproportional stratified sampling, the researcher may want to weigh the responses for each stratum. This is accomplished by using a mathematical formula that statistically determines the proportion contributed by each stratum to the total value of all the strata.

The advantage of stratified random sampling is that it ensures the representation of a particular segment of the population. The disadvantage of stratified random sampling is that it requires extensive knowledge of the population under study to stratify it accurately. Depending on the use of proportional or disproportional stratified sampling, knowledge of advanced statistical methods and/or assistance of a sampling consultant will be needed.

Two other disadvantages of stratified random sampling are that (1) a complete list of the target population is needed, and (2) it can quickly become very complex. For example, when studying some aspect of nursing students, two sexes, three types of nursing programs, and four sections of the country lead to 24 segments.

Cluster Sampling

Often the population the researcher plans to study is so large that it would take an enormous amount of time and money to set up a sampling frame for simple random sampling. For example, in a large-scale national study of all registered nurses, the state boards for all 50 states would have to be contacted for a list of current registered nurses in each state. After random sampling, the sample itself may only consist of two or three RNs per state. Then depending on the data collection method used, the researcher may have to contact them by long-distance telephone or travel to interview the participants, which could be very expensive. An alternate method of sampling is cluster sampling.

Cluster sampling takes place in stages. The researcher begins with the largest, most inclusive sampling unit, then progresses to the next most inclusive sampling unit until the final stage is the selection of the elements or participants in the study. Because of the different stages involved, this method is often called multistage sampling. Cluster sampling differs from stratified random sampling in that in the latter every stratum is sampled and data are collected from each stratum. In cluster sampling, data are not collected from each cluster; instead only the final elements derived from among the clusters are tested.

First, the researcher identifies the population to be studied, such as all registered nurses in the United States. A sampling frame is developed. For this example the most inclusive sampling unit would be all

50 states. From this sampling frame a cluster is randomly selected. In this case that could be all registered nurses in three states. If the researcher stops here, the type of cluster sampling used would be a simple one-stage cluster.

If the researcher chooses to continue, the researcher could contact the state board of nurse examiners from the three states and ask for a list of RNs according to districts or counties. The researcher would again randomly select a cluster of three districts or counties from each state. The final participants would be all the RNs on a comprehensive list from those nine districts or counties. If the researcher stops here, the type of cluster sampling used would be a two-stage cluster.

If the researcher chooses to continue, the researcher could identify all the hospitals located in the previously selected nine districts or counties. The researcher again randomly selects a cluster of three hospitals from each district or county for a total of nine. The final participants would be all the RNs listed on a comprehensive list working in those nine hospitals. This would be a multistage cluster because successive groups are randomly selected until the final sample of elements has been reached (see Figure 13-2 for a visual illustration of the above example).

Jackson, Taylor, and Pyngolil (1991) used a multistaged cluster sampling technique to study climacteric status and health symptoms in African-American women. Climacteric was defined in the study as the transition stage from biological reproductivity to nonreproductivity. The following is a description of the sampling technique:

> The sample of 522 25- to 75-year-old African-American women was drawn from nine neighborhoods selected randomly from a universe of 27 predominantly black

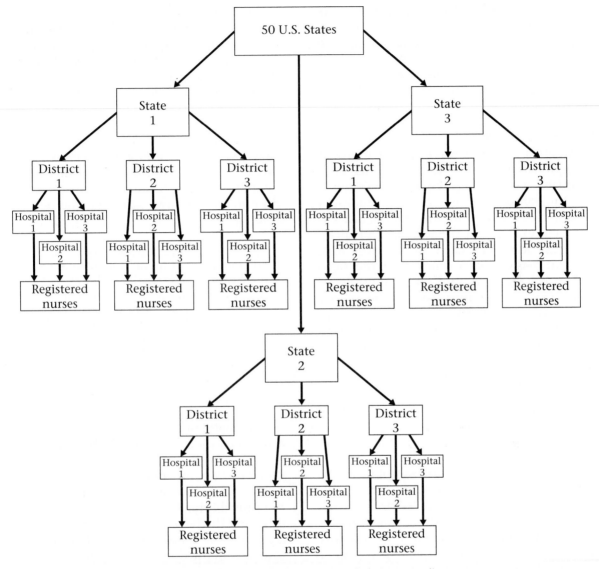

Figure 13-2. Example of multistaged cluster sampling.

neighborhoods in a large eastern city. Within these nine targeted neighborhoods, which included three senior citizen high-rise buildings, five enumerators identified over 7000 residential units. Estimating that one person would be eligible and agreeable for 2.5 households contacted, 1500 households were randomly selected from these subuniverses of addresses. A proportional cluster sampling technique was used to apportion these 1500 cases to each neighborhood. Under these procedures we found that the ratio of sampling error for clustering over the sampling error for a random sample was well within acceptable limits. (pp. 2-3)

The advantages of cluster sampling are that (1) it is economical and time saving, and (2) it allows probability sampling for a population that is not easily listed in a sampling frame. The disadvantage is the possibility for sampling error at each stage of the sampling process.

Systematic Sampling

Systematic sampling can be a probability or nonprobability sampling design. To be a probability sampling design, the elements in the sampling frame need to be listed randomly. If placed in any order, a bias exists. For example, if the RNs on a medical-surgical unit were listed and if every fifth person was a charge nurse and the sampling interval was five (or a multiple of five), the charge nurse would be picked every time or not at all.

Next the first element is chosen at random from the sampling frame. Then every kth element in the sampling frame is systematically chosen to be in the sample (k being a constant). The sampling interval, k, is determined by

$$k = \frac{N}{n}$$

In this equation, k is the sampling interval used in the sample selection, "N" is the accessible population, and "n" is the sample size. Using this fraction, the interval can be determined by dividing the accessible population by the sample. For example, a population list of 5000 with a sample size of 500 would yield an interval of 10. The starting element is obtained by randomly selecting a number from 1 to 10. The researcher would then systematically include every tenth element into the sample.

Another way to use this formula is to (1) decide on the sample size, (2) find out how many elements are in the population, (3) divide the sample size into the population

to give an interval width. The interval width is the number of units between each sample element. For example, a sample of 100 from a population of 1000 would yield an interval width of 10. The researcher would make a random start and count every tenth element to be included in the sample.

Gross, Rocissano, and Roncoli (1989) used systematic sampling in their study on "Maternal confidence during toddlerhood: comparing preterm and fullterm groups." They described their sampling method as follows:

> The full-term population consisted of 4000 mothers of toddlers born in a large northeastern metropolitan hospital between 1984 and 1986, who were full terms delivered vaginally or by cesarean section and products of single births with no known congenital anomalies. Systematic random sampling of hospital chart codes was used to identify a target population of 146 mothers to contact for participation. (p. 3)

Systematic sampling may also be used as a nonprobability sample. If the researcher chooses a method in which every element does not have an equal chance of being selected, then the sample becomes one of nonprobability. A common situation is one in which the telephone directory is used as a population source. If residents in a local area are defined as the population, it is often assumed that the telephone book will supply the names of all those residing in the area. The problem is that the telephone directory is in alphabetical order and does *not* list all residents in an area. Many residents choose to be unlisted in the directory, and some do not have telephones. A large section of the population is overlooked using this source.

The advantages of systematic sampling

are that it is a fast, easy, and inexpensive way to draw a probability sample. Because of its simplicity, error may be reduced. The disadvantage is that the elements listed in the sampling frame must be randomized. Also, if the elements have been placed in some kind of order, systematic bias may exist, and the results will not be representative of the population of study. In addition, estimating the sampling error is difficult using systematic sampling design.

Random Assignment
Random assignment is a term often confused with random selection. Random assignment is a method of assigning participants to either a control or treatment group. Random selection is not a prerequisite for random assignment to take place. In fact, random assignment is often used to provide at least some degree of randomness when random selection is impossible

An illustration of the random assignment is diagrammed in Figure 13-3. First the researcher chooses the target population. The sample elements are then selected to participate. After sample selection, the elements are randomly assigned to either a control or experimental group. The researcher uses a table of random numbers to assign the participants into the groups.

Smith, Hathaway, Goldman, Ng, Brunton, Simor, and Low (1990) used random assignment in "A randomized study to determine complications associated with duration of insertion of heparin locks." Over a 20-month period, 301 patients on 15 medical, surgical, obstetrical, and rehabilitation units were selected to participate in the study based on the following selection criteria: The participant had a heparin lock; therapy was expected to continue; the IV insertion site was free of complications; continuous infusions were not received through the lock; venous access was readily available for IV rotation; each participant maintained an appropriate mental status; and none had been entered in the study previously. Since all patients selected had to meet all criteria, random selection was not possible.

The participants were then randomly assigned to either a control group or a treatment group. The control group had their heparin locks changed every 72 hours. The treatment group had their heparin locks left in place for up to 168 hours. A table of random numbers was used to assign the sample to the two groups.

NONPROBABILITY SAMPLING
Nonprobability sampling is an alternate approach to probability sampling. Because random selection is not used, each element or participant in the study does not have an independent chance (or probability

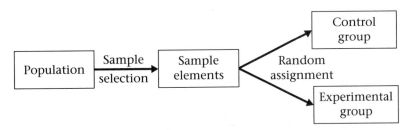

Figure 13-3. Model of random assignment.

greater than zero) of being included in the study. In addition, some elements have no chance of being included in the study. The disadvantages of using nonprobability sampling become obvious. The sample may not be representative of the larger population, and thus the results can not be generalized beyond the sample studied. In addition, the sampling error or the degree of departure from representation cannot be estimated. One means of overcoming these disadvantages is replication of the study. The advantages of nonprobability sampling are that it is less expensive and less complicated, and it allows the researcher to be more spontaneous when a research situation arises.

Nonprobability sampling is used in nursing research because often it is not feasible, economical, timely, or ethical to collect a random sample of the population under study. For example, Stewart, Fahs, and Kinney (1991) conducted a study to "determine whether alternate sites were effective in accomplishing the goals of low-dose heparin therapy (5,000 units) and to identify any differences in bruising at the injection site" (p. 204). Data were collected on 105 medical/surgical patients. The subjects were not randomly selected. All candidates that met the criteria for inclusion in the study were used. The researchers measured activated partial thromboplastin time (APTT) to determine the difference in the subcutaneous sites. In addition, the Institutional Review Board of the hospital evaluated the ethical considerations of the study.

Looking at this sample, it is easy to see why the researchers chose a nonprobability sampling approach. How feasible would this project have been had the researchers found it necessary to randomly select from all patients in the United States? Even if this were possible, the cost involved and time needed to complete the project would have greatly increased. In addition, the researcher needs to consider the ethical considerations. How ethical is it to give injections in sites that have not previously been proven in regard to bruising and absorption? Are those patients more at risk for the development of thrombophlebitis?

Three types of nonprobability sampling are convenience sampling, quota sampling, and purposive sampling. Examples of all three types of nonprobability sampling designs as seen in the literature are presented in Table 13-2.

Convenience Sampling
Convenience sampling uses participants who are easily accessible to the researcher and who meet the criteria of the study. For example, a nurse researcher might have easy access to an emergency department. If the population under study consists of family members of trauma patients, the most available family members willing to be interviewed and who meet the criteria of the study would be included in the sample. This is why it is commonly called accidental sampling.

Hill and Aldag (1991) describe the convenience sample used in their study of insufficient milk supply syndrome:

> The study sample was restricted to English-speaking mothers, able to read and write, and who initiated breast-feeding within 24 hours after delivery of a single infant. The mother did not have to be breast-feeding at the time of data collection. Women who met study criteria were approached for participation in the study if their infant was between 8.1 and 14 weeks of age when they visited the pediatrician's office or health department. The convenience sample consisted of 384

Table 13-2
Nonprobability Sampling

Sampling Procedure	Research Article Example	Description of Method
Convenience sample	Hill, P., & Aldag, J. (1991). Potential indicators of insufficient milk supply syndrome. *Research in Nursing & Health, 14,* 11-19.	A convenience sample of 384 mothers who initiated breast-feeding within 24 hours after delivery were selected for the study. Two private pediatrician offices and 17 WIC agencies in the Midwest were the locations of the study sample.
Quota sample	Noelker, L. (1987). Incontinence in elderly cared for by family. *The Gerontologist, 27*(2), 194-200.	The three major strata of the sampling framework were divided into substrata: geographic area of residence (urban, suburban, rural), race (black, white), and generational configuration (one-, two-, and three-generation household). Quotas were established for the substrata. The quotas were estimated based on the study's hypotheses and the area's population. From 120 sources, 614 caregiving households were selected to meet sampling quotas.
Purposive sample	Aroian, K. (1990). A model of psychological adaptation. *Nursing Research, 39*(1), 5-10.	To evaluate the emotional status of migration over time, a purposive sample of 25 Polish immigrants was divided into 3 comparison groups that varied in the length of time they resided in the United States.

mothers: 190 mothers who participated in WIC programs and 194 mothers who did not participate in WIC. (p. 13)

The advantages in using a convenience sample are the ease in carrying out the research and the savings in time and money. The disadvantages are the potential for sampling bias, the use of a sample that may not represent the population, and the limited generalizability of the results.

Snowball sampling or network sampling is a particular type of convenience sam-

pling. It is useful for studies in which the criteria for inclusion in the study specify a specific trait that is difficult to find by ordinary means. To accomplish this the researcher networks with a small sample of accessible participants and uses them to assist in identifying other participants with that specific trait.

Examples of participants with a specific trait are individuals with a rare disease, IV drug abusers, or prostitutes. The researcher may have access to a small sample of these individuals and may use them to act as informants to identify other potential participants. As these people are contacted and become participants in the study, they in turn can act as informants and identify even more potential participants. The soliciting of participants can be continued until the desired sample size is achieved.

Quota Sampling

Another method of nonprobability sampling is quota sampling. This method is similar to stratified random sampling in that the participants are divided into strata based on specified characteristics to provide representativeness of different groups within the population. Quota sampling differs from stratified random sampling in that the participants are not randomly selected from each strata.

The researcher first determines which strata are to be studied. A stratum can be an attribute variable or an independent variable of the study. Common variables are age, gender, race, and geographic location. The researcher then computes a quota (or number of participants) needed for each strata. The quota is computed proportionally or disproportionally to the population under study. Once the quota for each strata is determined, the subjects are solicited via a convenience sampling method (unlike stratified random sampling).

If the researcher wanted the sample to be proportional to the population under study, information would have to be obtained on the composition of the population. For example, if ethnicity was the variable under study, the proportion of individuals of Hispanic descent in one geographic location may be 20%, while the other 80% is of European descent. If the sample consisted of 100 participants, the quota for the strata of Hispanic descent would be 20 participants and the quota for those of European descent would be 80 par-

ticipants. This step ensures that all areas of the population are represented.

For example, Noelker (1987) used proportional quota sampling in her study of family caregivers. She described the sampling method as follows:

> . . . the sampling frame was stratified into three major substrata: geographic area of residence, (urban, suburban, rural), race (black, white), and generational configuration (one-, two-, three-generation household). Quotas were established for each of the substrata to ensure a sufficient number of households with specific combinations of racial, geographic, and generational characteristics relevant to the study's hypotheses and the area's population.
>
> Over 2000 referrals from approximately 120 sources were screened to obtain the 614 caregiving households necessary to meet sampling quotas. (p. 195)

Disproportional quota sampling occurs when the number of elements in each stratum is not proportional to the number in the target population. In the above example, the researcher may want the proportion to be 50/50 instead of 20/80. The researcher may choose a disproportional approach in this example to get a larger proportion of a minority group to be sure that they are adequately represented. If the sample consisted of 100 participants, the quota for the strata of Hispanic descent would be 50 participants and the quota for those of European descent would also be 50 participants.

Purposive/Theoretical/Judgmental Sampling

Purposive sampling, sometimes called judgmental or theoretical sampling (Glaser & Strauss, 1967), is another type of nonprobability sampling. The researcher, based on knowledge and expertise of the subject, selects or "handpicks" the elements of the study. The elements chosen are thought to best represent the phenomenon (or topic) being studied.

Purposive sampling is commonly seen in qualitative research, but can also be used in quantitative research. The researcher makes a judgment regarding the type of subjects needed to provide the most useful information about the phenomenon being studied. Both a focal group and a comparison group of subjects are selected, and sampling is a continuous selection process until data saturation occurs—that is, until the researcher sees information being repeated and a pattern emerging. The researcher does not know how many subjects are needed prior to data collection. Instead the determinant of the sample size is the saturation of the categories based on the phenomenon under study.

Using grounded theory as a basis for her research, Aroian (1990) describes her sample:

A purposive sample of 25 Polish immigrants, who resided in the Seattle area and had been in the United States ranging from 4 months to 39 years, was obtained for this study. Purposive sampling involved stratifying study participants according to three historically distinct waves of Polish migration (Sxulc, 1988), yielding three comparison groups of subsamples. Breakdown of the sample by wave of migration was as follows: Subsample 1 (post-World War II era) (n = 6), Subsample 2 (mid to late 1970s) (n = 5), and Subsample 3 (1980 to 1988) (n = 14). . . . Study participants' initial and changing experiences of migration and resettlement were inductively explored and testable hypotheses regarding psychological adaptation to migration and resettlement were generated. Cross-sectional sampling and retrospective reports provided documentation of changes in the experience of migration and resettlement over time. Stratifying the sample according to three distinct waves of migration also fulfilled the criteria for maximum variation or "theoretical" sampling recommended for grounded theory methodology. This sampling allowed making case comparisons among the three wave subsamples with respect to differences in their experiences of and their adaptation to both migration and resettlement. (p. 6)

Purposive sampling is also used in quantitative research. An example is the Delphi technique, which gathers experts' opinions on a specific topic. The experts are selected based on criteria determined by the researcher.

The advantage to purposive sampling is its allowance for the researcher to "handpick" the sample based on knowledge of the phenomena of study. The disadvantage is the potential for sampling bias, use of a sample that does not represent the population, and the very limited generalizability of the results.

DEVELOPING AND IMPLEMENTING A SAMPLING PLAN

A sampling plan is formulated in advance so the researcher can anticipate the cost, feasibility, and precision in sample selection. By using a systematic approach to sample selection, the researcher can increase representativeness of the sample, thus decreasing the sampling error and sampling bias (see box).

IDENTIFYING THE TARGET POPULATION

One of the first decisions the researcher must make in the sampling process is to identify the target population for the study. When the overall topic of study is decided, the researcher usually has some ideas about the target population based on

IMPLEMENTATION: STEPS IN IMPLEMENTING A SAMPLING PLAN

1. Identify the target population of interest.
2. Determine the accessible population.
3. Detail the inclusion and exclusion criteria.
4. Identify elements in the population to be studied.
5. Choose a sampling approach.
   - a. Probability
     - (1) Simple random sample
     - (2) Stratified random sample
     - (3) Cluster sample
     - (4) Systematic sample
   - b. Nonprobability
     - (1) Convenience sample
       - (a) Snowballing
       - (b) Network
     - (2) Quota sample
     - (3) Purposive sample
     - (4) Systematic nonprobability sample
6. Determine the sample size.
7. Contact the sample.
8. Evaluate the sampling approach.

an area of interest. A review of the literature reveals what target populations have been studied in the past and how they relate to the topic. In addition, the conceptual framework explains the relationships between or among variables, but the final choice of a target population is made when the researcher identifies the problem and purpose of the study.

The problem statement describes the area of concern and the purpose of the study. It clarifies the problem by stating the variables, population, and setting. Like the target population, the problem and purpose are derived from the conceptual framework and the review of the literature.

DETERMINING THE ACCESSIBLE POPULATION

After the target population is identified, the researcher determines the accessible population. The question of feasibility needs to be addressed: Based on the available resources, what population is accessible to the researcher for this research project? Money, time, location, and willingness of the participants to cooperate are a few areas to consider.

For example, Marchette et al (1991) state their target population in the formal stated purpose of their study: "The purpose of this research was to determine during unanesthetized circumcision the effects of pain reduction interventions (music, intrauterine sounds, pacifiers, music plus pacifiers, and intrauterine sounds plus pacifiers) versus no pain reduction intervention on neonatal pain" (p. 241). The target population is neonates. The accessible population is stated under Method in the article: "The accessible population included all full-term neonates who were born between November 1987 and July 1989, were scheduled for circumcision at a large southeastern medical center, had an uncomplicated vaginal or cesarean birth, had an Apgar score of at least 6 at 1 minute and 5 minutes of age, and had not undergone surgery" (p. 241). The accessible population is much more feasible to study than all neonates in the universe.

DETAILING THE INCLUSION AND EXCLUSION CRITERIA

The researcher specifies the characteristics of the population under study by detailing inclusion and exclusion criteria in the study. Inclusion criteria are characteristics that each sample element must possess to be included in the sample. Exclusion criteria are characteristics that a participant may possess that could confound or contaminate the results of the study. If the participant possesses a characteristic identified in the exclusion criteria, she or he would be disqualified and not able to be a part of the study.

Derdiarian (1990), in her study of cancer patients, specified the inclusion and exclusion criteria in the following description of the sample:

The sample included 223 cancer patients; they were included in the study if they were diagnosed as having cancer for the first time; were 18 to 70 years of age; had been diagnosed 6 to 20 months prior to participating; had received a major treatment for cancer 6 to 24 months prior to participation but were not undergoing treatment(s) at the time; had no other serious physical or mental disorders; did not have amputation of a limb or breast or surgery for head and neck cancer; were not terminally ill; did not experience a stressful life-event such as a divorce, death of a loved one, loss of a job and the like during the year before participation; could read and speak English; and consented and were able to participate. (p. 221)

IDENTIFYING THE ELEMENTS IN THE POPULATION

The elements in the accessible population must be identified. These are the individuals participating in the study. To begin, a sampling frame or a list of all the participants in the accessible population is made. Also, a list of sampling units or settings is formed.

Gay, Edgil, and Rozmus (1989) explain the sampling frame and sampling unit for their study of nursing journals read and assigned most often in nursing doctoral programs: "Invitations to participate in the study were extended to each dean of the 45 schools listed in *Doctoral Programs in Nursing 1986-87*" (National League for Nursing, 1987) (p. 246). From this statement the reader deducts that the sampling frame is the list of deans in the 45 schools and the sampling units are the 45 schools listed in the doctoral programs in Nursing 1986-87.

The researchers go on to say how they selected the elements in the population: "The deans who consented to participate were requested to select randomly five doctoral faculty for inclusion in the study" (p. 246). The elements or participants for the study were the doctoral faculty.

CHOOSING THE SAMPLING APPROACH

The researcher needs to decide the sampling approach to be used in the research study. The purpose of using a sampling approach is to increase representativeness, decrease bias, and decrease sampling error. There are several choices available to the researcher.

As discussed earlier in this chapter, the two basic approaches to sampling are probability and nonprobability sampling. Probability sampling is a method of random sample selection that promotes optimum representativeness in the sample selection process. With this optimum representativeness, the results can be generalized to the target population. This approach also reduces sampling error and minimizes the opportunity for sampling bias to occur.

Nonprobability sampling does not use random sample selection. Without the use of random selection, the researcher must look at other methods of achieving representativeness of the target population. In addition, caution must be taken to minimize sampling bias and sampling error. On the other hand, nonprobability sampling is less expensive, less time consuming, and the researcher can be more spontaneous in the research process.

The decision to choose probability or nonprobability sampling may be based on the researcher's ability to obtain a probability sample. However, in some cases, the researcher may be willing to sacrifice some population representativeness for more detailed information about a small select group versus obtaining superficial information about a larger, more representative group.

In nursing research the predominant approach to sampling is nonprobability sampling. This is largely because of the type of population and the ethical considerations associated with the use of that population. For example, Earp et al (1991) investigated the relationship between pulmonary artery and urinary bladder temperatures during rewarming in 14 adult patients in the intensive care unit after cardiopulmonary bypass surgery. The target population was composed of first-time, immediately postoperative, coronary artery bypass graft (CABG) surgery patients. To obtain a random sample, the researcher would have to make a list of all first-time CABG surgery patients and randomly select those to be included in the study prior to surgery. The list itself would be difficult to construct. The researcher would have to know in advance all the scheduled CABG surgeries plus be assured that the hospitals had the equipment to take urinary bladder and pulmonary artery temperatures. For the Earp et al (1991) study, in a four-month period only 14 patients met the criteria and all were included in the study. The time needed for this study would have greatly increased if a random sample had been required.

Both sampling approaches have their advantages and disadvantages. The researcher needs to weigh the advantages and disadvantages based on the type of research project to determine the desired sampling approach.

DETERMINING THE SAMPLE SIZE

A common question asked by researchers is, "How large a sample is needed for this study?" The answer is the larger the sample, the more representative of the target population it will be. Also, the larger the sample, the smaller the sampling error and the less chance of incorrectly accepting or rejecting the null hypothesis. An exception to this would be in the use of nonprobability sampling designs. If researcher bias is innate in the sampling design used, a large sample will not compensate for the faulty design.

Many factors interplay in deciding the appropriate sample size for a chosen study. Time, money, and availability of subjects are just a few. The goal of the researcher is to obtain a large enough sample to show statistical significance (when there is significance), yet be expedient and economical at the same time. The researcher needs to weigh the advantages and disadvantages of a large versus a small sample. Is it worth sacrificing the reliability and representativeness of a large sample for the convenience and economy of a small sample? In deciding the sample size, the researcher must examine each of these factors: the purpose of the study, the nature of the population, the number of variables, the sampling procedure used, the precision of the data collection instrument, and the type of data analysis.

Purpose of the Study
The purpose of the study will provide direction as to the sample size needed. If the purpose of the study is to explore trends and describe phenomena, the sample size will be small. Case studies, pilot studies, and exploratory qualitative and quantitative studies look for new knowledge in an

area. A small sample would permit more depth in these research designs. A large sample would be needed to analyze trends for a research design using surveys.

If the purpose of the study is to clarify concepts or examine relationships between variables, a larger sample is needed. Correlational studies frequently look at multiple variables. The more variables being examined in the study, the more subjects needed.

If the purpose of the study is to determine cause-and-effect relationships between variables, the sample size will decrease with the increased control of the setting. Experimental research design takes place in a highly controlled setting, whereas a quasi-experimental design has varying degrees of environmental control. The more control in the research study, the smaller the sample needed. Conversely, if several variables are examined, a large sample is needed even if the study is well controlled.

Nature of the Population
The nature of the population will help determine how many subjects are needed. A heterogeneous target population will have a wide range of characteristics. If the sample is small, the researcher runs a high risk of missing many of the differences seen in the population. If the population is homogeneous, a smaller sample could easily represent the target population because of their similarities. Still, the researcher needs to be aware that generalizability decreases as sample size decreases.

Attrition and Response Rate
Various study designs will require a larger sample because of attrition and low response rate. Attrition is a reduction in sample size caused by the failure of participants to complete the study after sample selection. The type of study design used will have an impact on the type of attrition seen. A pretest-posttest design has a higher attrition rate because some participants may quit the study during the interval between the completion of the pretest and the administration of the posttest. Longitudinal studies have a higher attrition rate because of participants moving, dropping out of the study, or dying.

Response rate is the ratio of completed instruments as compared to the number of instruments sent out. Mailed surveys have varied response rates; they can be as low as 5% or as high as 50%. Unfortunately, the respondents who do not mail back the survey usually share some biasing characteristic such as not being able to read or understand English.

Attrition and low response rate can pose a serious threat to the validity of findings. This is especially true when the participants who drop out of the study differ on key variables from those who remain in the study. Statistical methods are available to determine whether the remaining sample differs significantly from the original sample on key variables (Waltz, Strickland, & Lenz, 1984; Cook & Campbell, 1979; Tabachnick & Fidell, 1989). In addition, researchers should report attrition and response rates and explain how the rates affected the study results.

Sampling Procedure
The type of sampling procedure used is also a factor in determining sample size. When the sample is divided into several subsamples such as in cluster sampling and stratified random sampling, a large sample is needed. The size of the subsample, rather than the total sample, is critical in estimating the sampling error.

Statistical Test
The type of statistical test chosen to analyze the data may specify the sample size.

For a factor analysis, Nunally (1978) recommends 10 times as many subjects as variables. Based on his criteria, if there were 10 variables being examined, the sample size should be 100 to compute a factor analysis on the data.

Effect Size

The effect size is the extent to which the phenomenon under study exists in the population. It is also called strength of association or treatment magnitude. It is the amount of association or the degree of relationship found in the population. When the effect size is small, the sample needs to be large to detect the pervasiveness of the phenomenon. Conversely, when the effect size is large, the sample size needed to detect the effect will be small.

Power Analysis

Power analysis is a method of determining the sample size prior to conducting the research. The more powerful a statistical test, the more likely it will yield statistically significant results and reject the null hypothesis. Sample size is a factor in determining the power of a statistical test. Cohen (1977) in his book *Statistical Power Analysis for the Behavioral Sciences* writes about power analysis and how to determine the sample size based on the statistical test used. Chapter 14, Data Analysis, provides a more detailed explanation of power and its relationship to effect size and sample size.

CONTACTING THE SAMPLE

The potential participants, who have been identified in the sampling frame, now need to be contacted and solicited to participate in the study. Questions the researcher must answer are (1) How will the participants be contacted? (2) What is the cost involved? and (3) What is the expected response rate based on the method chosen?

Face-to-face contact brings the best response rate. It is also the most time consuming and costly method. Other methods of contacting participants are by mail or by telephone.

In the past contacting potential participants by mail or telephone resulted in a lower response rate as compared to the face-to-face interview. Dillman (1978) discusses a method that has brought the response rate of telephone and mail surveys high enough to compete with face-to-face interviews. These methods are discussed in greater detail in Chapter 15.

EVALUATING THE SAMPLING PLAN

It is important to evaluate the sampling plan described in a research study, both as the primary researcher and as a consumer of research. The appropriateness of the sampling plan is critical in determining if the sample represents the target population. Several aspects of the sampling plan need to be systematically evaluated. A checklist for evaluating a sampling plan is presented in the box.

It is easy to determine what is missing from a sampling plan. The consumer of research then needs to decide how to use the study results if some of the sampling information is missing. Questions to be considered are (1) Is the omitted sampling information vital, and does it threaten the generalizability of the results? (2) Should the study be replicated before the findings can be utilized in practice? (3) Does researcher bias affect the generalizability of the study?

SUMMARY

- A population is a set of objects, places, events, animals, or individuals that pos-

EVALUATING THE SAMPLING PLAN

1. Are the target population, accessible population, and sample described?
2. Are the elements of the study defined? Do they represent the target population?
3. What type of sampling approach is used (probability or nonprobability)?
4. If a nonprobability sampling approach is used, how is representativeness accounted for in the sample?
5. What type of sampling design is used?

Does it seem appropriate to the purpose of the study?
6. What type of researcher bias could occur with this method?
7. Are inclusion and exclusion criteria listed?
8. Is the determination of the sample size discussed? Does it seem appropriate?
9. What effect does the sample have on the interpretation of the results?

sess specific features a researcher is interested in studying.

- Because of the feasibility and economics involved, total populations are rarely studied. Based on sampling theory, a sample is selected to represent the population.
- The two basic approaches to sampling are probability and nonprobability sampling. Probability sampling ensures that each element in the study has some chance of being selected into the study. The four most common probability sampling designs are simple random sampling, stratified random sampling, cluster sampling, and systematic sampling.
- Nonprobability sampling does not use randomization techniques, so all elements do not have a chance of being included in the study. The three most common nonprobability sampling designs are convenience sampling, quota sampling, and purposive sampling.
- Steps in the sampling plan are:
  - Identifying the target population of interest.
  - Determining the accessible population based on feasibility, time, and cost.
  - Specifying inclusion and exclusion criteria for an element's inclusion in the study.
  - Identifying the elements (group members). An element is a singular entity or unit from which data are collected and generalizations made to the target population.
  - Choosing the sampling approach.
  - Determining the sample size. Multiple factors interplay in determining the sample size needed, but a general rule is to have as large a sample as possible so that the target population is represented.
  - Contacting the participants. The cost and amount of time needed in soliciting participants need to be calculated when deciding which method to use. Face-to-face contact brings a higher response rate than telephone or mail contact, but is more costly.
- The overall sampling approach must be systematically evaluated both by the researcher and consumer of research to determine if the sample is representative of the target population and if generalizations can be made from the sample to the target population.

FACILITATING CRITICAL THINKING

1. As a researcher, you would like to study the effects of music on low-birth-weight infants.
   a. What would be your target population?
   b. What would be your accessible population?
   c. What sampling plan would you use?
   d. What are your inclusion and exclusion criteria?
2. Using the table of random numbers in Figure 13-1 and the local telephone book as a sampling frame, select a sample of 100 participants for a potential study. What kind of sample is this? Why?
3. Suppose you defined your target population as all students seeking a Bachelor of Science degree in Nursing.
   a. What is your accessible population?
   b. What factor played a part in your decision?
   c. What type of sampling plan would you use?
   d. How much time do you think it will take to select your sample?
   e. How long do you think it will take to collect data from this sample if a mailed survey were being used?
   f. Estimate your expenses.

References

CONCEPTUAL

SLAKTER, M., WU, Y., & SUZUKE-SLAKTER, S. (1991). *, **, and ***: Statistical nonsense at the .00000 level. *Nursing Research, 40*(4), 248-249.

TABACHNICK, B., & FIDELL, L. (1989). *Using multivariate statistics.* New York: Harper & Row.

SUBSTANTIVE

AROIAN, K. (1990). A model of psychological adaptation. *Nursing Research, 39*(1), 5-10.

DEDIARIAN, A. (1990). The relationships among the subsystems of Johnson's behavioral system model. *IMAGE, 22*(4), 219-225.

EARP, J., & FINLAYSON, D. (1991). Relationship between urinary bladder and pulmonary artery temperatures: A preliminary study. *Heart & Lung, 20*(3), 265-270.

FRANKS, F., & FAUX, S. (1990). Depression, stress mastery, and social resources in four ethnocultural women's groups. *Research in Nursing & Health, 13,* 283-292.

GROSS, D., ROCISSANO, L., & RONCOLI, M. (1989). Maternal confidence during toddlerhood: Comparing preterm and fullterm groups. *Research in Nursing & Health, 12,* 1-9.

HERTH, K. (1990). Relationship of hope, coping styles, concurrent losses, and setting to grief resolution in the elderly widow(er). *Research in Nursing & Health, 13,* 109-117.

HILL, P., & ALDAG, J. (1991). Potential indicators of insufficient milk supply syndrome. *Research in Nursing & Health, 14,* 11-19.

JACKSON, B., TAYLOR, J., & PYNGOLIL, M. (1991). How age conditions the relationship between climacteric status and health symptoms in African American women, *Research in Nursing & Health, 14,* 1-9.

LYNN, M., MCCAIN, M., & BOSS, B. (1989). Socialization of R.N. to B.S.N. *IMAGE, 21*(4). 232-237.

MACLURE, K., HAYES, K., COLDITZ, G., STAMPFER, M., SPEIZER, F., & WILLETT, W. (1989). Weight, diet, and the risk of symptomatic gallstones in middle-aged women. *The New England Journal of Medicine, 321*(9), 563-569.

MCCABE, B. (1989). Ego defensiveness and its relationship to attitudes of registered nurses toward older people. *Research in Nursing & Health, 12,* 85-91.

NOELKER, L. (1987). Incontinence in elderly cared for by family. *The Gerontologist, 27*(2), 194-200.

SMITH, I., HATHAWAY, GOLDMAN, C., NG, J., BRUNTON, J., & SIMOR, A. (1990). A randomized study to determine complications associated with duration of insertion of heparin locks, *Research in Nursing & Health, 13,* 367-373.

STEWART FAHS, P., & KINNEY, M. (1991). The abdomen, thigh, and arm as sites for subcutaneous sodium heparin injections. *Nursing Research, 40*(4), 204-207.

WILLETT, W., STAMPFER, M., COLDITZ, G., ROSENER, B., & SPEIZER, F. (1990). Relation of meat, fat, and fiber intake to the risk of colon cancer in a prospective study among women. *The New England Journal of Medicine, 323*(24), 1664-1672.

METHODOLOGICAL

COOK, T., & CAMPBELL, D. (1979). *Quasi-experimentation: Design & analysis issues for field settings.* Boston: Houghton Mifflin.

GIVEN, B., KEILMAN, L., COLLINS, C., & GIVEN, C. (1990). Strategies to minimize attrition in longitudinal studies. *Nursing Research, 39*(3), 184-186.

WALTZ, C., STRICKLAND, O., & LENZ, E. (1991). *Measurement in nursing research* (2nd ed). Philadelphia: F.A. Davis.

HISTORICAL

COCHRAN, W. (1953). *Sampling techniques.* New York: John Wiley & Sons.

COHEN, J. (1977). *Statistical power analysis for the behavioral sciences.* New York: Academic Press.

DILLMAN, D. (1978). *Mail and telephone survey: The total design methods.* New York: John Wiley & Sons.

GLASER, B., & STRAUSS, A. (1967). *The discovery of grounded theory: Strategies for qualitative research.* New York: Aldine.

NUNALLY, J. (1978). *Psychometric theory.* New York: McGraw-Hill.

CHAPTER 14

MEASUREMENT

ANNE G. PEIRCE

Research studies are designed to develop an understanding of a concept, phenomenon, or object of interest. The ways in which researchers conduct their studies vary, but all researchers want their results to reflect the truth (validity) and to be replicable (reliable). The process that guides qualifying or quantifying a phenomenon of interest is called *measurement.* Measurement is traditionally defined as the process of assigning numbers to objects, where the numbers represent the quantity of the attribute under study (Nunnally, 1978). Numbers are not always used to describe an object (as qualitative research uses words), but the measurement process remains important. The rules of measurement help ensure that the research results obtained are meaningful.

Measurement instruments do not always give meaningful results. The Holmes-Rahe Social Readjustment Rating Questionnaire (Holmes & Rahe, 1967) is a well-known measure of stress that has made its way into the popular literature. This instrument measures stress by assigning points to

events considered stressful. The subject then checks off all the events experienced within the last year. A stress score is calculated by adding up the points for each event.

The scale was developed to assess how stress was related to the onset of illness. In past research studies it was frequently given to sick individuals to ascertain how much stress they had experienced prior to the illness. When given to subjects after they became ill, there was a high correlation between the level of stress and illness. However, after a few years and many research studies, the instrument was used prospectively; that is, it was given to people who were not ill to see if those with high-stress scores would later become ill. The researchers who used the instrument in this way found no relationship between illness and stress points.

Since that time it has been determined that people who fill out the questionnaire after getting sick may be trying to determine a cause for their illness (attribution of blame). This means that the sick individuals mark more items as stressful than they might normally. Also many of the items included on the scale are related to illness, so just being ill yields a high score. Finally, other researchers have determined that certain personality types answer the questionnaire differently, which could also artificially inflate the scores (Costa & McCrae, 1980). Thus, it appears that the instrument may not be measuring what it was designed to measure.

ERROR

The end result of all measurement should be accurate results, yet all measurement contains the possibility of error (Nunnally, 1978). One need look only as far as a bathroom scale to see evidence of error. One scale can measure weight very differently from another, and moving the same scale around on an uneven floor surface can give very different readings. Two people who view the same scale at the same time may read different weight values as well if the viewing angles are different.

Researchers know that all methods of measurement contain the possibility of error. The researcher's task is to control for error and to reduce it, where possible, to the lowest possible level in the planning of the measurement methodology.

TYPES OF ERROR
Error is generally classified as either random error or systematic error. *Random* error is defined as that error caused by chance factors that influence the measurement of phenomena (Waltz, Strickland, & Lenz, 1991). This type of error is due to changing conditions in the subject, the environment, or the instrument. One example of random error is incomplete results when a

subject inadvertently skips a question on a questionnaire.

Systematic error is defined as the error that is a fundamental or integral part of the measuring device. An instrument that always overestimates or underestimates an attribute would demonstrate systematic error, such as a weight scale that always weighs 5 pounds heavier than the true weight. Although always important, systematic error is of most concern in cases where the absolute value of the variable is significant in diagnosing or categorizing results. No one would want the laboratory to consistently over- or underestimate blood chemistry levels. This type of error is less important if the value of the variable is used to indicate change, such as weight loss, or where contrasting groups of subjects are all measured using the same instrumentation.

SOURCES OF MEASUREMENT ERROR
There are many sources of error in research measurement. The most common are those caused by environmental factors, researcher factors, instrumentation factors, and subject factors.

Environmental Factors
Measurement is influenced by the conditions under which it occurs. Such common factors as room temperature, lighting, and ambient noise can all influence the error rate. To control error, the careful researcher ensures that the environment is conducive to testing. She also takes care to make all testing times and sites similar. The time of testing is particularly important in the measurement of phenomena that have daily (diurnal) rhythms such as certain blood values, body temperature, and sleep patterns, or where subjects become easily fatigued.

Researcher Factors

The researcher can influence the results of a study in many ways. For example, if a subject is aware of the researcher's observation the subject may act differently, thus biasing the results. Subjects may try to please or displease the researchers with their answers or actions. Researchers may also inadvertently influence results by body language or wording used to phrase questions. When research is reactive, that is, responsive to the researcher, it is important to reduce these influences as much as possible. The researcher may elect to use trained data collectors, who are not aware of the research hypothesis, to collect data. These data collectors would reduce the possibility of hypothesis guessing by the subjects. The researcher who wants to observe subjects may have an extended observation period so that the subjects become used to his or her presence and are therefore less reactive.

Instrumentation Factors

The instrumentation used in research can be influenced by many factors. Nunnally (1978) writes that an inadequate sampling of items (from the domain of interest) is the other common source of instrumentation error. Among the other common sources of error in self-report measures are directions or items that are unclear and so are not understood by the subjects. Instruments can also be put together poorly so subjects inadvertently skip over questions. Sometimes instruments ask questions about sensitive topics that result in what is called response set bias (this could also be considered a subject factor), where the subjects answer in a socially desirable manner. Thus the way questions are worded can influence results, as can the format (open-ended or closed-ended) of the questions. Even the order in which the questions occur or are asked can be a source of error. All other forms of instrumentation, such as observational techniques and biophysical measures, can also introduce error.

The researcher should carefully consider all the possible sources of error in the instrumentation chosen and eliminate them. A careful researcher will also do a small-scale (pilot) study to ascertain if other sources of error become apparent and will be vigilant during the actual study to ensure that instrumentation error is not introduced into the study.

Subject Factors

People are a common source of error. A subject who is tired, sick, angry, or confused may cause error in the instrumentation. In fact, any changing physical, emotional, or psychological state of the subject could introduce error into the measurement process. The careful researcher ensures that the factors that influence the subject and the subject's responses are controlled.

CLASSICAL MEASUREMENT THEORY

Classical measurement theory is based on the assumption that all measurement contains random error. The theory proposes that all data collected contain the true value of those data plus an error value. Error is assumed to be present but not always measurable or detectable.

According to classical measurement theory, it is virtually impossible to be certain of an individual's true score or value; it can only be estimated. Thus, researchers can only be certain of what can be measured or what is called the observed score or value.

Classical measurement theory provides the foundation for most of the modern work on measurement. To illustrate the assumptions of classical measurement theory, the following formula is used:

$$O = T + E,$$

where

O = observation
T = true score
E = error score

Consider the following example as an illustration of the classical measurement theory. Suppose the nurse wants to measure blood pressure (indirect) in a sample. The nurse is tired and distracted and inadvertently uses the wrong size cuff on a subject. The result is random error with a systolic blood pressure reading 20 points below the patient's true (indirectly measured) blood pressure. According to the formula, the error score is −20 points. There is a 20-point difference between the true score and the observed score, or:

$$O = T + E$$
$$110 = 130 + (-20).$$

Researchers strive to control the error rate in order to obtain an observed score close in value to the true score. A clinical researcher who wanted to measure blood pressure would take steps to ensure that the blood pressure readings used in the study were as accurate as possible. For example, the researcher may routinely recalibrate the machinery used, use the correct size cuff, and have the patients in a consistent position. Despite careful attention to the correct procedure for obtaining a blood pressure reading, there will probably be chance variations in the patient, the machinery, and technique.

Random error theoretically does not affect the true score of the population. Thus,

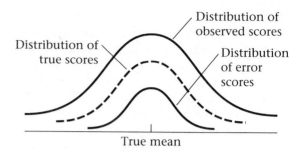

Figure 14-1. Distribution of blood pressure readings in a hypothetical study.

the total mean of the observed data is not affected if the sample is adequate. Rather, error around the mean affects the dispersion of scores or variance. The more random error there is in the measure, the more the scores will vary from the mean. Because the errors are assumed to be normally distributed, the mean of all the error scores would be zero (Figure 14-1).

RELIABILITY

Researchers try to estimate the amount of random error in a particular measure in order to determine if the results will show consistency, stability, and dependability. The assessment of these values is also called reliability. Thus, random error influences the reliability of measurement.

Researchers are interested in how people, objects, or events differ from one another; that is, their variance. Or in terms of classical measurement theory, the researcher is interested in how much of the variance is true variance and how much can be attributed to error or chance fluctuation.

Reliability is assessed by statistically estimating what portion of the instrument's total variance (a mathematical estimate of how scores vary around the mean) is true variance (Figure 14-1) and what is error. Reliability is most always assessed with correlational statistical procedures. The reliabil-

Table 14-1
Hypothetical Example of Random Error, Mean IQ (January–December) = 120, True IQ = 120

Month	Score	Month	Score
January	122	July	100
February	144	August	144
March	118	September	96
April	92	October	131
May	120	November	115
June	130	December	118

ity of any instrument will vary between zero (0.0), or no reliability, and 1 (1.0), or perfect reliability. The smaller the random error, the closer the reliability score will be to 1 (1.0). However, Goodwin and Goodwin (1991) caution that the error score should always be considered relative and multifaceted, not absolute.

For example, consider the hypothetical development of an Intelligence Quotient (IQ) test. The researcher wants to assess the reliability of the new instrument. Intelligence quotient (IQ) is considered a fairly stable attribute in adults, so the researcher would expect very little variance in the scores for any one person who took the test multiple times. In the following example, (see Table 14-1) one subject took an IQ test every month for 12 months. The individual's true IQ score is 120, yet only one of the hypothetical scores is equal to 120. However, the average of all the scores is equal to the true score.

The IQ test appears to have a tremendous amount of random error, as evidenced by the large distribution of scores, from 92 to 144, range of 52 points. The distribution of scores suggests that the IQ test may not have high reliability. Although the instrument would be the most com-

mon source of error in this example, the researcher would also look for other sources of error such as changing testing conditions.

When a researcher cannot rely on the results of measurement to be consistent, then the method is problematic. The researcher may decide that the instrument should not be used or should be used only after further evaluation and rectification of the identified problems.

VALIDITY

Validity is the appropriateness, meaningfulness, and usefulness of the inferences made from the scoring of the instrument (American Psychological Association, 1985). Validity is most influenced by the systematic error in the measure. The more systematic error present, the less valid the measure. Sources of systematic error include consistent characteristics of the subject, instrument, or environment that do not change from one testing to the next. A reliable instrument may or may not be valid, but because reliability is necessary to good instrumentation, an unreliable instrument will never be valid (Jennings & Rogers, 1989).

In the case of the IQ instrument, validity would not be possible given the measure's unreliability. As noted, an IQ test should measure a stable attribute, yet the test scores in the hypothetical example are anything but stable. The researcher would question whether the measure was giving a true picture of the individual's intelligence or was instead measuring another concept, such as readiness to learn.

LEVELS OF MEASUREMENT

In general, measurement can be defined as a "process that employs rules to assign numbers to phenomena" (Waltz, Strickland, & Lenz, 1991, p. 105). These rules are necessary in quantitative studies because many phenomena or subject characteristics do not normally lend themselves to number assignment but still need to be counted. Examples of such variables are hair color, gender, or religious preference.

Stevens (1946) developed a categorical system that serves as a guide in assigning numbers to objects of investigation. Stevens's four levels of measurement are labeled nominal, ordinal, interval, and ratio.

NOMINAL MEASUREMENT

Nominal variables are those that can only be categorized or sorted and are not truly measurable as they exist. Numbers are assigned to the variable in order to label or categorize (Nunnally, 1978) on the basis of defined properties of the variable that are mutually exclusive, exhaustive, and unorderable (Waltz et al., 1991). For example, many studies look at gender differences. Gender represents a categorical grouping and is classified as nominal because all study subjects can be placed in a category of male or female (exhaustive) and a subject will only fit one category (exclusive). To analyze a demographic variable such as gender with statistical procedures, numbers must be assigned, but the number assignment is arbitrary (unorderable). Gender may be assigned numbers such as female = 1, male = 2. In this case the number was assigned to the gender category and only makes sense in the context of the study. The numbers could easily be reassigned: male = 1, female = 2, and there would be no apparent difference in the number of male or female subjects or the results of the study. What is important to the nominal level of measurement is that the categories are exclusive, exhaustive, and unorderable.

The nominal scale of measurement allows the researcher to count objects or subject characteristics that are not normally countable. Traditionalists argue that only nonparametric statistical operations, such as frequencies, percentages, and chi-squares, should be used with nominal-scale measurement.

ORDINAL MEASUREMENT

Some variables demonstrate a natural or assigned rank order, but the divisions between the rankings are not consistent or equal. According to Nunnally (1978),

> An ordinal scale is one in which (1) a set of objects or people is ordered from "most" to "least" with respect to an attribute, (2) there is no indication of "how much" in an absolute sense, any of the objects possess the attribute, and (3) there is no indication of how far apart the objects are with respect to the attribute. (p. 14)

Thus ordinal-scale numbers are orderable, exclusive, and exhaustive.

Researchers use many ordinal-scale measurements in their studies. For example, an ordinal scale can be used to rank pain. The ranking of pain levels implies an order, but the ordering is not numerically absolute. A person who has pain that is ranked as intense may not have twice the pain as someone who ranks his or her pain as somewhat intense, even when 4 = intense and 2 = somewhat intense. Clinical rating scales may also represent ordinal scales of measurement, as do income and age groupings (see Figure 14-2). The figure shows a rank order, but there are no equal intervals between age categories. A person given a score of 1 is not exactly one half as old as a person given a score of 2. Because there is a rank order and the categories are exhaustive and exclusive, the scale is ordinal.

The researcher would take the ordinal level of measurement into account when deciding on the statistical analysis. Because

Please indicate the client's age by circling the number that applies			
Young adult	Adult	Mid-life adult	Older adult
21-29 years	30-44 years	45-64 years	65 and over
1	2	3	4

Figure 14-2. Example of an ordinal ranking.

the range of mathematical operations is theoretically restricted in ordinal scaling to the nonparametric, most researchers prefer to utilize the interval and ratio scales of measurement when possible. In the aforementioned example the researcher could easily ask for the person's age, thus obtaining a ratio-scale rather than an ordinal-scale measurement.

INTERVAL MEASUREMENT

Interval measurement involves categories that are exclusive, exhaustive, and orderable, with equal intervals between the numbers. However, in the interval-scale of measurement there is no absolute absence of the attribute because zero is assigned and represents an arbitrary point.

For example, a thermometer demonstrates the interval level of measurement. In the Celsius scale a temperature of 30° is 4° above a temperature of 26°, which in turn is 4° above a temperature of 22°. A temperature of 0°C does not indicate the absence of temperature. The assignment of zero to the scale represents the point between the state of liquid and solid water, not the absence of heat or cold. Temperature always exists on the Celsius scale.

Interval-scale measurement does not restrict the statistical procedures used with the data. The equal intervals between the

numbers allows the numbers to be added, subtracted, multiplied, and divided despite the absence of an absolute zero.

RATIO MEASUREMENT

The last level in Stevens's typology is the ratio scale. Ratio levels of measurement are exclusive, exhaustive, orderable, with equal intervals between numbers, as well as an absolute absence of the attribute or rational zero. Fluid volume provides an example of the ratio level of measurement. The fluid volume of urine is commonly measured in nursing practice. Because it is a ratio-scale of measurement a person can have an absence of urine or an absolute zero volume. In addition, every measurement of urine whether by liter or cubic centimeters (cc) provides an equal volumetric interval. A container with 200 cc of urine contains twice as much as a container with 100 cc (equal intervals), and the absence of any volume is truly a measure of zero (Table 14-2). The use of ratio-scale level of measurement permits the use of all mathematical operations.

However, the levels of measurement are not as clearly differentiated as it would appear by Stevens's rules. One major difficulty is that it is often unclear whether a variable has an absolute zero. For example, weight is classified as a ratio measurement, yet it is hard to conceive of an object that has an absolute absence of weight. For this reason, ratio and interval levels of measurement are often combined into one category. This results in three levels of measurement, not four, as shown in Table 14-3.

WHY ARE LEVELS OF MEASUREMENT IMPORTANT?

Because research requires the observation of multiple attributes, phenomena, and objects, investigators must often rely on numbers to represent the varied elements of interest. In order to share the results of a

Table 14-2
Deciding Between Levels of Measurement

Level	Nominal	Ordinal	Interval	Ratio
Can variable be put in an exclusive and exhaustive category?	Yes	Yes	Yes	Yes
Can variable be ranked?	No	Yes	Yes	Yes
Are the intervals between numbers equal?	No	No	Yes	Yes
Can there be an absolute absence of the variable?	No	No	No	Yes

Table 14-3
Levels of Measurement

Stevens's Categories	Revised Pragmatic Categories
Nominal	Nominal
Ordinal	Ordinal
Interval	Interval/ratio
Ratio	

quantitative study, the investigator must have a clear understanding of the nature of the study variables and represent them accurately with number values. The number representations do not always mean that all variables can be analyzed numerically. For example, it would be nonsensical to attempt to compute an arithmetic average (mean) using the values assigned to gender. Yet, numerical averages or mean scores are very appropriate for other variables such as test scores, subject height, blood pressures, and temperature. In these cases the numbers represent a level of measurement beyond that of the nominal scale. Therefore, the level of measurement for each variable of interest must be recognized before the statistical plan is developed.

The traditional view of measurement proposes that the level of measurement is important because it influences the choice of statistic. Like numbers, statistical operations have rules that govern their usage. For example, the Pearson product-moment correlation assumes that the data are measured at the interval (or higher) level. Traditionalists argue that the results of the statistical analysis may not be accurate if the assumptions, such as level of measurement, of the statistical test are not met. Pragmatists argue that most statistical procedures are not adversely affected by the level of measurement and that the ordinal level can be analyzed statistically just as accurately—perhaps even more accurately—than the interval or ratio levels. For further discussion on the controversy, see Knapp (1990, 1993).

MEASURING INSTRUMENTS AND LEVELS OF MEASUREMENT

Nurses measure variables of interest by a variety of methods. One consideration in choosing a method is the level of measurement yielded. An instrument that measures anxiety at the nominal level may not be as desirable as one based on an interval/ratio level because of the potential for statistical procedure restrictions. The most powerful statistics in discerning differences and similarities between subjects are held to be those that assume that the data are measured at the interval or ratio level. For this reason, researchers have allowed scale data, such as those yielded by Likert-type scales, to be used as interval level data rather than ordinal (Nunnally, 1978; Waltz, Strickland, & Lenz, 1991).

⚬ MEASUREMENT FRAMEWORKS

NORM-REFERENCED VERSUS CRITERION-REFERENCED MEASUREMENT

Two measurement frameworks, norm-referenced and criterion-referenced measurement, are commonly used in nursing research (Table 14-4). *Norm-referenced* measures compare each subject's performance or score relative to the others in a defined comparison or norm group (Martuza, 1977). Subjects in a study are compared to see how similar or dissimilar they are to one another and to others who may have been measured. For example, measurement of anxiety using Spielberger's State-Trait Anxiety Inventory (1983) would be classified as a norm-referenced measure. The researcher can use the measure to compare the anxiety levels of the subjects as well as

those of groups previously studied by the developer and other researchers.

Criterion-referenced measurement occurs when the subject's score or standing on a measure is compared to a preset standard or criterion. For example, the researcher may want to compare a subject's newly learned insulin injection technique to the known standards for insulin injection. In criterion-referenced measurement subjects are not compared to one another but rather to a criterion or standard.

The development of an instrument or assessment of a previously developed measure should take into account whether the research area of interest is norm- or criterion-referenced. The norm-referenced instrument should be used to compare individuals' levels of an attribute. Thus, norm-referenced instruments should be able to discriminate between levels of the variable. When the interested researcher is in mastery or achievement of a preset level or criterion, then a criterion-referenced measure should be used. A criterion-referenced instrument must be designed in such a way as to be able to discern mastery of knowledge or achievement of a standard.

Table 14-4
Norm-Referenced Versus Criterion-Referenced Measurement

	Norm	**Criterion**
Use	To evaluate the performance of subject relative to the performance of other subjects in a well-designed comparison (normative) group.	To determine if subject has acquired a set of target behaviors.
Key feature	Variance is critical. The instrument should maximally discriminate between subjects.	Variance is less critical. Discriminates between those who have acquired target behaviors and those who have not.
Results	Normally distributed. Interpreted in a relative sense (e.g., more or less of a variable, better or worse performance).	Skewed distribution. Interpreted in an absolute sense (e.g., met or unmet, pass or fail).

The following discussion of methods of assessing reliability and validity refers to norm-referenced measures.

RELIABILITY ASSESSMENT

Reliability is defined as the ability of the instrument to create reproducible results. Without the ability to reproduce results, no truth can be known, so reliability is considered a necessary, but not sufficient condition for validity. Reliability is never proven. Rather, it is considered situational and depends on the characteristics of the sample and the situation under which it is assessed.

Conceptually, reliability is the proportion of true variance to total variance in an instrument (Kerlinger, 1979). The reliability of any given measurement instrument may be determined statistically by comparing the variances of the true (estimated) and observed scores as follows:

$$\text{Reliability} = \frac{\text{True variance}}{\text{Total variance}}.$$

The choice of assessment method depends on the instrument's characteristics. When considering how to assess reliability, three attributes are important: stability, equivalence, and consistency. Each attribute is an important aspect of reliability, but not every attribute is relevant to all types of measures. For example, assessment of stability is not relevant for an instrument that measures a state of being, such as mood. Moods are not stable. Conversely, IQ should be stable, so an assessment of stability would be appropriate in assessing reliability.

The reliability values obtained are also influenced by the number of items on the instrument (in general the more items, the higher the reliability value obtained) and the heterogeneity of the subjects (the more homogeneous the subject pool, the lower the reliability values obtained).

STABILITY

The most common method of ascertaining stability of measurement is through the test-retest method. Test-retest reliability assumes that with a stable phenomenon, two testings of the same sample will yield approximately the same results. The statistical procedure used to ascertain test-retest reliability with interval-level data is the Pearson product-moment correlation.

When two testings of the same subject are measuring a stable attribute, the correlation between the two sets of scores should be close to 1 (1.00), as 1 represents a perfect correlation. Although there is some debate about what value represents an acceptable reliability score, many nurse researchers use Nunnally's (1978) standards, according to which a newly developed instrument should have a reliability score of at least 0.70 to be considered acceptable, whereas an established instrument should measure 0.80 or better.

CONSIDERATIONS IN USING THE TEST-RETEST PROCEDURE

As discussed, test-retest is only appropriate with stable phenomena. Thus, stability becomes the first consideration. Before using the test-retest technique, the researcher should also consider the potential learning effect that may occur from one testing to the next. In addition, some tests may sensitize the subject to the topic, causing them to find out more about the topic or undergo an attitudinal change. If either of these events occurs, then the outcome of the reliability assessment method will be adversely affected.

EXAMPLES OF STABILITY ASSESSMENT TECHNIQUE

Sideranko, Quinn, Burns, and Froman (1992) used test-retest in assessing the reliability of an instrument to measure the pressure of body weight on sacral and heel surfaces in subjects in the supine and semi-Fowler's positions. Using a fluid bag connected by catheter to a transducer, they measured the pressure at both sites in both body positions on two occasions. They determined that their instrument gave stable readings. The results for the different sites and positions over two testings ranged from $r = 0.71$ to $r = 0.92$

Source: Sideranko et al. (1992).

PROCEDURE

Test-retest reliability is ascertained by testing the same subjects on two separate occasions using the same instrument. The length of time between testing events is important. If the two sessions are too close in time, memory effects from the first testing could unduly influence the second. Testing sessions too far apart in time could result in a loss of subjects or unexpected changes in the variable. Waltz, Strickland, and Lenz (1991) recommend a 2-week interval between most testings, but the researcher should be guided by knowledge of the subject. The researcher should also keep the conditions of testing constant. Unequal testing conditions such as type or intensity of lighting, room comfort, noise, and time of day could cause changes in the error rate and affect the ultimate reliability score.

ANALYSIS

Once the results of the test-retest reliability computations are calculated, the researcher should examine the data for evidence of stability. If the instrument is stable, then the correlational analysis between the results of the two testings should reflect a score of 0.70 or higher. But even if the score is adequate, further analysis should be done. First, the means of each testing need to be examined. If the variable is truly stable, the means should be close in value (as reflected in the reliability score). They would rarely, if ever, be exactly the same because of the influence of the random error. Next, the researcher examines the standard deviation of each testing to get an indication of the variance of scores around the mean. If the standard deviations are very different from one another, the results should be carefully considered before the instrument is accepted as reliable. A decrease in variance on the second testing may provide evidence of sensitization. (See Tulman and Jacobsen [1989] for further discussion on variability.)

EQUIVALENCE

As noted, not all phenomena are stable, which restricts the use of test-retest as a form of reliability assessment. Reliability can also be assessed through equivalence. The most common form of equivalence reliability assessment is through parallel forms, also called alternative forms. Parallel forms reliability uses two versions of one instrument with one sample at one time (Martuza, 1977; Nunnally, 1978).

Equivalence of scoring can also be assessed by raters. These methods are called *inter-rater* and *intra-rater* reliability. In inter-rater reliability two raters are used with one rating instrument. Intra-rater reliability uses one rater to rate the same instrument or observation twice. In each instance, the assumption is that two ratings will be approximately equivalent.

PARALLEL FORMS

To assess parallel forms reliability, the researcher administers two forms of the instrument at the same time to one sample. To be considered parallel (or alternative) forms, the two instruments must be developed in an identical manner using the same objectives. The instruments must also have approximately equal standard deviations and means as well as equal correlations with a third variable found in the population under study (Martuza, 1977; Waltz, Strickland, & Lenz, 1991).

The researcher administers the two instruments to the sample at one time. The order in which the instruments are given should be varied to balance the error rate for fatigue or testing effects. Error can be introduced into a study when subjects become tired and inadvertently begin to make mistakes on an instrument. If the instruments are administered in different orders to different subjects, then the error rate is assumed to be equally distributed and so will not affect the reliability coefficient. The same is true of the testing effect.

After both instruments are scored, the scores from the two instruments are correlated. If the instrument measures at the interval level or above, the Pearson product-moment correlation is used. Again the researcher expects a reliable instrument to produce a reliability coefficient of $r = 0.70$ or higher.

The scores of each instrument at this testing should also be examined for compa-rable means and standard deviations. If the descriptive statistics are not similar, then the reliability of the instrument is probably not sufficient for use, despite the adequate reliability score and previous testing scores.

RATER RELIABILITY
Inter-Rater Reliability

With inter-rater reliability, two or more trained raters are asked to independently rate the same object or event at the same time using the same instrumentation or plan. The scores obtained are then used to obtain a percentage of agreement between the raters. If the rating instrument is reliable (assuming both raters received the same training in its use), then the scores obtained by the two raters should be comparable.

The researcher looks for a reliability assessment score of 70% agreement or higher. Percentage of agreement tends to overestimate reliability because the possibility of chance agreement is high. When the percentage of agreement is on the low side of acceptable, the researcher should be cautious in assuming reliability. See Topf (1987) for an interesting discussion about how and why inter-rater reliability may decline and what strategies can help eliminate the problem.

Other statistical procedures may also be used to assess inter-rater reliability. Brennan and Hays (1992) advocate the use of the kappa statistic for inter-rater reliability. Kappa indicates agreement beyond that expected by chance alone and so will generally give a more accurate indication of reliability. For further discussion about the appropriate use of kappa, see Brennan and Hays (1992). When there are three or more raters, the researcher may use Cronbach's coefficient alpha (alpha) (Waltz, Strickland, & Lenz, 1991).

EXAMPLE OF EQUIVALENCE ASSESSMENT TECHNIQUE

Conn (1991) studied how older adults cared for themselves when they had colds or influenza. The researcher developed a structured interview for the study. The results of the interviews were transcribed, and coding categories were developed. To assess the equivalence reliability of the coding, 10% of the interviews were coded by two different researchers. The results showed that there was a 97% agreement about coding categories between the two researchers.

Source: Conn (1991).

Intra-Rater Reliability

Intra-rater reliability relies on one rater to rate an object or event twice. For example, a videotape of a mother-infant interaction could be viewed and scored by the same person on two separate occasions. Again, the percentage of agreement is the most common method of statistical procedure to assess reliability. However, coefficient alpha could be used for more than two raters, or kappa could be used to reduce the effects of chance agreement.

HOMOGENEITY

Homogeneity indicates that the instrument is consistent within itself; that is, most of the items show a consistency of scoring. To illustrate the concept of internal consistency, consider a measure of anxiety given to students before a final exam. The assumption is that if subjects are highly anxious on one item of an anxiety measure, they would be expected to score as highly anxious on most other items as well.

Cronbach's Coefficient Alpha

The most common assessment method for homogeneity is Cronbach's coefficient alpha, hereafter referred to as alpha. Alpha assesses the internal consistency of the instrument by correlating each item with all other possible combinations of items, as follows:

$$\text{alpha} = \left(\frac{K}{K-1}\right)\left[1 - \left(\sum \frac{\text{var items}}{\text{var test}}\right)\right],$$

where

K = number of items on the measure
Var items = the sum of the individual item variances
Var test = the variance of the distribution of test scores

Nunnally (1978) states that an alpha should be obtained for all appropriate instruments, even if other reliability assessments are planned. Although alpha is the most popular method of assessing internal consistency, other methods exist. Ferketch (1990) outlines times when the omega or theta procedures may be a more appropriate choice.

Alpha is appropriate for instruments that use continuous, interval, or above-level data. In cases of dichotomous data there is a special form of alpha called Kuder-Richardson Formula (KR 20). Alpha and KR 20 generally yield scores that range from a low of 0.00 to a high of 1.00. See Knapp (1991) for a discussion of derived scores of less than 0.00.

Procedure

Because the alpha (and KR 20) compares all possible combinations of items, only one administration of one instrument to one sample is required. Once the scores are obtained, the alpha is quickly performed using a computer and appropriate statistical package. Alpha can also be estimated with a hand calculator.

Analysis

The computer printout provides the researcher with substantial information, including the alpha for the total instrument (Figure 14-3). The first column in the example tells the researcher what the mean score of the scale would be if the item was eliminated. In the example, the seventh item (Const4) appears to make a significant difference in the mean (compare 13.0158 to the other numbers shown). The second column tells the researcher about the item's contribution to the scale's variance. Again, the last item is very different from the others and appears to add substantially to the variance. The third and fourth columns give the researcher essentially the same information. Most researchers use the "Corrected Item-Total Correlation" column in their assessments. This column tells the researcher the correlation of that one item with the remaining items on the scale. Generally, if the item is correlated at 0.20 or less, the researcher carefully considers its inclusion in the scale. Again, the last item is the only item not to reach this level. Next, the researcher looks at the last column. This column tells the researcher what the scale's alpha would be if that item were deleted. In the example given, the fifth

Item-total statistics					
	Scale mean if item deleted	Scale variance if item deleted	Corrected item-total correlation	Square multiple correlation	Alpha if item deleted
CONST16	16.4926	30.3558	.5594	.4066	.6753
CONST15	15.5000	26.6355	.6796	.5602	.6294
CONST17	16.1574	29.9096	.4608	.2896	.6895
CONST8	16.4722	30.2329	.4674	.2664	.6889
CONST7	16.1944	29.4852	.4209	.2588	.6984
CONST6	15.5648	26.5967	.5654	.4332	.6601
CONST4	13.0158	34.9557	.0686	.0351	.6932
Reliability coefficients			7 items		
Alpha = .7261		Standardized item alpha = .7452			

Figure 14-3. Example of a computer printout reliability analysis using Cronbach's coefficient alpha.

(Const7) and seventh (Const4) items produce the highest alphas if eliminated, and the second item (Const15) causes the biggest drop.

Finally, the researcher then looks at the total alpha. Note that two scale alphas are given. The first alpha (0.7261) is the one most generally reported. The second alpha represents a value where the items are standardized by dividing each item by its respective standard deviation. It can also be used. In general, the two alphas are close in value.

Given all the information, the researcher must decide how to handle the items and the scale. First, the total scale alpha is 0.73 (when rounded off to the nearest hundredth). This alpha represents a respectable alpha for a newly developed scale but would be problematic if the scale was well established. In this example, the scale was a new one, and so the total alpha score was acceptable to the researcher. In the example, the total alpha is higher than any of the alphas given for a scale with item deleted (last column). This is not unexpected given that alpha is partly a function of test length. The researcher would also look at all the other information about the items. For instance, in this example item 7 (Const4) would be carefully reviewed. The researcher may or may not want to eliminate it or replace it with another item.

The alpha provides a good indication of internal consistency reliability as long as the items on the scale are all related to one concept. Heterogeneous items can result in the underestimation of alpha. For example, a researcher may want to assess the reliability of a measure that evaluates the functional ability of elders. The items may be very different (heterogeneous), with some items assessing physical function and others assessing cognitive function. In the case of heterogeneous items, an attempt should be made to put them into subscales through factor analysis or other means. The alphas for the subscales can then be determined. When using subscales, it is important to remember that alpha depends on test length. In general, the more items included in a scale, the higher the alpha.

The researcher should also assess total test variance and the distribution of scores. The coefficient alpha obtained will be higher if there is greater variance and distribution is normal than with a skewed distribution and low variance.

Split-Half Reliability

Another method of assessing homogeneity is the split-half technique. This technique was frequently used in the past but has not been commonly used since the advent of easily accessed computers. In the split-half method the items from the instrument are divided into 2, usually with the even-numbered items in one group and the odd-numbered in another. A correlation is then done between the scores of the two halves of the same instrument. Because this form of reliability somewhat depends on the number of items (all things being equal a longer instrument will have a higher reliability), the split reduces the reliability of the instrument. The loss of magnitude can be corrected through the use of the Spearman-Brown correction factor:

$$r^1 = \frac{2r}{1 + r}$$

where

r = reliability of split-half correlations
r^1 = estimated reliability if not split

If split-half reliability is 0.75, then one gets:

$$r^1 = \frac{(2)(0.75)}{1 + 0.75} = 0.86.$$

EXAMPLE OF HOMOGENEITY ASSESSMENT TECHNIQUE

Mahon and Yarcheski (1992) studied the situational and characterologic explanations of loneliness in adolescents of different ages. They measured loneliness with the Revised UCLA Loneliness Scale. To assess the scale's internal consistency, the researchers used Cronbach's coefficient alpha. They reported the results as follows:

Age Group	Coefficient Alpha
Early adolescent	0.87
Middle adolescent	0.87
Late adolescent	0.90

The researchers reported the alphas to be acceptable.

Source: Mahon & Yarcheski (1992).

The same standard of 0.70 for a new instrument and 0.80 for an established one can be used in assessing the reliability of the instrument for both the alpha and the split-half method.

✎ VALIDITY ASSESSMENT

Measurement validity is defined as the truthfulness of the measure in assessing the phenomenon of interest in a given sample or population. A valid measurement method should actually measure what it purports to measure. For example, an instrument designed to measure attitudes toward euthanasia could actually be measuring attitudes toward related variables, such as governmental or physician authority, religious beliefs, or the sacredness of life. To ensure that the instrumentation presents a true reflection, the researcher will assess validity. As was true of reliability, the validity of an instrument represents a given situation and sample and so needs to be reconsidered with every new use of the instrument.

The method(s) chosen to assess validity should be based on the researcher's knowledge of the variable of interest and related design issues, such as sample. There are three major approaches to validity: content validity, construct validity, and criterion-related validity. Some researchers claim that all validity assessment methods are forms of construct validity (Rew, Stuppy, & Becker, 1988).

Content validity, which is important to all instrumentation, assesses whether the instrument adequately measures the domain of interest or universe of concern (Nunnally, 1978). Content validity is evaluated before the instrument is used. Construct validity is a process that assesses the instrument in terms of the "degree to which an individual possesses some hypothetical trait or quality presumed to be reflected by performance" (Waltz, Strickland, & Lenz , 1991, p. 172). Criterion-related validity is used when the researcher wants to predict a subject's present or future standing, related to a topic not directly measured by the instrument. For example, standardized tests are often used to predict future success in college or graduate school. As noted by the American Psychological Association (1985), these categories, or types of validity, are useful labels. However, as labels they should reflect the instrument's validity as a whole, not the validity of one type or another.

STEPS IN INSTRUMENT DESIGN

1. Explication of objectives.
2. Blueprinting or test-item matrix.
3. Careful construction of the measure.
4. Check content validity—have a panel of experts rate each item.

5. Administration of instrument in a pilot.
6. Item analysis.
7. Revision.

CONTENT VALIDITY

Content validity assesses the instrument's ability to measure what is says it purports to. To be accurate, the instrument must assess the whole domain of interest. Thus, content validity is concerned with the congruence of the operational and conceptual definitions of the variables of study. For example, suppose a student is taking a research (domain of interest) class and is told to expect a cumulative (conceptual definition) final but finds it only contains questions on sampling (operational definition). The student would be right to complain that the final examination did not assess the whole domain of interest. This exam would not have content validity.

Sometimes content validity is confused with face validity. Face validity means that the researcher looks at the instrumentation and decides visually that the respondents will agree it measures the domain of interest. Face validity represents an opinion and should not be used in discussions of content validity. It is generally considered nothing more than the first preliminary step toward deciding what instrumentation to use in a given situation. The researcher needs a more in-depth analysis of how well and how completely the instrument was designed and how it will be accepted by the subjects. Although Thomas, Hathaway, and Arheart (1992) present convincing arguments for at least considering face validity, it should not be used to replace content validity.

Procedure

According to Waltz, Strickland, & Lenz (1991), the steps that are important in instrument design (see box) are also essential to achieve content validity. A correctly designed instrument is one that considers the total domain of interest. The first step is to list the objectives that guided the instrument's development or governed the choice of that instrument. Next, the researcher lists all the items or measuring points, along with any explanation of terms or concepts. The researcher should also clearly define the concept. For example, stress may be defined in many different ways.

This package of information—objectives, definition of terms, and items—is then given to a panel of experts. The minimum number of experts needed is two but could be as high as 20 (Gable, 1986). The experts are chosen based on their practical or academic knowledge, or both, of the domain of interest. The experts are asked to rate each item's relevancy to the objectives provided. They are also asked to comment on whether the scope of items truly covers the domain of interest or whether items need to be added.

EXAMPLE OF CONTENT VALIDITY ASSESSMENT

Blenner (1993) assessed the content validity of a scale developed to assess individual differences in ability to absorb stimuli. The 77 items, theoretically divided into four subscales, were developed from a conceptual framework of stimuli modulation and from the surrounding literature. The items, conceptual definitions, and scoring directions were given to a panel of six experts, three psychologists and three doctorally prepared nurse clinicians. Using Cohen's kappa to assess agreement, Blenner found that there was a 0.78 inter-rater agreement between the experts as to the appropriateness of the items. The researcher used the experts' suggestions to reword some items and add others to the scale.

Source: Blenner (1993).

The researchers are generally asked to rate each item on a four-point scale. A commonly used scale, developed by Waltz and Bausell (1981), reads as follows:

1 = Not relevant
2 = Somewhat relevant
3 = Quite relevant
4 = Very relevant

Lynn (1986) recommended that the wording be expanded to add clarity and be changed to the following:

1 = Not relevant
2 = Unable to assess relevance without item revision, or item is in need of such revision that it would no longer be relevant
3 = Relevant but needs minor alteration
4 = Very relevant and succinct

Analysis

To ascertain content validity, a content validity index can be obtained. If there are two experts, the researcher ascertains a percentage of agreement about the relevancy of the items. In looking at agreement between experts, the researcher expects that with valid instrument most items will be rated as 3s or 4s. If the experts agree that 80% of the items are relevant (scores of 3 or 4), the content validity index score will be 0.80 (Waltz et al., 1991). The level of agreement should be high (Gable, 1986).

CONSTRUCT VALIDITY

Constructs represent ways of thinking, talking, and or writing about nontangible variables such as personality types. Thus, they may vary depending on the theory and instrument used. Testing assumptions about the construct will give the researcher a sense of the instrument's validity. Construct validity is an ongoing process, as is all validity testing, with several studies needed before the researcher can assert the instrument's construct validity with a given population. The methods used to assess construct validity are listed in the box.

Contrasted or Known Groups Validity

Depending on the theory behind the construct, the researcher may identify groups of subjects who should obtain significantly varied scores on a given instrument. For example, in a study on anxiety the researcher may predict that students waiting to take a final exam will have higher levels of anxiety than students on a normal class day.

> **CONSTRUCT VALIDITY**
>
> - Contrasted (or known) groups
> - Hypothesis testing
> - Factor analysis
>
> - Multitrait-multimethod
>   Convergent validity
>   Divergent validity

Each group of students would be given the instrument designed to measure anxiety. The scores of the two groups could then be analyzed with a statistical procedure appropriate to ascertaining differences, such as a *t*-test or analysis of variance (ANOVA). If the instrument was a valid measure of anxiety, the researcher assumes that the "examination day" group would have higher anxiety scores than the "class day" group. A significant finding would indicate that the instrument appeared to have some validity with the sample as a measure of anxiety. As with all measurement assessment, the researcher always retains some skepticism as the instrument could be validating other constructs such as anger or fear.

Hypothesis Testing

A similar approach to validity assessment involves the testing of hypotheses. In this approach the researcher also tests assumptions about the variable of interest using hypotheses. If the assumption(s) is upheld, then there is some evidence of validity. For example, the construct of anxiety can be examined as a state or a trait. If the instrument is designed to examine anxiety as a trait, the researcher's hypothesis could assert that two administrations of the test to one group should show similar scores. A correlation done between the scores would reveal a correlational score close to 1 (1.0) if the instrument has some evidence of validity.

Multitrait-Multimethod Validity

The multitrait-multimethod (MMTM) assessment of validity was developed by Campbell and Fiske (1959). It represents a very complete way of assessing validity.

To assess MMTM validity, certain requirements must be met:

1. The research must reflect two (or more) different concepts of interest. For example, the study may include both anxiety and well-being. The two concepts are not expected to closely correlate, but instead they will "diverge" from one another. The researcher assesses the divergent validity of the two concepts as part of the MMTM.
2. The researcher must have two or more different ways of measuring each concept. For example, physiologic and self-report measures of well-being and anxiety would represent two very different methods. The two methods of measuring the same concept should correlate highly and will indicate convergent validity to the researcher.
3. The subjects must be willing to take four or more tests at one sitting.

The different scores from each of these measures are put into a correlation matrix (see Figure 14-4). The researcher then systematically examines each element, starting with the reliability estimates for each instrument. Only if the reliability estimates

| | | Method 1 (self-report) | | Method 2 (physiological) | |
		Anxiety	Well-being	Anxiety	Well-being
Self-report	Anxiety	A			
	Well-being	C1	A		
Physiological	Anxiety	B	C2	A	
	Well-being	C2	B	Cl	A

A = Reliability diagonal
B = Convergent validity
C = Divergent validity
    1 = heterotrait-monomethod
    2 = heterotrait-heteromethod

Figure 14-4. Example of a correlation matrix for assessing multitrait-multimethod validity.

are sufficient does the researcher proceed. Next, the researcher ascertains the convergent validity by reviewing the monotrait-heteromethod (one concept, two methods) diagonals. The researcher expects high correlations between different measures of the same trait, although the values should not be as high as the reliability estimates.

Finally, the researcher examines the matrix for evidence of discriminant validity. *Discriminant validity* is a three-step process. The first step is to look at heterotrait-monomethod diagonals (two concepts, one method). There should be some shared method variance evident in the correlation scores. The next step is to look at the heterotrait-heteromethod correlations (two concepts, two methods). These should be very low. Finally, the researcher looks at the different trait measure methods. The scores should show similar patterns if the trait relationships remain con-

stant (Campbell & Fisk, 1959). The results can also be analyzed with ANOVA and confirmatory factor analysis. For further discussion, see Lowe and Ryan-Wenzer (1992).

The methodology of multitrait-multimethod assessment reflects a very comprehensive way to examine validity. When possible, it is a method of choice for nurse researchers. However, its very comprehensiveness sometimes makes it hard to use. Besides the obvious problems of time, money, and expertise, other limitations exist. These include the visual nature of decisions based on the matrix, the heterogeneity of methods required, and the need for high reliability of measurement (Lowe & Ryan-Wenzer, 1992; Waltz et al., 1991).

Factor Analysis
The statistical method of confirmatory factor analysis can provide support for instru-

ment validity. Many theories or constructs have identifiable subconcepts. The instrument that measures the theory or construct should also reflect these subconcepts. For example, an instrument that evaluates the concept of coping must contain items on several different types of coping subconcepts such as denial and knowledge-seeking coping strategies. If the subscales truly reflect the theory, then the items related to each subconcept should cluster when subjected to factor analysis. For example, the researcher would expect the denial-type coping strategies to form one cluster and the knowledge-seeking–type strategies to form another. In factor analysis, each cluster of related items is called a factor.

To perform a factor analysis the instrument is given to a pilot sample. Because factor analysis is a numerically intensive procedure, the sample must be large enough to support factor analysis. A rule of thumb is to use 10 subjects per item, thus 10 items would require 100 subjects.

It is hoped that the items related to the various subconcepts will cluster into factors. If the factors support the researcher's or theories' conceptualization, then there is some evidence for validity. If there are identifiable clusters but they do not reflect the theory, then the researcher must carefully reexamine both the theory and the instrument. If there are no identifiable clusters or factors, then the researcher must be very concerned that the instrument is problematic.

CRITERION-RELATED VALIDITY

Many instruments used in research predict the present or future standing on a variable or criterion (standard). For example, standardized educational exams are used to predict success in school or college. The tests give the colleges an estimate of success. Such instruments require the use of criterion-related assessments of validity.

Criterion-related validity consists of two types: predictive and concurrent. Concurrent validity is concerned with the subjects' current status with regard to the variable, and predictive validity is concerned with future standing.

Concurrent Validity

To perform a concurrent validity assessment, the researcher must first identify predictor and criterion variables. Predictor variables are those expected to foretell the standing on the other variable. Knapp (1985) writes that concurrent validity requires that the criterion variable should be a higher-order conceptualization of the predictor variable, not simply another variable. For example, social network size

---

EXAMPLE OF CRITERION-RELATED VALIDITY ASSESSMENT

Keresztes et al. (1993) used concurrent validity assessment in their study of the functional ability of patients with coronary artery disease. The researchers wanted to assess the validity of the Specific Activity Scale, which measures the patients' perception of their level of symptom-free activity. The score obtained from the instrument was correlated with symptom-free treadmill exercise time. Keresztes et al. found a 0.68 correlation between the perception of ability (instrument score) and actual ability (treadmill score).

Source: Keresztes et al. (1993).

---

might be used to predict social support. A person whose social network measure showed many friends might be expected to show evidence of high social support on the social support measure.

Procedure

The researcher chooses measures to assess both variables. The availability of a reliable and valid measure of the criterion variable is critical to the assessment process. These two measures are administered to one group of subjects at one time or within a short time. The two sets of scores are then analyzed with correlational statistics or regression analysis (Waltz et al., 1991). The measure of the predictor variable is said to be valid if the two instruments (predictor and criterion) are highly correlated.

Predictive Validity

Predictive validity is a variation of concurrent validity. The difference between the two is the timing of the data collection. Predictive validity is used to measure future performance; therefore, the criterion instrument must be administered some time after the predictor instrument. For example, schools of nursing like to predict how well their graduates will do on the licensure exam. Because they are unable to administer the licensure exam, they must rely on other means of predicting success.

Procedure

To predict performance on the examination, the school could use another measure of nursing knowledge. In both cases the construct of interest is "knowledge of nursing" with the licensure exam reflecting the higher-order construct. A school may elect to use GPA of nursing courses, a standardized test, or clinical performance to predict passage of the licensure exam. The scores of the predictor measure are correlated with the pass rate of the licensure exam using the appropriate statistical analysis technique. If the predictor instrumentation is valid, then the correlation between the two measures should be close to 1 (1.0).

Interpreting Criterion-Related Validity

The most important factor to consider in interpreting criterion-related validity is the representativeness of the sample. Perhaps more than the other measures of validity, criterion-related validity is very dependent on sample characteristics. Unless the sample used in the validity testing truly represents the population of interest, then criterion validity is problematic.

The changing nature of samples makes criterion-related validity hard to repeat. The sample used for testing must be representative of the population for which the instrument is designed, preferably chosen by probability means. Also the mortality rate (those who stop participating) during the study and the characteristics of those who chose not to participate should be considered, as this can fundamentally alter validity.

Other Considerations

All measures should be assessed for reliability. Nonreliable instruments should never be utilized because they can never reflect validity. The researcher should also realize that criterion-related validity tends to overestimate validity, and so borderline results should be carefully considered before use (Waltz et al., 1991).

❧ MEASUREMENT CONSIDERATIONS WITH QUALITATIVE RESEARCH

Qualitative research generally uses words rather than numbers to describe the phenomena of research interest. Although classical measurement theory applies only to quantitative measures, the notions of reliability and validity are important to all research. There are many different approaches to qualitative research, and so reliability and validity assessments may vary. As pointed out by Kahn (1993), qualitative research's use of the word *validity* (and one would assume *reliability*) remains conceptually undeveloped. The following represents a general discussion; for reliability and validity assessments specific to a particular type of qualitative research, the reader is directed to Munhall and Oiler (1986).

RELIABILITY

Kirk and Miller (1986) describe three types of reliability: quixotic, diachronic, and synchronic.

Quixotic Reliability

Quixotic reliability "refers to circumstances in which a single method of observation continually yields an unvarying measurement" (Kirk & Miller, 1986, p. 41). This form may present a false sense of reliability as answers and observations generally give varying results in both qualitative and quantitative studies. As an example of this reliability, consider the answer given to the question, "How are you doing in school?" The vast majority of answers received will be "fine." Yet, not all those queried are really doing "fine."

Diachronic Reliability

This form of reliability refers to the stability of answers over time (Kirk & Miller, 1986). Diachronic reliability can be assessed by examining the results of two qualitative studies done at separate times for similarity of answers. As with any reliability that assesses stability, this form is only useful when the phenomena do not change over time.

Synchronic Reliability

Synchronic reliability assesses the similarity of qualitative measurement within the same time period. The researcher may use field notes from two separate observers to assess synchronic reliability.

VALIDITY

Validity is also important for the qualitative researcher who wants to achieve accurate results that reflect the true state of the phenomena under study. Miles and Huberman (1984) recommend that researchers present evidence of the following strategies before claiming validity.

Checking for Representativeness

The researcher must remember that the people (cases) in the study may be those who are easier to contact and may not be representative. The researcher should assume that the sample is nonrepresentative and set about to prove otherwise by increasing the number of cases, looking for contrasting cases, sorting the cases and trying to sort out weak cases, or by trying to sample randomly.

Checking for Researcher Effects

Researchers must remember that they influence the research site and the research site influences them and that both situations result in bias. There are many ways to help control the biases, including using unobtrusive methods when possible, interviewing off-site, spending some time away from the site, or showing field notes to another researcher.

Triangulating

Triangulation supports validity by indicating that other measures show similar, or noncontradictory, findings. This may include checking archival records, talking with other researchers, and using multiple sources and methods to collect data.

Weighting the Evidence

Some data are stronger or more valid than others. Researchers may find some informants to be stronger because they are more knowledgeable or articulate. The circumstances of the data collection can also be important to validity. Firsthand observations are stronger than second-hand, and volunteered information is stronger than that which is prompted.

Making Contrasts/Comparisons

The researcher should check for validity by consciously looking for contrasts and comparisons.

Checking the Meaning of Outliers and Extreme Cases

Researchers should look for and closely examine the exceptions to provide evidence for validity and to reduce bias.

Ruling Out Spurious Relations

When two variables appear to be related, researchers should always look carefully for an alternative explanation provided by a third, intervening variable.

Replicating a Finding

It is important that the researcher either replicate the findings with new informants or at a new site or have another researcher attempt replication.

Checking Out Rival Explanations

Researchers should try to entertain several different explanations as they progress through data collection and analysis to avoid premature closure.

Looking for Negative Evidence

The researcher should purposely examine the data for contradictory or negative evidence.

Getting Feedback from Informants

The informants can serve as expert judges for the conclusions drawn from the data. The informants may not be accurate either, but they do provide another test of validity.

❧ EVALUATING THE MEASUREMENT PLAN

It is very important to evaluate the measurement methods described in a research study. The thoroughness and appropriateness of the measurement assessment are critical to the results of the study. A checklist for evaluating the measurement aspects of the study is presented in the box.

Consumers of research need to decide how to use the research results if the measurement information is missing or is inappropriate. Questions to be considered are:

MEASUREMENT EVALUATION

1. Are the conceptual and operational definitions of the concepts appropriate and strongly related?
2. Is the level of measurement appropriate to the study and the statistical procedure?
3. How did the researcher assess the reliability of the instrumentation? Is the method or methods appropriate to the study?
4. How was validity assessed? Was the method, or methods, appropriate?
5. Were the statistical procedures used to assess the reliability and validity of the study reported in enough detail for the reader?
6. Are the values reported for the reliability and validity assessments adequate?

---

(1) Does the missing information threaten the validity of the findings? (2) If an inappropriate measurement method was used, does it seriously affect the results? (3) Does the researcher provide any explanation for the missing or inappropriate information?

SUMMARY

- Measurement is traditionally defined as the application of numbers to phenomena.
- All methods of measurement contain the possibility of error. Error may be classified as systematic or random.
- Sources of measurement error are environmental factors, researcher factors, instrumentation factors, and subject factors.
- Classical measurement theory is based on the assumption that all measurement contains random error. It proposes that all data collected contain the true value of those data plus an error value.
- The four levels of measurement used in research are nominal, ordinal, interval, and ratio.
- The *nominal* level of measurement is used for those variables that can only be categorized or sorted but not ordered in a meaningful way.

- The *ordinal* level of measurement is used for those variables that can be rank ordered, but the rankings do not indicate distance between the variables.
- The *interval* level of measurement is used for those variables that can be rank-ordered with equal distances between the variables but with no absolute absence of the variable.
- The *ratio* level of measurement is used for those variables that can be rank-ordered, with equal intervals between the numbers and with an absolute zero point.
- Two measurement frameworks commonly used in nursing research are norm-referenced and criterion-referenced measurement.
- Reliability is the ability of an instrument to produce reproducible results. Factors to consider in reliability assessment include stability, equivalence, and homogeneity. Reliability is assessed by test-retest, parallel forms or measures, or internal consistency.
- Validity is the truthfulness of a measure; that the instrument actually measures what it purports to measure. Types of validity include content validity, construct validity, and criterion-related validity.
- Although classical measurement theory

is not applicable to qualitative research, reliability and validity are important to all types of research.

• The thoroughness and appropriateness of the measurement assessment are critical to the results of the study.

FACILITATING CRITICAL THINKING

1. What are the steps in instrument development? Describe how error can be reduced in this process.
2. Compare and contrast norm-referenced and criterion-referenced instruments.
3. Name and describe the validity measures used with norm-referenced instrumentation.
4. Describe the decision process used when deciding how to assess reliability. What factors influence reliability scores?
5. Explain what the multitrait-multimethod measure of construct validity will measure.
6. Describe the fundamentalist argument over use of statistics with each level of Stevens's classification scheme. Name one statistic appropriate for use with each level.

References

SUBSTANTIVE

BLENNER, J. L. (1993). Development of the Stimulus Intensity Modulation Scale. *Journal of Nursing Measurement, 1*(1), 5-18.

CONN, V. (1991). Self-care actions taken by older adults for influenza and colds. *Nursing Research, 40*(3), 176-181.

GIVEN, C. W., GIVEN, B., STOMMEL, M., COLLINS, C., KING, S., & FRANKLIN, S. (1993). The caregiver reaction assessment (CRA) for caregivers to persons with chronic physical and mental impairment. *Research in Nursing and Health, 15,* 271-283.

KERESZTES, P., HOLM, K., PENCKOFER, S., & MERRITT, S. (1993). Measurement of functional ability in patients with coronary artery disease. *Journal of Nursing Measurement, 1*(1), 19-28.

MAHON, N. E., & YARCHESKI, A. (1992). Alternate explanations of loneliness in adolescents: A replication and extension study. *Nursing Research, 41*(3), 151-156.

SIDERANKO, S., QUINN, A., BURNS, K., & FROMAN, R. (1992). The effects of position and mattress overlay on sacral and heel pressures in a clinical population. *Research in Nursing and Health, 15,* 245-251.

SPIELBERGER, C. D. (1983). Manual for State-Trait Anxiety Inventory. Palo Alto, CA: Consulting Psychologists Press.

CONCEPTUAL

BRENNAN, P. F., & HAYS, B. J. (1992). The Kappa Statistic for establishing interrater reliability in the secondary analysis of qualitative clinical data. *Research in Nursing and Health, 15,* 153-158.

FERKETICH, S. L. (1990). Internal consistency estimates of reliability. *Research in Nursing and Health, 13,* 437-440.

GOODWIN, L. D., & GOODWIN, W. L. (1991). Estimating construct validity. *Research in Nursing and Health, 14,* 235-243.

JENNINGS, B. M., & ROGERS, F. (1989). Managing measurement error, *Nursing Research, 38,* 186-187.

KAHN, D. L. (1993). Ways of discussing validity in qualitative nursing research. *Western Journal of Nursing Research, 15*(1), 122-126.

KNAPP, T. R. (1985). Validity reliability and neither. *Nursing Research, 34*(3), 189-192.

KNAPP, T. R. (1990). Treating ordinal scales as interval scales: An attempt to resolve the controversy. *Nursing Research, 39*(2), 121-123.

KNAPP, T. R. (1991). Coefficient alpha: Conceptualizations and anomalies. *Research in Nursing and Health, 14,* 457-460.

KNAPP, T. R. (1993). Treating ordinal scales as ordinal scales. *Nursing Research, 42*(3), 184-186.

LOWE, N. K., & RYAN-WENGER, N. M. (1992). Beyond Campbell and Fiske: Assessment of convergent and discriminant validity. *Research in Nursing and Health, 15,* 67-75.

LYNN, M. R. (1986). Determination and quantification of content validity. *Nursing Research, 35*(6), 382-385.

REW, L., STUPPY, D., & BECKER, H. (1988). Construct validity in instrument development: A vital link between nursing practice, research, and theory. *Advances in Nursing Science, 10*(4), 10-22.

SAX, G. (1980). *Principles of educational and psychological measurement and evaluation* (2nd ed.). Belmont CA: Wadsworth.

THOMAS, S. D., HATHAWAY, D. K., & ARHEART, K. L. (1992). Face validity. *Western Journal of Nursing Research, 14*(1), 109-112.

TOPF, M. (1987). Interrater reliability decline under convert assessment. *Nursing Research, 37*(1), 47-49.

TULMAN, L. R., & JACOBSEN, B. S. (1989). Goldilocks and variability. *Nursing Research, 38*(6), 377-379.

WALTZ, C. F., & BAUSELL, R. B. (1981). *Nursing research: Design statistics, and computer analysis.* Philadelphia: F.A. Davis Company.

METHODOLOGICAL

AMERICAN PSYCHOLOGICAL ASSOCIATION, COMMITTEE TO DEVELOP STANDARDS. (1985). *Standards for educational and psychological testing.* Washington, DC: Author.

GABLE, R. K. (1986). *Instrument development in the affective domain.* Boston: Kluwer-Nijhoff.

KIRK, J., & MILLER, M. L. (1986). *Reliability and validity in qualitative research.* Newbury Park, CA: Sage.

MILES, M.B., & HUBERMAN, A. M. (1984). *Qualitative data analysis: A sourcebook of new methods.* Newbury Park, CA: Sage.

MUNHALL, P. L., & OILER, C. J. (1986). *Nursing research: A qualitative perspective.* Norwalk, CT: Appleton-Century-Crofts.

WALTZ, C. F., STRICKLAND, O. L., & LENZ, E. R. (1991). *Measurement in nursing research* (2nd ed.). Philadelphia: F.A Davis.

HISTORICAL

CAMPBELL, O. T., & FISKE, D. W. (1959). Convergent and discriminant validation by the multitrait-multimethod matrix. *Psychological Bulletin, 56*, 81-104.

COSTA, P. T., & MCRAE, R. R. (1980). Somatic complaints in males as a function of age and neuroticism: A longitudinal analysis. *Journal of Behavioral Medicine, 3*, 245-258.

HOLMES, T. H., & RAHE, R. H. (1967). The social readjustment rating scale. *Journal of Psychosomatic Research, 11*, 213-218.

KERLINGER, F. N. (1979). *Behavioral research: A conceptual approach.* New York: Holt, Rinehart & Winston.

MARTUZA, V. R. (1977). *Applying norm-referenced and criterion-referenced measurement in education.* Boston: Allyn & Bacon.

NUNNALLY, J. C. (1978). *Psychometric theory.* New York: McGraw-Hill.

STEVENS, S. S. (1946). On the theory of scales of measurement. *Science, 103*, 677-680.

CHAPTER 15

MEASUREMENT INSTRUMENTS

ANNE G. PEIRCE

Research studies conducted by nurses examine almost every conceivable phenomenon. To understand the phenomenon and to communicate findings to others in a concise and expedient manner, the phenomenon must be measured. There are many ways to measure, including methods that use self-reports, observations, and physiologic markers. Within each of these methodologies are hundreds if not thousands of measurement tools and instruments. The task of the researcher is to choose or develop instruments that accurately, precisely, and sensitively measure the variable(s) of interest. Carefully chosen instruments are critical to good research since they augment control and thus reduce error.

Despite the large number of instruments available, it is sometimes difficult to locate the exact instrument needed for a research study, and this has led to the development of new instruments by nurse researchers. Besides describing the characteristics of the various types of instrumentation, this chapter will discuss important considerations in using a previously developed instrumentation method, as well as the strategies for developing new ones. The reader is referred to Chapter 14 for discussion of the measurement characteristics of instruments.

SELF-REPORT INSTRUMENTS

The most common form of instrumentation involves directly asking the respondents about the study variables; hence the name self-report. Self-report instruments include questionnaires, scales, surveys, and interviews. These methods are very effective when the purpose of the study is to obtain information about attitudes, knowledge, feelings, and other information that cannot easily be observed or measured physiologically.

The type of self-report method chosen depends on the research purpose and the sample. Verbal methods such as interviews and written methods such as questionnaires, surveys, and scales have different strengths and weaknesses. These aspects are taken into account when the instrumentation is chosen. For example, the cost of the instrumentation and the time involved differ between verbal and written methods. In general, written instrumentation is less costly and quicker to administer than an interview. Interviews, on the other hand, generally provide a more in-depth view of the research topic and allow the researcher (or data collector) to clarify the questions being asked. Telephone interviews and group interviews or focus groups may reduce the cost in terms of money and time while still allowing the researcher to obtain information similar to that obtained from individual face-to-face interviews.

QUESTIONNAIRES

The most familiar self-report instrumentation is the questionnaire, where the respondent writes his or her answers in response to printed questions on a document. Questionnaires are commonly used to obtain demographic information. In addition, they can be used to test and explore relationships and validate assumptions. While paper documents are the most common, questionnaires may also be administered via computer.

Questionnaires allow the gathering of large amounts of information from a large sample relatively quickly and inexpensively. Because questionnaires do not ask for identifying information, they also can provide for confidentiality or anonymity when dealing with sensitive topics.

A major consideration in deciding to use a questionnaire includes the influences imposed by the questionnaire's structure. The structure is beneficial when it helps to ensure that the information being sought is obtained. However, the only information obtained is what is asked, so there is always the possibility that important unknown dimensions can be overlooked.

A well-designed questionnaire is easy for the respondent to fill out and is easy for the researcher to administer and score. Yet a good questionnaire is difficult to develop; each aspect, from the items themselves to the color of the paper used, can influence the responses of the respondents.

Developing Questions

Researchers frequently develop questionnaires. The development of a new questionnaire allows the researcher to tailor the questions to the research topic. Even if the main research instrument is well established, it is often necessary to develop questions or items. For example, the researcher may want to obtain additional demographic information not found on the original questionnaire from the respondents. The following points are important to question development:

Clear Understanding of the Purpose of the Research. A thorough understanding of the relevant literature is essential to question development. From that knowledge the researcher can develop a specification matrix that outlines the information needed for the study and approximately how many questions are needed for each aspect. This ensures that all aspects of the phenomena important to the research study are addressed by the instrumentation. For example, if the researcher is interested in knowledge of, and attitudes toward, restraint use with the hospitalized elderly, the specification matrix might look as follows:

	Chemical restraints	Mechanical restraints
Knowledge	10	10
Attitude	10	10

STEPS IN DEVELOPING A QUESTIONNAIRE

1. Understand the purpose of the research
2. Determine the structure of the questions
   Closed-ended questions
   Open-ended questions
3. Carefully phrase the questions and remember to:
   Consider the reading level
   Consider the clarity of the terminology
   Avoid ambiguous wording
   Avoid leading questions
   Avoid questions with more than one answer
4. Consider the total length of the questionnaire
5. Consider the following aspects of question arrangement:
   Group similar questions together
   Ask interesting and easier questions first
   Ask for sensitive information last
   Arrange questions from the general to the specific
6. Review newly developed items carefully

This specification matrix directs the researcher to develop 10 questions for each cell for a total questionnaire length of 40 questions. From this matrix we know that the researcher considers all the elements equally important.

Structure of Questions. All questionnaires have some structure by virtue of their printed nature. Structure is provided by the rules of administration and the type of question chosen. For example, questions may be closed-ended or open-ended. It is not unusual to find both within one questionnaire.

The researcher looks carefully at the pros and cons of each type of question before deciding on the question format. The format and wording can influence the results. Consider the following:

Closed-ended
Should marijuana use be legalized?
_____ yes   _____ no

Open-ended
Are there any circumstances under which the use of marijuana should be legal-

ized? (Please respond in the following space)

Each question asks for essentially the same information, yet the second question allows the respondent to qualify an answer. Positive answers to the two questions can provide very different impressions to the researcher. Someone who answers no to the first question, could conceivably answer yes to the second. For example, someone might answer "Yes, when there is clear evidence of medical benefit."

Researchers may also decide to use a mixed approach. Questions can be written in such a way that it combines closed- and open-ended responses. For example, the researcher may give the respondents several alternatives, but adds that they are free to supply a different answer.

CLOSED-ENDED QUESTIONS. Closed-ended questions, also called fixed alternative, are worded in such a way that only a limited response is possible. For example:

"Are you a male or female?" While certain respondents may qualify the answer, the answer can realistically only be yes or no.

The closed-ended question requires the

researcher to include all possible responses and to make sure that the responses are mutually exclusive. Consider the following hypothetical example: Please indicate your annual income level for the previous year:

1. $0.00 to $10,000.00
2. $10,001.00 to $35,000.00
3. $35,001.00 to $50,000.00
4. $50,001.00 and above

The choices reflect all possible income levels. Notice that the choices start with $0.00 and go to $50,001.00 and above. The categories are also mutually exclusive, only one answer is possible for a given respondent. There are no overlapping categories of income.

CONSIDERATIONS. The closed-ended question limits the answers to those options provided by the researcher. This has several advantages to the researcher; first, it facilitates the coding and analyzing of data; second, it ensures that the researcher obtains the desired information; and third, it can increase the reliability of the study.

Because only selected bits of information are collected, other equally important information may not be retrieved. Also some respondents become frustrated with the limited responses and expand their answers. Any experienced researcher who has used questionnaires can relate instances where respondents wrote lengthy answers on the margins or the back of the questionnaire to a seemingly simple yes or no question.

Also, with questionnaires designed to measure knowledge, it is hard to know if the respondent guessed the response or actually knew the material. Also, if an item is not answered, it is difficult to know if the respondent purposely did not answer or if it was inadvertently missed.

OPEN-ENDED QUESTIONS. Open-ended questions are appropriate when the re-searcher wants more information than a closed-ended questionnaire can provide. This form is also useful when the answers cannot be anticipated or when there are so many possible answers that the form would be unwieldy. Examples could include the names of natural medicines used by alternative medicine providers or the names of courses taken by college students.

Open-ended questions do not supply the response alternatives to the respondent. Each individual may answer as they desire. The open-ended question generally provides richer, more diverse data than can be obtained with closed-ended questions. These questions are also easier to construct, although they still require considerable effort. However, the very diversity of the answers makes it more difficult for the researcher to code and analyze the data.

Phrasing of the Question

READING LEVEL. The reading level of the questionnaire can influence the accuracy of the findings. The questions should be phrased so that the least able reader in the sample can comprehend the material. Several reading assessment methods are available for the researcher.

CLARITY OF THE TERMINOLOGY. The researcher must be careful to avoid terms that the average respondent would not know. It is easy to forget that the everyday language of the researcher and nurse is different from that of other groups. Even such common words as urine and blood pressure may not be familiar to all respondents (e.g., children). If any unknown words are used, the researcher should supply a definition. Also, respondents whose native language is not English may be unable to participate unless the instruments are translated.

AVOIDANCE OF AMBIGUOUS WORDING. A pilot study will often reveal ambiguous wording. For example, Peirce (1987) found that the word "couple" can have regional variations in meaning. In some areas couple means two only; in other parts of the country couple can mean up to three or four.

Avoidance of Leading Questions. Items and format can "clue" the respondent to what is expected. This results in bias, negating the usefulness of the findings. The researcher should try to avoid items or formats that suggest answers or trigger socially desirable answers. For example, consider the wording of the following question: "Do you think health care reform should occur at any cost?" The phrasing leads the respondent to consider that the researcher probably thinks that there are limits to what should occur with health care reform. The phrasing may influence the respondent to answer in a way that pleases the researcher.

Avoidance of Questions with More than One Answer. Consider the question, "Should cost and personal preference be considered in choosing a health care provider?" A respondent could conceivably think that one, but not both, aspects, should be considered. The response obtained will be meaningless for the researcher without further clarification.

Total Length of the Questionnaire. The questionnaire must be long enough to obtain the necessary information but not so long that it fatigues the respondent.

Question Arrangement. The arrangement of the questions in a questionnaire is critical. All questions must be arranged in a way that appears logical and relevant to the respondent. Various strategies exist to help the researcher decide how to arrange the questions.

1. *Group similar questions together.* In general, questions that ask for similar information should be grouped together. For example, the researcher who studies AIDS patients' knowledge of the disease might group together questions about transmission into one section and treatment into another.

2. *Ask interesting and/or easier questions first.* Response rates are usually higher if the more interesting questions are asked first, followed by the less interesting and/or more difficult questions. For this reason demographic information is generally asked last.

3. *Ask for sensitive information last.* Questions that ask for sensitive information are generally placed at the end of the questionnaire. It is thought that by placing the sensitive questions at the end the respondent is more likely to answer them. By the time the respondent comes to the end, he or she is more "committed" to answering the questionnaire. Also the data from respondents who do not answer certain questions can still be revealing. Placing sensitive questions at the end will allow the researcher to collect the bulk of the data. For example, consider a research study designed to examine how the health beliefs of women influence choice of birth control. The researcher might decide to place sensitive questions about sexual activity last. If a significant number of women chose not to answer the questions, the researcher could examine the data to see if there were significant differences between the health beliefs of those women who answered the questions and those who did not. While this type of information is not directly tied to the research question, the information gained could prove invaluable in designing future studies.

4. *Arrange questions from general to specific.* Finally, researchers generally arrange questionnaires so that questions that ask for general information are followed by those that ask for the specific. This sequencing helps avoid biasing by reducing the suggestion of appropriate answers. The same is true of open-ended questions preceding closed-ended.

Review of Newly Developed Items. Because of the importance of item construction, the researcher should have multiple reviewers for any newly developed items. The reviewers should consider sequence, wording, cultural bias, disciplinary and other forms of bias, social desirability, readability, and so forth.

In item review it is important that both experts and lay people be used. The measurement and content experts can give thoughtful reviews based on professional knowledge, while the lay expert can give meaningful insights based on insider knowledge of the topic and the sample.

Administration

Questionnaires can be administered in a variety of ways. They can be mailed, hand delivered, given in groups or one-on-one, or even given by computer. Each administration method has its own considerations. Whatever the decision, it is important that the administration of the questionnaire be the same for all respondents. The conditions under which a questionnaire is administered influence its error rate. The researcher tries to reduce these variations to gain as much consistency as possible.

Mailed Questionnaires. Mailed questionnaires are commonly used when the researcher wants to reach a large sample in a relatively short time. Mailed questionnaires

are sent to the respondents' homes or work addresses, but not to both to reduce variation in stimuli when the questionnaire is answered. The researcher decides where to send it based on the subject matter and on knowledge of the work or home environment and of the respondents. Unknown differences will still occur as individual's work and home environments differ as do unforseen events in both. Also respondents may move the questionnaire form one site to another before answering.

Considerations. With a mailed questionnaire an adequate response rate probably should be 60% or more. However, according to Waltz, Strickland, and Lenz (1991) a 30% response rate is not unusual.

A low response rate is problematic for many reasons. The most important consideration is that differences exist between those respondents who answer the questionnaire and those who do not. Respondents and nonrespondents may vary in their interest in the topic, ability to understand and answer, time available, and so forth. All these factors will influence the results, yet the researcher is generally unable to discern why a questionnaire is not answered.

The researcher should try to discover how representative the obtained sample was relative to the projected study sample. For example, it may be possible to determine demographic similarities and differences using census data.

Improving Response Rates. To help improve the response rate of mailed (and other) questionnaires a variety of techniques are suggested. First, the questionnaire should be well designed. A professional-appearing questionnaire, with easy-to-read directions and items, is more likely to be answered than a sloppy or confusing one. A well-written cover letter that explains the general purpose of the questionnaire, how the data will be used and its importance, can also influence return rates. The cover letter replaces the verbal explanation of the research and so should include all the pertinent information plus motivate the respondent to answer. Also important is the presence of a stamped, self-addressed return envelope.

A follow-up system is also recommended. For example, one system may be to follow up the first mailing with a reminder postcard or telephone call at a predetermined time, such as 2 weeks. This can be followed by other reminders and even a second or third copy of the questionnaire. A very complete and systematic method for handling questionnaires is suggested by Dillman (1978).

Other Forms of Questionnaire Administration

Group Administration. Group administration of a questionnaire is also common. Group administration has many benefits. The researcher can be present to answer questions that may arise. The return rate is usually high and a significant number of completed questionnaires can be obtained at once. To obtain a good response the researcher must ensure that there is enough space to write, that everyone has writing utensils, and that the room is comfortable and free from distractions.

The researcher must also make provisions to protect the confidentiality or anonymity of the respondents. This might be accomplished by having a return box at the back of the room or by asking one of the respondents to collect the questionnaires. Respondents should not feel coerced into answering. The researcher must make sure that any respondent who chooses not to answer can do so without undue attention.

Computer Administration. Computer administration of questionnaires is becoming more common. Computers have many advantages. The questionnaire is easily programmed and can be designed so that questions can be individualized. For example, questions that do not pertain to a certain respondent can be skipped by the computer. The computer can also be programmed to have the important benefit of being able to code and analyze the data without intermediate steps by the researcher!

Considerations in computer administration include getting respondents to computers, as well as the small number of computers generally available for use at any one time. Also, many people are still uncomfortable with computers and may find them difficult to use correctly.

SCALES

Scales can be considered a variant of the questionnaire format and a useful and effective method of ascertaining the affective domain and other attributes. A scale is composed of a set of numbers, letters, or symbols that have rules and that can be used to locate individuals on a continuum. For example, if scale scores for anxiety rise as anxiety increases, respondents with higher scale scores would be presumed to have a higher anxiety level than respondents with lower scores.

Scales are composed of a stem statement that directs the respondent, anchor words, and a series of scale steps (see below). The scale steps usually are composed of numbers, for example, 1 to 5 or 1 to 7, but can also be symbols or letters. The values obtained are treated as interval level data, although technically the intervals between answers may not be equal.

Labor is:

Pleasant ----Unpleasant	- **stem statement**
1 2 3 4 5 6 7	- **anchor**
	- **scale steps**

TYPES OF SCALES

Semantic differential	Likert scale
Rating scales	Guttman scales
Summated rating scale	Visual analogue scale

Semantic Differential

Semantic differentials measure attitudes toward a concept by asking the respondent to rate qualities such as evaluation, potency, and activity on a 5- to 9-point scale anchored by the bipolar adjectives (Osgood, Suci, & Tannenbaum, 1957).

Development. First, the researcher picks a concept. The concept can be designated through a word, picture, symbol, phrase, or sentence. The researcher may also have the sample respond to more than one concept for comparison purposes. For example, pregnancy could be contrasted with childbirth.

Next the researcher chooses the adjectives to describe the concept. Osgood, et al. (1957), using factor analyses of many semantic differentials, found that most adjectives fit into three factors that they labeled evaluation, potency, and activity. In the example seen in Figure 15-1, adjective pair 16 could represent evaluation, pair 2 potency, and pair 9 activity.

While the same adjective pairs can be used to describe many concepts, the researcher must ensure that all word pairs are appropriate for the concept under study. In the example given the researcher interviewed 30 women to obtain a list of appropriate adjectives.

Scoring. To score a semantic differential the scores are added up to form a composite overall score, a scale score, or both. Gen-

erally, the adjective pairs are randomly placed as far as the negative and positive being on the left or the right. For example:

hard------------easy	positive value
1 2 3 4 5 6 7	to the right)
good------------bad	(positive value
1 2 3 4 5 6 7	to the left)

If the researcher decides that higher numbers represent a positive word value, the negative, high-score items are "flipped." So an item score of 7 for the adjective pair "good-bad" would be scored as a 1 when it was summed, and the pair "hard-easy" would remain as a score of 7. In most cases if the items are not flipped, the total score would be meaningless.

The scores from semantic differentials can be used in many ways. Respondents can be compared, scales can be compared, subscales can be compared, and so forth. Factor analysis may reveal important differences and add to the theoretical development of the concept.

Rating Scales

Rating scales are the most basic of the scaled instruments. Rating scales consist of a stem and scale steps. The scale steps are an ordered set of categories of the variable. Each of the categories is given a number that implies more or less of the variable (see Fig. 15-2). This form of scale is relatively easy to construct, and most respondents are familiar with the format. It is very

Labor/delivery construct scale

Below is a list of paired words women have used to describe childbirth. Please look at each pair of words and circle the number on the scale which you feel most accurately describes your labor and delivery.

1. Painful   **Not painful**
1   2   3   4   5   6   7

2. Easy   **Hard work**
1   2   3   4   5   6   7

3. Pleasurable   **Uncomfortable**
1   2   3   4   5   6   7

4. Not scary   **Scary**
1   2   3   4   5   6   7

5. Anxiety producing   **Not anxiety producing**
1   2   3   4   5   6   7

6. Beautiful   **Awful**
1   2   3   4   5   6   7

7. Lonely   **Shared**
1   2   3   4   5   6   7

8. Exciting   **Not exciting**
1   2   3   4   5   6   7

9. Slow   **Fast**
1   2   3   4   5   6   7

10. Long   **Short**
1   2   3   4   5   6   7

11. Short wait   **Long time coming**
1   2   3   4   5   6   7

12. Controllable   **Uncontrollable**
1   2   3   4   5   6   7

13. Prepared   **Unprepared**
1   2   3   4   5   6   7

14. Unknown   **Known**
1   2   3   4   5   6   7

15. Satisfying   **Unsatisfying**
1   2   3   4   5   6   7

16. Rewarding   **Unrewarding**
1   2   3   4   5   6   7

17. Relieving   **Burdening**
1   2   3   4   5   6   7

Figure 15-1. Example of a semantic differential scale. (From Peirce, A. G. [1987]. Event review in the coping process of parous women, Doctoral dissertation, University of Maryland, Dissertation Abstracts International, 42, 705-B).

1. Advanced practice nurses should provide first level primary care:
   a. never
   b. sometimes
   c. always

2. Advanced practice nurses should provide all primary care:
   a. never
   b. sometimes
   c. always

3. Advanced practice nurses should work closely with a physican:
   a. never
   b. sometimes
   c. always

4. Advanced practice nurses need close physician supervision:
   a. never
   b. sometimes
   c. always

Figure 15-2. Example of rating scale questions.

common to use rating scales in everyday interaction; for example, "How would you rate your summer vacation—the best ever, the worst ever, or somewhere in between?"

Use with Observation Data. Rating scales allow a quantitative approach to observation data and are often used to structure observational studies. The scales also help to ensure that the researcher obtains the wanted information either at the time of observation or afterward. For example, the researcher might look at angry behaviors in a toddler playgroup and rate the intensity of the anger observed.

Summated Rating Scales
Summated rating scales consist of a series of scaled items where each item is scored in approximately the same way. The scale scores are added to derive a total score; hence the name.

The scale's reliability is dependent to a substantial degree on a sufficient number of items and scale steps. According to Waltz, Strickland, and Lenz (1991) 10 to 15 items with five to six scale steps is adequate. There sometimes is disagreement among researchers about whether to have an odd or even number of scale steps. It is more common to have an uneven number of steps. This uneven number allows what is called the "middle alternative" or a neutral response. However, when researchers want to force the respondent to respond either positively or negatively, they supply an even number of scale steps.

Likert Scale
Likert scales are a form of summated rating scales used to ascertain opinions or attitudes. They consist of a declarative statement that forms the stem and scale steps (Figure 15-3).

Please circle the number which most closely corresponds to whether or not you agree that this is a coping strategy that you used to deal with childbirth. The numbers have the following meanings:

1 = strongly disagree
2 = disagree
3 = undecided
4 = agree
5 = strongly agree

1. Went over in my mind what I did from the time it all started

1   2   3   4   5

2. Reviewed everything in my mind

1   2   3   4   5

3. Talked with other people about what had happened to me

1   2   3   4   5

4. Talked about it with people who were willing to listen

1   2   3   4   5

5. Thought about each aspect of the event and what it meant to me

1   2   3   4   5

6. I found myself needing to talk about what had happened

1   2   3   4   5

7. Thought about my response to the event

1   2   3   4   5

8. Went over what I thought happened

1   2   3   4   5

9. I went over and over the event

1   2   3   4   5

10. I reviewed each step

1   2   3   4   5

11. Tried to explain my response to the event

1   2   3   4   5

12. I kept bringing the event to mind

1   2   3   4   5

13. I told other people about why I decided to do what I did

1   2   3   4   5

14. I kept picturing what happened in my mind

1   2   3   4   5

Figure 15-3. Example of a Likert type scale. (Adapted from Peirce, A. G. [1987]. Event review in the coping process of parous women, Doctoral dissertation, University of Maryland, Dissertation Abstracts International, 42, 705-B.)

The original scale used a five-point scale of "strongly disagree," "disagree," "uncertain," "agree," and "strongly agree." Now other types and numbers of scale steps are seen. In fact, a "Likert-type" scale is often used to refer to any scale that uses a declarative stem followed by a scale with several steps. A Likert scale question is as follows:

I think nurses should practice therapeutic touch in patient care situations:

Strongly disagree	Disagree	Uncertain	Agree	Strongly agree
1	2	3	4	5

While Likert and Likert-type scales are commonly used in American research, Flaskerud (1988) raises the possibility that Likert scales are culturally biased. She reports that both the Hispanic and the Asian groups studied preferred a dichotomous (yes, no) response to a scaled response.

Guttman Scales

Guttman scales, also called cumulative scales, are used to assess attitudes toward a singular concept. In this form of scale each item is related in an incremental way to the prior item. Thus the person who answers a question positively is assumed to also be in agreement with the item before it but not necessarily with the item that follows.

The items, usually only four or five, are arranged in order of intensity. The respondent is asked to agree or disagree with each item and receives a cumulative score from a tool. For example, a researcher may list five health care packages that could be offered in a national health care plan (Figure 15-4).

Reproducible results are important to Guttman scales. To assess the reproducibility of the scale, researchers use scalogram analysis. The analysis helps the researcher determine the unidimensionality of the scale by determining if knowledge of a person's score correctly identifies their standing on each item. For example, if a person receives a score of three (for three items marked agree), the researcher should know that they agreed with items 1 to 3 but not with 4 or 5. If the scale does not predict with accuracy, it is probably not measuring a unidimensional concept.

The main advantage of Guttman scales is their scalability. Relative standings can be simply determined from the scores. The major disadvantage is the difficulty of constructing a good cumulative scale. Also Guttman scales generally include a small number of items, reducing their ability to discriminate between individuals.

Visual Analog Scale

A visual analog scale is a particularly useful scale for assessing perception of physical stimuli such as pain, sleep quality, and shortness of breath. The visual analog scale consists of a linear scale, most frequently 100 mm in length, anchored by two words or phrases. Because of its length, the scale allows for fine numerical discrimination between respondents.

The linear scale may be either horizontal or vertical. However, vertical lines may be preferable to many respondents. The word anchors are chosen by the researcher to reflect the totality of the concept. For example, with pain the anchors might be "no pain" and "pain as bad as it could be."

The respondent is asked to read the item (or items) and then to place an X or other mark on the line. The mark indicates the intensity of their response in relation to the two words. For example, a visual analog scale could be used to assess discomfort during selected activities for arthritic clients (Figure 15-5).

The score is obtained by measuring the

Please indicate the level of health care which should be provided under a national plan.

1. Medical and surgical care for acute, potentially fatal problems.
   Prenatal care

2. Medical and surgical care for acute, potentially fatal problems.
   Prenatal care
   Well-infant and child care

3. Medical and surgical care for acute, potentially fatal problems.
   Prenatal care
   Well-infant and child care
   Medical and surgical care for nonfatal chronic problems

4. Medical and surgical care for acute, potentially fatal problems.
   Prenatal care
   Well-infant and child care
   Medical and surgical care for nonfatal chronic problems
   Non experimental fertility care, including invitro-fertilization

5. Medical and surgical care for acute, potentially fatal problems.
   Prenatal care
   Well-infant and child care
   Medical and surgical care for nonfatal chronic problems
   Non-experimental fertility care, including invitro-fertilization
   Experimental treatments and therapies

Figure 15-4. Example of a Guttman scale.

Please make a X on the line to indicate the amount of discomfort you have right now with your arthritis.

Discomfort as bad as it can be

No Discomfort

Figure 15-5. Example of a visual analog scale.

distance between the low end of the scale and the mark made by the respondent. Because of the differences in the shape of the mark made by different respondents, the researcher often chooses a consistent place to measure, such as where the two lines of the X intersect. Because the scale produces at least interval level data, and with some experts claiming ratio level data, it is particularly appealing to researchers who wish to use certain parametric statistical procedures.

Considerations. The visual analog's advantages are that it is relatively easy for researchers to develop and for respondents to use. The scale allows the respondent the widest possible range of expression without the limitations sometimes imposed by numbered scale steps.

The disadvantages include concerns with reliability and validity. Test-retest reliability has been used successfully with visual analog scales. However, test-retest is only appropriate when the scale measures a stable trait. Changeable states result in low correlations. Internal consistency assessment is not possible because there generally is only one question, or one question per topic; thus items cannot be rated against one another. Interrater or intrarater reliability is important to ensure that the obtained measurement score is accurate.

Other Scaling Methods
Other types of scales exist, and readers interested in other methodologies are referred to the measurement texts listed in the chapter reference list.

SURVEYS
The term *survey* is used in a variety of different ways. To survey means to ask questions, and the survey can be used to describe the design of the study. A survey can also mean any questionnaire or interview used to collect information from a sample.

Uses
Surveys are used to collect information on a wide variety of topics. For example, surveys are used to ascertain knowledge, opinions, attitudes, values, buying habits, political views, and so forth. The questions that can be asked are limited only by what respondents will answer. Along with content questions surveys ask demographic questions. The demographic questions allow the researcher to ascertain how the sample represents the population.

Descriptive surveys collect selected information from a sample to develop a concept and or to estimate its occurrence in the total population. Along with the instrument used to collect the data, the sample chosen is critical to the success of the survey. In most cases the sample should closely resemble the population and should be large enough to allow estimation of population parameters. For specific information about sample selection see Chapter 13.

Longitudinal, descriptive surveys are also important when there is an interest in following a topic over a period of time. In a longitudinal survey there are repeated times of measurement. The instrumentation should be carefully developed so that it remains relevant over the period of time in which the data is collected.

Format
Most surveys use a questionnaire format and are conducted through interviews, either personal or by telephone, or mailed questionnaires. The format chosen is based on the knowledge of the sample and the research question.

Considerations. Surveys are a wonderful vehicle for obtaining a large amount of information in a short amount of time. Because of their nature they are generally not the best method for obtaining an in-depth analysis of a given topic; rather they represent a broad overview. Also, little can be inferred about cause and effect since surveys are not well controlled.

Delphi Survey Technique

The Delphi survey technique uses a panel of experts and multiple rounds of surveys to achieve consensus on a topic of interest. Delphi surveys are often used when the topic of interest is policy issues, historical data, or program development. They can provide a comprehensive means of achieving consensus, assessing priorities, and forecasting long-range goals. Because the respondents are generally surveyed by mail or by electronic means, it is possible to reach a geographically diverse group. The methodology also reduces the influence a powerful or well-known person may have on the group's opinion during a meeting.

Procedure. The first step in a Delphi survey is to identify an appropriate group of experts. To be effective the experts should not be homogeneous in their thinking; diversity is needed. It has been suggested that other forms of diversity are also important such as their region, gender, and so forth.

Next the participants are given the first round of questionnaires (or other instrumentation). It is important to the survey that participants not communicate with one another during the survey process.

With the first round completed, the results are tabulated and sent back to the expert sample. Also a statistical summary usually is sent. The respondents are asked to examine the data again and to comment appropriately. For instance, they may be asked to choose the 10 most important nursing policy issues out of the 50 identi-

fied in the first round. Again the results are analyzed and tabulated. Other rounds may occur until consensus is achieved. The researcher then reports the final round as the research findings.

Considerations. While the Delphi is an important method in garnering expert opinion, it is not without its drawbacks. It can be an expensive and time-consuming method.

Delphi surveys can be difficult for the researcher who must quickly compile the surveys between the rounds. The compilation of the surveys is critical. The results must be completely and thoughtfully analyzed; otherwise the results are not meaningful, and any further rounds, or the final report, will be compromised.

INTERVIEWS

Interviews are the verbal exchanges between researcher (or surrogate) and respondent to obtain information from the respondent. The interview need not be face to face; it can also occur by telephone and other electronic means.

Interviews are the most direct method of obtaining facts from the respondent. They can also be useful in ascertaining opinions, attitudes, and knowledge. Unlike questionnaires, in most cases the interviewer is available to clarify a question or to help the client expand on a theme. Interviews are also useful for those who cannot read and write or for other reasons cannot use pen-and-paper questionnaires.

Interview Formats

Interviews are generally classified as either structured or unstructured. Structured interviews are formalized so that all respondents hear the same questions in the same order. The unstructured interview may be more free flowing with its structure limited only by the focus of the research. However, both structured and unstructured interviews have many degrees of structure.

Structured Interviews. Structured interviews use a script and set questions for the interview. The questions are devised, placed in order, and generally pilot tested before the research study begins. The structured interview provides the most control for the researcher. The United States census is a formally structured interview with little or no variation allowed in the way the interviewer approaches the respondent.

Structured interviews vary in the interviewers' ability to probe and clarify. In the most structured of interviews the interviewer must adhere strictly to the given script of questions and probes. Some very structured interviews even provide the respondent with a list of possible answers. The only clarification that can be given is an approved part of the questionnaire. Other structured questionnaires are less rigidly designed, and the interviewer is allowed to clarify the questions or answers and devise individualized probes.

Unstructured Interviews. Unstructured interviews leave the wording and organization of questions, and sometimes even the topic, to the discretion of the interviewer. The degree of structure varies from completely unstructured to somewhat structured.

The somewhat structured interview may include an agenda, a list of representative questions, and certain goals. The interviewer, however, determines how the desired information is obtained and in what order. Clinical admission interviews provide an example of the more structured of unstructured interviews. The primary nurse generally needs to obtain certain information, but the order and the way in which the questions are asked is generally left to the nurse.

At the other end of the interview spectrum are the completely unstructured interviews. While unstructured interviews have few if any format rules, most have a topic or a focus. For example, the interviewer may be interested in health concepts regarding hypertension in the urban poor. The interviewer tries to explore the respondents' beliefs. The unstructured interview allows the interviewer to individually determine the question pathways while still keeping the end point in mind.

Types of Questions
Question development, sequencing, and wording considerations are similar to those discussed under questionnaire development and should be reviewed prior to the interview. In addition, all interview schedules should be pretested and assessed for reliability and validity.

Interview Administration
The time and place of interview administration is important. All interviews should occur at a time that is mutually convenient for the researcher and respondent. Allowing adequate time is crucial to completion of interview schedules.

The site of administration is also important. Interviews may occur in a variety of settings from the respondent's home to a laboratory. The home setting is the least controlled, but may provide the most natural response. The laboratory setting provides more control but may make the respondents more anxious. The site of the interviews should be decided beforehand and should remain consistent throughout the study.

The gender, ethnic origin, and even dress of the interviewer can also influence the interview results. In most cases researchers try to match the interviewer characteristics to those of the sample.

The method of recording the interview results is also important. Interview data can be recorded during the interview by note, tape or video recorder, or after the interview. When the recording occurs during the interview, it may influence the results. This factor must be balanced against the loss of interview information that will occur if the results are recorded after the session. In either case the interview results are transcribed and usually analyzed by content analysis.

Training interviewers is critical to the success of any research study. The training includes practice sessions where questions and possible answers are rehearsed. Problem areas should be anticipated by the researcher and possible strategies developed. Videotapes of practice sessions can give the trainee important insights into the verbal and nonverbal behaviors that may influence results.

Considerations. Interviews can provide the researcher with rich data about a given topic. The format also provides flexibility and generally the means to really explore a topic, clarify thinking, and confirm answers. For these reasons interviews can also be time consuming and costly in terms of manpower.

The interview does not usually work as well as a questionnaire when the topic is a very sensitive one such as sexual activity. Some individuals are understandably reluctant to discuss such things as sexual activity face to face but are more comfortable when asked on an anonymous questionnaire.

The interview is also very sensitive to biasing activity by the interviewer, whether intentional or unintentional. It is very hard for interviewers to maintain neutral body and facial language if there is an expected or hoped for outcome to the interviews.

PHYSIOLOGIC MEASURES

Because of the strong connection of physiologic measures to the clinical practice of nursing, there has been an increased use of physiologic measures in nursing research. These add an important dimension to many studies, as well as nursing care in general. They not only supply the important biometric dimension to the research study, but they also are valued for their objectivity, precision, and validity. In addition, the resultant data is generally measured at the ratio level allowing the use of sophisticated statistical measures.

Among the most familiar physiologic measures used are blood pressure values, blood values, urine values, and electrocardiograms. There are also a myriad of less familiar measures used by nurse physiologists and other nurse researchers.

Physiologic measures are considered among the most reliable and valid of measurements. However, as with all forms of measurement, physiologic methods are still subject to error. False-positive or false-negative tests results are only one example of the many types of error found.

Physiologic measures can be broken into two classifications. These are (1) biophysical, (2) biochemical/microbiologic.

BIOPHYSICAL
The biophysical methods measure physical characteristics of living organisms. Examples of biophysiologic measurement instruments include electrocardiograms, ultrasounds, and magnetic resonance imagery. Physiologic values may also be assessed

with more commonly used equipment such as the sphygmomanometer, the reflex hammer, or the ophthalmoscope.

Considerations. All biophysical measurement must be assessed for reliability and validity, more commonly called precision and accuracy. Nurse researchers want the biophysical measures used to provide consistent, reproducible results. To ensure precision the researcher carefully designs each portion of the study to avoid preanalytic problems such as those that occur with specimen collection errors, analytic problems such as those that occur with undependable machinery, and postanalytic problems such as transcription errors (Noe, 1985).

Using blood pressure measurement as an example of biophysical measures, the considerations are as follows (Cromwell, 1973):

1. *Not all variables can be directly measured.* Blood pressure is at best an indirect measure of cardiac status.
2. *Human beings are variable, and so are the variables measured from them.* Blood pressure varies from moment to moment, and at best the researcher can only talk in averages.
3. *The instrumentation used can influence the measurement.* Placement of the blood pressure cuff or size of the cuff in relationship to the size of the extremity can influence the reading.
4. *Extraneous signals can cause error.* In listening for the blood pressure, extraneous noise can influence the reading recorded.
5. *Instrumentation can damage people.* Blood pressure measurement damage may be limited, such as bruising or pain. Other instruments may inflict more serious damage.

BIOCHEMICAL/MICROBIOLOGIC MEASUREMENTS

The laboratory measurement of the chemical constituents of body fluids and tissues represent biochemical measurement. When the purpose is to assess the presence of microorganisms such as bacteria or to assess body tissue, then it is microbiologic or microscopic.

Considerations. The most obvious advantage of laboratory methodology is its high level of objectivity. These measures are probably the most objective and least influenced by respondent or researcher. On the negative side biophysiologic methods are expensive, often invasive, and can require a lot of time. They also require extensive training by those who perform them.

With laboratory testing care must be taken to reduce error to a minimum. The first step is proper collection and storage of the specimen. The laboratory procedures must also be carefully done, including the care of the machinery and correct use and calibration. The results should also be recorded and interpreted correctly. Because most physiologic measures are norm-referenced, it is important for the researcher to know if the norms are appropriate to the sample under study. A value normed on men may not be appropriate to women or to children. There are other influences as well, including circadian rhythms, body position, external influences, and so forth.

Q METHODOLOGY

Q methodology is a comparative rating system that retains the individual subjective response (Dennis, 1990). Using this method allows the researcher to examine commonalities among individuals who share certain characteristics. According to Dennis (1990), Q methodology allows the researcher to explore what dimensions of a phenomenon are important to the respondent and then to examine statistically how these dimensions are the same or different among respondents. Q methodology compares the respondent's subjective response in an objective, orderly, and scientific manner (Dennis, 1985).

Unlike standard methods that examine the statistical variance between individuals in terms of the average, Q methodology does not assume an average. Rather the whole range of possible responses becomes important (Brown, 1980).

METHOD

There are different methods employed in designing the sort. In one of the methods employed the researcher first must determine the items that will comprise the Q sort. The choice of item is critical to the method and must be truly representative of the domain of interest. The items become the study population as individuals are "loaded" onto items rather than items being loaded onto individuals. They also should be items that vary among individuals, such as the need for information during hospitalization.

The researcher chooses 25 to 75 items, preferably randomly, from a larger pool of items (Dennis, 1985). The selected items, usually in the form of descriptive statements, are then placed on $3'' \times 5''$ index cards.

The respondent is asked to sort the cards into 9 to 11 categories. The choice of categories is also important and is determined by the researcher. Dennis (1990) used a forced Q-sort distribution, with categories scored from -5 (most unimportant) to $+5$ (most important). There are generally preset limits on how many cards can be placed in any one category.

The sort forces the respondent to decide about the relative ordinal ranking of items. Obviously this can be hard for respondents, and they must be carefully taught how to perform the sort. Some earlier researchers advocated unforced sorting, but studies did not show it to be advantageous (Block, 1961).

Once the data are collected, the scored items are factor analyzed. The difference between the Q-sort analyzing and other factor analysis is that with the Q sort the factor loadings are the respondents, not the items. Thus in Q sort the researcher looks at how respondents relate to an item.

PSYCHOLOGIC TESTING

PROJECTIVE TECHNIQUES

Many psychologic tests are based on projective techniques where the individual is given an ambiguous item to respond to, with the assumption that the individual's concept of self will be projected onto the ambiguous item. One of the most familiar of these tests is the Rorschach Inkblot Test, in which the respondent is shown 10 inkblots and asked to describe what he or she sees. The answers are then interpreted by a trained researcher and are used to describe personality characteristics.

In general, most projective techniques test subjective responses and thus require extensive training by the researcher in administration and interpretation. Those nurse researchers interested in the use of standardized projective techniques should refer to the specific guidelines for each test.

INTELLIGENCE, DEVELOPMENTAL, AND ACHIEVEMENT TESTS

Intelligence, developmental, and achievement tests are frequently used by nurse researchers to classify the pool of respondents.

The tests are generally standardized and can be used in a wide variety of situations.

The reliability and validity of such standardized tests are often reported for a normative group. Each new use should still include some minimum level of measurement assessment and if used on a new group or in a new way, more extensive assessment is mandatory.

DIARIES

Diaries are an appropriate form of instrumentation when the researcher wants to measure the ongoing reflections or behaviors of the respondent. In this method the respondents are asked to keep diaries on the topic of interest. The diaries are then analyzed by the researcher.

The major advantage of the diary is that the respondent is asked to write daily (or more or less often) on the topic of interest. The diary is apt to be more reflective of valid feelings than asking the respondent to look back in time. Butz and Alexander (1991) report that diaries reduce recall bias but that the data can be hard to analyze.

Considerations include fatigue on the part of the respondents, resulting in failure to complete the diaries. Recording a diary can also sensitize the respondent to the topic and thus result in bias.

VIGNETTES

Vignettes are short, descriptive paragraphs that set up a situation to which the individual responds. The vignette helps control responses by standardizing the story. For example, respondents may be given a vignette about the ethics of euthanasia and asked to answer a series of questions about the vignette situation. The main disadvantage of the vignette is that it presents a somewhat artificial situation.

DEVELOPING A RESEARCH INSTRUMENT

The development of a good instrument is an intensive task and should only be undertaken when an adequate, previously developed instrument cannot be found. However, it is often the case that instruments need to be developed by the researcher. While the process of instrument development will vary (see Waltz, Strickland, & Lenz, 1991), the following represents a generic outline of what is required.

STEP 1. IDENTIFY THE CONCEPT TO BE MEASURED

The most critical step in instrument development is the identification and specification of the research concept. The researcher should be thoroughly familiar with all the literature on the concept of interest. This thorough familiarity with the knowledge base will allow the researcher to determine if a suitable or adaptable instrument exists. It will also ensure that all the dimensions of interest are tested.

Once the researcher has determined the parameters of the concept, an outline should be developed. For example, the researcher might be interested in the concept of lies. Lying has been examined from many different viewpoints. An inclusive instrument would address each of these different approaches. An outline might be as follows:

1. Philosophical aspects of lying
2. Ethical aspects of lying
3. Moral aspects of lying
4. Religious aspects of lying
5. Professional aspects of lying

STEPS IN DEVELOPING A RESEARCH INSTRUMENT

1. Identify the concept to be measured
2. Determine the format of the instrument
3. Develop the items
4. Sequence the items
5. Write the directions
6. Develop a draft instrument and supporting materials
7. Review and pretest
8. Revise

EXAMPLE OF INSTRUMENT DEVELOPMENT

Keresztes, Holm, Penockofer, and Merritt (1993) noted that determining the functional ability of patients with heart disease had been limited to asking clients about the presence of anginal pain (or other symptoms) or to measuring the onset of symptoms using a treadmill machine. The ability to accurately measure function, not just the onset of symptoms, was important because interventions are often based on functional ability. Yet there was no measurement method to ascertain functional change, either improvement or decline, related to changing symptomatology.

To measure the level of symptomatology and the extent that it compromised functional ability, the researchers developed an instrument called the symptom scale. The rating scale, with three subscales, asked the respondent to rate the severity of symptoms, the symptoms' interference with function, and the method used to treat the symptoms. The total score was achieved by adding up each subscale score. Low scores indicated that there was a high level of functional ability, and high scores indicated a low level. The researchers reported the Cronbach's alpha for each subscale. Concurrent validity was assessed by noting that the instrument correlated in the expected direction with the treadmill achievement level.

From Keresztes, P., Holm, K., Penockofer, S., & Merritt, S.: Measurement of functional ability in patients with coronary artery disease. *Journal of Nursing Measurement,* 1(1), 19-28.

STEP 2. DETERMINE THE FORMAT OF THE INSTRUMENT

The researcher's knowledge of the concept and of the respondents will influence the choice of format. The researcher will also want to consider how the information obtained will be handled and what results are needed. For example, an unstructured interview will result in transcripts of words that will have to be content analyzed. This will mean a rich data set, but one that is probably measured at the nominal level. A questionnaire on the same topic may mean less rich data, but can quickly give data measured at the interval/ratio level. As previously noted, each instrument has advantages and disadvantages.

STEP 3. DEVELOP THE ITEMS

Using the previously developed outline of the concept and knowledge of the format, the researcher next develops the items. If the items are in the form of questions, the researcher must decide between open-ended and closed-ended questions. Open-ended questions do not call for a specific response and allow the respondents to give any answer and as long an answer as they want. On the other hand closed-ended questions call for a specific response on the part of the respondent. Open-ended questions usually result in more information, while closed-ended questions result only in short answers to specific questions. This is balanced by the fact that closed-ended questions are easier to code and analyze.

The number of questions is also critical. Too few questions will not capture the concept; too many will tire the respondent, who will either fail to answer items or not answer them carefully.

The wording of the items is the next step to be considered. The researcher, who knows the topic well, needs to be able to translate that knowledge into items that are understood by the respondents. The items should be worded as simply and concisely as possible. The researcher should consider the reading level of the respondents if a pen-and-paper instrument is being developed.

The items should also be carefully phrased. It is very easy to inadvertently bias respondents' answers through wording or ordering of questions. Many researchers have noted these biasing effects and how they influence the information obtained.

STEP 4. SEQUENCE THE ITEMS

Questions that ask about sensitive topics, such as income or sexual habits, should generally be placed at the end of the instrument. Respondents may not answer these items and if they are placed at the end, researchers can salvage at least some of the data.

Many times there is a logical sequence: either from simple to complex, less sensi-

tive to most sensitive, or most interesting to least interesting. Questions about different topics are usually best asked together. If there is not a logical sequence, random ordering is often the best choice.

STEP 5. WRITE THE DIRECTIONS

Respondents need carefully constructed, clear directions if they are to complete the instrument correctly. This is also true for interview schedules.

Questionnaires also require a cover letter if they are to be mailed. The cover letter should clearly state the purpose of the study, information about confidentiality, what the respondent should do with the questionnaire when it is completed, and how the respondent may obtain further information.

STEP 6. DEVELOP DRAFT INSTRUMENT AND SUPPORTING MATERIALS

Once all the elements are ready the instrument should be assembled. The "look" of the instrument is especially important when it is to be given to respondents. Such things as spacing of questions and even the color of the paper can affect responses.

STEP 7. REVIEW AND PRETEST

The instrument should be reviewed by other knowledgeable researchers. The researchers should be asked to examine the instrument for completeness, clarity, and layout. Content experts (both lay and professional) should be asked to comment on the instrument. After making any changes needed, the instrument should be pretested.

Pretesting is done with a small sample of individuals who possess characteristics similar to those proposed for the larger study. The pretest should also occur under similar circumstances to the proposed study. The pretest will help the researcher to deter-

EVALUATING THE DATA-COLLECTION INSTRUMENT

1. *Content.* The content of the instrument should accurately and completely reflect the conceptual definition of the variable; that is, there should be a congruence between the conceptual and operational definitions.
2. *Efficiency.* The researcher wants an efficient instrument, one that collects the desired information as quickly and easily as possible.
3. *Sensitivity.* The researcher wants the instrument to be sensitive to the concept under study. Sensitivity allows the researcher to learn as much as possible.
4. *Population.* The population of interest is very important to consider when choosing a method of measurement. Physical, emotional, developmental, psychological, and other characteristics must all be considered. Elderly nursing home patients may not do well with a questionnaire with small print, while an interview would yield important results with this group.
5. *Administrative issues.* How the instrument is to be administered is important. Respondents who are to fill out questionnaires need pens or pencils and a desk or table. Interviews require quiet and some privacy. Physiologic measurers often require the respondent to come to the test site. The time required is also important.
6. *Reliability and validity*: Finally the researcher must be very concerned with the reliability and validity of the instrument. No instrument should be used without an assessment of reliability and validity.

mine if respondents can understand the items, if the directions are clear, and even if it has some preliminary reliability and validity. It is helpful to interview respondents after the pretesting to elicit their suggestions and opinions.

STEP 8. REVISE

Once the pretest is complete, the researcher should revise the instrument as indicated. If the researcher finds it necessary to make major revisions, a second pilot test should be performed.

☙ ELEMENTS OF A GOOD DATA-COLLECTION INSTRUMENT

Appropriate instrumentation is critical to good research. Study instruments should accurately and completely reflect the conceptual definition of the study variables. If possible researchers should try to use previously developed instruments in studies. The use of an existing instrument is less costly in terms of both time and money. Generally, most existing instruments also have been assessed for reliability and validity, and while these values are not sufficient, they do give the researchers some initial confidence that the instrument is a good one.

Various sources are available to help in locating existing instruments. Researchers may use computerized resources, networks and bulletin boards. Other sources include reference books, journals, and even other researchers.

In the case of either an existing instrument or a researcher-developed instrument, the elements listed in the box should be considered.

SUMMARY

- Self-report measures are used to ascertain the respondent's attitudes, opinions, or knowledge about a given respondent.
- Questionnaires are the most common form of self-report.
- Scales are a form of self-report. The respondent rates the variable on a continuum. There are several different forms of scales; the most common is the Likert.
- Interviews are a form of instrumentation that use verbal communication between researcher and respondent. Interviews can be structured or unstructured.
- Physiologic measures assess the respondents' biophysical, biochemical, or microbiologic standing.
- Many other forms of measurement exist. The researcher should use the method most appropriate to the variable of interest and sample.
- Instrument development may follow the following steps:
  1. Identify and develop the concept.
  2. Determine instrument format.
  3. Develop the items.
  4. Sequence the items.
  5. Write the directions.
  6. Develop the draft instrument.
  7. Review and pretest the instrument.
  8. Revise.
- When choosing or developing an instrument examine for efficiency, sensitivity, population, administrative issues, reliability, and validity.

FACILITATING CRITICAL THINKING

1. What are the steps in instrument development? Describe how error can be reduced in this process.
2. What are the advantages of self-report instruments?
3. What considerations must the researcher take into account when choosing self-report methods?

References

SUBSTANTIVE

BEDARF, E. W. (1986). Using structured interview techniques. Washington, DC: Program Evaluation and Methodology Division, U.S. General Accounting Office.

BRIGGS, C. L. (1986). *Learning how to ask: A sociolinguistic appraisal of the role of the interview in social science research.* Cambridge, U.K.: Cambridge University Press.

BROWN, S. R. (1980). *Political subjectivity: Application of Q methodology in political science.* New Haven: Yale University Press.

BUTZ, A. M., & ALEXANDER, C. (1991). Use of health diaries with children. *Nursing Research, 40*(1), 59-61.

DENNIS, K. E. (1985). A multi-methodological approach to the measurement of client control. Unpublished doctoral dissertation. Baltimore, University of Maryland.

DENNIS, K. E. (1990). Patient's control and the information imperative: Clarification and confirmation. *Nursing Research, 39*(3), 162-166.

DILLMAN, D. (1978). *Mail and telephone surveys: The total design method.* New York: John Wiley & Sons.

GIVEN, C. W., ET AL. (1992). The caregiver reaction assessment (CRA) for caregivers to persons with chronic physical and mental impairment. *Research in Nursing and Health, 15,* 271-283.

GOODMAN, C. M. (1987). The Delphi technique: A critique. *Journal of Advanced Nursing, 12,* 729-734.

GORDON, R. L. (1987). *Interviewing: Strategy, techniques, and tactics.* Chicago: Dorsey Press.

LINSTONE, H., & TUROFF, M. (Eds.). (1975). *The Delphi method: Techniques and applications.* Wellesley, MA: Addison-Wesley.

NOE, D. (1985). *The logic of laboratory medicine.* Baltimore: Urban & Schwartzenberg.

PEIRCE, A. G. (1987). Event review in the coping process of parous women (Doctoral dissertation, University of Maryland). *Dissertation Abstracts International, 42,* 705-B.

SWEETLAND, R. C., & KEYSER, D. J. (1983). *Tests: A comprehensive reference for assessment in psychology.* Kansas City: Test Corporation of America.

Waltz, C. F., Strickland, O. L., & Lenz, E. R. (1991). *Measurement in nursing research.* Philadelphia: F.A. Davis Company.

Wewers, M. E., & Lowe, N. K. (1990). A critical review of visual analog scales in the measurement of clinical phenomena. *Research in Nursing and Health, 13*(4), 227-236.

CONCEPTUAL

Flaskerud, J. H. (1988). Is the Likert scale format culturally biased? *Nursing Research, 37*(3), 185-186.

Keresztes, P., Holm, K., Penockofer, S., & Merritt, S. (1993). Measurement of functional ability in patients with coronary artery disease. *Journal of Nursing Measurement, 1*(1), 19-28.

Sax, G. (1980). *Principles of educational and psychological measurement and evaluation* (2nd ed.). Belmont, CA: Wadsworth Publishing Company.

METHODOLOGICAL

Block, J. (1961). *The Q-Sort method in personality assessment and psychiatric research.* Springfield, IL: Charles C Thomas.

Cromwell, L. (1973). *Biomedical instrumentation and measurements.* Englewood Cliffs, NJ: Prentice Hall

Norusis, M. J. (1983). *Introductory statistics guide: SPSSX.* New York: McGraw-Hill.

HISTORICAL

Nunnally, J. C. (1978). *Psychometric theory.* New York: McGraw-Hill.

Osgood, C., Suci, G., & Tannenbaum, P. (1957). *The measurement of meaning.* Urbana, IL: University of Illinois Press.

Stevens, S. S. (1946). On the theory of scales of measurement. *Science, 103,* 677-680.

CHAPTER 16

DATA ANALYSIS

B. GAYLE TWINAME

How nurses dress is an important part of who they are and how they are perceived. Nurses have been trying for decades to be perceived as professionals by other health care professionals and by their patients. However, dress codes are changing to allow nurses to dress with more flexibility and less professionally (Springhouse, 1987). Many nurses are now wearing multicolored uniforms, or scrubsuits and running shoes. How do administrators, other nurses, and patients perceive these uniforms? Do nursing dress codes really matter to their patients?

A recent study by Garrison, Lind, Mangum, Thackeray, and Wyatt (1991) attempted to answer these questions and found that dress does make a difference in how nurses are perceived. Utilizing the nurse image scale (NIS), the authors surveyed 100 patients, 30 nurses, and 15 administrators. The authors discovered that there was a significant difference between how dress affects patients and how it affects nurses and administrators. All three groups preferred a nurse in a pants uniform with a stethoscope as the nurse they would most like to have care for them. But here the opinions diverged. Patients next ranked the nurse in a dress with a cap, while administrators and nurses preferred the nurse in a dress with a stethoscope. Scrubsuits were least preferred by 45% of the patients, nurses, and administrators. Both patients and nurses would least like to have a nurse dressed in white pants with a colored top, a scrubsuit, or a lab coat over street clothes care for them. As nurses continue to strive for professionalism, image does matter (Kalish & Kalish, 1987), and what nurses wear may be perceived as unprofessional.

How did the researchers determine from the large amount of data collected that the results did indeed indicate a significant difference in perception of nurses based on dress? This was done through statistical analysis. The research process and proposed methodology guides the researcher in the selection of the appropriate data analysis technique. Decisions are dependent on the research question, the research design, and the level of measurement used.

This chapter discusses the steps necessary to choose the appropriate method of quantitative data analysis. Discussion will include procedures for data analysis, as well as descriptive and inferential statistics. The use of computer programs in data analysis, as well as a step-by-step plan for evaluating data analysis, is included.

✎ PURPOSE

Research can help us determine whether a relationship exists between two or more variables through the systematic observation and description of the characteristics or properties of people, objects, or events. Research can also help to describe, predict, and explain. Of paramount importance is the researcher's ability to develop generalizations that may be used to explain phenomena and to predict future relationships between variables.

Effective empirical research also relies on statistics to organize, summarize, and interpret numerical data generated by nurse researchers. Such measurement enables us to assign precise and universally accepted quantitative values to the properties of objects, people, and events. Finally, statistics provide measurement and evaluation of quantitative data.

✎ DESCRIPTIVE STATISTICS

Descriptive or univariate statistics are used to describe a particular sample or a particular individual within a sample. The data are limited to describing *only one* variable, group, or individual. Any conclusions that are made cannot be extended to anyone outside that particular sample. *Inferential statistics* can be used to make generalizations outside a particular sample (if certain criteria are met) and will be discussed later in this chapter.

Descriptive statistics provide us with an organized visual representation of data in a variety of ways, including shape, location, and spread. Imagine taking the pulse of every patient in a 500-bed hospital. Imagine viewing those numbers as they were initially recorded or rewritten from highest to lowest. Which would be easiest to comprehend? Even though both lists would contain the same data, the arrangement of the data would make a big difference in how well and how easily the data could be understood.

Research data yields a collection of numbers that must be organized into a more comprehensible manner. Shape is the easiest to understand and interpret and provides a visual representation of data through a frequency distribution and/or graphs. Shape can also be used to make comparisons to the normal distribution (bell curve) (Figure 16-1).

Shape is vitally important since a number of inferential statistical tests are based on the assumption that the variables under study are normally distributed or match the shape of the normal curve. If the shape of a distribution is not normal, certain statistical tests must be used that do not depend on the assumption of normality.

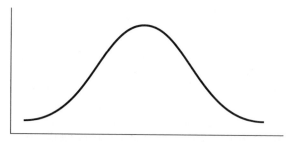

Figure 16-1. The normal or bell curve.

FREQUENCY DISTRIBUTION

Imagine that a nurse, Rosa, working on a medical floor for the past 2 years, noticed that patients over the age of 65 had more prescribed medications than any other patients on the unit. She was amazed by the number of different medications these patients were taking and concerned about the number of side effects these medications might cause. In some cases she believed that patients were prescribed more medication to counteract the side effects of other medications previously prescribed. Rosa wondered if all of these medications were necessary. She decides to keep track of the next 50 elderly patients and write down the number of medications taken by each one (Table 16-1).

Rosa wants to be able to tabulate her data so that she can better organize the information on the number of medications taken by patients over the age of 65 on her medical unit. She begins by tallying and recording the frequency (f) of medications (variable X) taken by her elderly patients (Table 16-2).

The data in Tables 16-1 and 16-2 are ungrouped data. Sometimes ungrouped data are difficult to work with because of a large number of responses or values. It is evident that when a distribution has a wide number or range of values, it is necessary to group data to provide all information in the most uncomplicated form.

To group Rosa's data we might consider grouping the number of medications from 0 to 4, 5 to 9, and so on as shown in Table 16-3. Choosing interval size is an arbitrary decision of the researcher to enable the most meaningful presentation of data possible. It is important when grouping data to be certain that the intervals include all possible values (are exhaustive), do not overlap (are mutually exclusive), and are equally spaced.

By viewing the data in this manner Rosa is quickly able to determine that the majority of elderly patients received between 10 and 19 medications, as the highest number

Table 16-1
Unorganized Listing of Medications

14	17	6	10	11	22	15	4	17	28
30	12	16	5	15	32	17	22	15	2
21	19	9	16	26	30	11	31	7	11
11	22	18	33	8	27	12	11	10	9
31	3	10	11	9	7	27	22	31	11

Table 16-2
Tally and Frequency Distribution of Number of Medications Taken

Medications (X)	Tally	Frequency (f)
2	I	1
3	I	1
4	I	1
5	I	1
6	I	1
7	I I	2
8	I	1
9	I I I	3
10	I I I	3
11	LHT I I	7
12	I I	2
14	I	1
15	I I I	3
16	I I	2
17	I I I	3
18	I	1
19	I	1
21	I	1
22	I I I I	4
26	I	1
27	I I	2
28	I	1
30	I I	2
31	I I I	3
32	I	1
33	I	1

Table 16-3
Grouped Frequency Distribution

Number of Medications	Frequency
0-4	3
5-9	8
10-14	13
15-19	10
20-24	5
25-29	4
30-34	7

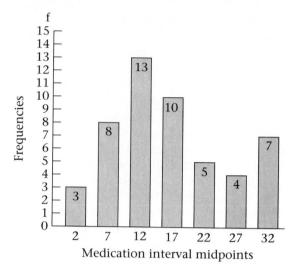

Figure 16-2. Bar graph: number of medications taken.

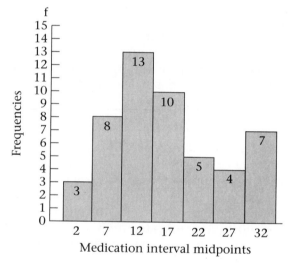

Figure 16-3. Histogram: number of medications taken.

are in categories 10 to 14 and 15 to 19. This data can also be represented in another visual manner as a graph. Graphs allow the reader to quickly grasp essential information in a short time. As such, they are often used as visual aids to enhance research reports and presentations.

When constructing a graph, it is common practice to label each interval by its midpoint rather than by the endpoints. Thus, in this example, the midpoint of the 10 to 14 category would be labeled on the horizontal axis as 12 and the midpoint of the 15 to 19 category would be labeled as 17. Since these labels are smaller, the graph will appear less cluttered and easier to read.

Bar Graph
A bar graph is a chart that represents the frequency of each class by a rectangle or bar. The values of the variable are depicted on the horizontal axis, and the frequencies of occurrence are depicted on the vertical axis (Figure 16-2).

Histogram
A histogram is also a chart that represents the frequency of each class by a rectangle or bar. A histogram differs from a bar graph in that in a histogram the bars do not have spaces between them, indicating the continuous nature of a variable (Figure 16-3).

Frequency Polygon
In a frequency polygon the vertical and horizontal axes of the graph are the same as in the bar graph and histogram. However, instead of using bars to indicate the frequency of medication interval mid-

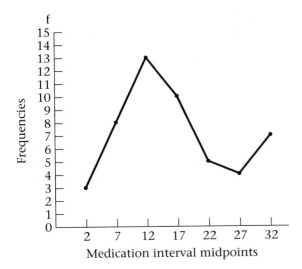

Figure 16-4. Frequency polygon: number of medications taken.

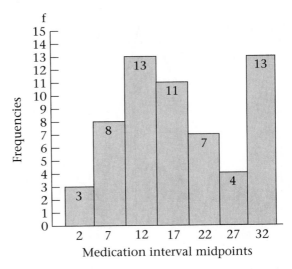

Figure 16-5. Bimodal histogram: number of medications taken.

points, points are used and then connected by straight lines (Figure 16-4).

There are a number of other graphic representations that may be used by researchers or seen by consumers when critiquing research articles. These include the stem and leaf diagram, the pie chart, and others.

MEASURES OF CENTRAL TENDENCY

After determining the shape of a distribution, it is possible to determine the location of the most typical values within that distribution. Location consists of determining the three most common statistical measures of central tendency: the mode, median, and mean.

Mode

The mode is the most frequently occurring value. In the above example Rosa determined that the mode of the grouped data for the number of medications received by patients over 65 on her medical unit was 10 to 14. This indicates that the greatest number of Rosa's patients received from 10

to 14 medications per day. The mode for her ungrouped data (Table 16-2) was 7; this distribution would have one mode and be referred to as unimodal. The mode can be used with all levels of measurement. Although it is not the best measure of central tendency, it is the best measure for nominal data.

It is possible for a distribution to have more than one mode. For example, if 13 of Rosa's patients were taking from 10 to 14 medications and 13 were taking from 30 to 34 medications, how would the distribution look? (Figure 16-5). This distribution is referred to as bimodal since it has two modes. It is also possible to have multimodal distributions (Figure 16-6).

In a bimodal or multimodal distribution the modes may or may not be equivalent. The normal curve is unimodal and symmetrical (see Figure 16-1).

Median

The median of a distribution is its midpoint. Half of the scores are above the median and half of the scores are below. The

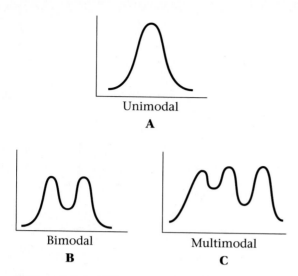

Figure 16-6. Different types of distributions. **A**, Unimodal; **B**, bimodal; **C**, multimodal.

median, in addition to being the actual middle value, is not affected by the actual values of the scores above and below it. The median is frequently used with ordinal level data. The median is very simple to calculate when there is an odd number of scores. Going back to our example, Rosa determines that the median for her ungrouped data (Table 16-2) is 15. Since she had an even number of scores (50), she determines that the midpoint is actually halfway between the twenty-fifth and twenty-sixth score when the scores are ranked from highest to lowest. Keeping in mind that scores must be ranked first, what is the median for the following scores?

5 4 2 7 10 12 2 14 (unranked)
2 2 4 (5   7) 10 12 14 (ranked)

The median in this data is equal to 5 + 7 divided by 2, or 6, because three scores lie above the 7 and three scores lie below the 5. What would happen if the top score was 612 instead of 14? The median would remain the same. This demonstrates that the

median is not sensitive to all of the scores in a distribution. For this reason the median is a better indicator of central tendency than the mode and it can be used with ordinal level data.

Mean
The mean is the arithmetical average of all the scores in a distribution and is represented by the symbol $\overline{X}$. The mean is equal to the sum (Σ) of all the scores (x) divided by the total number of scores (n).

$$\overline{X} = \frac{x}{n}$$

The mean is the most frequently used measure of central tendency; most tests of statistical significance are based on the mean. To calculate a mean, data must be at the interval or ratio level.

Is Rosa able to calculate the mean for her data? What level of measurement is her data? The level of measurement of number of medications is ratio. A total of 814 medications are taken by the 50 patients. Therefore the mean for her ungrouped data is 16.28. What if Rosa wanted to calculate the mean for her grouped data? The formula for this is a little different. The mean of grouped data can be calculated by (1) multiplying each interval's frequency by its midpoint, (2) adding these products together, and then (3) dividing the sum of these products by the number of measures. For example, let us find the mean for the following grouped data:

Number of medications	Frequency (f_i)	Midpoint (m_i)
0-4	3	2
5-9	8	7
10-14	13	12
15-19	10	17
20-24	5	22
25-29	4	27
30-34	7	32

For this sample the formula would be

$$\text{Grouped mean} = \frac{\Sigma f_i m_i}{n}$$

Grouped mean =

$$\frac{3(2) + 8(7) + 13(12) + 10(17) + 5(22) + 4(27) + 7(32)}{50}$$

or 16.6

(Note that there is a slight discrepancy between the means for the grouped and ungrouped data. This is to be expected, since the midpoints do not represent the true numbers perfectly.)

By calculating the mode, median, and mean we are able to determine if our distribution is normal or approximates the normal or bell curve. We have already determined that the normal curve is unimodal (see Figure 16-1). The normal curve is also symmetrical—if it was folded in half along the center line, each half would be exactly the same.

Where would the median and mean fall on the normal curve? The median would be located at the mode, since 50% of the scores would be above the mode and 50% of the scores would fall below the mode. The mean would also be located at the mode. In a normal distribution the mode, median, and mean are equivalent.

The portions of the curve to the left and right of the central area are called tails. It is important to note that the lines are not touching the horizontal axis. The tails would continue indefinitely, getting closer and closer to the horizontal axis, but never really touching it (Marzillier, 1990).

Not all distributions are symmetrical like the bell curve. Refer to Rosa's data in Figure 16-3. Is her distribution symmetrical? Not really; if that figure were folded in half, the two sides would not be equal. Her distribution is asymmetrical, or skewed. Distribu-

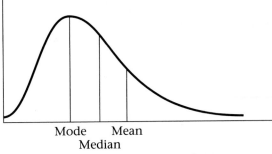

Mode   Mean
Median
A Positively skewed distribution

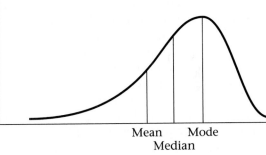

Mean   Mode
Median
B Negatively skewed distribution

Figure 16-7. Asymmetrical distributions. **A**, Positively skewed distribution; **B**, negatively skewed distribution.

tions provide us with information about the measures of central tendency. Distributions can be negatively or positively skewed, and the mean, median, and mode are all affected (Figure 16-7). Skewness interferes with the validity of data analysis. Distributions that are extremely skewed require the use of nonparametric statistical tests that do not rely on the assumption of normal distribution. It is important to note that skew is determined by the direction of the *tail* of the distribution, not the placement of the higher number of scores. At times this appears counterintuitive. It may be easier to remember simply that in a positively skewed distribution the tail points to the right and in a negatively skewed distribution the tail points to the left.

Table 16-4
**Means, Medians, and Modes for
Asymmetrical Data**

Scores	Mode	Median	Mean
2 4 5 5 6 8	5	5	5
1 5 5 5 5 9	5	5	5
5 5 5 5 5 5	5	5	5

Although the measures of central tendency provide a good idea of shape through modality and symmetry, how much information can really be obtained from the mode, median, and mean? Examine the three samples in Table 16-4. Even though these samples have very different values, their measures of central tendency are the same. So for these three samples measures of central tendency are not enough to fully describe a sample.

MEASURES OF VARIABILITY

Measures of variability, or spread, tell us how the data are distributed. In nursing we frequently refer to measures of variability to make decisions about our clients. We are all aware that 98.6°F has been generally accepted as the normal temperature for adults. If an adult client's temperature is 98°F, we will probably not notify the physician because we are already aware that this is a variation within the normal spread of adult temperatures. However, if the same client's temperature is 103°F, we know that this client needs further assessment and intervention. We are able to make this decision based on our knowledge of the spread or variability of the sample of normal adult temperatures.

The following measures of variability is discussed in this chapter: the range, the interquartile range, the variance, and the standard deviation. By determining these measures we are better able to understand just how varied the scores in a sample are.

Range
The range is the easiest of the measures of variability to compute. The range is computed by subtracting the lowest score from the highest. In our previous example of the three samples that had the same measures of central tendency, the ranges would be 6, 8, and 0. The range provides us with further data because it is sensitive to extreme scores. For example, in the following sample of 1, 2, 3, 4, 6, 10, the range would equal 10 − 1, or 9. If the highest score was changed to 77, the range would be 77 − 1, or 76. The range only takes into account the highest and lowest score, but gives us no information about the scores in between. What was the range for Rosa's data? The range was 33 − 2, or 31.

Interquartile Range. The interquartile range consists of the middle 50% of scores. Twenty-five percent of the scores are above the interquartile range and 25% of the scores are below it.

Although the interquartile range is not affected by extreme scores, it only takes into account 50% of the values. It requires a little more computation than the range, and it is good to use with ordinal level data. Just as the range included only the highest and lowest score and ignored the values in between, the interquartile range takes into account only the middle scores. The semiquartile range is sometimes reported in research studies and is obtained by dividing the interquartile range in half.

Variance
The variance is a descriptive statistic that examines how scores or values in a data set are distributed. It takes into account all of the scores in a distribution. To calculate

the variance it is necessary to first calculate the mean of the scores. For example,

5 8 14 15 22 23 24 30 34 35

$$\overline{X} = 21$$

The variance determines how the scores deviate or vary from the mean of the sample. If each score was subtracted from the mean of 21, we would get a deviation score (d). If all of the deviation scores were added together, the result would be zero. Squaring each number or deviation (d^2), whether positive or negative, gives a positive number that can then be added together (Figure 16-8).

For this sample the sum of the squared deviations is 970. To determine the variance this number must be compared to the sample size. The variance is equal to the sum of the squared deviations divided by the number of scores in a sample and is denoted by s^2.

$$\text{Variance } (s^2) = \frac{d^2}{n}$$

x	d	d^2
5	16	256
8	13	169
14	7	49
15	6	36
22	−1	1
23	−2	4
24	−3	9
30	−9	81
34	−13	169
35	−14	196
$\Sigma x = 210$	$\Sigma d = 0$	$\Sigma d^2 = 970$

n = 10

$\overline{X} = 21$

$s^2 = 970 \div 10$ or 97

Figure 16-8. Example of variance calculation.

If the data in this sample were more dispersed, the variance would be greater than 97; if less dispersed, smaller than 97. The variance of a total population is denoted by σ^2 and is calculated by dividing by the size of the entire population (N).

The variance is a good measure of variability or spread because it encompasses every score in a distribution. One drawback of the variance is that by squaring the deviations there is a resulting effect on the final calculation. For example, let us say that an architect is to design a new medication room as a prototype for the entire hospital. He or she might begin by measuring all of the medication rooms in the hospital and possibly other hospitals to get an idea of how different their sizes might be. To cal-

culate the variance the architect would begin by determining the mean number of linear feet per room, how each room deviated from the mean (in feet), and then squaring the deviations. The final number would be presented in square feet, not linear feet, and the variance would also be represented by square feet. This can present inaccuracies in interpretation. The standard deviation is a more precise measure of variability because it returns data to the original form of measurement. It is calculated by taking the square root of the variance.

Standard Deviation

The standard deviation for a sample is denoted by *s* and for a population it is denoted by σ. In the example in which measurement was recorded in linear feet and the variance was reported in square feet, the standard deviation would be reported in linear feet as in the original sample.

The standard deviation for the scores in Figure 16-8 would be the square root of 97, or 9.85. The great advantage in using the standard deviation as the measure of vari-

Table 16-5
Levels of Measurement for Descriptive Statistics

Level of Measurement	Central Tendency	Variability
Nominal	Mode	Range
Ordinal	Mode	Range
	Median	Interquartile range
Interval/Ratio	Mode	Range
	Median	Range
		Interquartile range
	Mean	Variance
		Standard deviation

ability is that it includes every observation and is reported in the same form of measurement as the original data.

Just as the mode, median, and mean are appropriate to specific levels of measurement, so are the range, interquartile range, variance, and standard deviation. Measures of central tendency and variability that can be used with nominal level data may also be used with higher levels of data. However, those descriptive statistics used at higher levels of data may not be used with lower levels (Table 16-5).

The standard deviation helps us to determine how individual scores differ from one another and can assist us in interpreting the scores of one individual within the distribution in relation to other scores. To understand the meaning of the standard deviation it is necessary to refer to the normal curve (see Figure 16-1).

As in any distribution, the area under the normal curve approximates 100%. Figure 16-9 gives the standard deviations and their percentages of the area under the normal curve. By calculating the standard de-

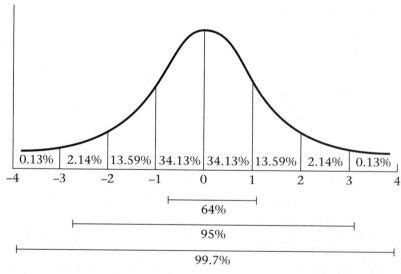

Figure 16-9. Standard deviations and percentages of the normal curve.

viation of any sample it is possible to determine what percentage of the sample lies within each of the standard deviations.

Standard Scores
Standard scores can be used to interpret how an individual's score in a sample relates to those of other individuals within the same sample. Imagine that you received a 65 on your last nursing exam. Most students would panic at the thought, but was this 65 a failing score? What if you received a 65, but the highest possible score was only 80? Furthermore, what if the mean was 48 and the standard deviation was 8.5? You could now determine how well you actually did on the exam. Since your score was 17 points above the mean, you could calculate how many *standard deviations* above the mean your score was as well. Your score would be two standard deviations above the mean. Your score was actually in the top 99% of the class, so it was not a failing grade.

The raw score of 65 in the example above was quite meaningless without additional information about the sample. After the entire sample was described, it was possible to determine how well you did in relation to the rest of the class. Standard scores can tell us how far from the mean of a group of measures the score falls and whether the score is above or below the average score (Johnson, 1989).

z-Scores
To convert a raw score to a z-score one must first determine the mean and standard deviation for the entire set of scores. To calculate the z-score, subtract the mean score for the sample from the individual's score (deviation score) and divide by the standard deviation for the sample.

$$z = \frac{X - \overline{X}}{s}$$

If the resulting z-score is negative, the individual score is that number of standard deviations below the mean. If the z-score is positive, the individual score is that number of deviations above the mean.

T-Scores
T-scores are derived from z-scores, but eliminate the need to work with negative numbers and fractions. The T-score is scaled to a distribution with a mean of 50 and a standard deviation of 10 (Johnson, 1989). To calculate a T-score, multiply the z-score by 10 and add 50 (Figure 16-10).

$$T = 10z + 50$$

In Figure 16-9 we looked at the standard deviations and percentages for the normal curve. z-scores and T-scores can also be depicted on the normal curve. By displaying z-scores and T-scores on the normal curve we can better understand how an individual's score relates to all of the scores in a distribution (Figure 16-11).

Percentiles
Percentiles are often used to allow people to compare their performance to others in a group. Percentiles are used frequently in the assessment of infants and children. The

	Peggy	Mary	Ruby
Individual scores	83	77	91
Sample mean = 55			
Standard deviation = 9			
z-score (z = $\underline{X - \overline{X}}$)	3.1	2.4	4
T-score (T = 10z − 50)	81	74	90

Figure 16-10. Example of z-score and T-score calculation.

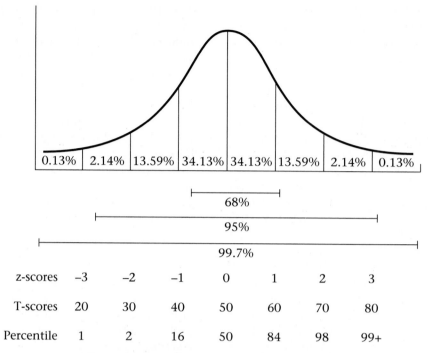

0.13%	2.14%	13.59%	34.13%	34.13%	13.59%	2.14%	0.13%

68%

95%

99.7%

z-scores	−3	−2	−1	0	1	2	3
T-scores	20	30	40	50	60	70	80
Percentile	1	2	16	50	84	98	99+

Figure 16-11. Standard scores and percentiles.

Denver II consists of certain activities that allow the nurse to compare a child's performance on certain developmental skills such as fine and gross motor development to a standard. By determining a child's percentile, the nurse is able to decide whether a child is developing within normal limits. Certain data collection instruments also use percentiles for reporting individual scores.

By referring to Figure 16-11 we are better able to understand the individual scores of Peggy, Mary, and Ruby. Peggy scored in the ninety-ninth percentile, Mary in the ninety-eighth percentile, and Ruby in the ninety-ninth percentile. So, even though the individual scores ranged from 77 to 91, all three girls scored at or above the ninety-eighth percentile.

BIVARIATE STATISTICS

As stated at the beginning of the discussion on descriptive or univariate statistics we have been examining single variables, whether groups or individuals. However, nursing research is often conducted to determine a relationship between two or more variables. This extended statistical analysis is referred to as bivariate statistics.

Contingency Tables

Contingency tables, or cross tabulation tables, are used to visually represent the relationship between two or more variables at the nominal level or at the ordinal level if there are not too many categories. Specifically, a contingency table is a way of combining the frequency distribution of these two or more variables and representing them in table form. Like graphs, contingency tables are easier to understand than a large number of individual scores.

Ann is interested in studying whether adult women who drink decaffeinated beverages are more likely to participate in exercise regularly than adult women who drink caffeinated beverages. She poses this question to 200 adult women and constructs a contingency table to present her data (Table 16-6). Ann places the number of women answering positively or negatively to each question in the corresponding cell, or box, and calculates the percentages for each cell. Contingency tables like Ann's consisting of two variables and two categories, are referred to as 2 × 2 contingency tables. If Ann had been interested in studying alcoholic beverages as well, she would have constructed a 2 × 3 contingency table. If she included a category for men and alcoholic beverages, she would have needed a 3 × 3 contingency table, and so on.

The data from Table 16-6 seem to indicate that the majority of women drink caffeinated drinks. However, women who drink decaffeinated beverages appear to exercise more regularly than women who drink caffeinated beverages. Although this may be the case, we cannot say that drinking decaffeinated beverages causes an individual to exercise regularly or vice versa. There are a number of other variables that Ann did not consider that may be involved in the decision to exercise on a regular basis, such as number of children, cigarette smoking, and weight.

Correlation

Another common bivariate statistic reported in nursing research articles is correlation. Correlation can show whether two variables are related and the degree of that relationship. To determine whether variables are correlated the level of measurement of both variables must be ordinal, interval, or ratio. Correlated variables tend to fluctuate together; as one increases, the other has a tendency to increase or decrease as well. For example, it would seem logical that nursing students with high GPAs would have a higher science GPA than nursing students with low GPAs. If this were true, then these two variables (nursing GPA and science GPA) would be positively correlated. In other words, the higher the nursing GPA, the higher the science GPA. With negatively correlated variables, higher values on one variable are associated with lower variables on the other. For example, weight and exercise may be negatively correlated: the more a person weighs, the less likely he or she exercises.

Statistical tests can provide the researcher with a correlation coefficient. Correlation coefficients vary from a magnitude of +1 (a perfect positive relationship) to −1 (a perfect negative relationship). Correlation coefficients in between +1 and −1 indicate an imperfect positive or imperfect negative correlation. Variables that are positively correlated are often said to be *directly* related to each other, while negatively correlated variables are *inversely* related. A correlation coefficient of zero indicates that the two variables are not re-

Table 16-6
Example of 2 × 2 Contingency Table

	Caffeinated Beverages	Decaffeinated Beverages	Total
Exercise regularly	20 (7%)	40 (80%)	140 (70%)
Do not exercise regularly	140 (93%)	10 (20%)	60 (30%)
Total	150 (75%)	50 (25%)	200 (100%)

lated, or are uncorrelated. Behavioral scientists may be quite satisfied with a correlation of between ±.50 and ±.70, believing that this correlation indicates a strong relationship between variables. However, physical scientists may believe that a correlation less than −.85 to +.85 is weak. It is rare to discover a perfect positive or negative relationship when humans are studied. The interpretation of correlation depends a great deal on the type of variables under study and the desired result.

Correlation can only reflect a *relationship* between two variables; it does *not* reflect a cause-and-effect relationship. Correlation is only the first hint that there is a possible causal link between variables, but it does not imply causality. It is possible for two variables to be highly correlated but have no causal relationship whatsoever. However, it is most likely that as the strength of a relationship between variables becomes greater, so does the plausibility of a causal link. If the researcher determines through correlation that no relationship exists, than a causal relationship is impossible.

Scatter Plot. The scatter plot, scatter diagram, or scattergram is a graphic representation of correlation. Scatter plots allow the investigator to visually represent the direction, shape, and magnitude of the relationship between two variables. The scatter plot enhances the interpretation of correlation coefficients and can assist the researcher in determining whether data meet the assumptions for inferential data analysis.

The researcher may make decisions based solely on a correlation coefficient, only to discover that the relationship between the variables looks quite different on a scatter plot. For example, the investigator may decide that two variables are uncorrelated only to discover on a scatter plot that they have a curvilinear relationship.

Like all graphs, scatter plots are diagrammed on a vertical and horizontal axis. The two variables under study are referred to as the X-variable, plotted on the horizontal axis, and the Y-variable, plotted on the vertical axis. Normally, the independent or predictor variable is plotted on the X axis, and the dependent or outcome variable is plotted on the Y axis. A single point on the scatter plot represents each pair of scores, one from the X-variable and one from the Y-variable (Figure 16-12).

Figure 16-12 illustrates a positive, but imperfect, correlation. Figure 16-13 illustrates examples of perfect positive, perfect negative, imperfect negative, curvilinear, and uncorrelated relationships. Note that a perfect correlation, whether negative or positive, is indicated by a straight line (linear), while imperfect correlations have some indication of a linear relationship. The closer the points come to representing a straight line, the more linear the relationship and the higher the degree of correlation between the two variables. The two most common correlation coefficients, the Pearson Product Moment Correlation and

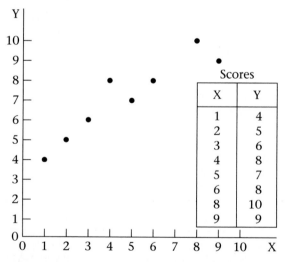

Figure 16-12. Scatter plot showing an imperfect positive correlation.

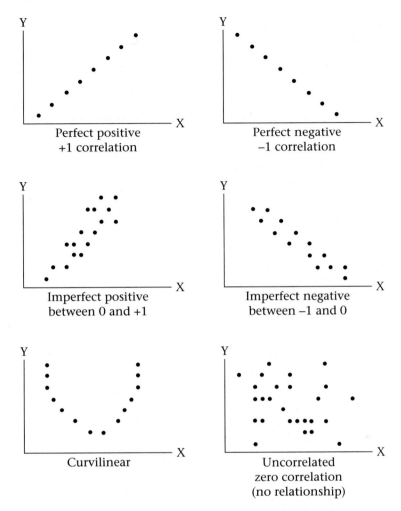

Figure 16-13. Correlation scatter plots.

the Spearman Correlation, will be discussed later in the chapter. We will also take a closer look at the linear relationship by studying linear regression.

∾ *INFERENTIAL STATISTICS*

Descriptive statistics assist the researcher in describing a particular sample under study. Inferential statistics help the researcher to do one or both of the following:

1. Estimate or predict a population parameter from a sample statistic.
2. Test a null or statistical hypothesis.

GENERALIZATION TO THE POPULATION

Inferential statistics and random selection of subjects assist the researcher in making generalizations from the sample under study to a larger, similar population that was not measured. When random selection of subjects is used, these statistics enable researchers to draw conclusions about much larger groups (populations) if the smaller group (sample) is accurately representative of the population.

For example, while studying the behaviors and attitudes of rural adolescents in Woodville, Texas, who are at risk for getting HIV disease, a researcher might discover that active involvement in extracurricular activities is associated with least-risky behaviors. This may be of interest to the other individuals living in Woodville, but would have little value for other rural areas unless the investigator was able to generalize such findings to these other communities. Inferential statistics would enable the researcher to make inferences from the sample of adolescents in Woodville to other rural adolescent populations if the sample was chosen at random. Nurses working with high-risk adolescents in other rural areas with similar characteristics could then apply the results of the study in their communities. By using subjects representative of the population as a whole (through random sampling), the researcher can make inferences from the representative sample back to the larger population.

Sampling Distributions

Sampling distributions are actually frequency distributions constructed to allow researchers to study the relationship between sample statistics and population parameters. What is a sample statistic? Sample statistics are characteristics of a sample. We calculated several sample statistics at the beginning of the chapter: the mode, median, mean, variance, and standard deviation were all sample statistics. A parameter is a characteristic of the entire population. Since it is unrealistic to study an entire population, population parameters are estimated from sample statistics.

Sampling Error

When a researcher selects a random sample from a population, every effort is made to select a representative sample. However, samples may still vary even though they are drawn randomly from the same population. This variation is called sampling error.

For example, Rhonda wants to study the effect of positive affirmations on the weight of school-age children in a metropolitan city. She decides to select a sample of 100 school-aged children from the rosters of all school-aged children in the city. When Rhonda obtains the mean weight of school-aged children in her sample (X = 115), she believes that her sample is representative of the population. What would happen if Rhonda decided to choose another 100 children in the same manner? Would she obtain the exact same mean? Probably not. If Rhonda chose 100 children over and over, there would be some variations in the sample mean (Figure 16-14). If Rhonda continued to obtain samples and averaged the means of all of the samples selected, the result would be the population mean. Since each individual sample Rhonda selected had different means, it is also possible to calculate the standard error of the mean or how much the sample

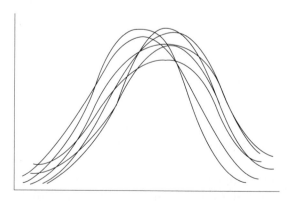

Figure 16-14. Standard error of the means.

means deviated around the population mean. The lower the standard error of the means, the more precise the parameter estimates will be. Since it is doubtful that Rhonda, or anyone else, has the time, money, and other resources to continue to select and study sample after sample, the standard error of the mean can be estimated by using the following formula:

$$\text{Standard error of the mean (SEM)} = \frac{s}{\sqrt{n}}$$

The standard error of the mean is equal to the standard deviation of the sample (s) divided by the square root of the sample size (n). It is apparent from this formula that the larger the sample size, the smaller the standard error of the mean and the more accurate the estimation of the parameter. This certainly makes sense because the more people included in the sample, the more likely the sample will be representative of the population.

Estimation of Parameters

Point Estimation. Estimating parameters is a common example of inferential statistics. Point estimation allows the investigator to make a "best guess" of a single population parameter from a representative sample statistic. Point estimation can provide the researcher with a close approximation of the population mean, median, variance, or standard deviation from the corresponding sample statistic. Although point estimation is possible, it is not always accurate.

Consider an experiment where we observe 72 successes in 100 trials. Now suppose that we obtain 7200 successes in another experiment with 10,000 trials. In these two experiments the point estimate (.72) is the same, and there is no way to distinguish one experiment from the other.

However, one could guess that the accuracy of the second point estimate is 10 times more reliable than the first, given the larger sample size. Unless we can add a specific statement about the degree of accuracy of a given point estimate, we do not know whether an estimate is highly accurate or totally inaccurate. A good example of the use (or abuse) of point estimation is the public opinion poll. One never knows the accuracy of a public opinion poll because there is never any discussion of the accuracy of their point estimate.

Interval Estimation. Interval estimates are preferable to point estimates, although they are similarly derived. Interval estimates indicate that a population parameter lies somewhere in the interval, but does not give a precise point. Interval estimates are also called confidence intervals and consist of a range of values calculated to estimate a population parameter from a random sample with a stated degree of confidence.

For example, Rhonda might estimate with 100% confidence that all the school-aged children in the school district weighed between zero and 500 pounds. Rhonda might even be more daring and suggest that 100% of the children weighed between 30 and 300 pounds. Anyone would probably agree with Rhonda and could have made the same guess with 100% confidence as well. But what does the information tell us about the population? Not much. To provide any truly practical and significant information, Rhonda needs a much narrower interval. Unfortunately, Rhonda cannot choose as narrow an interval as she might want. As the interval narrows, the less confident Rhonda can be that the actual parameters lie within that interval. Rhonda can be 100% certain that the average weight of all school children in the city is between 0 and 500 pounds, but she is also 0% certain that the exact mean is 123 pounds.

Confidence intervals require a sample size of at least 30, are based on the normal distribution, and can be calculated using a modification of the z-score formula. Recall that earlier we determined that the normal distribution has certain percentages that correspond to standard deviations and z-scores (see Figure 16-11). Actually, a confidence interval gives the researcher the ability to state the probability of a parameter lying within the percentages of the normal curve. It is a common practice to predetermine confidence intervals at 90%, 95%, and 99%. The 95% confidence interval corresponds to ± 1.96 standard errors or z-scores from the mean. To obtain a confidence interval, the upper and lower limits must be calculated as follows:

$$\text{Upper limit} = \overline{X} + (z)(\text{SEM})$$
$$\text{Lower limit} = \overline{X} - (z)(\text{SEM})$$
$$\text{where SEM} = \frac{s}{\sqrt{n}}$$

The z in the equation equals 1.65 for the 90% confidence interval, 1.96 for the 95% confidence interval, and 2.58 for the 99% confidence interval. Suppose that you wanted to calculate a 99% confidence interval when the $\overline{X} = 20$, $s = 2.88$, and $n = 45$. What would z be in this example? For a 99% confidence interval $z = 2.58$. The formula would be:

$$20 \pm (2.58)\frac{2.88}{\sqrt{45}}$$

The upper limit would be 21.24 and the lower limit would be 18.76. This tells you that you can be 99% certain that the true mean (population parameter) for this sample lies between 21.11 and 18.89. If you wanted a 90% confidence interval, the upper limit would be 20.71 and the lower

limit would be 19.29. You can see that as the confidence level increases, so does the width of the interval.

HYPOTHESIS TESTING

Inferential statistics are not only used to estimate parameters from a sample statistic. A more common use of inferential statistics in nursing research is hypothesis testing. It is important to remember that researchers make inferences based on the principles of negative inference. How is the hypothesis stated prior to data collection related to the hypothesis currently being tested? In hypothesis testing the focus turns from the original hypothesis to a statistical hypothesis that can be tested. Researchers typically state two hypotheses, a statistical or null hypothesis (H_0) and a research or alternate hypothesis (H_a). The research hypothesis states what the researcher believes will be the outcome of the study, and the null hypothesis is for statistical purposes. The H_0 always states that there is no relationship between the variables.

For example, Ginny wants to study the effect of weather on the number of admissions to psychiatric inpatient facilities. Ginny believes that more patients are admitted during periods of extreme weather than during periods of calm weather with little variation. Ginny states her research hypothesis as follows: There is a relationship between weather patterns and the number of admissions to inpatient psychiatric facilities. Ginny's null hypothesis would be: There is no relationship between weather patterns and the number of admissions to inpatient psychiatric facilities.

To reach a conclusion about whether the difference is the result of changes in the variables or the result of chance the researcher must test the null or statistical hypothesis. The steps involved in testing the null hypothesis are listed in the box on page 335.

STEPS IN TESTING THE NULL HYPOTHESIS

1. Check the assumptions associated with the statistical test to be sure they can be met.
2. Establish the null (H_0) and alternative (H_a) hypotheses.
3. Specify the test statistics.

4. Specify a level of significance.
5. Determine the decision rule.
6. Compute the value of the test statistic.
7. Make a conclusion based on your calculations in comparison to table values.

Checking Assumptions
There are different assumptions underlying statistical tests, depending on which class of statistical test is used, parametric or nonparametric.

Parametric Tests. Parametric tests of significance require that the sample frequency distribution match the normal curve and a level of measurement on at least an interval scale. These tests also require the estimation of at least one parameter for the population from the sample. If the sample frequency distribution does not match the normal curve, the accuracy of hypothesis testing is seriously jeopardized.

Nonparametric Statistical Tests. Nonparametric tests of significance, as the name implies, do not rely on estimating parameters. They can be used with both nominal and original level data. Nonparametric tests, sometimes referred to as distribution-free statistics, are used when normally distributed sample data fall below the interval/ratio level of measurement. These tests are easier to understand and can be applied under a wide range of conditions. Most nonparametric tests require ranks or ordering rather than numerical values of the observations. Common nonparametric tests include the following: Wilcoxin matched-pairs signed rank test, Mann-Whitney U test, Kruskal-Wallis test, and the chi-square test.

Nonparametric tests require the same basic steps in hypothesis testing as parametric tests. The null hypothesis for ranked tests is based on whether the ranks are normally distributed among the experimental groups. In such cases the alternate hypothesis suggests that subjects in one group tend to rank higher than those in the other.

Stating the Null Hypothesis
The null hypothesis states that there is no relationship between variables and therefore any observed relationship is the result of chance fluctuations in samples. If a theory has been previously established, this theory should be designated as the null hypothesis. If a new theory is being tested against an established one, it should be designated as the alternative or research hypothesis. The researcher usually desires to reject the null hypothesis (that changes in the variables were the result of chance) in favor of the research hypothesis. Although this is somewhat biased toward the null hypothesis, it requires that enough evidence is present to accept an alternative theory. Suppose that there is no cure for multiple sclerosis (MS), and a drug company develops a drug that they claim will cure MS. Now the company's sample evidence, presented to the Federal Drug Administration (FDA), must clearly indicate that the null hypothesis (that there is no cure for MS) can be rejected in favor of the

alternate hypothesis (that drug X can cure MS). This is a built-in protective mechanism that helps investigators be certain that an alternative treatment is better than existing treatments. In this way the researcher must show that the results obtained in the study were caused by the impact of the independent variable on the dependent variable and not caused by chance alone.

While it is never possible for the investigator to show that the research hypothesis is true, it is possible through the use of inferential statistics to state that the null hypothesis has a high probability of being incorrect. It is important to remember that the researcher is actually comparing a mathematical ideal (the population that matches the normal curve) to the sample selected in the hope that the sample differs enough from the mathematical ideal to say that the data is different as a result of the independent variable or treatment.

In a recent study Stewart, Fahs, and Kinney (1991) established three hypotheses in the null format. One of the null hypotheses was stated as follows:

> There is no difference in the occurrence of bruising at injection site with low-dose heparin when administered in three different subcutaneous sites.

Although no research hypothesis was stated by the authors, it might read:

> There is a difference in the occurrence of bruising at injection site with low-dose heparin when administered in three different subcutaneous sites.

The authors were unable to show that there was any difference in bruising, other than that which occurred by chance, so they accepted the null hypothesis. If they had been able to reject the null hypothesis,

they would concur that differences in bruising were related to changes in site.

One-Tailed and Two-Tailed Tests. Significant knowledge about a phenomenon is required before being able to designate hypothesis direction. For that reason, most nursing research is conducted using a two-tailed test. In a two-tailed test the significance level specifies the critical or improbable values at both ends of the distribution where values are not likely to occur. If a significance level of .05 is established using a two-tailed test, then each tail would contain 2.5% of the 5% area, as shown in Figure 16-15.

Occasionally an investigator may know

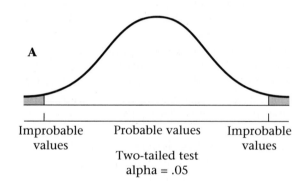

A

| Improbable values | Probable values | Improbable values |

Two-tailed test
alpha = .05

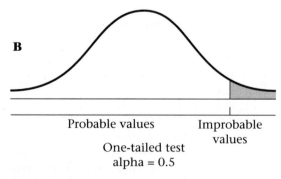

B

Probable values   Improbable values

One-tailed test
alpha = 0.5

Figure 16-15. Critical value range for **A**, two-tailed, and **B**, one-tailed tests.

enough about a phenomenon to designate a directional hypothesis. Or if previous research has been conducted to indicate that there is sufficient knowledge about the relationship between variables, a directional hypothesis can be stated. A directional hypothesis requires the use of a one-tailed statistical test and places all of the critical values at one end or the other, depending on the stated direction. Figure 16-15 shows the one-tailed test with a significance level of .05. In using a one-tailed test, the critical region of .05 covers a larger region of the specified tail, which causes the one-tailed test to be less conservative. It is also easier to reject a null hypothesis using a one-tailed test. This causes the risk of a type I error to increase.

Specifying the Test Statistics
To decide which statistical test is appropriate for your data, it is necessary to first consider the following questions:

1. How many variables do you have? Are you interested in one or two, or do you have more than two?
2. At what level of measurement are your variables (nominal, ordinal, interval, or ratio)?
3. Are the variables normally distributed?
4. How many groups do you have? Are they independent or dependent? Are they of equal size?
5. What do you want to measure? Are you measuring the difference between the groups (i.e., pretest, posttest), or are you interested in the strength of the relationship between two or more variables?

All of these questions can help guide your choice of an appropriate statistical test. By answering each question you nar-row the possible tests that can apply to your data. In some research studies more than one type of statistical test will be used to answer all of the research questions or hypotheses. For example, most studies use a combination of descriptive analysis and one or more inferential tests. Table 16-7 provides a quick overview of which statistical tests might be appropriate for different research designs and variables.

Specifying the Level of Significance
It is crucial to establish a level of significance prior to data analysis. In nursing research significance levels are usually selected at the .01 or .05 level. This means that for a .01 significance level the researcher has a 99% chance of reaching a correct conclusion based on data analysis. With a .05 significance level the researcher expands the probability of error to 5%. Significance levels are denoted by the Greek letter alpha (α) and may also be referred to as a *p* value or probability value of making an erroneous decision.

Type I and Type II Errors. In drawing a conclusion about a hypothesis there is the possibility of making one of two different errors. In designing a statistical test the researcher predetermines the risk (significance level) of rejecting the null hypothesis when it should be accepted—a type I error. For example, Miriam decides to study the relationship between estrogen levels and breast density in postmenopausal women. Prior to data collection she establishes a significance level of .05, so Miriam predetermines that she is willing to accept a 5% risk of making a type I error. The probability of making a type I error is always the same as the significance level and is specified by the researcher.

A type II error occurs when the researcher accepts the null hypothesis when

Table 16-7
Guide to Choosing a Statistical Test

Number of Groups	Level of Measurement	Parametric (P)/ Nonparametric (NP)	Test Statistic
ONE GROUP			
z-test			Z
Single sample t-test			t
TWO DEPENDENT GROUPS			
McNemar's chi-square	Nominal	NP	χ^2
Sign test	Ordinal	NP	Z
Wilcoxin matched-pairs signed-ranks test	Ordinal	NP	Z
Friedman ANOVA for ranks	Ordinal	NP	χ^2
Dependent t-test	Interval/ratio	P	t
TWO OR MORE DEPENDENT GROUPS			
Friedman two-factor ANOVA by ranks	Ordinal	NP	χ^2
TWO INDEPENDENT GROUPS			
Chi-square	Nominal	NP	χ^2
Mann-Whitney U	Ordinal	NP	U
Kendall's tau	Ordinal	NP	tau
Kruskal-Wallis	Ordinal	NP	k
Spearman rho rank correlation	Ordinal	NP	(rs) rho
t-test for independent groups	Interval/ratio	P	t
ANOVA	Interval/ratio	P	F
Linear regression	Interval/ratio	P	y
Pearson product-moment correlation	Interval/ratio	P	r
TWO OR MORE INDEPENDENT GROUPS			
Chi-square	Nominal	NP	χ^2
Kruskal-Wallis one-way ANOVA by ranks	Ordinal	NP	H
ANOVA	Interval/ratio	P	F

it should be rejected. Suppose Miriam discovers that there is a relationship between estrogen levels and breast density in postmenopausal women. Miriam would make a correct decision if she rejected the null hypothesis that there is no difference between the two variables. Miriam would make a type II error if she accepted the null hypothesis that there is no difference between the two variables. The probability of rejecting the null hypothesis when it should be rejected (making a correct decision) is called the power of the test. Power depends on the "degree of falseness" of the null hypothesis. A powerful study usually means a power of .80 or greater and is equivalent to stating that the researcher is willing to take only a 20% risk of committing a type II error. Power is established by the investigator, or it can be calculated using the following formula:

$$\text{Power} = 1 - \beta \text{ (beta)} \quad \text{or} \quad \text{(beta) } \beta = 1 - \text{Power}$$

The probability of committing a type II error can be assessed by the computation of the power curve or power function of a test (power analysis). By reducing the probability of a type II error, the power of the test is increased.

In reality we try to achieve a balance between alpha levels and power by keeping a moderately low alpha level of .05 or less and increasing the power by using large samples. It is important to observe that as you decrease the risk of a type I error, you increase the possibility of a type II error and vice versa.

For example, John established a null hypothesis that there is no difference in mean diastolic blood pressure of menstruating and nonmenstruating female patients. For John to reject the null hypothesis (H_0) he determined that a difference of 20 mm Hg was required. He also knew that he would be able to accept the research hypothesis

(H_a) if he was able to show a difference between the means. John was concerned that he would make a type I or type II error. The possible error associated with John's decision making is depicted in Figure 16-16.

Power Analysis. Power is, in essence, a measure of sensitivity, the ability to detect small differences among the groups that were studied. Cohen (1977) determined that there are four parameters of power: significance level, sample size, effect size, and power. Using a power analysis formula, it is possible to calculate any one of these parameters if we already know the other three. One can increase power by increasing the sample size, increasing the alpha level, or using a one-tailed test if warranted.

Most studies provide information about alpha level and sample size, but often do not indicate effect size (ES). Effect size is the strength of effect the independent variable has on the dependent variable (Polit & Sherman, 1990). For example, if a researcher wanted to measure depression (dependent variable) before and after diagnosis of a fatal illness (independent variable), prior to diagnosis we would expect a small effect size and after diagnosis a larger effect size (more depression). If everything else is equal in a study, as the effect size increases, the power will increase and the needed sample size will decrease (Polit & Sherman, 1990). In other words, smaller effect sizes require larger samples. Effect size is difficult for the researcher to control; its value can be estimated (Polit & Sherman, 1990).

Power analysis allows the investigator to determine what significance level and sample size are needed to yield the most powerful study. As stated previously, .80 is an acceptable standard for power, and .05 or .01 is an acceptable significance level. So, if we already know the significance level and the

Population situation

John's decision based on his sample	$H_o \leq 20$ mm hcg H_o is TRUE H_a is FALSE	$H_a > 20$ mm hcg H_o is FALSE H_a is TRUE
ACCEPT H_o	No error correct decision 1 −alpha	Type II error (accept H_o when H_o is FALSE) beta
REJECT H_o	Type I error (reject H_o when H_o is TRUE) alpha level	No error correct decision power or 1−beta

Figure 16-16. Possible error associated with John's decision about his hypothesis that there is no difference in mean diastolic blood pressures of menstruating and nonmenstruating females.

power, and if we could estimate the effect size, we could determine what size sample we would need to have a powerful study.

Effect size can be estimated in several ways, although in nursing research the most common way is through a pilot study or through an estimate based on prior research and clinical experience. Sometimes investigators can review similar research studies in which power analyses have been calculated to find an acceptable effect size. Effect size is usually estimated as small for new areas of research and medium or large if the expected relationship is substantial (Cohen, 1977). Cohen (1977) noted that each statistical test has a different formula for estimating the effect size (Table 16-8).

Power analysis is vital to expanding the knowledge base in nursing research and can be used in two ways. First, the investigator can calculate a power analysis prior to conducting a research study to determine what sample size is needed to pro-duce a specific level of power. Second, power analysis can be done following the completion of the research and data analysis to assist the consumer in applying the findings.

Power analysis is also important to the consumer of nursing research. If an investigator makes a claim that two variables are strongly related, it would be nice to know that there is some truth to this claim. What happens if the power of the study is only .30? There would be a 70% chance that the two variables were not related. For example, suppose that a study showed that immersing a person with Alzheimer's disease in an ice bath for an hour three times a day would cure the disease. Before immersing someone, or for that matter before someone tried to immerse *you* in that tub, you would probably want to know whether there was a 30% chance or an 80% chance that this were true! Similarly, it is important to know what the power of a study

Table 16-8
Formulas for Effect Size and Definitions of Levels of Effect Size for Five Statistical Tests

Test	Effect Size Population Parameter	Effect Size Values*		
		Small	Medium	Large
t-test for 2 group means	$d = \dfrac{|\bar{X}_1 - \bar{X}_2|}{\sigma}$	.20	.50	.80
F-test for *k* independent means	$f = \dfrac{\sigma_{mi}}{\sigma}$	.10	.25	.40
r (r ≠ 0)	*r*	.10	.30	.50
F (*R²* ≠ 0)	$f^2 = \dfrac{R^2}{1 - R^2}$	.02	.15	.35
(Multiple regression)				

From Polit, D., & Sherman, R. E. (1990). Statistical power in nursing research. *Nursing Research, 39* (6), 365-369.
*The definitions of effect size values are based on Cohen (1977).

was before accepting or rejecting new treatments based on research that may or may not have been sufficiently powerful.

How powerful are nursing research studies? Polit and Sherman (1990) found that the average power for small effect studies was <.30 and for medium effect studies was .70 and that it was very high for large effect studies. Unfortunately, they also discovered that only 15% (n = 62) of all of the studies had adequate power for all of their analyses. The authors concluded that power analysis should be conducted prior to undertaking a research study and that it should be required when requesting funding for any quantitative research (Polit & Sherman, 1990).

Research requires a great deal of time, effort, and expense, so it would stand to reason that an investigator would want some assurance (through power analysis) that the study is worth conducting. Similarly, it would stand to reason that nurses owe themselves and their clients the assurance that the treatments recommended and used are better than any other treatments currently, or previously, available. Statisti-

cal computer software packages are available that are capable of calculating a power analysis.

Determining the Decision Rule
How do you decide when to accept or reject the null hypothesis? Is it an arbitrary decision made by the researcher? Absolutely not! The researcher must decide when to accept or reject the hypothesis based on regions of acceptance or rejection for each of the test statistics. To formulate a decision rule, the researcher must determine the degrees of freedom specified for each statistical test. Degrees of freedom is a statistical concept that refers to the number of sample values that cannot be calculated from knowledge of other values and a specific statistic. The concept of degrees of freedom is difficult to understand, but the calculation is relatively easy. Normally, the degrees of freedom require the use of *n* or the number of values in a sample. For most statistical tests degrees of freedom (df) equal *n − 1*, although for tests with two groups, df may equal *n − 2*. Most statistical tests will provide a formula for the degrees

of freedom as well, or they will be incorporated into the test statistic. To determine the table value for a test statistic one must use the degrees of freedom.

After the investigator establishes the degrees of freedom and the level of significance, a critical value can be found on a table of values for the statistical test specified (Table 16-9). Each statistical test has a corresponding table of values. It is important to be certain that the correct table is used for each of the statistical tests. Statistical tables are contained in the Appendix.

Computing the Sample Value
The researcher calculates the value for the appropriate test statistic using the data from the sample. Each statistical test uses different formulas and requires differing statistical skill levels. A number of nurse researchers rely on computers for statistical computations, and at times the assistance of a statistician can be invaluable.

Drawing a Conclusion
Based on the calculations of the sample value, it is now possible to determine whether to reject the null hypothesis. Normally if the calculated value is equal to or greater than the critical (table) value in the corresponding table, the null hypothesis is rejected. There are a few tests where the

calculated value needs to be equal to or less than the table value. Suppose that we calculated a chi-square of 7.0 with df = 2 and $\alpha = .05$. By looking at the table values in Table 16-9, we would determine that our calculated value of 7 is larger than the table value of 5.99. Therefore we are able to reject the null hypothesis (H_0).

USING DATA FROM AN INDEPENDENT SAMPLE TO MAKE INFERENCES ABOUT A SINGLE POPULATION

Chi-Square Goodness-of-Fit Test
The chi-square goodness-of-fit test is the most basic form of chi-square and is used to test for differences between observed and expected values. The chi-square statistic (χ^2) is used to test the hypothesis that the observed frequencies are not different from the frequencies to be expected if no association existed between the variables. In actuality the researcher is trying to assess whether the two variables are associated or independent of one another.

The chi-square statistic is computed by comparing two sets of frequencies: those that were observed and those that would be expected under conditions of no association. Expected frequencies are calculated so that

$$f_e = \frac{f_r f_c}{N}$$

where
  f_e = expected frequency in a cell in the table
  f_r = observed frequency for the row
  f_c = observed frequency for the column
  N = total number of participants in the study

The chi-square statistic is computed from the formula

$$\chi^2 = \Sigma \frac{(f_o - f_e)^2}{f_e}$$

Table 16-9
Sample Table of Critical Values for Decision Making (Chi-Square Test)

df (k −1)	Probability Levels				
	.90	.95	.975	.99	.995
1	2.71	3.84	5.02	6.63	7.88
2	4.61	5.99	7.38	9.21	10.6
3	6.25	7.81	9.35	11.3	12.8
4	7.78	9.49	11.1	13.3	14.9

where f_o = observed frequency for a cell and f_e = expected frequency for a cell. The chi-square statistic is compared to a table of values with df = (R − 1) where R = number of rows.

Gaynor (1990) studied the effects of giving long-term care at home to a medically disabled relative on short- and long-term caregivers and on a control group. Gaynor measured physical health subjectively using three questions from the Structural Model of Self-Reported Physical Health Scale.

Using the chi-square statistic, Gaynor was able to show that the long-term care group had significantly more illnesses than the other groups (Table 16.10). Short-term caregivers averaged 3.0 years of caregiving, while the long-term group averaged 7.5 years of caregiving. The long-term group gave an average of 4.5 hours of direct patient care, while the short-term group averaged only 1.8 hours of care daily.

t-Test

The t-test allows investigators to look at differences in group means. There are two types of t-tests, one for independent samples and the other for dependent (paired, matched, or related) samples. The t-test for independent samples is used to compare two different samples. For example, an independent t-test might be used to compare an experimental and control group, or a group of ICU nurses and a group of psychiatric nurses. The t-test for dependent samples compares the same sample over time, for example, a group of subjects who were given a pretest and posttest.

A t-test is used to compare data at the interval or ratio level and must meet the assumptions of normal distribution. A t-test may be used for both directional and nondirectional hypotheses. A directional hypothesis would require a one-tailed t-test, while a nondirectional hypothesis would require a two-tailed t-test.

Table 16-10
Mean Physical Health Measures with Standard Deviation

	Long-term Caregivers		Short-term Caregivers		Control Group		X	p
	X	s	X	s	X	s		
Ill days in last 6 months	2.9	(11.8)	1.0	(2.9)	.6	(2.1)	4.0	.13
Meds	2.1	(1.9)	1.7	(2.0)	1.9	(1.7)	2.7	.25
Diagnoses	1.9	(1.5)	1.5	(1.5)	1.6	(1.4)	3.3	.19
MD visits for (husband) in last 12 months	59.1	(221.0)	30.1	(166.0)	1.1	(2.7)	25.7	.001*
MD visits for own health in last 6 months	2.2	(2.3)	1.1	(1.3)	1.8	(1.5)	8.2	.01*

From Gaynor, S. E. (1990). The long haul: The effects of home care on caregivers. *IMAGE: Journal of Nursing Scholarship,* *22*(4), 208-212.
*$p \leq .01$.

When using a t-test for small samples, it is necessary to first meet the assumption of homogeneity of variances. In other words, there must be some equality between the two groups; if a difference does exist it must not be statistically significant. To determine whether samples meet the criterion for homogeneity of variance, the following F-test is used

$$F = \frac{S^2 \text{ (Larger variance)}}{S^2 \text{ (Smaller variance)}}$$

The F ratio is never less than 1 because the larger variance is always divided by the smaller variance. To determine the critical value of F one must use an F table. If the calculated F value is equal to or higher than the F table (critical) value, it can be assumed that the variances are homogeneous and the difference between the groups is not significant. In this case the separate variance formula is used, and if H_0 is acceptable, the pooled variance formula is used.

The t-test for independent samples is both a popular and powerful statistical test. The t-test does not directly address itself to the degree of the relationship between the dependent and independent variables; rather it tests for differences between the means of the two samples. To calculate the t-test one must first determine which formula to use based on the results of the F test. There are two formulas for the independent t-test: the pooled variance formula and the separate variance formula. These formulas are as follows:

Pooled variance:

$$t = \frac{\overline{X}_a - \overline{X}_b}{\sqrt{\left(\dfrac{\Sigma \overline{X}_a^2 - \Sigma \overline{X}_b^2}{n_a \; n_b}\right)\left(\dfrac{1+1}{n_a \; n_b}\right)}}$$

where $\overline{x}_a$ and $\overline{x}_b$ are the respective sample means, Σx_a^2 and Σx_b^2 are the respective sum of squares, and n_a and n_b are the sample sizes.

Separate variance:

$$t = \frac{\overline{X}_a - \overline{X}_b}{\sqrt{\dfrac{s_a^2}{n_a} + \dfrac{s_b^2}{n_b}}}$$

where $\overline{X}_a$ and $\overline{X}_b$ are the respective sample means, s_a^2 and s_b^2 are the sample variances, and n_a and n_b are the sample sizes.

Let us use the t-test for independent samples (separate variance formula) on a group of boys and a group of girls to determine whether there is a significant difference in their weight ranges. The null hypothesis is that there is no difference between the two group's weight ranges. Let us assume that the study meets the assumptions required for the t-test and that we were able to reject H_0 using the F test (Step 1).

$$\text{Step 2: } H_0: \overline{X}_1 - \overline{X}_2 = 0$$
$$H_a: \overline{X}_1 - \overline{X}_2 \neq 0$$

The null hypothesis is that the mean of group 1 minus the mean of group 2 will equal zero or that there is no difference between the two groups. The alternate hypothesis states that there will be a difference between the two means or that they will not equal zero.

Step 3: We have decided to use a t-test for independent groups (separate variance formula).

Step 4: We will choose a significance level of $\alpha = .05$, degrees of freedom $n - 2$.

Step 5: Establish the decision rule by checking the table in Appendix B.

Reject H_0 if the calculated t is ≤ -2.819 or ≥ 2.819

Accept H_0 if calculated t is $-2.819 < t > 2.819$

Step 6: Compute the critical value of the test statistic.

First, we must calculate the standard error of the mean of both groups. You may recall we did this earlier in the chapter. There are 12 girls and 12 boys in the class. For group 1, $n = 12$, $s = 13.6$, and $\overline{X} = 134.5$. For group 2, $n = 12$, $s = 10$, and $\overline{X} = 127$.

Using the formula for t for separate variances we can calculate the critical value.

$$\frac{134.5 - 127}{\sqrt{\dfrac{13.6}{12} + \dfrac{10}{12}}} =$$

$$\frac{7.5}{1.9663} = 3.814$$

$$t = 3.814$$

Step 6: $-2.819 \geq 3.814 \geq 2.819$. We reject the H_0, meaning that there is a significant difference between the two groups or that the boys and girls had a significant difference in weight.

Let us apply our knowledge of power analysis to determine what the power was in this study. By referring to Table 16-8 we can find the formula for effect size for the t-test for independent samples. The formula is:

$$d = \frac{X_1 - X_2}{s}$$

Based on data from the previous example, the effect size would be:

$$d = \frac{134.5 - 127}{10*} = .75$$

---

*Either of the standard deviations can be used since one of the assumptions is that they are about equal.

We could then refer to the appropriate power table in the Appendix using an n of 12, a two-tailed test, and a power of .75. The probability of committing a type II error is 59%, so we would most likely want to repeat the study with a larger sample of boys and girls.

The pooled variance formula can also be used to calculate the t statistic. Suppose that a cardiac rehabilitation nurse wanted to test the effectiveness of two different aerobic exercise programs. Group A would train by using a treadmill, and group B would train using stair climbers. At the end of 10 weeks the cardiac nurse would test for their perceived fitness level. Hypothetical data for this study is shown in Figure 16-17.

Calculating the t statistic may seem rather overwhelming at first, although the actual calculations are fairly easy with a calculator.

What if 1000 people were included in the sample? Most researchers would use a computer to calculate a t-test for a sample of that size. A computer printout for an independent t-test is shown in Table 16-11. Note that the computer program indicates whether a t value is significant and at what level. In this example the test was significant at the .05 level.

How is a t-test used in an actual research study? Algase (1992) studied cognitive discriminants of wandering among nursing home residents and used an independent t-test for a portion of her data analysis. Although she did not state a hypothesis, she stated that the study "was undertaken to identify cognitive factors differentiating wandering from nonwandering . . ." (Algase, 1992). She divided her subjects into wanderers and nonwanderers and administered the Everyday Indicators of Impaired Cognition Scale (EIIC). The EIIC yields numerical data at the ratio level. Algase used

Treadmill group (a)	Stair climber group (b)
27	22
25	24
26	23
28	24
27	24
24	26
26	21
24	20

$$na = 8 \qquad\qquad nb = 8$$

$$\overline{X}a = 25.88 \qquad\qquad \overline{X}b = 23.00$$

$$\Sigma xa^2 = 14.88 \qquad\qquad \Sigma xb^2 = 26.00$$

F test for homogeneity of variance:

$$sa^2 = \frac{14.88}{7} = 2.13$$

$$\frac{3.71}{2.13} = 1.74 \le 3.79$$

$$sb^2 = \frac{26.00}{7} = 3.71$$

The calculated value of F $\le$ the critical value of F 3.79 so we accept the H_o that there is no difference and we can use the pooled variance t-test.

Pooled variance t formula:

$$t = \frac{25.88 - 23.00}{\sqrt{\left(\frac{14.88 + 26.00}{8 + 8 - 2}\right)\left(\frac{1 + 1}{8 \quad 8}\right)}}$$

$$t = \frac{2.88}{\sqrt{\left(\frac{40.88}{14}\right)\left(\frac{2}{8}\right)}} = \frac{2.88}{\sqrt{0.73}} = \frac{2.88}{0.85} = 3.39$$

At 14 degrees of freedom, assuming $\alpha = .05$, using a two-tailed test and assuming that there is no difference in the two programs, we are able to reject H_o because the calculated t 3.39 is $\ge$ the table value of 2.145. Therefore there is a difference in the two exercise programs. It would appear that the treadmill resulted in higher scores.

Figure 16-17. Example of t statistic calculation.

an independent two-tailed t-test (because she compared wanderers and nonwanderers or two different groups of people, and she had a nondirectional hypothesis) to test the difference between the two groups (Table 16-12). All four subscales of abstract thinking, judgment, language skills, and spatial skills were significantly different between the wanderers and nonwanderers. The wanderers scored higher on all of the EIIC subscales, indicating greater impairment than the nonwanderers. In other words, she was able to reject the null hypothesis and conclude that the differences in the two groups were not a result of chance alone.

Table 16-11
Sample Computer Printout of a t-Test for Independent Groups

t-Tests for Independent Samples of SKOL
GROUP 1 - SKOL EQ 1
GROUP 2 - SKOL EQ 2

Variable	Number of Cases	Mean	Standard Deviation	Standard Error	F Value	2-Tail Prob.
ATOT						
GROUP 1	767	34.9752	5.285	.191	2.55	.000
GROUP 2	1833	22.5957	3.309	.077		
D15						
GROUP 1	767	2.9296	1.341	.048	1.53	.000
GROUP 2	1833	2.6470	1.085	.025		
D16						
GROUP 1	767	2.0443	1.099	.040	2.04	.000
GROUP 2	1833	1.8554	.769	.018		
D17						
GROUP 1	767	3.0039	1.397	.050	1.23	.001
GROUP 2	1833	2.8129	1.259	.029		
D18						
GROUP 1	766	3.3982	1.673	.060	1.04	.525
GROUP 2	1833	3.5117	1.706	.040		

Table 16-12
Descriptive Statistics and t-Tests on Everyday Indicators of Impaired Cognition EIIC Subscales

Subscale	Wanderer			Nonwanderers			
	M	SD	Range	M	SD	Range	t Value
Abstract thinking	4.46	2.12	0-6	3.06	2.12	0-6	−2.69*
Judgment	1.88	1.71	0-4	0.81	1.16	0-4	−3.64**
Language skills	2.26	2.60	0-7	0.48	1.28	0-7	−5.61**
Spatial skills	2.18	2.21	0-5	0.82	1.42	0-5	−4.14**

From Algase, D. L. (1992). Cognitive discriminants of wandering among nursing home residents. *Nursing Research, 41*(2), 78-81.
df = 161.
*p < .01.
**p< .001.

Spees used an independent t-test to test the hypothesis that "there would be a significant difference between *nurses' perception* of clients' and families' knowledge of medical terms and their *actual* knowledge of medical terms" (1991). Nurses working in a surgical unit expected clients and families to understand 50 terms that were approved for client education. Using a t-test to determine if clients and families actually understood these terms, Spees found that clients and family members comprehended medical terms at a lower rate than the nurses expected (t = 6.3, p = .001). In other words, the family members understood fewer of the terms than the nurses believed they would.

Mann-Whitney U Test

The Mann-Whitney U test is a nonparametric test equivalent to the t-test. This test is used to determine whether two groups are significantly different when scores from two sets of data are ranked and compared. The test can be used with continuously distributed variables that are at the ordinal level of measurement or higher. The ranked scores are always used. It may also be used when two random samples are drawn from a population and both samples receive different treatments, as with control and experimental groups. The Mann-Whitney U test is a powerful alternative to the t-test and, unlike the t-test, it can also be used with small samples (under 20 in each group).

The Mann-Whitney U statistic (U) is calculated by totaling the number of times that scores of group 1 preceded the scores of group 2. Suppose that Hospital "A" has determined that it needs to close one of its two medical units to cut costs. Since Hospital "A" has a strong belief in providing quality patient care, the administration decides to have a convenience sample of the next 14 patients admitted to unit 1 and the next 14 patients admitted to unit 2 fill out a questionnaire ranking quality of nursing care on a scale of 0 to 100, with 100 being the best possible nursing care. These are the results of the survey:

Group a		Group b	
Unit 1	Rank 1	Unit 2	Rank 2
76	16	91	25
42	9	98	28
39	7	92	26
82	19	15	1
66	15	86	22
46	13	84	21
28	4	97	27
29	5	22	2
25	3	83	20
43	10	81	18
77	17	30	6
44	11	40	8
45	12	89	24
49	14	88	23

$$\Sigma Rk_1 = 155 \quad \Sigma Rk_2 = 251$$

Step 1: $H_0: U_a = U_b$
$H_a: U_a \neq U_b$

Step 2: Significance level .05 two-tailed test

Step 3: Reject H_0 if calculated $U \leq 55$

Step 4: $U_a = n_a (n_b) + n_b \dfrac{(n_b + 1)}{2} \; \Sigma Rk_b$

$$14 (14) + \frac{14 (15)}{2} - 251 = 50$$

$$U_b = n_b (n_a) + n_a \frac{(n_b + 1)}{2} - \Sigma Rk_a$$

$$U_b = 14 (14) + \frac{14 (15)}{2} - 155 = 146$$

Step 5: Use whichever calculated number is smaller and reject H_0 since $50 \leq 55$. There is a difference in the quality of nursing care between the two units as measured by patients.

Once again a table is used to determine whether a U value of this size or smaller could occur at a prespecified level of significance. The H_0 is rejected if the calculated value of U is equal to or smaller than the table U. If a U table is not available, further calculations can be done to obtain a z score.

Sisney (1993) recently studied the relationship between social support and depression in recovering chemically dependent nurses. Depression was measured at the ordinal level and ranked from not depressed to extremely depressed. Social support data were analyzed with a different statistical test because social support was measured at the interval/ratio level. As part of her extensive statistical analysis Sisney used the Mann-Whitney U test to determine whether there was a significant difference between males and females on measures of depression. Using a one-tailed Mann-Whitney U test ($z = -1.628$, $p = .05$), she was able to show that females were significantly more depressed than males

Analysis of Variance

The analysis of variance (ANOVA) is a parametric test for differences among two or three groups made by comparing two or more population means. The ANOVA is similar to a t-test, but it can test differences between the means in two or more groups. You might wonder why one could not just do two t-tests rather than an ANOVA. Remember, though, that the t-test relies on the independence of groups. If we had three groups (A, B, and C), we would have to do a t-test for groups A + B, B + C, and A + C. In repeating the t-test for the third group we would violate this assumption and increase the chances of committing a type I error. If an investigator has only two groups, either a t-test or an ANOVA could

be used, and both would yield the same results.

The ANOVA compares the variability in a data set attributed to chance with the variability caused by systematic differences in the population under study. The ANOVA assists us in addressing a research question in which the investigator wants to show that the variability in scores is caused by the independent variable(s). The researcher would state the following research question: "Can a significant part of the variability in the dependent variable be caused by changes in the independent variable?"

The ANOVA separates the total variability of a set of scores into two components: (1) the variability resulting from the independent variability (variance between groups) and (2) the variability resulting from other things, such as measurement error and individual differences (variance within groups). The statistic computed for the ANOVA is called the F ratio statistic. Computing the F ratio is more difficult than computing t because we have added to the complexity of the t-test by adding more groups. It is important not to confuse the ANOVA F ratio with the F-test that we used previously to test for homogeneity of variances. These are two different procedures, and each one leads to different conclusions.

The ANOVA actually has several models, but we will address only the one-factor or one-way ANOVA and the two-factor or two-way ANOVA.

One-Factor Analysis of Variance. The one-factor analysis of variance (ANOVA) is used to test the relationship between one independent and one dependent variable. For example, a self-esteem test was administered to four randomly selected groups of patients with rheumatoid arthritis, multiple sclerosis, cancer, and diabetes. Were the mean test scores of each of the four groups significantly different from one another? To answer this question the null hypothesis would state that the means of the four groups are equal.

To calculate the ANOVA it is necessary to first determine the variance of the scores for the four groups of patients and combine them into one composite group. This variance is known as the combined groups variance or *total groups variance* (V_t). Next the mean value of the variances of *each* of the four groups is computed separately; this is known as the within groups variance or V_w. The difference between the total groups variance and the within groups variance or ($V_t - V_w$) is known as the between groups variance. The F ratio is computed as follows:

$$F = \frac{V_b = \text{Between groups variance}}{V_w \text{ Within groups variance}}$$

The within groups variance represents the sampling error between the distributions, while the between groups variance represents the influence of the independent variable. If the between groups variance is not substantially greater than the within groups variance, the investigator concludes that the difference between the means is caused by sampling error. Once again, the investigator uses a table, in this instance the F table, to determine whether or not the results are significant. If the F

ratio is equal to or larger than the table value, then the researcher concludes that the variance was probably too great to be a result of sampling error alone and thus the null hypothesis is rejected.

In a recent study Twiname (1992) compared HIV disease classification with the severity of depression and incidence of suicidal intent. Twiname used a one-factor ANOVA to test which classification of subjects (HIV+ asymptomatic, HIV+ symptomatic, or those with AIDS) as more depressed. Results of the ANOVA are presented in an ANOVA table (Table 16-13) and indicate that there was a significant difference at the .03 level between the three groups.

MULTIPLE COMPARISON OR POST HOC TESTS. We now know that the means of depression scores among the three groups were significantly different, but there is still a problem. How can we tell which classification or rather which group had higher means and therefore more depression? To determine which group or groups had more depression the investigator must follow the ANOVA with a post hoc test. The post hoc test determines which significant differences between or among the means is significant and in which direction. Twiname (1992) decided to use a Tukey's post hoc test to help determine which group or groups had significantly higher depression (Table 16-14).

The results of the Tukey's HSD post hoc test indicate that there was a significant dif-

Table 16-13
Analysis of Variance for HIV Classification and Depression

Depression	SS	df	MS	F	P
Between groups	997.3895	2	498.6948	3.6769	.03
Within groups	10443.5824	78	135.6309		
TOTAL	11440.9719	80			

Table 16-14
Tukey HSD Post Hoc Procedure

	HIV+	**ARC**	**AIDS**
HIV+ (M = 14.8421)	—	8.311*	8.2862*
ARC (M = 23.1538)		—	0.0252
AIDS (M = 23.1286)			—

*$p = .01$.

ference between subjects with ARC (X = 23.1538, n = 26) and AIDS (X = 23.1286, n = 35), and subjects who were HIV+ (X = 14.8421, n = 19). This test indicated that subjects with ARC and AIDS were significantly more depressed than asymptomatic subjects who were HIV+. There are a number of post hoc comparisons that can be used. The five post hoc tests or *a posteriori* procedures that are commonly used in nursing research are the Fisher's least significant difference (LSD), the Duncan's new multiple range test, the Student Newman-Keuls procedure, the Scheffé test, and the Tukey's honestly significant difference (HSD).

These post hoc tests differ in their precision and sensitivity, and there tends to be a hierarchy with regard to which test is best. The Tukey's HSD test is preferred for comparing the means of two samples of equal size. The Scheffé test is most frequently used and suitable under most other circumstances. The Scheffé is not limited by samples of equal size and can be used with simple paired or multiple comparisons. One problem with the Scheffé test is that it is the most conservative of the five methods and is very likely to miss detecting a real difference when one exists. The Fisher's LSD is the least exact of the post hoc tests and provides the highest risk of making a

type I error. The Duncan's test is similar to Fisher's; although it is slightly more conservative, there is a 95% agreement between the two. The Student Newman-Keuls is more conservative than Fisher's or Duncan's. Most researchers rely on the other two post hoc tests for comparisons.

Two-Factor/Multifactor Analysis of Variance. The two-factor or two-way ANOVA and the multifactor ANOVA can add more independent variables or treatments that might influence the dependent variable. For example, let's say that a family nurse practitioner is interested in finding out whether patients with chronic low back pain and patients with chronic neck pain respond differently to treatment with heat or cold therapy.

The two-way ANOVA uses differences in rows and columns. In other words, is there a difference in the two row differences (or treatments) (in this example heat or cold application), or in the column differences (in this example chronic low back or chronic neck pain). These two tests of difference between rows and columns are called the tests of main effects. The third test is called a test of the interaction effect or whether there is any systematic influence on the dependent variable that cannot be explained by the row and column (main) effects. If there is not an interaction effect or a main effect, then the results are caused by random error only.

To successfully find the two-way ANOVA one must work through three different calculations. Most researchers rely on a computer to calculate this test. The calculations required are the row effect and column effect (main effects), and the interaction effect.

To test for main effects it is necessary to begin by testing for column effects where the H_0 states that all column means are equal and the H_a states that at least two of the column means are not equal. F = mean square columns; that is, mean square between *columns,* not groups divided by mean squares error or mean squares within. In this calculation the mean squares between is exactly the same as in the one-way ANOVA, but the mean squares within may be smaller because of the interaction between rows and columns. One must then calculate the row effects in which the H_0 states that all row means are equal and the H_a asserts that at least two of the row means are not equal. The row effects are divided by the interaction effects or mean squares between.

Finally, the interaction between rows and columns, or the interaction effect, is calculated. The interaction effect is any systematic influence on the dependent variable that is not explained by the two main effects (columns and rows). Any interaction effect will in turn lower the random error. Actual calculations for the two-factor ANOVA are beyond the scope of this text, but the interested reader may consult a statistics text for more information.

How might a two-factor ANOVA be used within the context of a research study? Suppose that we are trying to determine how individuals with chronic lower back pain and individuals with chronic neck pain respond to heat application and cold application. We could design a study in which these two groups are randomly assigned to receive either heat or cold therapy and then measure the amount of perceived pain at the end of the experimental period.

As stated earlier there are several steps in analyzing this research. First of all, we want to know whether either heat or cold therapy is a more effective method of treating chronic pain (row effect). Second, we want to know if people with chronic neck pain or chronic lower back pain have changes in their perceived pain depending on which type of treatment they receive (column effect). We also want to know whether there was a difference between the effects of the two treatments on individuals with chronic lower back pain and chronic neck pain (interaction effect). One way that these data might be presented is in table form (Table 16-15).

By looking at the data in Table 16-15, it is possible to make the following general observations: (1) subjects who had cold applied experienced less pain than those who had heat applied ($\overline{X} = 27$, $\overline{X} = 18$); (2) subjects with low back pain experienced less pain than subjects who had neck pain ($\overline{X} = 21$, $\overline{X} = 24$); and (3) both groups of subjects (low back pain and neck pain) responded better to cold therapy than to heat therapy. In an actual two-factor ANOVA an F ratio would be calculated that could be compared to the F table to determine whether the null hypothesis could be rejected.

The multifactor ANOVA is more complex than the two-factor ANOVA, but it can also look at a greater combination of more variables. The multifactor ANOVA or MANOVA is frequently used in data analysis in nursing research. The MANOVA is commonly used with multiple dependent variables, while the two- and three-way ANOVA is frequently used with multiple independent variables.

Kruskal-Wallis Test

The Kruskal-Wallis test is a nonparametric alternative to the one-factor analysis of variance. The Kruskal-Wallis test makes no assumptions about normal distribution or homogeneity of variance and can be used with ordinal level data from a continuously distributed population. It is based on a test statistic calculated from ranks established by pooling the observations from c independent, simple, random samples, where $c > 2$.

The null hypothesis for the Kruskal-Wallis test is that the populations are identically

Table 16-15
Two-Factor ANOVA

Factor B—Type of Pain	Factor A—Type of Treatment*		
	Heat (1)	Cold (2)	
Low back pain (1)	14 24 19 31 $\overline{X} = 16$ 21 12 17 10 30	12 16 32 19 $\overline{X} = 25$ 40 38 26 17 29	Low back pain $\overline{X} = 21$
Neck pain (2)	17 13 22 30 $\overline{X} = 19$ 24 21 14 19 11	33 18 28 27 $\overline{X} = 28$ 36 39 26 15 31	Neck pain $\overline{X} = 24$
	Treatment 1 $\overline{X} = 18$	Treatment 2 $\overline{X} = 27$*	

*Numbers have been rounded off.

distributed or, alternately, that the samples were drawn from identical populations and therefore have equal means. The investigator is able to reject the null hypothesis if the Spearman coefficient is equal to or larger than the tabled value. The Kruskal-Wallis test can be used with two or more samples. When testing with only two samples, however, the Mann-Whitney U, an equivalent test, may be preferred because of its versatility for both two-tailed and one-tailed tests.

Chi-Square Test of Independence

The chi-square test of independence is a joint frequency distribution for two or more variables. The chi-square test determines if one variable is independent of the other. The first step in computing the chi-square is to develop a contingency or cross-tabulation table. Let us consider the following two variables, ethnic group and health care delivery setting preference, by stating the following hypothesis: There is no difference among ethnic groups for preference of health care delivery setting.

Ethnic group	Hospital	Clinic	Private Dr.	Total
Black	22	30	16	68
White	20	25	10	55
Other	12	15	34	61
Total	54	70	60	184

Let us pretend that we have established a hypothesis that there is no difference in the observed and expected frequencies at α = .01.

The formula for chi-square is:

$$\chi^2 = \frac{(o_1 - e_1)^2}{e_1} + \cdots + \frac{(o_m - e_m)^2}{e_m}$$

Where:

o_1 = observed frequencies
e_1 = expected frequencies
o_m = observation of m number of probabilities
e_m = expectation of m number of probabilities

Step 1 is to calculate the expected frequencies:

	Hospital	**Clinic**	**Private Dr.**
Black	$\dfrac{68 \times 54}{184}$	$\dfrac{68 \times 70}{184}$	$\dfrac{68 \times 60}{184}$
	= (19.9565)	= (25.8696)	= (22.1739)
White	$\dfrac{55 \times 54}{184}$	$\dfrac{55 \times 70}{184}$	$\dfrac{55 \times 60}{184}$
	= (16.1413)	= (20.9239)	= (17.9348)
Other	$\dfrac{61 \times 54}{184}$	$\dfrac{61 \times 70}{184}$	$\dfrac{61 \times 60}{184}$
	= (19.9022)	= (23.2065)	= (19.8913)

Next, a cell-by-cell calculation is required to determine the cumulative contribution of each cell to the value of χ^2.

$$\chi^2 = \frac{(22 - 19.965)^2}{19.965} + \frac{(30 - 25.8695)^2}{25.8697} +$$
$$\frac{(16 - 22.1739)^2}{22.1739} + \frac{(20 - 16.1413)^2}{16.1413} +$$
$$\frac{(25 - 20.9239)^2}{20.9239} + \frac{(10 - 17.9348)^2}{17.9348} +$$
$$\frac{(12 - 17.9022)^2}{17.9022} + \frac{(15 - 23.2065)^2}{23.2065} +$$
$$\frac{(34 - 19.8913)^2}{19.8913}$$

χ^2 = 0.2074 + 0.6595 + 1.7190 + 0.9225 + 0.7940 + 3.5106 + 1.9459 + 0.9225 + 10.0072

$$\chi^2 = 22.69$$

With degrees of freedom = (R − 1)(C − 1) or (3 − 1)(3 − 1) or 4, the critical value

at 4 df with α = .01 is 13.277. Our calculated value of 22.67 is greater than the table value, so there is a difference among ethnic groups for choice of health care delivery settings.

How is the chi-square used in an actual research study? Kalafat and Elias (1992) were interested in determining male and female adolescents' knowledge of and experience with suicidal peers. The adolescents responded to questions with a yes or no answer (nominal level). Table 16-16 represents their results. Kalafat and Elias were able to determine that there was a significant difference in the percent of males versus females (higher number of females) who knew someone who had attempted suicide, who had talked to someone who might have considered suicide, and who had talked to someone who was definitely considering suicide.

The appropriate use of the chi-square statistic depends on meeting several requirements. All observations must be independent; therefore the data from a pretest and a posttest given to the same subjects cannot be analyzed by means of the chi-square test for independence. However, McNemar's (1969) test for matched samples would work, given that the observations are independent and the expected frequency in any cell is not 0. In addition, expected frequencies of less than 1 may not occur in more than 20% of cells at any time.

USING DATA FROM REPEATED MEASURES OF AN INDEPENDENT SAMPLE TO MAKE INFERENCES ABOUT TWO OR MORE TREATMENTS

Repeated Measures t-Test

Let us test the following hypothesis using the dependent t-test: Guided imagery affects test scores of nursing students. A nondirectional hypothesis was used because there is little information available

Table 16-16
Male and Female Adolescents' Knowledge of and Experience with Suicidal Peers

	Percent Responding Yes			
Variable	**Females**	**Males**	**Total**	χ^2
Know someone who has attempted suicide	66.87	41.45	54.10	19.529**
Know someone who has committed suicide	15.38	10.56	12.87	1.407
Talked to someone who might have considered suicide	63.69	40.63	52.05	16.897**
Talked to someone who is definitely considering suicide	38.85	22.30	30.60	9.979*

From Kalafat, J., & Elias, M. (1992). Adolescents' experience with and response to suicidal peers. *Journal of Suicide and Life-Threatening Behavior, 22* (3), 315-320.
*$p < .01$.
**$p < .005$.

about the possible effects of guided imagery on test scores. A sample of 16 students were given a pretest, practiced guided imagery for 3 weeks, and then took a posttest. Table 16-17 shows the pretest and posttest scores of the students.

The formula for the dependent t-test is:

$$t = \frac{\overline{X}_1 - \overline{X}_2}{\sqrt{\dfrac{s_{12} + s_{22} - 2r(s_1)(s_2)}{N}}}$$

Where $\overline{X}_1$, and $\overline{X}_2$ are the respective groups, means s_{12} and s_{22} are the group variances

s_1 and s_2 are the group standard deviations

r is the correlation between the two groups of data

N is the sample size (number of pairs of scores)

The df for the dependent t-test is n − 1 (the same people are in both group) so df = 14. We will use α = .05 and a two-tailed

test because we are unsure of how guided imagery might affect the test scores. According to Appendix B, the critical value is 2.145. Our calculated value of 5.38 ≥ 2.145 so we can reject H_0. Therefore the guided imagery did have an effect on test scores.

Refer back to our previous discussion of Algase's study on wanderers versus non-wanderers. If Algase (1992) had been interested in testing whether there is an improvement in wandering following an intensive, daily, one-on-one intervention with a particular caregiver, she would have done a preintervention and postintervention test and used a dependent (related) t-test instead of the independent t-test.

Wilcoxin Matched-Pairs Test
Wilcoxin matched-pairs signed-rank test is a nonparametric alternative to the t-test for two related samples. In this simple test positive and negative signs are assigned to the differences between a pair of scores, depending on whether the X or Y variable is larger. The difference between the scores is obtained and the absolute difference is

Table 16-17
Pretest and Posttest Scores

Student	Pretest X_1	$X_1{}^2$	Posttest X_2	$X_2{}^2$	$X_1 X_2$
1	26	676	20	400	520
2	28	784	21	441	588
3	26	676	20	400	520
4	19	361	20	400	380
5	17	289	12	144	204
6	29	841	24	576	696
7	25	625	27	729	675
8	21	441	15	225	315
9	24	576	20	400	480
10	28	784	29	841	812
11	25	625	20	400	500
12	26	676	26	676	676
13	18	324	15	225	270
14	25	625	25	625	625
15	24	576	22	484	528
Σ	361	8879	316	6966	7789

$$\overline{X}_1 = 24.06 \qquad \overline{X}_2 = 21.06$$

$$\Sigma x_{12}{}^2 = 8879 - \frac{(361)^2}{15} = 191$$

$$\Sigma x_{22}{}^2 = 6966 - \frac{(316)^2}{15} = 309$$

$$\Sigma x_1 x_2 = 7789 - \frac{(361)(316)}{15} = 184$$

$$s_1{}^2 = \frac{191}{15} = 12.7 \qquad s_2{}^2 = \frac{309}{15} = 20.6$$

$$s_1 = 3.56 \qquad s_2 = 4.54$$

$$r = \frac{184}{(191)(309)} = .76$$

So:

$$t = \frac{24.06 - 21.06}{\sqrt{\dfrac{12.7 + 20.6 - (2)(.76)(3.56)(4.54)}{15}}}$$

$$= \frac{3}{\sqrt{\dfrac{32.6 - 24.56}{15}}} = \frac{3}{0.56} = 5.38$$

ranked. The Wilcoxin matched-pairs test is used to test the hypothesis that plus and minus signs are randomly assigned. All rank tests use ordinal data or higher-level data that have been transformed from a numerical scale to rank data. The following example demonstrates how the Wilcoxin matched-pairs test can be calculated. A researcher wants to know whether a class on human sexuality affects nurses' attitudes toward sexual assessment (Table 16-18).

Table 16-18
Wilcoxin Matched-Pairs Signed-Rank Test

Matched Pairs	Experimental	Control	d	Rank
1	47	40	7	9
2	43	48	5	5
3	36	42	−6	−7*
4	38	25	13	12
5	30	29	1	1
6	22	26	−4	−4
7	25	16	9	11
8	21	18	3	3
9	14	8	6	7
10	12	4	8	10
11	5	7	−2	−2
12	9	3	6	7

*Carry over any sign from d whether positive or negative.
  Sum all − ranks: −4 + −7 + −2 = −13.
  Sum all + ranks: 9 + 5 + 12 + 1 + 11 + 3 + 7 + 10 + 7 = 65.
  If any pair has a d score of 0, it should be dropped from the computation.
  Value = 13. Always use the smallest number without regard to sign as your value (similar to Mann-Whitney U). Reject H_0 if the calculated value is ≤ the table value. The test is always two-tailed.
  Table value = 14. Thus there is a significant difference between the experimental and control groups. In other words, a class on human sexuality affects nurses' attitudes toward performing a sexual assessment.
  If there is a larger number of positive scores, the experimental group did better than the control group. So in this instance the group that had a class on human sexuality did better than the group that did not have the class.
  If there is a larger number of negative scores, then the control group did better than the experimental group.

The investigator used experimental and control groups to answer the question.

Analysis of Variance with Repeated Measures
In the repeated measures ANOVA the same subjects are measured again using three or more observations. This test is similar to the dependent or repeated measures t-test where subjects are taking pretests and posttests. The repeated measures ANOVA can also be used with three or more matched groups. Matched groups are hand-picked by the investigator in an attempt to pick individuals who closely resemble one another based on the characteristics to be measured.

BIVARIATE STATISTICAL METHODS
Sometimes a researcher is concerned about the extent of one variable's association with another variable. Many studies have indicated that there is an association between smoking and lung cancer. Other studies indicate that there is an association between repressed hostility and certain chronic illnesses. There are several ways to test for association; we will discuss the chi-square test and correlation coefficients.

Pearson Correlation
As you recall, correlation is measured from -1 to $+1$; the closer to 1, the more perfect the correlation between two variables. The Pearson Product-Moment correlation coefficient is the most popular and the most widely used of all the correlation coefficients. It is obtained by determining the mean of the z-score products of two paired variables.

The Pearson correlation will be larger for heterogeneous groups than for homogeneous groups, so it is important for the sample to be well described in any research study where the Pearson is used. The Pearson is based on the assumption that the relationship between the two variables is linear. To determine whether a relationship is linear it is important to first construct a scatterplot. If the scatterplot indicates a nonlinear relationship between the variables, it will invalidate the use of the Pearson correlation. The Pearson also relies on the two variables having a similar distribution, so it is important to first consider shape, location, and spread through descriptive statistics.

The Pearson correlation yields a correlation coefficient r. Once again, the investigator uses a table to determine if the obtained r value is equal to or greater than the table value at a specified level of significance. The Pearson also yields r^2, the coefficient of determination, which is used to explain what percentage of the variability in one variable is responsible for variability in the other variable. r^2 like r has a range of 0 to $+1$, or from 0% to 100%. If r equals 0.82, then r^2 would equal 0.67, which would mean that variable X explains 67% of the variance in variable Y. It is important to understand that just because one variable "explains" a variation in the other, it does not specify a cause-and-effect relationship.

For example, suppose that a gerontologic nurse, Katy, decided to compare the weather with the number of falls at her nursing home. Surprisingly, Katy discovers that the number of falls and rainy days were positively correlated and significant at the .05 level. Did the rainy weather cause the falls? Or did the falls cause the rainy weather? Although most people would not believe that the weather changed because a number of elderly patients were falling, they might consider that perhaps the floor was wet from visitors and therefore more patients fell. Either way, it is difficult to imply causation with this example even though the two variables were correlated. It is better to assume that high correlation does not demonstrate a cause-and-effect relationship until proven otherwise.

Cohen (1991) studied self-care actions taken by older adults for influenza and colds. Using the Pearson r, she was able to show that there was a positive correlation between cold duration and the number of self-care actions taken by the adults ($r = .28$, $p = .0004$). She also discovered that the number of cold self-care actions was significantly associated with the age of the subjects ($r = -.17$, $p = .03$). Note that whenever a statistical value is stated, the significance level (either p or alpha) is reported as well.

The calculation of r is not really that difficult, although the formula is rather long.

$$r = \frac{N \Sigma XY - (\Sigma X)(\Sigma Y)}{\sqrt{[N \Sigma N^2 - (\Sigma X)][N \Sigma Y^2 - (\Sigma Y)]}}$$

Spearman's Rho Rank Correlation Coefficient
Spearman's rho is the nonparametric equivalent of the Pearson product-moment coefficient of correlation and can be used when one or both variables are measured at the ordinal level. The Spearman correlation coefficient is calculated in the same manner as the Pearson correlation coefficient except that the ranks of individuals are substituted for individual scores. The Spearman correlation coefficient is much easier to calculate than the Pearson coefficient and is sometimes used to approximate the Pearson. As with the Wilcoxin matched-pairs signed-rank test, the Spearman relies on the assumption that no two people will have the same rank, so if a number of tie scores occur, its use may be questioned. An example of correlation using both the Pearson r and the Spearman rho can be found in Figure 16-18. The example is provided to show how similar the two tests are in their calculations and in their results. It is clear that the Spearman rho is not as powerful a

test as the Pearson r because the calculated r value of the Spearman rho is higher (less sensitive) than the r value of the Pearson (more sensitive).

In this example the Pearson r is computed with an attitude score (ratio level), and the Spearman rho is calculated with ranks (ordinal).

Sisney (1993) used the Pearson r and the Spearman rho to determine whether there was a relationship between social support and depression in recovering chemically dependent nurses. One of her hypotheses was that this would be an inverse relationship. Using the Pearson r ($r = -.643$, $p = .001$) and the Spearman Rho (rho $= -.4699$, $p = .000$), she was able to show that a significant inverse relationship did exist between the two variables. In applying the results of both the Pearson and the Spearman rho, it is once again possible to see that the Pearson is a more powerful test than the Spearman rho.

Linear Regression
Do you recall the scatter plot that we developed before we did inferential testing to determine whether the variables were normally distributed? We also considered whether the lines that the points made on the graph were linear or nonlinear. This method for determining existence of a linear relationship is not particularly accurate, especially if there are a large number of scores to plot. We can make a better prediction of a linear relationship using the formula for a straight line or the formula for linear regression.

Correlation helps determine the degree of linear relationship between two variables that are related to each other in a linear fashion, as we saw earlier by looking at the relationship between variables on a scatter plot. Each variable was diagrammed on a different axis, and points were made where an intersection of the two variables oc-

Subject	Attitude score 1	X	Attitude score 2	Y	Rank 1	XY	Rank 2	d	d²
1	34	1156	28	784	1	952	6	−5	25
2	33	1089	40	1600	2.5	1320	1.5	1	1
3	33	1089	40	1600	2.5	1320	1.5	1	1
4	28	784	31	961	4	868	4	0	0
5	25	625	29	841	5.5	725	5	.5	.25
6	25	625	36	1296	5.5	900	3	2.5	2.25
7	24	576	27	729	7	648	7	0	0
8	22	484	23	529	8	506	9	−1	1
9	21	441	22	484	9	462	10	−1	1
10	20	400	21	441	10	420	11	−1	1
11	19	361	26	676	11	494	8	3	9
12	15	225	19	361	12	285	12	0	0
	299	7855	352	10302		8900		0	45.5

To calculate Spearman Rho

$$\text{rho} = \frac{1 - 6\Sigma d^2}{n^3 - n} = \frac{1 - 6(45.5)}{12^3 - 12} \quad \frac{1 - 273}{1716} \quad \text{rho} = .841$$

To calculate Pearson r

$$r = \frac{12(8900) - 299(342)}{\sqrt{[12(7855) - 299]\,[12(10302) - 352]}}$$

$$r = \frac{4542}{\sqrt{4859\,(6680)}} = \frac{4542}{\sqrt{32360940}} = \frac{4542}{5688.66} = r = .7985$$

If we used a significance level of .05, the table value would be 0.5324. In this example, both the results of the Spearman Rho and Pearson r would be significant. However, let us suppose the tabled value was 0.8143., the Spearman Rho would be significant, but not the Pearson r, which illustrates the sensitivity (and lower power) of the Spearman Rho.

Figure 16-18. Example of Spearman and Pearson correlation.

curred. Linear regression allows us to develop an equation with one variable as a linear function of the other. In other words, it can help us make predictions about one variable based on another. We already know how to determine how much of one variable can be explained by the variation in another variable through the coefficient of determination (r^2). If we know the value of one variable, we should be able to predict a value for the other variable with greater accuracy.

The first step in linear regression is calculating the slope-intercept with the formula $Y' = a + bX$. In this formula Y' is the dependent variable, and X is multiplied by a constant (b) and added to another constant (a). These concepts are not new, and a number of formulas rely on the same type of constants. Recalling the conversion from Celsius to Fahrenheit temperature (F = 32 + 1.8C), pretend that F is the dependent variable and Y the independent variable. The value of F depends on the value of C in this equation and can easily be calculated (Johnson, 1989). Let us use six arbitrarily chosen temperatures to demonstrate the equation (Table 16-19). An important concept in linear regression is the slope of the line. The next step in linear regression is to plot the six pairs of variables on a scattergram and draw the line of best fit. Slope occurs as a result of plotting the pairs of variables. In this example, if we moved up one

Table 16-19
Celsius and Corresponding Fahrenheit Temperatures

Celsius	Formula	Fahrenheit
0	32 + 1.8(0)	32
15	32 + 1.8(15)	59
35	32 + 1.8(35)	95
55	32 + 1.8(55)	131
70	32 + 1.8(70)	158
90	32 + 1.8(90)	194

degree in Celsius temperature, we would have to move across 1.8 degrees in Fahrenheit temperature. This would give a step-like progression up each degree and then over. This rise from one variable to another (slope) can be calculated using the formula

$$b = \frac{\Sigma xy}{\Sigma x^2}$$

The slope of the line from Celsius to Fahrenheit temperature is 1.8. Since other variables could also be related on a line that has a slope of 1.8, more information is needed.

The intercept is the point at which the *value* of the dependent variable intersects the axis that *represents* the dependent variable. In Figure 16-19 what is the intercept? The dependent variable line intersects the dependent axis at 32. The intercept is a constant and is represented by *a* in the equation Y = a + bX. The slope in this

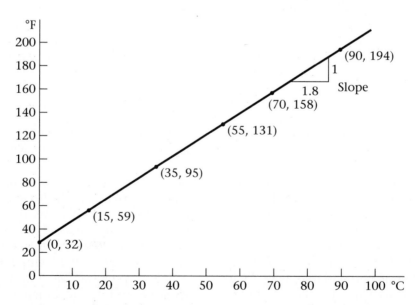

Figure 16-19. Scatter diagram and line of best fit for temperature.

equation is b. The scatter plot in Figure 16-19 represents the correlation between Celsius and Fahrenheit temperatures and shows a 1+ positive correlation. The scatter plot shows us the line of regression caused by the plotting of the dependent and independent variables. Unfortunately, in most instances the variables do not have a perfect linear correlation, so it is also important to calculate the least-squares criterion.

If X and Y do not have a perfect relationship (±1), then the scatter plot will not show a perfectly straight line; some points will not fall on the line (refer to our discussion of the scatter plot for a pictorial demonstration). In this case we could predict the values of Y from the values of X. These predicted values are denoted by Y' (or Y prime) and may or may not be equal to the actual values of Y. The difference between the actual score of Y and Y' is called e (error) and is equal to Y − Y'.

Consider an example of linear regression where we attempt to predict a score on the Y variable from a known score on the X variable (Table 16-20). Suppose that we have six sets of scores from students who took both microbiology and pathophysiology. We are interested in developing a way to predict how other students will do in pathophysiology based on these other six students. Somehow we have to determine what a and b will be in our regression equation. To do this we must first calculate the regression coefficient (b) as follows.

$$b = \frac{\Sigma xy}{\Sigma x^2} \qquad a = Y - bX$$

In this formula: a is the intercept constant; Y is the mean of variable Y; X is the mean of variable X; x represents the deviation scores from X; and y represents the deviation scores from Y; and b is the slope constant. As shown in Figure 16-20, the data may be used to develop a scattergram and line of best fit.

How correct are we in our prediction?

Table 16-20
Example of Simple Linear Regression

X	Y	x	x²	y	y²	xy	Y'	e	e²
2	4	−2	4	−4	16	8	3.2	.8	.64
6	7	2	4	1	1	2	8.8	−1.8	3.24
1	5	−4	16	−1	1	4	1.8	−.8	.64
3	3	−1	1	−3	9	3	4.6	−1.6	2.56
5	8	1	1	2	4	2	7.4	−2.4	5.76
7	9	3	9	3	9	9	10.2	−3.2	10.24

mean	mean								
X = 4	Y = 6		Σx² = 20		Σy² = 40		Σxy = 28		Σe² = 23.08

$$b = \frac{28}{20} = 1.4 \qquad \Sigma e = 10.24$$

$$a = 6 - 1.4\,(4) = .4$$

$$Y' = a + bX \qquad Y' = .4 + 1.4(X)$$

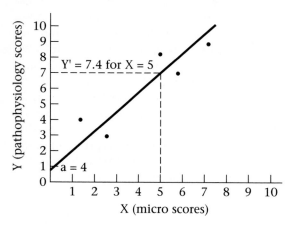

Figure 16-20. Scattergram and line of best fit for the data shown in Table 16-20.

Once we predict a score, the difference between the actual score and the score we predicted is called the error of estimate. This discrepancy between the known scores Y and predicted scores Y' can be seen in Table 16-20 under column *e* (error).

Let us calculate the standard error of the estimate (SEe) for these scores.

$$\text{SEe} = \frac{\Sigma e^2 =}{\Sigma y^2 =} \frac{23.08}{40} = .577$$

In this example 57% of the proportion of the total sum of squares for Y is accounted for by error.

How does one use this information? Suppose we only had scores on the microbiology test and we wanted to predict scores on the pathophysiology test. If someone scored a 2 on the microbiology test, then Y' = .4 + 1.4(2), or 3.2. In Table 16-20 we predicted Y' from each of the X scores (ignore the Y, Y', and xy columns), and we also looked at the error (*e*) or residuals. In this way we could determine the SEe or the standard error of the estimates to see how much error we might have made in our prediction of the pathophysiology test scores.

USING COMPUTERS IN DATA ANALYSIS

Most quantitative research studies use both descriptive statistics and one or more inferential statistical tests. With large samples, calculating these tests by hand can be very time consuming and frustrating even with a calculator. The number of mistakes possible when calculating tests by hand can be significantly decreased by using computers. Most researchers today rely on computers to assist with data analysis.

Figure 16-21 gives examples of the computer printouts for a frequency distribution and Pearson correlation. Figure 16-22 shows a computer printout from a crosstabulation table.

To use a computer for data analysis, data must first be coded on a coding sheet and then entered (loaded) onto a data file. While it is possible to make errors when coding data, more errors are typically made when calculating tests by hand. Figure 16-23 shows an example of a coding sheet and Figure 16-24 a computer data file. Once a data file is loaded, a program needs to be written to apply the correct statistical analysis. Table 16-21 shows a command file for a one-way ANOVA. Following this analysis the computer printout has to be reviewed and results interpreted. Computer printouts may appear overwhelming to the novice researcher; however, they are quite easy to interpret once they are understood. Individuals who are already computer literate may find using computers for data analysis simply a matter of translating computer literacy to a different form. Those who dread learning computer skills may need to overcome a number of obstacles before they feel confident in their computer ability.

Computer literacy and familiarity, as well as time, energy, and money, may affect whether one uses a computer for data

FILE:

SCORE

VALUE LABEL	VALUE	FREQUENCY	PERCENT	VALID PERCENT	CUM PERCENT
	3	1	10.0	10.0	10.0
	4	1	10.0	10.0	20.0
	5	3	30.0	30.0	50.0
	6	1	10.0	10.0	60.0
	7	1	10.0	10.0	70.0
	8	2	20.0	20.0	90.0
	9	1	10.0	10.0	100.0
	TOTAL	10	100.0	100.0	

MEAN	6.000	STD ERR	.615	**B** MEDIAN	5.500
MODE	5.000	STD DEV	1.944	VARIANCE	3.778
KURTOSIS	−1.067	S E KURT	1.942	SKEWNESS	.113
S E SKEW	.687	RANGE	6.000	MINIMUM	3.000
MAXIMUM	9.000	SUM	60.000		

VALID CASES   10   MISSING CASES   0

--- P E A R S O N   C O R R E L A T I O N

NLN

LEAGUE   0.8667
         (16)
         P = .000

Figure 16-21. Sample computer printouts.

analysis. One major decision factor is the complexity of the analysis, and another is the size of the sample. If a sample size is larger than 100, chances are a computer is the best option. For samples less than 100, a calculator may actually be cheaper and easier than a computer, depending on the complexity of the analysis.

CONSULTING A STATISTICIAN

Whether you are a novice or an experienced researcher, it sometimes helps to consult a statistician who can help guide the data analysis. This requires that you contact a statistician early on in the planning and design of the data analysis. Often the statistician can code and load the data, as well as provide insight into the important aspects of interpretation. Cultivating a relationship with a good statistician can certainly be helpful throughout the research process. How much you decide to rely on a statistician may depend on how familiar and comfortable you are with de-

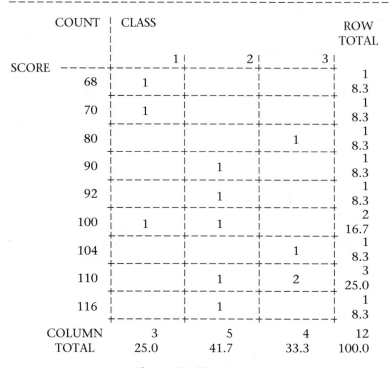

Figure 16-22. Computer printout of cross-tabulation table.

scriptive and inferential data analysis. In some ways developing a relationship with a statistician is rather like developing a relationship with a financial planner. Some people decide to turn over all of their decision-making power to someone else to do all of the work, checking their progress now and then. Others prefer to do their own financial management, but rely on a financial planner to give advice and keep an eye on the overall investment strategy. Still others feel comfortable without any advice, confident in their knowledge level and in their ability to make independent decisions.

Most universities have a statistician available for consultation. It is important to remember that statisticians may be more familiar with certain disciplines than others. If you are lucky enough to be able to locate a nurse who is also a statistician, you will probably receive the best possible advice. Since there are relatively few nurse statisticians, most nurses rely on statisticians from psychology, math, or business to assist with data analysis. If possible, try to find someone who is also familiar with computer data entry and analysis.

Statisticians usually charge an hourly fee for their services. Hourly fees vary depending on the area of the country and the level of expertise, but expect to pay at least $20 per hour or more for statistical advice. Graduate students are normally provided

FORTRAN CODING FORM

PROGRAM: SPSSX / AIDS DATA
PROGRAMMER: G. Twiname DATE: 5/19/94

| COMM | STATEMENT NUMBER | CONT | FORTRAN |

| 1 | 2 3 4 5 | 6 | 7 8 9 10 11 12 13 14 15 16 17 18 19 20 21 22 23 24 25 26 27 28 29 30 31 32 33 34 35 36 37 38 39 40 |

```
1 2 4 3 2 1 4 3 2 4 3 2 2 0 0 1 0 2 0 3 0 5 0 3 0 4 0 8 8 2 1 2 4 3 3 2 1 2 2
2 1 3 2 1 4 3 2 2 4 3 2 0 1 1 2 1 2 0 3 0 4 3 2 1 0 3 6 2 4 2 1 2 3 3 2 2 1 0
3 1 3 3 3 3 2 0 2 0 0 2 2 1 1 1 1 1 1 4 3 3 2 2 2 0 1 1 2 2 4 3 2 1 1 0 1 1 2
2 2 1 1 3 4 3 2 3 3 4 4 2 2 1 3 3 7 3 4 2 3 4 5 3 2 1 2 2 3 2 3 2 1 2 2 4 3 2
2 2 4 3 3 4 3 3 2 1 2 2 4 3 2 1 0 0 1 2 2 4 3 3 5 2 4 3 2 4 4 2 2 1 1 0 0 0 0
3 2 1 0 1 1 4 1 3 2 2 1 0 0 1 0 0 2 0 0 3 0 0 1 0 0 2 0 0 4 0 0 3 0 0 2 1 1 2
2 2 2 1 1 4 0 1 3 4 3 2 1 0 0 2 3 3 2 3 3 1 3 3 2 3 3 4 3 3 2 1 2 0 2 2 1 2 2
1 1 1 1 1 4 3 2 1 2 2 1 2 2 2 4 4 3 2 1 1 0 2 2 3 0 0 1 0 0 2 1 0 0 3 2 3 0 4
2 3 2 2 1 2 3 2 4 3 0 1 0 0 3 2 3 3 2 4 2 2 1 1 0 4 0 0 3 0 4 0 4 0 3 0 4 2 2
0 0 1 2 3 4 3 0 0 2 4 5 0 3 2 4 3 4 3 3 0 0 0 3 2 0 0 2 0 0 2 2 4 4 4 4 4 3 2
3 2 0 4 0 2 1 1 1 1 0 0 1 0 1 3 3 0 2 2 2 2 1 0 2 2 3 3 3 3 1 1 1 3 4 3 2 2 1
1 2 2 4 0 3 0 0 2 0 2 1 2 2 3 2 2 1 0 0 1 0 0 2 2 3 2 1 0 0 4 4 3 4 3 2 2 1 0
1 3 3 5 4 4 3 2 1 2 2 3 3 3 4 0 0 1 3 4 2 4 3 3 2 1 0 0 0 1 1 4 4 3 2 1 2 1 4
3 3 2 4 0 2 0 2 1 0 4 3 2 2 1 4 3 2 2 1 1 2 1 2 1 4 3 4 3 2 4 3 3 2 2 2 2 1 0
2 2 3 3 0 0 0 0 0 0 1 2 3 3 3 2 2 2 2 2 1 0 1 0 1 2 2 1 2 1 0 2 0 3 0 4 3 3 3
1 0 1 0 1 0 2 0 3 0 2 3 2 3 2 2 1 1 0 1 1 4 4 4 3 1 0 0 1 0 3 2 3 3 4 0 4 0 3
1 3 3 2 4 1 4 3 3 2 1 4 1 4 3 1 2 3 3 2 2 5 2 6 2 1 2 2 3 0 3 4 3 3 4 2 4 4 3
4 1 1 2 4 1 3 2 2 0 3 4 1 4 4 2 4 3 2 4 2 3 2 1 0 2 0 3 3 3 2 1 0 2 2 4 3 3 2
3 2 2 4 1 1 4 5 4 3 4 3 3 2 3 2 3 2 3 2 3 3 2 2 4 2 1 0 2 2 4 3 3 4 3 2 2 1 0
4 4 2 2 3 2 3 3 3 3 4 2 1 2 2 1 1 0 0 0 1 3 0 2 1 0 1 0 2 3 2 1 0 0 3 2 1 0 4 0
2 1 2 2 3 2 1 1 0 2 1 0 0 0 1 1 4 3 0 0 0 0 4 0 3 2 2 2 2 4 2 1 4 3 3 2 1 1 0
2 2 0 0 2 2 1 1 1 1 2 2 1 0 2 1 2 3 3 2 0 0 0 1 0 4 3 2 2 3 1 0 2 0 0 3 0 0 4
0 0 2 2 1 3 2 2 2 1 3 3 2 1 0 2 2 1 2 2 2 1 2 2 0 2 1 2 2 4 4 3 2 2 1 0 2 2 3
2 2 1 0 0 2 1 0 0 2 0 1 3 3 4 2 3 3 2 4 2 4 3 4 3 3 2 2 2 0 2 3 3 4 3 2 1 2 2
```

| 1 | 2 3 4 5 | 6 | 7 8 9 10 11 12 13 14 15 16 17 18 19 20 21 22 23 24 25 26 27 28 29 30 31 32 33 34 35 36 37 38 39 40 |

Figure 16-23. Sample data coding sheet.

```
AAABAABABCBCAABBBBBAAABBAACCCEBDAEAABBBBAAAABA
BABBAAADBCBAAABCAABAABBCAAABADCAABAABBBBBABEBA
EBEDCABDBCBCBABBAABAAABBAABBBCBCACBBBBBBADEBA
CABBAAAEBDBAAABBBBBAACBBABBBCDCBACAABBBBAAAABA
ABABAAABBCBAAABBAABAACBBACCBCBDBADAABBBBBBCEBA
BABBAABEECBCAABCBBBAABBBABACBDDCAEAABBBAAAABA
ABBBAAAAECBAAABBAABAACBBAABACDEDAEAABBBBCCCEBA
CBCBBBBDDCBAAABBBBBAAABBAAABAECBABAABBBBCBBEBA
AAABAAAEBCBAAABBABBAAABBABBABDECADBBBBBBBBBEBA
BBCBAABAEDBAAABBBBBAACBBAAABAEAAADAABBBBAAAABA
ABAEAAADBCBAAABBBBBAABBBAACAECDDADAABBBBBBBEBA
DBDBCCAADDBAAABBBBBAACBBAAABBEDDBCAABBBBECCECA
ABBBAAAACDBAAABBBBBAABBBAAAAAACCDABBBBBBCBBBBA
BBBBAAAADCBACABBBCBAACBBAADACDDCADAABBBBDBCECA
EBECBBBEECBAAABBAABAAABBAAAAAAEEAAEAABBBBCBEEBA
EACABAABECBAAABCBBBAACBCDEDADAABBBBBBBBBAAEBA
CADBAABCDCBAAABBBBBAACBBAAABACDCAEAABBBCBCEBA
BBBBABADDCBAAABBBBBAAABBAAABAEDDAEAABBBBCACEBA
ABABAAAAECBBBABACBCAACBCAABBAECBCABBBBBAAAABA
CBDBAABABDBAAABAAABAAABCABEEEEBDAEBBBBBBCBEBBA
DBCBAAAACBAAABBBBBAACBBAAAAAAEEBAEAABBBBBBBEBA
DBCBAABCBCBABABCABBAACBBABABAECBADAABBBBCACEBA
ABBBAAACCCBAAABBABBAABBBABDAEBAAADBBBBBCBCBBA
EBCBAAADBCBAAABBBBBAABBBBAAADCDCAACAABBBAAAABA
BBBBAABACCBABABBBBBAAABBBABBBCDBAABAABBBBABEBA
CABBAAAAAABAAABACBAABBBCAAABBDDBAEAABBBBBABEBA
CBCBAABBBCBAAABBBBBAABBBBAABCBEDBAEBBBBBBECBBBA
ABBBAAAEBCBAAABBBBBAAABBAABBBCCBABAABBBBCBBBBA
AAABAAAADCBAAABBABBAABBBAAAABEECAEAABBBBCCBBBA
ABABAAAABBBABABBBBBAABBBBAAEBEECBACAABBBBBBEBBA
AABBAAADCCBAAABBBBBAACBBABCDCDCDAAAABBBDCDEBA
ABABABBDCCBCBABBCBBAACBBAABABDCECDBBBBBBCCCBBA
CBCBAACABCBAAABBBBBAAABBBACBCBEECABBBBBBCCDEBA
BABBAAAACBCCABCBBBAABBBAAAAAEBBACBBBBBBAAAABA
BBBBAABABCBAAABBBBBAACBBBAABADDAAAEBBBBBBECDBBA
BABBAAADDCBACABBBBBAACDDAAAAAEDBADAABBBBAAAABA
AAABAAAEECBAAABBACCAABBCABBBBDCBAEBBBBBBAAAABA
DBCBAAACBABAAABBBBBAABBBBABAABCCAADAABBBBCCDEBA
BBBBAABAECBAAABBBBBAACBBACBBAECAAEBBBBBBCBCEBA
AAABAAACDCBAAABAAAAACCBACABAECDAEAABBBBCCCECA
DACBAAAABCBAAABBBBBAAABBABCCDCCCAEAABBBBBABEBA
DACBBABDDCAAAABBBBBAACCBAAABAEDEBDAABBBBDCCEAA
EBDBAABDBCBAAABBAABAAABAAAEAEAAAAEAABBBBAAAABA
CBBAAACACCBACABBBBCAACBBAACABCBAAEAABBBAAAABA
BADBCABAABAAAABBBBBAABBBAABABDDAACAABBBBCBEBCA
ABABAABABABBBABAABBABAABBAACCACBBBBBBBBABEBA
BBBBAAABBCBAAABCBBBAAABBBABBBBCDAACAABBBBAAAABA
CADBBABABCAAAABBBBBAABBBAAAAAAECAACAABBBBECEEBA
AABBAAACBCBCAABBBBBBACCBBAAACBDCBACBBBBBAAAABA
AAABAACECCBBBCBCBBBAACCBAEABADCAAEAABBBBBBCEBA
```

Figure 16-24. Sample computer data file.

the use of a statistician as part of their student fees, and most universities subscribe to a number of statistical software packages.

Software packages usually available on a university mainframe computer include SPSS or the Statistical Package for Social Sciences, BMDP or Biomedical Data Package, and SAS or Statistical Analysis System. There are also a number of statistical soft-

Table 16-21

BMDP Computer Command File for One-Way ANOVA

/PROBLEM	TITLE IS 'ONE WAY ANOVA'.
/INPUT	VARIABLES ARE 2.
	FORMAT IS '(F1.0,F2.0)'.
	FILE IS 'COMP.3DAT'.
/VARIABLE	NAMES ARE GROUP, INTERACT.
	GROUPING IS GROUP.
/GROUP	CODES (1) ARE 1,2,3,4.
	NAMES (1) ARE, A,B,C,D.
/DESIGN	DEPENDENT IS INTERACT.
/END	

(This is a sample command file used with BMDP statistical software for a one-way ANOVA.)

ware packages available for use with personal computers (PCs). Some of the more popular PC statistical software packages include Abstat by Anderson-Bell Corp., A-Stat by Rosen Grandon Associates Inc., BMDP-PC by BMDP Statistical Software Inc., Number Cruncher Statistical Systems, and SPSS-PC by SPSS Inc. PC software packages range in price form $100 to $1500. Some university departments have PC packages available for use on PC computers. Purchasing a software package is probably not necessary unless you plan to do research on a continuing basis. Otherwise, you should be able to find a good statistician and all the computer resources you need on a college campus. The use of computers for data analysis is discussed in detail in Chapter 26.

☙ EVALUATING THE DATA ANALYSIS

Critiquing the data analysis section of research reports is extremely important. Some students (and other nurses) prefer to avoid the statistical portion of an article and move on to the findings and discussion. Unfortunately, without understanding the data analysis, the reader is blindly accepting that all research is done perfectly. Remember that financial planner? Just as an intelligent investor would not blindly accept that a financial planner is handling his or her money in the best way possible without ever checking to see if this were true, it is important to check on how the research is conducted and how it is reported. Factors to consider when critiquing data analysis are summarized in the box.

Critiquing a statistical analysis begins with the hypothesis. The hypothesis indicates what type of statistics need to be used. Descriptive statistics will be used to summarize data and should be presented for each variable stated in the hypothesis. Research studies that are exploratory in nature may *only* use descriptive statistics, and other studies may use descriptive statistics to test certain hypotheses. Correlation will be used if an investigator is interested in whether a relationship will be found between two variables. Tests of differences between the means are used when the investigator is interested in whether there are differences between the groups under study.

The methods section of the report should include an indication of the levels of measurement used for each of the variables under study. If no levels of measurement are stated, it should be possible to determine them from either the hypothesis or operational definitions. The descriptive statistics should match the level of measurement for each variable. If the variable is at the nominal or ordinal level, then expect to see mode, median, or frequency distributions and nonparametric tests. If the variables are interval or ratio level, expect to see the mean, range, variance, and standard deviation, as well as parametric inferential tests. If a statistical test that is be-

EVALUATING THE DATA ANALYSIS

1. Are the statistical methods described clearly?
2. Does the researcher give enough information to determine if the correct statistics were used?
3. Are the statistics appropriate and applicable to the hypothesis?
4. What levels of measurement were chosen for the important variables under study?
5. How many groups were there?
6. Do the levels of measurement suggest use of nonparametric or parametric testing?
7. Is the significance level established prior to data collection and applied throughout the entire study?
8. Are all the underlying assumptions for inferential analysis met?
9. Are there any other threats to the validity of the statistical conclusions?
10. Are statistical results accurately calculated?
11. Does the author discuss how missing data are handled?
12. Was data clearly presented in the tables and do the tables match the text?
13. Was a power analysis performed? What was the result?
14. Are effect size (ES) values included, as well as values of the test statistics, degrees of freedom, and correlations?
15. Are the results of each hypothesis presented?
16. Are you able to understand the results?

yond the scope of this chapter was used, it may be necessary to consult a statistics textbook for additional information.

The size of the sample will also affect which tests can be used. Recall that as the sample size increases, it is less likely that any one extreme score will affect the descriptive statistics. Also recall that one of the assumptions for certain inferential tests is a sample size greater than 20.

The results section of the report should provide enough data to allow the reader to understand how each hypothesis was analyzed. The data analysis section should be presented at an understandable level; the reader should not need an advanced degree in statistics to understand it. If tables are used, they should be referred to in the body of the report and should be clearly labeled and identified. Most reports will include a table stating the descriptive analysis and another covering the inferential analy-

sis. Other tables may be added, depending on the complexity of the analysis. Tables should be used to enhance material presented in the text, not merely to repeat it. All tables should agree with data presented in the context of the paper and accurately represent what statistics were used and what statistical procedure was done. For example, if an author states that 15 people in a study weighed over 400 pounds, this same number should be reflected in any frequency distribution. If an author states a significance level of .05 was used, it should be applied consistently throughout all of the analysis.

Another important aspect of data analysis evaluation is power. Did the author use power analysis? If not, is there enough information to be able to do it yourself?

Remember, data analysis can only be viewed as an extension of the hypothesis, design, data collection, and sample. Just as the nursing process relies on the accuracy of the assessment, nursing diagnosis, and goals, so does the research process rely on the accuracy of its many components. Taking just a short-term goal from a nursing care plan for a patient without viewing the patient holistically provides little pertinent information. Similarly, taking one piece of data from a research study without looking at the entire study provides little pertinent information.

Another factor to remember is that data can be interpreted in many ways. Occasionally an investigator who has spent years on a research study is so intent on showing significant results that less than rigorous statistical analysis may be applied. For example, if you review a study in which ratio level measurement is used and all of the assumptions for parametric testing can be met, you would expect the investigator to use parametric testing. However, what if a nonparametric test was used? Were the results perhaps significant with nonparametric testing because the test was more lenient (less powerful)? It takes many hours and much effort to do research and sometimes nonsignificant results are viewed as failure. Remember: although changing data analysis to obtain the desired result is unethical, it is sometimes done. If nothing else, remember that data can lie!

SUMMARY

- Quantitative data analysis is a vital component of nursing research and can be divided into two main categories, *descriptive* and *inferential.*
- Descriptive statistics describe a distribution and can be further divided into *measures of central tendency* (the mean, median, and mode) and *measures of variability* (range, interquartile range, semi-quartile range, variance, and standard deviation).
- Graphs are often used to present information about frequency distributions. Some commonly used graphs are the *histogram, bar graph,* and *frequency polygon.*
- An understanding of the normal curve is essential to inferential statistics and includes an understanding of *symmetry, skewness,* and *standard scores.*
- Inferential statistics are used for two main reasons, *estimating parameters* and *testing hypotheses.*
- Estimating parameters can be accomplished through *point estimation* and through more accurate interval estimation.
- Confidence intervals can be used to establish a high level of probability that estimations are accurate.
- *Parametric tests* are the most powerful inferential tests and require variables to be at the interval level or above. *Nonparametric tests* can be used with lower-level data.
- Inferential tests have certain assumptions that must be met such as sample size and level of measurement. These assumptions may vary depending on the type of test used.
- *Hypothesis Testing* consists of seven steps:
  1. Check the assumptions associated with the statistical test to be sure they can be met.
  2. Establish the null (H_0) and alternate (H_a) hypotheses.
  3. Specify the test statistic.
  4. Specify a level of significance.
  5. Determine the decision rule.
  6. Compute the test statistic.
  7. Make a conclusion based on your calculations in comparison to table values.
- In drawing conclusions about a hypoth-

esis it is possible to make either a *type I or type II* error. A type I error can be controlled by establishing the level of significance and means that there is a predetermined risk of rejecting the null hypothesis when it should be accepted. A type II error occurs when the researcher accepts the null hypothesis when it should be rejected. The ability to make a correct decision is called the power of the test.

- *Power analysis* is an essential part of nursing research and can be conducted prior to or following data collection and analysis. The four parameters of power are *significance level, sample size, effect size (ES),* and *power*.

- Inferential tests that use data from an independent sample to make inferences about a single population include independent measures t-test, the chi-square test of independence, the Mann-Whitney U test, and the independent measures ANOVA (both single-factor and two-factor).

- Inferential tests that use data from repeated measurements of an independent sample to make inferences about two or more treatments include repeated measures t-test, the Wilcoxin matched-pairs signed-rank test, and the repeated measures one-factor ANOVA.

- Bivariate statistical methods include Spearman correlation, the Pearson correlation, and linear regression.

- The use of a statistician and a computer may be invaluable during data analysis. Although each of these can be very helpful, it is important to have an understanding of statistics to ensure that all aspects are carried out appropriately.

- The entire approach to data analysis must be viewed as an integral part of the research process. It must be systematically evaluated not only by the investi-

gator but by consumers of research as well.

FACILITATING CRITICAL THINKING

1. If 10 points were added to each score in a distribution, how would it change the following:
   a. Range
   b. Mean
   c. Median
   d. Mode
   e. Variance
   f. Standard deviation

2. Collect data from your classmates on a topic of your choice and develop a frequency distribution and graph of the data.

3. Given a score point located 1.42 standard deviations above the mean in a normal distribution, compute the following:
   a. The proportion of the area between the mean and the score.
   b. The proportion of the area to the left and right of the score.
   c. The percentile equivalent.

4. In a normally distributed set of raw scores with a mean of 60 and a standard deviation of 5, a raw score of 72 would convert to the following:
   a. A standard z score of _____
   b. A standard T score of _____
   c. A percentile of _____

5. A random sample of 75 patients were asked to rate the food in the hospital cafeteria on a scale of 1 to 30. The sample mean was 28, and the sum of squares (Σx^2) was 1024.
   a. Calculate s, the standard deviation statistic.
   b. Calculate the standard error of the mean (SEM).
   c. Determine the limits of a 95% confidence interval.

6. Describe a research study where each of the following statistical tests might be used.
   a. Independent t-test
   b. Repeated measures (dependent) t-test
   c. Chi-square test of independence
   d. Mann-Whitney U test
   e. Pearson product-moment correlation
7. An investigator is studying the relationship between hopelessness and job satisfaction. She administers a job satisfaction inventory and a hopelessness inventory to 100 nurses and compares the results. The mean score on the hopelessness inventory was 65.8, and the mean score on the job satisfaction inventory was 72. What statistical test would she use? What would the degrees of freedom be? What is the critical table value for a significance level of .05?
8. Using the power table for a one-tailed t-test with α = .05, determine what the power would be for a study with 24 subjects and decide whether you need to increase the power.
9. As investigator you obtain significant results in a study in which 60 patients taking allergy shots either cleanse the injection site with alcohol or do nothing to the site. Following a power analysis you discover that for a small effect size the power is .47. Would you recommend that your allergy patients use alcohol? If not, how could you increase the power when the study is replicated?

References

SUBSTANTIVE

ALGASE, D. L. (1992). Cognitive discriminants of wandering among nursing home residents. *Nursing Research, 41*(2), 78-81.

CONN, V. (1991). Self-care actions taken by older adults for influenza and colds. *Nursing Research, 40*(3), 176-181.

GARRISON, C., LIND, C., MANGUM, S., THACKERAY, R., & WYATT, M. (1991). Perceptions of nurses' uniforms. *Journal of Nursing Research, 23*(9), 127-130.

GAYNOR, E. G. (1990). The long haul: The effects of home care on caregivers. *IMAGE: Journal of Nursing Scholarship, 22*(4), 208-212.

KALAFAT, J., & ELIAS, M. (1992). Adolescents' experience with and response to suicidal peers. *Suicide and Life-Threatening Behavior, 22*(3), 315-320.

KALISCH, P. A., & KALISH, B. J. (1987). *The changing image of the nurse.* Menlo Park, CA: Addison-Wesley.

SISNEY, K. F. (1993). The relationship between social support and depression in recovering chemically dependent nurses. *IMAGE: Journal of Nursing Scholarship, 25*(2), 107-112.

SPRINGHOUSE CORPORATION. (1987). *The nurse and apparel.* Uniform Marketing Division, Springhouse, Pa: Author.

STEWART FAHS, P., & KINNEY, M. R. (1991). The thigh, abdomen, and arm as sites for subcutaneous sodium heparin injections. *Nursing Research, 40*(4), 204-207.

TWINAME, B. G. (1992). The relationship between HIV disease classification and depression and suicidal intent. Doctoral Dissertation, Ann Arbor MI: UMI.

CONCEPTUAL

BEST, J. W. (1981). *Research in education.* Englewood Cliffs, NJ: Prentice-Hall.

BRIGHTMAN, H. J. (1986). *Statistics in plain English.* Cincinnati: South-Western Publishing.

DAVIES, O. L. (1958). *Statistical methods in research and production.* New York: Hafner Publishing.

HAMBURG, M. (1987). *Statistical analysis for decision making* (4th ed.). San Diego, CA: Harcourt Brace.

JOHNSON, D. M. (1989). *Probability and statistics.* Cincinnati: South-Western Publishing.

LARSON, R. J. (1975). *Statistics for the allied health sciences.* Columbus, OH: Charles E. Merrill.

MARZILLIER, L. F. (1990). *Elementary statistics.* Dubuque, IA: Wm. C. Brown Publishers.

NOETHER, G. E. (1971). *Introduction to statistics* (2nd ed). Boston: Houghton-Mifflin.

PETRIE, A. (1978). *Lecture notes on medical statistics*. London: Blackwell Scientific Publications.

METHODOLOGICAL

KIMBLE, G. A. (1978). *How to use (and misuse) statistics*. Englewood Cliffs, NJ: Prentice-Hall.

POLIT, D. F., & SHERMAN, R. E. (1990). Statistical power in nursing research. *Nursing Research, 39*(6), 365-369.

ROSCOE, J. T. (1975). *Fundamental research statistics for the behavioral sciences* (2nd ed). New York: Holt, Rinehart & Winston.

HISTORICAL

COHEN, J. (1977). *Statistical power analysis for the behavioral sciences*. New York: Academic Press.

KILPATRICK, S. J. (1973). *Statistical principles in health care information*. Ann Arbor, MI: Ann Arbor Press.

MCNEMAR, Q. (1969). *Psychological statistics*. New York: Wiley.

CHAPTER 17

ADVANCED STATISTICAL METHODS

GAIL C. DAVIS • MICHAEL C. ROBINSON

To assume that heart disease is the result exclusively of cholesterol and that any other variables (e.g., genetic predisposition, smoking, obesity, hypertension, and sedentary life-style) are not important contributing factors would clearly be erroneous. Prevention programs or treatment based on such a claim would obviously be mistaken. Most clinical studies address such complex "real-world" situations that involve more than two variables, thus requiring the use of multivariate analysis procedures. These procedures are an outgrowth of attempts to compensate for the artificiality of many univariate or bivariate research designs.

Multivariate analysis techniques allow the researcher to investigate complex interactions between a number of contributing variables and to determine the relative significance of each variable's contribution. Within this perspective, multivariate analysis includes not only multiple numbers of variables but also multiple combinations of and interactions between those variables.

In its broadest terms, multivariate analysis may be viewed as a series of analytical procedures based on (1) the degree of dependence assumed between variables, (2) the number of variables assumed to be dependent, and (3) the way in which the variables are measured. Although all multivariate procedures are useful in conducting nursing research, an examination of reported nursing studies reveals that the multivariate techniques most often used are multiple regression, multivariate analysis of variance, and factor analysis. Because these are used most often, they will be described in detail. Other methods that might also be considered for addressing clinical, educational, and administrative research questions include multiple discriminant analysis, cluster analysis, canonical correlation analysis, multidimensional scaling analysis, logistic regression, and structural equation modeling. This last technique is growing in popularity. Before further examining these representative multivariate techniques, an understanding of some of the basic concepts is important.

CONCEPTS BASIC TO SELECTING AN ADVANCED STATISTICAL METHOD

Research data may be categorical (non-metric) or continuous (metric) in nature. Data that represent features or properties of a variable, identifying or classifying it along a descriptive dimension, are categorical. Examples of such data include gender, ethnicity, or the presence or absence of some characteristic. Continuous data are quantitative measurements that reflect the degree or quantity of some characteristic of the variable (e.g., age, weight, temperature, level of anxiety, or intensity of fatigue). Although continuous data are generally used in multivariate analysis, sometimes variables represented by categorical data are relevant to the study. Attention must be given, therefore, to selecting an analysis technique that is compatible with the data collected.

Multivariate statistics are generally used in an attempt to achieve one or more of the following goals: (1) describe and summarize the data collected during research, (2) establish the nature and degree of the relationships between different variables, and (3) determine a possible causal or predictive relationship between variables. To achieve this, it is necessary to distinguish between the cases and the variables in a data set. The *cases* are the individual stimuli that provide the data. These stimuli may be individual subjects, observations, items, events, or other discrete objects. *Variables* are those measurable characteristics that identify each case or distinguish one case from another; they may represent a condition, feature, attribute, or behavior that can be observed or controlled. In describing or summarizing the variables in a data set, univariate statistical procedures are used to establish the central tendency (mean) and variance (standard deviation)

of each variable across cases. Multivariate procedures are used to investigate the relationships between these same variables.

When a causal relationship is hypothesized, one must further distinguish between those variables that are presumed to represent the cause and those that represent the effect. The presumptive causal variables are known as *independent* or *predictor variables,* and those that indicate the effect are called *dependent* or *criterion variables.* In most instances it is assumed that changes in the independent variables are reflected by some changes in the dependent variable. In other words, the relationship between the independent variables and the dependent variable is linear. It must also be assumed that the distribution of values of the dependent variable for any given value of the independent variable is normal. This means that for each value of the independent variable, the value of the dependent variable will have a different mean but the same variance.

MATCHING THE STATISTICAL METHOD AND THE RESEARCH QUESTION

In most experimental paradigms, the study design assumes that a causal relationship exists between the variables studied. Implicit in this approach is the additional assumption that values of some of the variables depend on values of others. In other words, there are one or more dependent (criterion) variables and two or more independent (predictor) variables. Multiple regression, canonical correlation, multiple discriminant analysis, and multivariate analysis of variance are multivariate versions of bivariate techniques used to explore such dependence relationships.

Other methods address the interdependence of variables rather than causal relationships. Factor analysis, cluster analysis, and multidimensional scaling analysis exemplify such techniques that examine underlying relationships among the variables. The actual method(s) selected for any investigation depends of course on the research question to be addressed.

This chapter is intended to help the nurse investigator select the statistical method that is congruent with the research question. It provides an overview of selected data analysis techniques from which one might select when studying a complex multivariate problem or situation, as well as some basic information related to the selection and use of these techniques. Although the nurse investigator will most often work with a statistician, a basic working knowledge of what can be accomplished through the application of various techniques is important, for both the researcher and the consumer of research.

Examples of studies from the nursing and health care literature will be cited throughout the chapter to illustrate the application of multivariate techniques. These references are intended to help the reader better understand concepts basic to multivariate methods and related terminology.

MULTIPLE REGRESSION

Multiple regression is used when there is a single continuous dependent variable and two or more continuous independent variables. The major goals of a multiple regression analysis are to predict changes in the dependent variable from changes in the independent variables, determine which of the independent variables are useful predictors of the dependent variable, and ascertain the proportion of change in the dependent variable attributable to each independent variable. For example, a multiple regression analysis would be appropriate for examining the predictive role of age, weight, daily sodium intake, and level of perceived stress on systolic blood pressure. The analysis would examine the contribution of each independent variable in "explaining" the variance in the measured blood pressure.

The regression analysis tests a linear equation to determine the contribution of each independent variable in predicting the criterion variable. This linear regression equation takes the following form:

$$Y' = a + b_1x_1 + b_2x_2 + b_3x_3 + \cdots + b_kx_k,$$

where Y' represents the predicted value for the criterion variable, the constant a is the intercept of the regression line on Y, b_1 to b_k are the regression coefficients computed for each of the multiple independent variables, and x_1 to x_k are the independent variables.

One potential problem in performing multiple regression arises from the variation in the scaling of the independent variables. In most instances the variables (x_1 to x_k) that predict the dependent variable may represent entities measured along significantly differing scales. Consider for example, the attempt to predict systolic blood pressure by the following independent variables: age in years, weight in pounds, daily sodium intake in milligrams, and level of perceived stress as rated on a scale of 0 to 100. In such cases when the scaling is so different, the variables are scaled to z scores so that the distribution of each variable has a mean of 0 and a standard deviation of 1. This facilitates the comparison of the variables.

When the variables are used in their original raw score format, the corresponding regression coefficient is called a b weight; when scaled to standard scores, the coefficient is called a beta weight (β). The beta weight is the regression coefficient generally used for interpreting the contribution of the independent variable to the prediction of the dependent variable.

The R^2 statistic, or coefficient of determination, can be interpreted as the percentage of the variance in the dependent variable explained by the independent variables. This explained variance is called the *regression variance,* and the remaining variance is referred to as the *residual variance.* Residual variance most likely accounts for systematic or random measurement error and specification error. The latter error is associated with the theory underlying the analysis. It may indicate that an independent variable is highly associated with the dependent variable or that a variable that should be included in the regression analysis is missing from the equation. The goal of a regression analysis is to maximize the regression (i.e., explained) variance and minimize the residual variance. An F statistic can be computed from these two variances, which is essentially the same as the F ratio in an analysis of variance (ANOVA) and may be interpreted in a similar fashion. As the regression variance gets larger and the residual gets smaller, the size of the F statistic will increase. The larger the computed F value, the greater is the probability that the equation will significantly predict values of the dependent variable. A table of F values can be used to determine significance.

These concepts might best be understood by looking at a simple hypothetical example. A researcher would like to investigate the possible prediction of chronic pain experience (i.e., response to persistent pain) by several theoretically related independent variables: current pain intensity, depression, and social support. The dependent variable (Y') is the chronic pain experience. Essentially, the study's intent is to estimate the amount (i.e. percentage) of the variance explained by the independent variables; R^2 is the computed statistic representing this. In this example a computed R^2 of .52 would indicate that slightly over half of the variability of the chronic pain experience is explained by these three variables. Other variables not included in the present equation could also add to the explanation or could account for some of the unexplained variance. The researcher might want to add additional variables for further testing; however, this should be done only if they are theoretically relevant. The magnitude and significance of each beta weight is examined to determine the importance of each independent variable as a predictor. The F ratio provides a test of significance. It is important to note that although the standardized regression coefficient (β) indicates the weight of the independent variable and whether it is a positive or negative relationship, the R^2 indicates only magnitude (i.e., 0 to 1). The adjusted R^2 is the statistic generally reported, because it compensates for overestimation error (Schroeder, Sjoquist, & Stephan, 1986).

The use of multiple regression analysis in nursing and health care studies is increasing because it does allow for the inclusion of a greater number of variables that better mirror real-world situations. Studying a greater number of variables also requires a greater number of study subjects. Generally, the number of subjects per variable recommended is 5 to 10. The suggested rule of thumb is to use as large a study sample as possible (Kerlinger, 1986) and to keep the sample size equal for the different variables measured, if possible.

There are a number of variations in the use of multiple regression. The approach most commonly used is stepwise regression, which takes all the independent variables and considers them simultaneously.

These variables are then "stepped" into the equation according to the ability to predict R^2. A popular theory-based technique is staged regression analysis, or path analysis. This allows the researcher to enter and study the variables as guided by a theoretical model (Asher, 1983; Pedhazur, 1982).

Table 17-1 provides several examples of studies using multiple regression. In addition, a number of references demonstrate a variety of applications (Braden, 1990; Grey, Cameron, & Thurber, 1991; Mercer, Ferketich, & DeJoseph, 1993; Smith et al., 1990). In reviewing these studies special attention might be given to the researcher's theoretical selection of independent variables to predict a criterion variable (e.g., support of the selection by a conceptual explanation and the comprehensiveness of the selection), the approach to analysis (e.g., backward elimination and stepwise forward estimation), the sample size, and the interpretation of the statistical results, especially the explanation of the obtained R^2. A number of methodological references provide a discussion of the general approaches and underlying assumptions to regression analysis (Berry & Feldman, 1985; Ferketich & Verran, 1984; Fox, 1991; Hair, Anderson, & Tatham, 1987; Neter, Wasserman, & Kutner, 1985; Pedhazur, 1982; Verran & Ferketich, 1984, 1987).

MULTIVARIATE ANALYSIS OF VARIANCE

As discussed in Chapter 16, ANOVA deals with one dependent variable, which is continuous, and more than one independent variable. The goal of using multivariate analysis of variance (MANOVA) is similar to the application of ANOVA, for both are

Table 17-1
Examples of Studies Using Multiple Regression

Study Purpose	Sample	Independent Variables	Dependent Variable	Source
To identify correlates of fatigue in rheumatoid arthritis (RA)	Adults with RA ($n = 133$)	Demographics (age, gender, education), pain, sleep quality, physical activity, number of comorbidities, functional status, duration of disease	Fatigue	Belza, Henke, Yelin, Epstein, and Gillis (1993)
To examine the predictive abilities of selected factors in predicting self-care agency	Nursing home residents ($n = 87$)	Race, previous occupation, morale, perception that nursing home promotes dependency (*note:* dummy coding used for variables measured nominally)	Self-perception of self-care agency	Jirovec and Kasno (1993)
To test a theoretical model predicting the relationships among four concepts	Mothers of acutely ill, hospitalized children from 1 to 24 months of age ($n = 45$)	Predictability of events, control, anxiety	Coping effort	Schepp (1991)

useful in exploratory designs that determine the effects of independent variables on a dependent variable (ANOVA) or variables (MANOVA).

The difference in the null hypotheses representative of each method is exemplified as follows:

- ANOVA null hypothesis: A cardiovascular educational program offered at four different sites (i.e., to four unmatched groups) will have no impact on knowledge of health practices that could potentially reduce the risks of cardiovascular disease.
- MANOVA null hypothesis: A cardiovascular educational program offered to four unmatched groups will have no impact on (1) the knowledge of health practices that could potentially reduce the risks of cardiovascular disease, and (2) the belief in the ability to perform these health practices.

The MANOVA F test provides the measure of significance between groups. It provides a test of group differences across the dependent variables for a given probability of significance. Other equivalent methods available for making group comparisons include Hotelling's T^2 and Wilks's lambda. When the statistic obtained by any of these methods (F, T^2, or lambda) is significant, the null hypothesis is rejected. This means that there are significant differences between the means of the dependent variables in each of the groups. When the null hypothesis of no group differences is rejected, the univariate F tests on the dependent measures are examined to determine which of the multiple dependent variables are the major contributors to the significant difference between the groups being compared.

Table 17-2 highlights some studies that have used MANOVA. Additional studies (Beckmann, 1990; Champion & Scott,

Table 17-2
Examples of Studies Using MANOVA

Study Purpose	Sample	Independent Variables	Dependent Variables	Source
To test the effects of a nonoscillating waterbed flotation on indicators of energy expenditure: motor activity, heart rate, and behavioral state	Preterm infants (n = 22) with a stable medical condition	On-waterbed and off-waterbed treatment; off-waterbed and on-waterbed treatment	Motor activity, heart rate, and behavioral state	Deiriggi (1990)
To determine if quality of life varies as a function of disease status	Adults with a confirmed diagnosis of HIV infection who know their HIV classification (n = 95)	Disease status: HIV positive, AIDS-related complex, and AIDS	Quality-of-life measures, e.g., sleep and rest, emotional balance, and body care management	Ragsdale and Morrow (1990)

1993; Robinson et al., 1991) may be examined for examples of other applications of this statistical technique.

MULTIPLE ANALYSIS OF COVARIANCE

The multiple analysis of covariance (MANCOVA) procedure is essentially the same as MANOVA, except that it allows for the use of metric covariates. This may decrease the variance in the dependent variable associated with one or more of the covariates. The designation of a dependent variable as a covariate may be especially useful when it is thought to be highly correlated with another dependent variable but not with the independent variables.

FACTOR ANALYSIS

Factor analysis is an interdependence technique by which a large number of variables may be examined for interrelationships, combined into a smaller number of correlated variables, and then conceptually interpreted in terms of those correlations. It is useful, therefore, to reduce the volume of data. The procedure requires a large number of subjects if the researcher's goal is to identify factors that can be generalized to population factor structures (Aleamoni, 1973). Nunnally (1978) recommends 10 subjects per variable, but Gorsuch (1983) believes that five is an acceptable number. Arrindell and van der Ende (1985), however, suggest that subject-to-variable ratio has little effect on factor stability.

The researcher must make several decisions when selecting the appropriate factor analysis procedure. Initially, decision making involves selecting either principal components or common factors analysis. *Principal components analysis* is generally applied to a study's measured data when relationships between the variables are to be explored for the occurrence of underlying components or factors. *Common factors analysis* is applicable when factors have

been hypothesized and the researcher would like to estimate these factors from available data. Both approaches are highly conceptual, and determining which method is appropriate is not always easy. Nunnally (1978) points out that in most instances both methods lead to the same solution; but the investigator needs to be aware that there can be misleading results when principal components analysis is incorrectly selected.

A decision tree is provided by Ferketich and Muller (1990) (Figure 17-1) for guiding this selection process. This model and the related discussion provide a good reference to explain the process further. It begins with determining whether the measurement model is classic or neoclassic. The *classic model* is based on the belief that the measurement error is random and thus, all variance is unique to an individual item. The *neoclassic model* is based on the belief that measurement error is composed of random and systematic error and that, therefore, common variance exists among items. When the researcher is unable to adequately control for systematic error, as in the case of using available data set(s), common factors would be the more appropriate choice. Ferketich and Muller (1990) point out that the decision may be reduced to a philosophical one, based on the researcher's belief about the nature of measurement error.

Principal components is the most commonly used method; its resulting components are gleaned from the measured data and are called "real" factors (Nunnally, 1978, p. 332). Common factor analysis, in contrast, results "in factors that are extensions of the data and represent unmeasured or latent variable(s) discerned from the data" (Ferketich & Muller, 1990, p. 60). Because the resulting factors are estimated from the data rather than directly gleaned from measured data, the resulting common

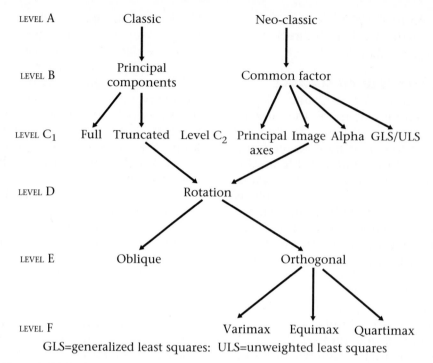

LEVEL A   Classic   Neo-classic

LEVEL B   Principal   Common factor
           components

LEVEL C$_1$ Full   Truncated   Level C$_2$ Principal   Image   Alpha   GLS/ULS
                                                axes

LEVEL D   Rotation

LEVEL E   Oblique   Orthogonal

LEVEL F   Varimax   Equimax   Quartimax

GLS=generalized least squares: ULS=unweighted least squares

Figure 17-1. Factor analysis decision tree. (From Ferketich, S. L., & Muller, M. (1990). Factor analysis revisited. *Nursing Research, 39,* 59-62.)

factors are called *hypothetical* (Nunnally, 1978, p. 332).

Because factor analysis is concerned with the interdependence of variables, differentiation between independent and dependent variables is not required; rather, all of the variables in the data set are considered simultaneously. The purpose of factor analysis is to summarize all of the information contained in a data set and present it in a more manageable form with minimal loss of information. Essentially, this is accomplished by identifying latent relationships (i.e., factors) that underlie the original variable set. Meaningful interpretations by the researcher must be guided by theory.

The basic assumption in factor analysis is that any complex phenomenon contains underlying traits or factors. In other words, a large number of similar descriptive variables may be related among themselves; by using this procedure, latent relationships among them may be determined. Obviously there should be a strong theoretical basis for performing such an analysis.

To accomplish factor analysis, the values of all the variables in a data set are intercorrelated with one another. *Communality* is the term used to describe the amount of variance that one variable shares with the others. Those subsets of variables that are most highly correlated are assumed to be related and are treated as separate factors or dimensions. The analysis then compares various linear combinations of correlated variables to establish the amount of total variance for which each combination accounts. The linear combination that explains the most variance is designated as the first factor (Factor I), the linear combination explaining most of the remaining variance is Factor II, and so on. The measure of how much variance a linear combination explains is called an *eigenvalue*. Only factors with an eigenvalue equal to or greater than 1 are generally acknowledged as being of sufficient importance to be included in the final factor model of the data. The scree test is another method often used in combination with this in making the decision about the final number of factors to be retained; for further discussion, see Cattell (1966).

The actual computation of factors is quite complex (Gorsuch, 1983). Very basically, the process involves plotting the variables, drawing axes through those variables which evidence the greatest interrelationships (i.e., the factors), and then rotating these factors. The researcher may select either an orthogonal or oblique rotation strategy. The *orthogonal rotation* assumes that the resulting factors are independent of each other. The *oblique rotation* is the appropriate choice when the factors are not assumed to be independent. The selection of the appropriate procedure can be a complex process. Nunnally (1978) suggests that if a clear solution is provided by one method, the same solution will likely result

from other approaches as well. In practice, if the researcher is not sure about the assumption of independence, it is wise to perform both analyses. When the orthogonal rotation is used, several approaches (e.g., varimax, equamax, and quartimax) are available in most statistical packages; varimax is the most frequently used. This rotation maximizes a variable's loading on one factor and minimizes its loadings on all others; this makes interpretation clearer.

A number of criteria are used when making decisions about variables to be retained in a data set. Two of the most commonly suggested stipulate that (1) the variable have a loading of at least .40 on a factor, and (2) there be a difference of at least .15 in a variable's loading on any two factors (Kerns, Turk, & Rudy, 1985). In instrument development, for example, these criteria may be used to make decisions about retaining items and whether or not to continue the data-reduction process. This process may be repeated until the researcher feels that the best empirical and theoretical explanation of the data has been reached. The application of theory is an important part of this data-reduction technique.

Table 17-3 provides examples of studies

Table 17-3
Examples of Studies Using Components and Factor Analysis

Study Purpose	Sample	Variables	Type of Analysis	Rotation	Source
Development of the Parental Stressor Scale: neonatal intensive care unit (PSS:NICU)	Parents (*n* = 190) of infants hospitalized in five NICUs	Forty-six items identified from pilot test of PSS: NICU	Principal components	Orthogonal (Varimax)	Miles, Funk, and Carlson (1993)
To assess the subscale structure of the Maternal Fetal Attachment Scale (MFAS)	Two groups of women (Group A = 371; Group B = 310) comprised two study samples	Twenty-three items of the MFAS	Common factor (principal axes)	Orthogonal (Varimax)	Muller and Ferketich (1993)

that use principal components and common factors analysis. Additional applications (Champion, 1993; Gulick, 1991) may also be reviewed. However, give special attention to the purpose (e.g., instrument development and testing construct validity of an instrument), sample size, type of analysis (i.e., principal components and common factors), and type of rotation. Using Figure 17-1 as a guide, note whether the authors have explained why they made each of the decisions guiding their analysis.

OTHER PROCEDURES
Discriminant Analysis
Discriminant analysis is a technique used when the dependent variable is categorical and the independent, or discriminating, variables are continuous. It is appropriate when the dependent variable can be divided into distinct classes of two or more. The term *multiple discriminant analysis (MDA)* is generally used when three or more classifications are identified.

Discriminant analysis has two major areas of application: interpretation and classification. As noted, discriminant analysis is useful in determining the linear combination of variables that maximize the group differences once the MANOVA procedure has demonstrated that there are group differences. This represents interpretation. In addition to interpreting the differences between groups, it is often used to classify cases into groups. When the research focus is classification, the focus is on deriving mathematical equations (i.e., discriminant functions) that "combine the group characteristics in a way that will allow one to identify the group which a case most closely resembles" (Klecka, 1980, p. 9).

This application finds a linear combination of independent variables that will discriminate between the groups or categories of the dependent variable. The discriminant function maximizes the variance between groups while minimizing the variance within groups, thus providing for maximum separation between them. This relationship is expressed as the ratio of between-group to within-group variance. Meaningful group separation is demonstrated if the between-group variance is large in relation to the within-group variance.

The first step in using this procedure is to specify the dependent and independent variables, focusing on the number of groups to be identified for the dependent variable (DV). For example, the researcher might be interested in creating a profile of chronic pain patients who are most likely to experience various levels of depression (i.e., high, moderate, and low). As with multiple regression, the independent, or predictor, variables are identified based on their theoretical relevance to the dependent variable; in this case those identified are level of education, current pain intensity, duration of pain, perceived family support, and the perceived helpfulness of current pain management. All of the variables may be analyzed at the same time (i.e., simultaneous entry), or they may be entered one at a time (i.e., stepwise). The procedure looks for the best linear combination of independent variables to discriminate between the specified groups of the dependent variable (high, moderate, or low levels of depression). This involves computing discriminant scores (z scores) and then averaging these scores for all individuals in a group (i.e., group centroid). The statistical significance of the discriminant function is determined by the distance between the group centroids and the degree of overlap of the group distributions. If the overlap is small, the function is a good discriminator between the groups. Conversely, if the

---

EXAMPLE OF DISCRIMINANT ANALYSIS

Title of Study: The influence of family support on chronic pain

Study Purpose: To determine the variables that most accurately predict perception of family support.

Sample: Chronic pain patients; 233 described their families as always supportive, and 275 noted some family support.

Results: Nine of 19 variables were identified as differentiating best between patient groups: those from supportive or nonsupportive families. The variables correctly classified 69.8% of the cases.

Source: Jamison and Virts (1990).

---

overlap is large, the function is a poor discriminator between groups.

Discriminant analysis is a technique suited to a variety of clinical research applications. The results of such analysis might be applicable, for example, in assisting with the determination of a patient's diagnosis, identifying persons at risk for certain specified conditions, or planning a treatment program. An example of discriminant analysis is provided in the box. Additional examples of clinical research using this procedure (Davidson & Neufield, 1974; Klein et al., 1985) may be reviewed, giving special attention to the specific application, selection of variables, sample size, and methods of reporting the results. The sample size recommended is 10 times the number of independent variables plus the number of treatment groups (McLaughlin & Marascuilo, 1990). In general, research reports include the coefficient of significance between the group means (F or U) and the percentage representing classification accuracy.

Cluster Analysis

Cluster analysis refers to a variety of procedures used for classification. These procedures allow the researcher to take information from a data set and empirically form groups or clusters that are very similar (i.e., highly correlated). Such analysis, including the choice of variables to be selected from a data set, should be guided by theory (Aldenderfer & Blashfield, 1984). Like factor analysis, these are data-reduction techniques concerned with the interdependence of variables, not with the examination of independent and dependent variables.

A brief comparison to factor analysis might be helpful. Factor analysis looks for underlying commonalities or dimensions among variables. These commonalities suggest that some variables belong together, and they are referred to as *factors*. In cluster analysis the relationships among cases are examined in a manner very similar to the method used in factor analysis. The focus here, however, is to look for relationships among cases rather than among variables. Consequently when cases are analyzed in this manner, clusters of similar cases will emerge that may reflect subgroups of subpopulations. If, for example, measures of height, weight, daily sodium intake, and perceived level of stress were obtained for a group of patients in a clinic, clusters of similar cases might emerge that suggest subgroups of a larger group composed of individuals diagnosed as being hypertensive.

One subgroup might be overweight and have a high sodium intake; another might be within the normal weight range and have a high level of perceived stress. On the other hand, factor analysis would determine only which of the variables, if any, showed interdependence or formed possible underlying factors of hypertension.

In cluster analysis all members of a population are measured according to two or more variables and then divided into distinct subgroups on the basis of their degree of similarity. Hair, Anderson, and Tatham (1987) describe the analysis as having three major stages: partitioning, interpretation, and profiling. Once the analysis has identified clusters (i.e., partitioning), the distinguishing characteristics are studied, and an appropriate name is given to each subset (i.e., interpretation). Profiling then focuses on describing the characteristics of the clusters.

This technique may be clinically useful when the researcher is attempting to make sense out of a large data set that includes a variety of variables. For example, a survey of older adults experiencing depression might show that emotional instability, chronic illness, low self-esteem, insomnia, irregular eating habits, inability to make decisions, and persistent suicidal ideations are commonly occurring characteristics. A cluster analysis of these measured variables might segregate the study population into four groups, each showing emotional instability and low self-esteem. In addition, Group 2 might show significant eating and sleeping difficulties; Group 3, an inability to make simple decisions; and Group 4, suicidal ideations. On the basis of the analysis, sample participants could be classified as being mildly, moderately, severely, or profoundly depressed. The characteristics of each classification provide a useful profile.

Clustering methods are useful in health care research, for they can assist in developing diagnostic classifications, forming hypotheses about commonly associated variables that one sees recurring among patients, and testing these hypotheses. Because such analysis involves a high degree of theoretical knowledge and interpretation, its application in clinical research is best made by one who is very familiar with the area of study. This theoretical base is combined with statistical methods (e.g., correlation coefficients and distance measures). When used, the type of clustering method should be carefully selected and reported; the various methods are explained in more detailed discussions of the procedure (Aldenderfer & Blashfield, 1984; Hair, Anderson, & Tatham, 1987).

Canonical Correlation

Canonical correlation analysis is used when there are multiple dependent and independent continuous and categorical variables. The goal of this procedure is to extract sets of both the dependent and independent variables that maximize the correlation between the two sets. In other words it provides a measure of strength of the relationship between the linear combinations of the independent and dependent sets of variables. This might be conceptualized as a bivariate relationship between the two linear composites.

Given an example of the older adult with diagnosed osteoporosis and related chronic pain, canonical correlation analysis would be appropriate for determining the best relationship between the independent variables (level of physical activity, amount of calcium supplement taken, and self-care abilities) and the dependent variables (bone density, pain intensity, and personal response to pain). Because clinical situations often involve a multiple number of independent and dependent variables, this technique has many potential applications in nursing and health care research. Redeker (1992) provides one example.

Multidimensional Scaling Analysis
Multidimensional scaling analysis is designed to transform individual evaluations of similarity or individual preferences into composite distance measures, or measures of proximity; it does not involve independent and dependent variables. Multidimensional scaling spatially represents the interrelationships that exist among measured stimuli (e.g., objects, items, and concepts). Once the assessments of each measured stimulus have been converted to distances, the stimuli can be plotted in multidimensional space to provide a graphic representation of the spatial relationship between each of the stimuli. For example, if the nursing staff of a hospital were asked to compare five different plans for rehabilitating stroke patients, they would compare each of the plans against all of the others for similarity of effectiveness. A correlation of the comparisons gives a matrix of distances between each pair of plans based on the perceived similarity between pairs. A multidimensional scaling analysis of the matrix would reveal the number of dimensions (axes) of similarity, and each dimension (axis) could then be interpreted in terms of stimulus characteristics to show specific features on which the comparisons were made. In this instance the distribution of the stimuli along each axis might suggest that one dimension reflects the amount of interaction between patient and nurse, another dimension might be seen as reflecting the volume of paperwork associated with each plan, and another dimension might be the perceived cost of each plan. This type of analysis is particularly useful when the researcher wishes to determine cognitive or perceptual dimensions of

evaluation without specifying this as an overt goal of the experiment. Dimensional representation may also be very helpful when the investigator is attempting to explain a concept theoretically, for it allows exploration of the dimensions and their relationships to one another. For a more detailed discussion of this procedure and reference to computer programs, see Kruskal and Wish (1978).

Structural Equation Modeling
Structural equation modeling may be used to analyze a causal model that may include a variety of exogenous (i.e., not influenced by other variables in the model) and endogenous (i.e., influenced by other variables in the model) variables. In causal analysis, both recursive and nonrecursive relationships may be examined. Path analysis, or staged multiple regression, deals only with recursive models; that is, models in which a theoretical one-way causal relationship may be tested. Structural equation modeling has the advantage of testing nonrecursive models; thus it permits the analysis of reciprocal relationships among variables, and it allows for the interplay of theory and data (Asher, 1983). Although theory is obviously important in any model testing, the fact that this procedure permits the analysis of all relationships that are deemed important makes it an attractive choice. Using this technique, both latent (unobserved) and manifest (observed) variables may be included in the model to be tested.

Other references (Hayduk, 1987; Pedhazur, 1982) provide a detailed discussion of structural equation modeling. Two computer programs available for model analysis are LISREL (*Li*near *s*tructural *rel*ations) (Hayduk, 1987; Joreskog & Sorbom, 1989) and EQS (Bentler, 1983). The use of these procedures requires a basic understanding

---

EXAMPLE OF LOGISTIC REGRESSION

Title of Study: Predicting alcohol use in rural children: A longitudinal study.

Study Purpose: To predict alcohol use versus nonuse in grades 6 and 7 from sociodemographic and personality and attitude measures obtained in grades 3 and 4.

Sample: Two hundred and fifty-four children in sixth and seventh grades who had initially been tested in grades 3 and 4.

Independent (Predictor) Variables: Personality/attitude and sociodemographics.

Dependent (Criterion) Variables: Categories of "User" and "Nonuser."

Results: Children who in grades 3 and 4 had a negative self-concept and a negative attitude toward school were more likely to be users in grades 6 and 7. Those who in grades 3 and 4 had either positive self-concept or attitude toward school but not both were more likely to be users in grades 6 and 7.

Source: Long and Bolk (1993).

---

of matrix algebra computations. In addition, some knowledge of the specific symbols used by LISREL is necessary.

The number of nursing studies using structural equation modeling is growing, for it provides a mechanism for studying the kind of multivariate models typical of those needed to guide practice and research. An exploration of Pender's Health Promotion Model provides an excellent example of its application (Johnson, Ratner, Bottorff, & Hayduk, 1993).

Logistic Regression Analysis

Logistic regression analysis is mentioned because it provides a way for studying the prediction of a criterion variable when the independent variables cannot be assumed to have a normal distribution. It is therefore a nonlinear regression model (Neter, Wasserman, & Kutner, 1985). A study by Long and Bolk (1993) provides an example of its application (see the box).

SELECTING THE APPROPRIATE ANALYSIS PROCEDURE

Some procedures, such as multiple regression, MANOVA, multiple discriminant analysis, canonical correlation, and logistic

regression analysis, allow the researcher to explore causal relationships between independent and dependent variables. Others, such as factor analysis, cluster analysis, and multidimensional scaling analysis, provide a way to examine interrelationships among variables when no independent or dependent variables are identified.

Since there are numerous choices for analyzing the kind of complex problems that involve questions of either causal relationships or interrelationships among variables, the research consumer needs to ask questions regarding the appropriateness of the techniques used. The box contains guidelines for evaluating the use of advanced statistical methods.

SUMMARY

- Multivariate analysis refers to a class of statistical procedures used to examine the interrelationships between three or more variables in a data set. These techniques allow the investigation of complex interactions that reflect most clinical situations.

- Multivariate analysis may be viewed as a series of analytical procedures based

EVALUATING THE MULTIVARIATE DATA ANALYSIS

1. Are the statistical methods clearly described?
2. Does the researcher give information for determining whether appropriate statistical techniques were used? For example,
   - Do these these techniques directly address the research questions or hypotheses?
   - Are the techniques appropriate for the level(s) of data?
   - Are the techniques appropriate for the type of data (i.e., continuous or categorical)?
3. Is the sample size appropriate for the number of variables studied?
4. Is the assumption of a linear relationship among the study variables met?
5. Are the independent and dependent variables clearly identified when appropriate?
6. Are the criteria for making analysis decisions explained?
7. Does the research report present results for each hypothesis or research question?
8. Are the results clearly presented and understandable?
9. Do the results support the conclusions drawn by the researcher?
10. When the statistical technique used is multiple regression analysis, is the approach (e.g., stepwise forward estimation and backward elimination) explained?
11. When the statistical technique used is factor analysis,
    - Does the researcher note the method (i.e., common factors or principal components) and the rotation used and why these were selected?
    - Is there an explanation of the decision made about the number of factors to be retained?

upon (1) the degree of dependence assumed between variables, (2) the number of variables assumed to be dependent, and (3) the way in which the variables are measured.

- Multivariate statistics are generally used in an attempt to achieve one or more of the following goals: (1) describe and summarize the research data collected, (2) establish the nature and degree of the relationships between different variables, and (3) determine a possible causal or predictive relationship.
- Most experimental designs assume a causal relationship between variables. This assumption implies that the values of some variables depend on the values of others (i.e., that there is a linear relationship).

- Multiple regression is used when there is a single metric dependent variable and two or more independent variables and when the goal is to predict changes in the dependent variable from changes in the independent variables, determine which of the independent variables are useful predictors of the dependent variable, or determine the proportion of change in the dependent variable attributable to each independent variable.
- Multivariate analysis of variance (MANOVA) tests the equality of two or more nonmetric independent variables on multiple metric dependent variables.
- Factor analysis examines a large number of variables for interrelationships and combines them into a smaller number of correlated variables that can then be

conceptually interpreted. Principal components analysis is the most commonly used method of factor analysis; it results in components that are gleaned from the measured data.

- Discriminant analysis is the method used when the dependent variables represent one or two a priori categories. Multiple discriminant analysis is the technique used when there are three or more a priori defined categories.

- Multiple discriminant analysis is used when the independent variable is non-metric and represents three or more a priori designated categories and when the independent variables are metric. It finds a linear combination of independent variables that will discriminate between a priori classifications of the dependent variable.

- Cluster analysis provides clinically useful data-reduction techniques that require a strong theoretical base. It provides a way to determine clusters of cases (i.e., sub-populations) that might emerge within a set of measured variables.

- Canonical correlation analysis determines the best relationship between two or more independent and two or more dependent variables. It provides a method that is useful in clinical situations involving numerous dependent, as well as independent, variables.

- Multidimensional scaling analysis spatially represents the existing interrelationships among variables. A numerical index (such as a correlation coefficient) provides a measure of proximity.

- Structural equation modeling allows for analysis of models with multiple indicators of latent variables, reciprocal causation, and correlated residuals. Two computer programs available for analysis of structural equation models are LISREL and EQS.

- Logistic regression analysis provides an alternate multivariate procedure that is useful when it cannot be assumed that the independent variables have a normal distribution.

FACILITATING CRITICAL THINKING
What method of multivariate data analysis should be used when the researcher would like to:

1. Identify the underlying dimensions of the construct of patient satisfaction.
2. Determine which of five measured variables are the best predictors of the hospitalized patient's satisfaction with nursing care. (Hint: All measured variables are metric.)
3. Determine the similarity of the effectiveness of various pain-management techniques by studying the spatial relationship among ratings of their effectiveness by persons with a medical diagnosis of rheumatoid arthritis.
4. Determine whether the outcome (client's knowledge of health-promoting behaviors related to cardiovascular disease) is significantly different for four client groups taught in four different settings.
5. Determine whether any specified variables (educational level, age, and economic level) significantly predict the program outcome in item 4 (i.e., client's knowledge of health-promoting behaviors related to cardiovascular disease).
6. Determine whether a combination of demographic variables classifies the participants in the cardiovascular teaching program as high, moderate, or low achievers on a knowledge pretest.
7. Test a causal model of reciprocal relationships among variables that theoretically explain the diabetic teenager's adherence to prescribed treatment.
8. Determine whether persons with a

medical diagnosis of rheumatoid arthritis who are (1) in remission or (2) not in remission perform significantly differently on measures of physical function, participation in social activities, and pain response.

9. Use a data-reduction technique as one of the approaches to developing a clinically useful instrument for measuring patient satisfaction.

10. Test a reciprocal causal model with staged variables theoretically identified as predictors of self-efficacy for the person with a medical diagnosis of chronic obstructive lung disease.

References

SUBSTANTIVE

BECKMANN, C. A. (1990). Postterm pregnancy: Effects on temperature and glucose regulation. *Nursing Research, 39,* 21-24.

BELZA, B. L., HENKE, C. J., YELIN, E. H., EPSTEIN, W. V., & GILLIS, C. L. (1993). Correlates of fatigue in older adults with rheumatoid arthritis. *Nursing Research, 42,* 93-99.

BRADEN, C. J. (1990). A test of the self-help model: Learned response to chronic illness experience. *Nursing Research, 39,* 42-47.

CATTELL, R. B. (1966). The scree test for the number of factors. *Multivariate Behavioral Research, 1,* 245-276.

CHAMPION, V. L. (1993). Instrument refinement for breast cancer screening behaviors. *Nursing Research, 42,* 139-143.

CHAMPION, V., & SCOTT, C. (1993). Effects of a procedural/belief intervention on breast self-examination performance. *Research in Nursing & Health, 16,* 163-170.

DAVIDSON, P. O., & NEUFIELD, R. W. J. (1974). Response to pain and stress: A multivariate analysis. *Journal of Psychosomatic Research, 18,* 25-32.

DEIRIGGI, P. M. (1990). Effects of waterbed flotation on indicators of energy expenditure in preterm infants. *Nursing Research, 39,* 355-360.

GREY, M., CAMERON, M. E., & THURBER, F. W. (1991). Coping and adaptation in children with diabetes. *Nursing Research, 40,* 144-149.

GULICK, E. E. (1991). Reliability and validity of the Work Assessment Scale for persons with multiple sclerosis. *Nursing Research, 40,* 107-112.

JAMISON, R. N., & VIRTS, K. L. (1990). The influence of family support on chronic pain. *Behavior Research and Therapy, 28,* 283-287.

JIROVEC, M. M., & KASNO, J. (1993). Predictors of self-care abilities among the institutionalized elderly. *Western Journal of Nursing Research, 15,* 314-326.

JOHNSON, J. L., RATNER, P. A., BOTTORFF, J. L., & HAYDUK, L. A. (1993). An exploration of Pender's Health Promotion Model using LISREL. *Nursing Research, 42,* 132-138.

KLEIN, L. E., ROCA, R. P., MCARTHUR, J., VOGELSANG, G., KLEIN, G.B., KIRBY, S. M., & FOLSTEIN, M. (1985). Diagnosing dementia: Univariate and multivariate analyses of the Mental Status Examination. *Journal of the American Geriatrics Society, 33,* 483-488.

LONG, K. A., & BOLK, R. J. (1993). Predicting alcohol use in rural children: A longitudinal study. *Nursing Research, 42,* 79-85.

MERCER, R. T., FERKETICH, S. L., & DEJOSEPH, J. F. (1993). Predictors of partner relationships during pregnancy and infancy. *Research in Nursing & Health, 16,* 45-56.

MILES, M. S., FUNK, S. G., CARLSON, J. (1993). Parental Stressor Scale: Neonatal Intensive Care Unit. *Nursing Research, 42,* 148-152.

MULLER, M. E., & FERKETICH, S. (1993). Factor analysis of the Maternal Fetal Attachment Scale. *Nursing Research, 42,* 144-147.

RAGSDALE, D., & MORROW, J. R. (1990). Quality of life as a function of HIV classification. *Nursing Research, 39,* 335-360.

REDEKER, N. S. (1992). The relationships between uncertainty and coping after coronary bypass surgery. *Western Journal of Nursing Research, 14,* 48-68.

ROBINSON, S. E., ROTH, S. L., KEIM, J., LEVENSON, M., FLENTJE, J. R., & BASHOR, K. (1991). Nurse burnout: Work related and demographic factors as culprits. *Research in Nursing & Health, 14,* 223-228.

Schepp, K. G. (1991). Factors influencing the coping effort of mothers of hospitalized children. *Nursing Research, 40,* 42-46.

Smith, C. E. Marien, L., Brogdon, C., Faust-Wilson, P., Lohr, G., Gerald, K. B., & Pingleton, S. (1990). Diarrhea associated with tube feeding in mechanically ventilated critically ill patients. *Nursing Research, 39,* 148-152.

Yarcheski, A., Mahon, N. E., & Yarcheski, T. J. (1992). Validation of the PRQ85 social support measure for adolescents. *Nursing Research, 41,* 332-337.

METHODOLOGIC

Aldenderfer, M. S., & Blashfield, R. K. (1984). *Cluster analysis.* Newbury Park, CA: Sage.

Aleamoni, L. M. (1973). Effects of size of sample on eigenvalues, observed communalities, and factor loadings. *Journal of Applied Psychology, 58,* 266-269.

Arrindell, W. A., & van der Ende, J. (1985). An empirical test of the utility of the observations-to-variable ratio in factor and components analysis. *Applied Psychological Measurement, 9,* 165-178.

Asher, H. B. (1983). *Causal modeling* (2nd ed.). Beverly Hills, CA: Sage.

Bentler, P. M. (1983). Theory and implementation of EQS, a structural equations program. Los Angeles: BMDP Statistical Software.

Berry, W. D., & Feldman, S. (1985). *Multiple regression in practice.* Newbury Park, CA: Sage.

Ferketich, S. L., & Muller, M. (1990). Factor analysis revisited. *Nursing Research, 39,* 59-62.

Ferketich, S. L., & Verran, J. A. (1984). Residual analysis for casual model assumptions. *Western Journal of Nursing Research, 6,* 41-60.

Fox, J. (1991). *Regression diagnostics.* Newbury Park, CA: Sage.

Gorsuch, R. L. (1983). *Factor analysis* (2nd ed.). Hillsdale, NJ: Erlbaum.

Hair, J. F., Anderson, R. E., & Tatham, R. L. (1987). *Multivariate data analysis* (2nd ed.). New York: Macmillan.

Hayduk, L. A. (1987). *Structural equation modeling with LISREL: Essentials and advances.* Baltimore: The Johns Hopkins University Press.

Joreskog, K., & Sorbom, D. (1989). *LISREL 7: User's reference guide.* Mooresville, IN: Scientific Software.

Kerlinger, F. N. (1986). *Foundations of behavioral research* (3rd ed.). New York: Holt, Rinehart & Winston.

Kerns, R. D., Turk, D. C., & Rudy, T. E. (1985). The West Haven-Yale Multidimensional Pain Inventory (WHYMPI). *Pain, 23,* 345-356.

Klecka, W. R. (1980). *Discriminant analysis.* Newbury Park, CA: Sage.

Kruskal, J. B., & Wish, M. (1978). *Multidimensional scaling.* Beverly Hills, CA: Sage.

McLaughlin, F. E., & Marascuilo, L. A. (1990). *Advanced nursing and health care research: Quantification approaches.* Philadelphia: Saunders.

Neter, J., Wasserman, W., & Kutner, M. H. (1985). *Applied linear statistical models* (2nd ed.). Homewood, IL: Irwin.

Nunnally, J. C. (1978). *Psychometric theory.* New York: McGraw-Hill.

Pedhazur, E. J. (1982). *Multiple regression in behavioral research: Explanation and prediction* (2nd ed.). New York: CBS College Publishing.

Schroeder, L. D., Sjoquist, D. L., & Stephan, P. E. (1986). *Understanding regression analysis: An introductory guide.* Newbury Park, CA: Sage.

Verran, J. A., & Ferketich, S. L. (1984). Residual analysis for statistical assumptions of regression equations. *Western Journal of Nursing Research, 6,* 27-40.

Verran, J. A., & Ferketich, S. L. (1987). Testing linear model assumptions: Residual analysis. *Nursing Research, 36,* 127-130.

CHAPTER 18

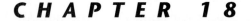

INTERPRETATION OF THE FINDINGS

MARYANN F. PRANULIS

Interpreting findings is one of the most challenging and least structured steps in the research process. Both novice and more seasoned researchers are often heard lamenting: "I've got all these data and all these computer printouts. Now, what do I do with them?" Interpreting research findings is challenging because it demands creativity, critical thinking, and courage.

Interpreting, rather than just reporting, research findings requires the investigator to be *creative* because it necessitates: (1) detecting patterns that may not be patently obvious, and (2) finding or assigning meaning to patterns or to the absence of anticipated patterns. Interpreting findings requires *critical thinking* because it necessitates continuous comparison and contrast between and among the findings at large, subsections within the findings, the findings of others, theory, and practical experience. Interpreting research findings requires *courage* because it demands a willingness to go beyond and even to *challenge* established explanations for reality. Results may be met with doubt and disdain from peers and the larger scientific community. However, the rewards inherent in discovery, whether on a purely personal level or when significant contributions are made to the advancement of knowledge, provide strong motivation.

Interpreting research findings is often conceived of as "unstructured" when each research problem is viewed as being unique and without precedent or outside of an established scientific paradigm. Established paradigms provide structure by determining the phenomenon of interest within the discipline. They guide the formulation of acceptable research questions, methods to address those questions, and criteria or guidelines for analyzing and interpreting empirical findings.

In nursing, as in most emerging scientific disciplines, research precedents and paradigms are lacking or are ill-defined. However, although scientific paradigms and structures for conducting research and interpreting the findings may be unavailable, a disciplined approach is still needed to meet the challenges of deriving a conceptually valid interpretation.

Interpreting research findings can overwhelm even seasoned researchers. However, investigators can increase their abilities to meet the challenges to their creativity, critical thinking, and courage by (1) regularly exercising personal creativity and critical thinking, and (2) developing a plan for data analysis and interpretation of the findings *prior* to beginning data collection. The purpose of this chapter is to facilitate an investigator's abilities to interpret findings by presenting (1) methods to expand personal creativity and critical thinking, and (2) guidelines for systematically interpreting empirical findings. Creativity and critical thinking are defined, and methods for developing and nurturing them are presented. Guidelines for systematically interpreting findings are then discussed.

∾ CREATIVITY AND CRITICAL THINKING

WHAT IS CREATIVITY?

Creativity is the ability to look at the same thing others are looking at and to see it differently—to do the same thing as others do and to do it differently. Webster's dictionary (1980) defines creativity as the ability to create—to produce something through imaginative skills or to bring something new into existence.

Creativity and Science
When asked to think of someone creative, one imagines artists or sculptors creating two- and three-dimensional images of how they view and interpret reality. But how can a quantitative scientist be creative? Are there not rules for using the scientific method to which the investigator must adhere rigorously to produce valid and reliable results?

Many say, "Using one's *imagination* pro-

duces art not science." Yet some of the most notable scholars, such as Leonardo da Vinci and Albert Einstein, who made significant contributions to the advancement of empirically based knowledge were truly creative geniuses. A broader view of creativity is presented by von Oech (1990), who in a lighthearted monograph on building creativity stated:

> Creative thinking requires an attitude that allows you to search for ideas and manipulate your knowledge and experience. With this outlook, you try various approaches, first one, then another, often not getting anywhere. You use crazy, foolish, and impractical ideas as stepping stones to practical new ideas. You break the rules occasionally, and explore for ideas in unusual outside places. In short, by adopting a creative outlook you open yourself up to both new possibilities and to change. (p. 6)

Creativity in science allows one to discern patterns and explanations for the patterns or lack of anticipated patterns in observations and measurements of external, objective reality. Only the creative investigator is able to go beyond the obvious and make discoveries that expand the horizons of knowledge. Thus, creativity born of the union of imaginative risk taking and systematic scientific observations is the hallmark of brilliant scientific research rather than its antithesis.

Developing and Nurturing Creativity
The first step in developing and nurturing creativity is to be *open* to alternatives to scientific ways of knowing and scientific or empirically based knowledge. In addition to the scientific method, intuition, tradition, experience, and authority are ways of receiving, developing, and communicating knowledge. In addition to scientific knowl-

edge, personal, ethical, and spiritual knowledge and other forms of knowledge are also valid (Carper, 1978; Watson, 1981). The limitations of nonscientific ways of knowing lie in the difficulties inherent in testing the universality and reproducibility of knowledge generated through these methods; the ability to test universality and generalizibility through its reproducibility is a strength of the scientific method.

By being open to alternative ways of knowing, the scientist may facilitate obtaining insights or seeing the meaning in findings that may not be readily apparent by using only scientific procedures. The insight or meaning can then be tested against the empirical findings (using scientific methods and critical analysis) to determine the extent to which they support each other.

The second step is to *practice* creativity (frequently but not universally thought of as a predominantly right-brain function) as energetically and regularly as one might practice deductive logic (which is viewed by many as a predominantly left-brain function). This step is based on the assumption that creativity is a *skill* like any other psychomotor skill. In order to develop and maintain a skill, it is necessary to practice it. Then, when the skill is needed, it can be called upon and demonstrated with ease, efficiency, and effectiveness.

The Pranulis IPPET model (Immersion, Play, Practice, Exercise, Transfer) (Pranulis, 1993) for developing and nurturing creativity consists of a set of exercises or activities designed to enhance creativity. Although the model has not been tested empirically, practical experience has demonstrated its usefulness. The model consists of a series of activities that build on one another. The first set of activities involves *immersion* in the creative works of others such as literature, poetry, music, art, dance, drama, and comedy. Immersion requires the observer to experience the creative work rather than to analyze it. This is often difficult for highly cognitive, analytical people because it requires turning off cognitive processing. When the observer steps back from the "experiential" realm and begins to analyze the elements such as the use of light and shadow and the artist's techniques, a leap has been made from an exercise in creativity to an analytical exercise. Doing so is appropriate when attempting to establish a balance between experiential and cognitive modes of knowing.

Immersion in the creative works of others can be likened to passive exercise. Active creativity exercises begin with *play*—engaging in pattern-recognition games such as puzzle construction or square dancing. The main consideration when moving into the play stage is that the activity should be pleasurable and relaxing. Goal attainment such as winning or becoming skilled requires work and should not be the motivating force driving the activity at this stage.

When creativity exercises become sufficiently habitual through play, it is time to move into the next stage: *practice*. This stage requires work, but it can still be enjoyable if engaged in as a leisure-time activity. It is during the practice stage of creativity building that analytical skills are invoked—when one's creative abilities and skills are subjected to evaluation and either correction or reinforcement in order to refine the skill. When the skill has been sufficiently developed so it can be called upon at will, then it is time to begin *exercising* the skill regularly in order to maintain it. The final stage, *transfer,* occurs when there is a demand for the skill in another situation such as when a creative solution is needed for resolving a problem. This can occur in a variety of ways and situations. What is transferred is the ability to see what others see but to see it differently.

WHAT IS CRITICAL THINKING?

Scientific method and critical thinking are both processes built on skepticism and entail an examination of what is known and of how things are done. Both involve identifying assumptions underlying knowledge and actions. And both entail questioning or challenging the validity of these underlying assumptions, their roots, and their manifestations by comparing and contrasting the assumptions for their correspondence with evidence derived from empirical observations of an external reality. However, the scientific method is systematic, whereas critical thinking, although often systematic, is not such a formalized process.

Critical thinking is a cognitive process (rather than a product) that, as Brookfield (1991) points out, has been widely examined in the twentieth century. It is a process of questioning, discerning discrepencies or inconsistencies, and identifying similarities or consistencies. Critical thinking employs and even demands creativity that, as described, defies logic and formalization. Critical thinking involves seeing what is and conceiving of (or envisioning) what could be (the creative component). It involves examining knowledge or actions in their current context and in alternative contexts and mentally trying alternative explanations or actions. It entails repeatedly asking, "Why?" and "Why not?" All of these activities are essential mental tasks in the scientific method. However, the end point of critical thinking per se is personal enrichment and, ultimately, enrichment of society through increasing awareness and acceptance of diversity and improved understanding of universal truisms. The end point of the scientific method is the uncovering of universal truths.

KNOWING WHEN TO USE CREATIVITY VERSUS CRITICAL THINKING

The question arises, "How can a scientist develop and nurture creativity and still practice rigorous science?" The first step is to know when it is appropriate to adhere to the "rules" for scientific ways of knowing and when is it appropriate to use other ways of knowing. For example, creativity is needed to identify and analyze a researchable problem, to generate researchable questions, to propose interventions that might resolve the problem, to identify patterns or lack of patterns, and to find or ascribe meaning when *interpreting* the findings. It is advisable to adhere rigorously to the rules of science for planning methodology, sampling, collecting and processing data, and analyzing data. However, expert scientists often extend the boundaries and use more than one way of knowing in each stage of their research process. The brilliance of their endeavors is revealed in the "fit" between various components of the investigator's research process and product.

Logical coherence, congruence, and internal consistency are used as three tests of "fit" between process and product. The research is said to be *logically coherent* if an uninvolved or objective reviewer can rationally deduce the relationships between and among the following: the research problem, questions, definitions of terms, methods to measure variables, methods to address the question(s) and resolve the problem(s), and the findings or outcomes of the study.

The research is said to be *congruent* if the *parts* of the research are in harmonious agreement. For example, if stress is defined as a *biologic* phenomenon (one part), then in order to meet the criteria of congruence, measures (another part of the research) of biologic or physiologic processes, such as heart rate, blood pressure, or serum catecholamines, will be used. If stress is defined as a *psychosocial* phenomenon, then measures of psychosocial phenomena, such as mood state and self-reports of distress, will be used. A study of the effects of extreme environmental temperature on healthy human subjects' biologic functions would be said to demonstrate congruence if it includes measures of environmental temperature and the subject's core temperature, skin temperature, and thermal regulating mechanisms such as heart rate. These examples demonstrate congruence because the *individual parts* of the research are in harmonious agreement.

The criteria of congruence and internal consistency are similar in that both revolve around "agreement." However, consistency is a more precise criterion used to examine the sameness, or agreement, between and among the parts and the whole. For example, a study would be internally consistent if the method for measuring heart rate (e.g., number of beats felt in an apical pulse in 60 seconds) described in the methods section is the same as what is reported in the findings (beats per minute). It would lack internal consistency if the methods called for measuring heart rate in apical beats per minute but if in the findings section the investigator reported the averaged r-r time intervals derived from an electrocardiographic recording, even though both methods measure heart rate. If a study of *biologic* stress in healthy, *unmarried* human subjects concludes that *marital* discord (a psychosocial phenomenon among married people) reflected biologic stress, the study lacks both congruence and consistency. Every scientist should examine the scientific process and emerging product for logical coherence, congruence, and internal consistency repeatedly throughout the research process. Satisfaction that these criteria have been met as the scientist moves between creativity and critical thinking lends credence to the soundness of the findings' interpretation. However, creativity and critical thinking do not substitute for the systematic analysis and interpretation of data.

GUIDELINES FOR SYSTEMATICALLY INTERPRETING FINDINGS

Five steps carried out sequentially facilitate the systematic analysis and interpretation of data. They are listed in the box and discussed in the following paragraphs.

ORGANIZING FINDINGS

One of the most challenging tasks facing an investigator is to organize the data in a coherent manner. This step cannot be separated from (and should be carried out simultaneously with) preparations for conducting statistical analysis. This step is simplified if the investigator has developed or utilized a conceptual and operational diagram of the variables of interest as part of the research planning. Suggested analytical strategies follow.

Sample and Population Characteristics
The characteristics of the total sample should be examined and compared with those of the population from which the sample was drawn. The characteristics of persons who were invited to participate in the study but declined or subsequently withdrew should also be examined. The examination should include demographic factors and any antecedent variables that

STEPS IN INTERPRETING THE FINDINGS

1. Organize the data in a consistent manner.
2. Evaluate the data to determine its adequacy.
3. Explore the findings to assign meaning.
4. Evaluate the importance and generalizability of the findings.
5. Identify the implications of the results for theory, research, education, and practice.

may make a difference on the study variables and about which data are available. Population characteristics may be derived from published census data for the geographic region or from the administrative or clinical data banks maintained at the study site. Access may be limited for the study site sources, and institutional guidelines regarding seeking Institutional Review Board approval should be followed. If the sample's characteristics differ substantially from the population or from the characteristics of the nonparticipants or dropouts, then the findings cannot be generalized beyond the study sample.

Between Group Differences

If the study was designed with more than one group of subjects (e.g., experimental and control, men and women, adults and children), the next step is to compare and contrast the characteristics (demographic and antecedent variables) of the groups. This is especially important for studies that introduce an experimental intervention. It is also important in studies involving a "natural" experiment (an event such as a flood, earthquake, economic setback, or other life event that occurs and is not under the control or manipulative abilities of the investigator). An example of natural experiment would be a study of the long-term health impact of the Midwestern floods of 1993 (intervention not subject to the investigator's manipulation) on subjects who were displaced from their homes (nonrandomized group A) and those who were not (nonrandomized group B).

The groups should be similar for the most influential characteristics (antecedent variables) before intervention if random methods were used for group assignment. If the groups differed *before* intervention, then the internal validity of the study is compromised (see Chapter 11 for design validity issues). The investigator cannot determine whether any postintervention differences were a result of the intervention or of preintervention differences. If the groups were similar, then it is more likely that any postintervention differences were related to the intervention.

Searching for Covariables

A search for variables that change in relation to the dependent variable(s) should be performed before testing the hypotheses. For many studies the theory or previous research on which the current study is based will suggest or delineate important covariables. However, the search can also be carried out by performing simple tests of correlation between antecedent and intervening variables, antecedent and dependent variables, and intervening and dependent variables for the *total* sample. If any of the variables are (statistically) significantly related to the dependent variable(s) and are clinically and/or theoretically important, then multiple regression and/or analysis of covariance (ANCOVA) techniques should be used to test the hypotheses.

However, ANCOVA analysis is complicated, and its merits are controversial. The risks of finding statistical significance in nonsignificant findings increases with the number of variables. Therefore, caution should be used when deciding to carry out the search for covariables before testing the hypotheses or as an exploratory step in an effort to explain unclear findings after primary analysis has been completed.

It is not uncommon to find differences in how time and a covariable affects groups differently in response to the independent variable. Viewing findings with objectivity, creativity, and critical thinking helps discern the meaning of the patterns that emerge and address the question, "Why does A affect one group differently in the presence of B from the other group?"

Evaluating Intervention Consistency
It has long been a mark of rigor in laboratory studies to have objective data to describe and document the consistent application of the experimental manipulation. For example, continuous recording of room, incubator, or refrigerator temperatures is required for studies in which environmental temperature is an important experimental or intervening variable. However, such rigor has been lacking in nursing studies and in psychosocial intervention studies in a variety of other disciplines. This led to describing nursing studies as a "black box" experiment: Something was done, but it is not clear exactly what.

Dumas's (1963) study of the effect of preoperative nursing intervention on the incidence of postoperative vomiting is an example of one of the early nursing studies that did not rigorously control and systematize the experimental intervention. Although this landmark study was the first published study to demonstrate that preoperative nursing intervention made a statistically significant difference on patient outcomes, it was not known whether the findings were the result of a particular *process* of interaction, of the informational *content* of the communication, or of the investigator's charismatic *interpersonal style.* Knowledge about the specifics of the intervention is needed to replicate the study and, if the results are supported, to teach the intervention to others.

Subsequent studies sought to control the *content* of the instructional component of preoperative preparation for surgery by communicating structured information (Pranulis, Johnson, & Dabbs, 1975; Wolfer & Visintainer, 1975). However, the interpersonal style of the nurse delivering the intervention was not controlled. Johnson subsequently controlled and manipulated the content and the process of patient preparation for stressful events by using structured communication, prerecorded instructional materials that were presented to patients (Johnson, 1972; Johnson & Lauver, 1989; Johnson, Lauver, & Nail, 1989). Johnson's rigor in controlling and monitoring the consistency of the experimental intervention in repeated studies was instrumental in developing an empirically based, "self-regulating theory" that serves as a paradigm for research and clinical practice in preparing patients for stressful events.

In many clinical or experimental nursing interventions, more than one nurse performs the intervention. In studies of this nature it is important to have some method for evaluating the comparability of the interventions both between intervention nurses and by each nurse over time. Training of the intervention nurses, detailed protocols, and periodic observation/ supervision and retraining enhance consistency and rigor. For interaction studies randomly tape recording or video recording interventions and analyzing them help in evaluating consistency.

The internal validity of an intervention study is jeopardized when the intervention is not consistent (see Chapter 14 for threats to the study validity). The study's internal validity is suspect when intervention consistency is not documented. Even if there have been rigorous consistency checks, it cannot be stated without reservation that the intervention was responsible for any changes observed in the postintervention measures. The most that can be stated is that the hypotheses about the effect of the experimental manipulation (intervention) were either supported or refuted.

EVALUATING THE ADEQUACY OF THE DATA

Evaluating the adequacy of the data is carried out in three stages: (1) a priori determination of what constitutes a usable data set, (2) data processing, and (3) psychometric testing of data-collection instruments. Steps 1 and 2 are performed prior to data analysis; step 3 is carried out prior to testing hypotheses.

Usable Data

Incomplete data sets are a fact of research life even in the most rigorous studies. Unanswered interview or questionnaire questions, failure to follow instructions for recording or reporting data or ratings, incomplete medical progress notes or diagnostic tests, illegible handwriting, unintelligible audio- or videotaped data, and numerous other human, mechanical, or electronic failings contribute to this research nightmare. It thus behooves an investigator to anticipate such problems and to devise a plan—before beginning data collection—to avoid such pitfalls.

For standardized questionnaires, rating scales, and interview guides, the developer's instructions are the first recourse for deciding what constitutes "complete" data. For example, Maslach (1986) states that *all* questions on the Human Services Survey (measuring three components of burnout) must be answered for the questionnaire to be considered valid. Thus only complete questionnaires would be processed.

However, many instrument developers do not specify what constitutes an adequate level of completion. In this situation the investigator cannot make an a priori decision but must process the data, carry out psychometric testing, and rely on the results of the internal consistency analysis of the data set. In this event the first questions to explore are, "What is the level of internal consistency for this data set?" (this is discussed more fully in Chapter 14); "Is the internal consistency in this study similar to (consistent with) published reports?" If the instrument's internal consistency is lacking or differs from published reports, the investigator must explain the differences.

Second, address the following questions: "To what extent does each question/rating contribute to the total score?" "How and to what extent would the total score and the internal consistency be affected if the item were missing?" It is possible to use the data if the missing items are "filler" items and do not contribute significantly to the total score or affect the internal consistency of the instrument.

In order to derive scientifically sound meaning from the findings, an adequate data set is essential. Deriving interpretations from inadequate data (incomplete data or data lacking validity and/or reliability) is equivalent to relying on alternative methods of knowing rather than on the scientific method.

Data Processing

Preparing (coding) raw data for analysis, entering data on the computer, and proofreading data sets all require rigor in order to maintain the *integrity* of the data. A quiet environment is essential; errors occur even when distractions are minimal. Error rates also are affected by fatigue—general fatigue and fatigue from working at the computer, mental acuity, and mood state. Thus in addition to a conducive environment, a rested state and unaltered cognitive functions are important. The complexity of the coding and data-entry processes also affects accuracy. Statistical programs that require minimal or no coding of data reduce the probability of coding errors and facilitate proofreading.

There are a variety of methods for proofing the data set. The quickest and simplest is to run summary statistics for each variable. The results are first examined for the total sample size and the number of subjects for each group for each variable to check that no subjects were dropped. Then the actual range of scores is compared to the potential range based on the characteristics of the instrument. For example, if the scores on a pain-rating scale range from 0 (no pain) to 10 (worst pain imaginable), then the actual range of scores *must* fall between 0 and 10. A score in excess of 10 is an *outlier* indicating an error. The computerized data for that subject has to be verified against the raw data.

Although reviewing the summary statistics for each variable is an important step in preparing statistical analysis, relying solely on this method to determine the adequacy of the data is not enough to ensure accurate (error-free) data processing. For example, a computer-entered score can fall within the potential range of scores and still be transcribed wrong. It is easy to enter a score of "10" when the intended score is "01." Errors of this nature can seriously affect the mean scores and the outcomes of the other statistical tests.

Another method, especially when sample sizes and/or data sets are large, is randomly to select a sample of data to proofread against the raw data. It is possible for one person to proofread. However, it is most helpful to have two people proofing: One reads the computer printout of the data, and the other reads from the raw data. The most rigorous method for proofing is to have *all* of the data, rather than a randomly selected subset, double-proofed. Two people who did *not* enter the data into the computer compare the raw data to the coding sheets (if used) and to the hard copy of the data set.

Three criteria are used for evaluating the adequacy of the data *before and in addition* to psychometric testing: completeness, integrity, and accuracy. If these three criteria are not met, the results of the psychometric testing and of any subsequent analysis are questionable.

Psychometric Testing of Data Collection Instruments

As described in Chapter 14, data must be reliable and valid before any scientifically valid meaning can be drawn from or attached to the findings. Tests of internal consistency, stability over time for stable variables (test–retest reliability), and inter-rater reliability (when there is more than one data collector) provide information about the accuracy of the data. Content, construct, and predictive tests and other forms of validity provide information about the truthfulness of the data in relation to the variables, factors, or concepts of interest.

If, when tested, the data do not meet preassigned levels of acceptable reliability and validity, the investigator must ask the following questions: "Do the instruments adequately measure the phenomenon of interest?" "Are the instruments appropriate for the sample?" For example, some questionnaires developed in the United States may not be appropriate in another country because the cultures may be different. The reading abilities of the study subjects must also be consistent with the reading level required for using the instrument.

Additional questions include: "Is the phenomenon being studied stable or variable?" "How, to what extent, and under what conditions does the phenomenon vary?" Rigorous preparatory work when selecting instruments addresses these issues and helps prevent or overcome some of these problems. However, because science is self-correcting knowledge without absolutes, even the most rigorous instrumentation efforts may not address the new knowledge uncovered in a research effort.

Preparing and organizing the data for analysis and evaluating the adequacy of the data are cornerstones of rigorous research. These are time-consuming, tiresome, and often tedious tasks. However, attempting to test hypotheses and to find patterns and meaning in the findings is a premature—and often wasted—effort if the preliminary steps are not completed to satisfaction. Many researchers who have taken shortcuts and bypassed these steps have found that they must return to them after the fact, which is even more painful. Unfortunately, some have learned this lesson after presenting a paper or submitting a manuscript for publication.

FINDING AND/OR ASSIGNING MEANING

Being able to find meaning in the results of statistical analysis requires performing the appropriate level of analysis, objectivity, critical thinking, and creativity. The steps described in the preceding pages are re-

ferred to as *preliminary analysis* (or preparation for hypothesis testing). The next step, *primary analysis,* begins to yield results in the search for meaning.

For studies using a descriptive correlational or preexperimental design primary analysis and the search for meaning overlap with (and in fact consist of) the preliminary analysis and the exploration of summary statistics. For intervention studies using a quasi-experimental or experimental design, primary analysis involves testing the hypotheses after the summary statistics have been analyzed. If the investigator has carried out the primary analysis and met the basic assumptions underlying the statistical tests being used, then it can be assumed that the findings are ready for interpretation.

Exploring Statistically Significant Findings

The sequence for examining the findings is highly individualized. However, many investigators look first at the significance levels for the tests and highlight in some way those tests that are statistically significant (as determined by the pre-established alpha). However, the search for meaning does not stop with statistically significant findings. The next step is to reexamine the findings to ensure that the data did, indeed, meet the basic assumptions for the specific statistical test(s) and that the alpha and sample size provided sufficient power to detect differences. The investigator can have greater confidence that the statistically significant findings were not a result of chance under the following conditions:

1. The data did meet the assumptions.
2. The alpha and sample size provided sufficient power for avoiding a type I error (see Chapter 16).
3. The findings are consistent with, sup-

port, and/or expand theory and/or previous research.

4. The findings "make sense" or are understandable.

It is tempting to end analysis and interpretation when significant findings emerge, especially if the findings support the research hypotheses. However, doing so turns research into a mechanical and technical process (Meleis, 1992). The real challenge of research and scientific discovery of new knowledge lies in the next steps—reexploring the statistically significant *and* nonsignificant findings. In this step the investigator objectively and critically asks, "Why?" and "Why not?" for *every* finding that holds or was anticipated to hold statistical, theoretical, and/or commonsense (common knowledge gained through life experience) significance. This step merges with the next step, returning to theory (the conceptual framework underlying the study) and the literature.

The Role of Theory and of the Literature
Theory is a description and explanation of reality that facilitates predicting and controlling reality (Meleis, 1992). Theory provides a paradigmatic perspective about the phenomenon of interest, including assumptions, the types of questions that are appropriate for the paradigm, and the types of findings that are consistent with the paradigm. Study findings should be compared and contrasted with emerging/existing theory to facilitate uncovering explanations for the findings.

In a theory testing study the hypotheses are derived from theoretical propositions, and the findings should be consistent with and either support or illuminate the propositions. If the findings are inconsistent with or do not support the propositions, then the study *methods* (sample, unit of analysis, instruments, level, and methods of analysis), as well as the theoretical and study *assumptions,* must be objectively and critically reexamined for congruence between research and theory. The lack of supportive findings may result from errors in interpreting and applying the paradigm in research, flaws in the theory, or a combination of both. The investigator's critical thinking skills and objectivity are challenged extensively in this process.

If the study is theory generating or atheoretical (purely empirical), or if the findings are inconsistent with the theory on which the study was based, the findings should still yield propositions and hypotheses for future testing. The search for plausible explanations takes a two-pronged approach. First, the literature is reviewed, and the literature search is expanded. In this way the study findings are compared and contrasted with published reports of similar and/or related studies. When comparing the findings to theory, the investigator's critical thinking skills are used extensively. Second, the data are visually displayed, and the investigator's creativity is challenged.

Searching for Patterns: Displaying the Data
The use of scatterplots, contingency tables, line graphs, two- and three-dimensional models, diagrams, and other techniques for visually displaying data facilitates the demonstration of patterns or lack of patterns in the data. This provides an opportunity for the investigator to utilize creativity that has been developed, nurtured, and exercised, as described in the first section of this chapter.

One of the most productive ways to approach this effort is to "play" with the data. Sketching preliminary drafts of conceptual or statistical relationships, looking for patterns in scatterplots (likened to looking for shapes in clouds), and trying tables in one direction then another, all help discern spatial relationships, as well as separate foreground from background and light from shadow in the search for patterns and trends. When a possible pattern or trend emerges, the data are tested for "fit," that is, consistency and congruence. If a plausible explanation emerges, then the next step is to evaluate the importance and generalizability of the findings.

EVALUATING THE IMPORTANCE AND GENERALIZABILITY OF THE FINDINGS
Statistical and Clinical Significance
Two questions guide the objective evaluation of the importance of the findings: "So what?" and "Who cares?" (Smoyak, 1990). A finding may be statistically significant and bear little relevance for patient care. On the other hand, a statistically non-significant finding (because of sample size, small effect size, or inappropriate alpha) may have significant clinical impact. For example, the association between ice water ingestion and myocardial ischemia as measured by s-t segment displacement on the electrocardiogram may not be statistically significant; however, the occurrence of one major ischemic episode closely following ice water ingestion can have a significant impact on the patient experiencing it. This illustrates the difference between statistical and clinical significance (Kirchhoff, 1990).

Power and Error
It is difficult to overstate the importance of setting the alpha appropriately, obtaining a sufficiently large sample, and accurately estimating the effect size for enhancing statistical power to detect relationships and differences. Even with rigorous advance planning, it is important to review the findings and rerun a power analysis based on actual data. Doing so provides an esti-mate of the probability of a type I or a type II error in interpreting the findings (see Chapter 16 for a more extensive discussion). In clinical research it is always wise to err on the conservative side of interpreting the findings. The investigator must always consider what might happen if changes based on the findings are instituted and the findings are indeed inaccurate.

Cost, Quality, and Outcomes
The 1990s era of global economic problems demands that all research and health care innovations be evaluated in terms of cost, quality, and outcomes (NIH, 1992). Cost calculations should include both the direct and indirect costs of providing a service or intervention. Costs and charges may differ substantially within one health care facility and between facilities. Therefore estimates for the cost of all services/interventions should take into consideration time (costed out as actual time $\times$ hourly wages + pro-rated benefits, which include vacation, sick time, health insurance, and other benefits) spent by the researchers preparing, delivering the services, and engaging in follow-up activities. Cost estimates should also include purchasing costs for supplies and equipment, depreciation costs, and other overhead or administrative costs. The costs to the patient (e.g., in terms of time, special foods/clothes/environment, transportation) should also be considered. It should be noted that "cost" is differentiated from "charges" for services.

When evaluating two or more options, final cost should not be the only deciding factor. Quality and outcomes must also be considered. The short-term cost of a particular option may be more economical, but the long-term effect may not be as beneficial and may ultimately result in higher overall costs, such as rehospitalization.

Quality and outcomes indicators *that matter* need to be identified. This is a monumental task requiring the involvement, critical analysis, and consensus of groups of experts in the field. The National Institutes of Health, Agency for Health Care Policy and Research, is undertaking this task through a series of Patient Outcomes Research Trials (PORT) studies (NCNR, 1992). However, individual investigators can evaluate the importance of their findings by using techniques similar to those described.

Generalizability

If random sampling methods are used, there should be no *known* selection bias that prohibits generalizing the study findings to the population from which the sample was drawn. However, many studies rely on nonrandom or convenience sampling methods such as snowball sampling, representative sampling, proportional sampling, and other nonrandom methods. Both random and nonrandom sampling techniques may or may not yield a sample that is comparable to the target population. Thus the investigator must compare the characteristics of the study sample to the known characteristics of the target population (as described in the section on preliminary analysis) before meeting generalizability criteria. If the sample characteristics differ from any known influential antecedent variable, then generalizability is limited to the study participants. Even if the sample characteristics are similar to those of the target population, the investigator must use caution; it is not known whether and to what extent the sample might differ from the population on influential variables that were not measured.

IDENTIFYING IMPLICATIONS

No interpretation of study findings is complete until the implications of the study for theory, research, education, and practice (including health care delivery systems) are identified. A series of questions can be explored to facilitate this effort, as summarized in the following paragraphs. Identifying study implications is probably one of the greatest challenges to the investigator's objectivity and ability to divest ego involvement from the research. It is also a major challenge to the investigator's creativity (being able to envision something new) and critical thinking.

Theory

Some of the questions that help identify implications for theory follow. Did the findings support or contradict the theory on which the study was based? Did the findings add to or expand knowledge about the phenomenon of interest? Did the findings uncover contradictions or inconsistencies in the theory? Did the findings lend support to the assumptions underlying the theory? Did the findings suggest linkages between theoretical propositions? Between theories?

Research

Every study has implications for future research. Researchable questions emerge in at least four areas: existing knowledge base, measurement (instrument development and testing), developing or refining an intervention, and generalizability of the findings to other populations. By the time the investigator has reached the stage of interpreting the findings, it is easy to conclude that "the study needs to be replicated in other settings and with other populations." However, doing so short-circuits the flow of creativity. The best research ends with a greater number of questions and ideas for future research than the investigator envisioned when the study was initiated. No one researcher can undertake in one lifetime the number of projects that can result from a single well-conducted project. Therefore, in keeping with the scientific belief in the communal nature of knowledge, it behooves investigators to share the researchable questions and concerns that arise from their studies.

Education

As mentioned in the introduction, the research process does not end with personal discovery; scientific knowledge must be communicated (see also Chapter 27). Education is the process of communicating what is known. Thus all research has some implication for education: Are changes in the *substance* or *process* of generic professional education warranted? Are changes in specialty education warranted? What changes are desirable, needed, necessary? Do the study findings have implications for preventive health education, public education, patient education? What is the nature of the change, and what are the possible outcomes of not implementing the change? How would the educational change affect professional licensure and regulation?

Practice

Answers to the "So what?" and "Who cares?" questions addressed in analyzing the significance of the findings bear repeating to identify the study's implications for practice. In addition, questions that should be addressed include: What are the possible outcomes if changes in practice, based on the study, are introduced? What will (might) happen if no change is introduced? What is the potential impact on the patient, the patient's family or significant others, and society?

Testing Ideas

One of the underlying characteristics of scientifically generated knowledge is the belief that knowledge is communal. No one individual "owns" knowledge. In keeping with the spirit of this belief, investigators share ideas about the meaning of their findings with one another and "test" the extent to which their ideas "make sense." This scholarly exchange in which ideas are explored, challenged, and tested produces an energy that enables the visualization of trends and patterns that may not be patently obvious to the lone observer. It also produces a spirit of colleagueship that is priceless.

However, the rewards associated with the discovery of new knowledge (which include academic retention/promotion, patents, honorary recognition, and other financial rewards) often engender competition rather than cooperation among investigators. As a result, many investigators rush their findings to press before their findings or their interpretations of their findings are explored with others. This competition has resulted in the publication of erroneous (and at times fraudulent) findings, has created many ethical dilemmas, and has cast a shadow on the credibility of health care and biomedical research in the 1980s and 1990s.

EVALUATING THE INTERPRETATION OF THE FNDINGS

When reading a research report, the reader evaluates the researcher's interpretation of the findings by considering a series of questions (see box). These questions encourage the reader to think critically about how the interpretation of the data relates to the study's original intent. First, it is expected that a well-written report will include a logical organization of the findings, using appropriate statistics with tables and figures to show trends and a description of the study's sample. Second,

EVALUATING THE INTERPRETATION OF THE FINDINGS

1. Does the researcher organize the findings in a clear and logical fashion using the study's theory as a framework for presentation?
2. Does the discussion relate the findings to each hypothesis or research question?
3. Are tables and figures used to supplement and support the narrative report?
4. Is the presentation of the findings strictly a data-bound perspective?
5. Is there a clear association between the study's original purpose and the stated interpretation?
6. Are unexpected as well as expected findings discussed thoroughly?
7. Does the researcher identify the implications for theory, research, education, practice, and the health care delivery system?
8. Are the researcher's conclusions about the generalizability of the findings data-based?
9. Does the analysis of relationships enhance understanding and permit replication?

the adequacy of the data should be addressed through a discussion of the testing of each hypothesis. The presentation should be data-bound; i.e., it should be related closely to the actual data collected. Third, the researcher should find and/or assign meaning to the findings by associating the study's purpose with the final interpretation. Fourth, the researcher should evaluate the importance and generalizability of the findings in a way that facilitates replication and enhances understanding. Finally, the researcher should identify implications for theory, research, education, and practice.

SUMMARY

- Interpreting research findings requires creativity, critical thinking, and courage to challenge established explanations.
- The ability to interpret research results is enhanced by (1) regularly exercising personal creativity and critical thinking, and (2) developing a plan for data analysis prior to data collection.
- Creativity is the ability to look at the same thing others are looking at and see it differently.

- Creativity may be nurtured through the IPPET model of immersion, play, practice, exercise, and transfer.
- Critical thinking is a cognitive process of questioning, discerning discrepancies or inconsistencies, and identifying similarities or consistencies.
- The steps involved in interpreting research findings are (1) organizing the findings, (2) evaluating the adequacy of the data, (3) finding and/or assigning meaning, (4) evaluating the importance and generalizability of the findings, and (5) identifying the implications for theory, research, education, and practice.
- Organizing the findings involves examining the characteristics of the sample and population, looking for differences between groups, searching for covariables, and evaluating the consistency of the intervention.
- Evaluating the adequacy of the data includes determining the usability of the data, data processing, and determining the reliability and validity of the data.

- The search for meaning entails the exploration of both statistically significant and nonsignificant findings.
- Both statistical and clinical significance of the results must be considered; a finding that is statistically significant may have little relevance for patient care, whereas a statistically nonsignificant finding may have great clinical relevance.
- The characteristics of the study sample must be compared carefully to those of the target population to determine whether the results can be generalized to the population.
- The implications of the results for theory, research, education, and practice must be identified.

FACILITATING CRITICAL THINKING

Andersen, and Holland (1992) conducted a study to compare the patency of peripherally inserted central catheter (PICC) line in which one group was flushed with 10 units of heparin and a second group was flushed with 100 units of heparin. It was "hypothesized that 10 units of heparin would maintain the patency of the PICC line as effectively as 100 units" (p. 85). This retrospective study examined 46 patients in a home care environment. The tables on the following page present a summary of the data.

The researchers' conclusions are as follows: "Given the fact that this study was retrospective and uncontrolled, a statistical analysis was inappropriate; however, as a descriptive study, there appears to be evidence to support the original hypothesis. A controlled, blinded study must be performed to test the hypothesis statistically" (p. 84).

1. From the above synopsis, come up with alternative suggestions for interpreting the findings.

a. Compare the intent of the study to the discussion and interpretation of the findings. Are the findings within the context of the study? Can you think of alternative implications for this study? Does the discussion enhance understanding of the phenomena?

b. Examine the study's methodology and data analysis. Did the researcher's choice of methodology and data analysis influence the study results?

c. Look at the conclusions the researcher makes. What conclusions are drawn from this study? Based on the data presented, would you come up with the same conclusions?

d. Look for the implications related to nursing. Does the researcher discuss the implications for nursing related to theory, research, education, practice, and/or the health care delivery system?

e. Note the recommendations for further. Does the discussion promote replication through further research?

2. Listed are several research articles. Select one (or more) to read, then focus on the interpretation of the findings. Answer questions a thru e from question #1 as they relate to these actual research studies.

- Chen, H. (1994). Hearing in the elderly: Relation of hearing loss, loneliness, and self-esteem. *Journal of Gerontological Nursing, 20*(6), 22-28.
- Helberg, J. (1993). Patients' status at home care discharge, *IMAGE: Journal of Nursing Scholarship, 25*(2), 93-99.
- Koniak-Griffin, D. (1994). Aerobic exercise, psychological well-being, and physical discomforts during adolescent pregnancy. *Research in Nursing & Health, 17*(4), 253-263.

Summary Table of Patients Flushed with 100 μ/ml Heparin

	No. of Patients	Treatment Days	Average Treatment Days/Patient	Percent Days
Completed treatment	7	145	20.71	42.77
Clotted	2	18	9	5.31
Fell out	5	72	14.4	21.24
Pulled out by nurse				
Pain	2	5	2.5	1.47
Leaking	0	0	0	0
Phlebitis	0	0	0	0
Inability to tolerate	0	0	0	0
Infection	1	52	52	15.34
Expired	3	13	4.33	3.83
Hospital admission lost to follow-up	0	0	0	0
Replaced by Hickman catheter device	1	34	34	10.03
Still indwelling as of 3/1/91	0	0	0	0
Total	21	339	136.95	100

Summary Table of Patients Flushed with 10 μ/ml Heparin

	No. of Patients	Treatment Days	Average Treatment Days/Patient	Percent Days
Completed treatment	43	1188	27.63	61.81
Clotted	6	95	15.83	4.94
Fell out	4	45	11.25	2.34
Pulled out by nurse				
Pain	7	71	10.14	3.69
Leaking	4	86	0	4.47
Phlebitis	1	8	0	0.42
Inability to tolerate	0	0	0	0
Infection	0	0	0	0
Expired	4	66	16.5	3.43
Hospital admission lost to follow-up	4	44	0	2.29
Replaced by Hickman catheter device	0	0	0	0
Still indwelling as of 3/1/91	18	319	0	16.6
Total	91	1922	81.35	100

Reprinted with permission from Anderson, K., and Holland, J. (1992). Maintaining the patency of peripherally inserted central catheters with 10 units/cc Heparin. *Journal of Intravenous Nursing, 15*(2), 84-88.

- Melnyk, B. (1994). Coping with unplanned childhood hospitalization: Effects of informational interventions on mothers and children. *Nursing Research,* 43(1), 50-55.

References
SUBSTANTIVE
ANDERSEN, K., & HOLLAND, J. (1992). Maintaining the patency of peripherally inserted central catheters with 10 Units/cc Heparin. *Journal of Intravenous Nursing, 15*(2), 84-88.

DUMAS, R. G., & LEONARD, R. C. (1963). The effect of nursing on the incidence of postoperative vomiting. *Nursing Research, 12,* 12-5.

JOHNSON, J. E. (1972). Effects of structuring patient's expectation on their reactions to threatening events. *Nursing Research, 21,* 499-504.

JOHNSON, J. E., & LAUVER, D. R. (1989). Alternative explanations of coping with stressful experiences associated with physical illness. *Advances in Nursing Science, 1*(2), 39-52.

JOHNSON, J. E., LAUVER, D. R., & NAIL, L. M. (1989). Process of coping with radiation therapy. *Journal of Consulting Clinical Psychology, 57*(3), 358-364.

KIRCHHOFF, K. T., HOLM, K., FOREMAN, M. D., & REBENSON-PIANO, M. (1990). Electrocardiographic response to ice water ingestion. *Heart & Lung, 19*(1), 41-48.

PRANULIS, M. F., DABBS, J. M., & JOHNSON, J. E. (1975). General anesthesia and the patient's attempts at control. *Social Behavior and Personality, 3,* 49-54.

VON OECH, R. (1990). *A whack on the side of the head: How you can be more creative* (revised ed.) New York: Warner Books, Inc.

WOLFER, J. A., & VISINTAINER, M. A. (1975). Pediatric surgical patients and parents stress responses and adjustment as a function of psychological preparation and stress-point nursing care. *Nursing Research, 24*(4), 244-255.

CONCEPTUAL
BROOKFIELD, STEPHEN D. (1991). *Developing Critical Thinkers: Challenging Adults to Explore Alternative Ways of Thinking and Acting.* San Francisco: Jossey-Bass Publications.

MELEIS, A. I. (1992). On the way to scholarship: From master's to doctorate. *Journal of Professional Nursing, 8*(6), 328-334.

NATIONAL CENTER FOR NURSING RESEARCH (1992). *Patient outcomes research, examining the effectiveness of nursing practice.* Proceedings of the State of the Science Conference Sponsored by the National Center for Nursing Research, September 11-13, 1991. Rockville, MD: DPHS #93-3411.

WEBSTER'S NEW COLLEGIATE DICTIONARY. (1980). Springfield, MA: G & C Merriam Co.

METHODOLOGICAL
MASLACH, C. (1982). *Burnout—the cost of caring.* Englewood Cliffs, NJ: Prentice Hall, Inc.

MASLACH, C., & JACKSON, S. E. (1986). *Maslach burnout inventory manual,* (2nd ed.). California: Consulting Psychologists Press.

PRANULIS, M. F. (1993) "Creativity in Practice: A Race with Time." Unpublished keynote address presented at the *Seventh Annual Nursing Research Practice Conference,* co-sponsored by the Northport RMEC and the Northport Veterans Affairs Medical Center, Northport, L.I., New York.

SMOYAK, S. (1990). Personal communication, University of Utah College of Nursing.

HISTORICAL
CARPER, B. A. (1978). Fundamental patterns of knowing in nursing. *Advances in Nursing Science, 1*(1), 13-23.

SHERMIS, S. S. (1962). On becoming an intellectual discipline. *Phi Delta Kappa,* 84-86.

WATSON, J. (1981). Nursing's scientific quest. *Nursing Outlook, 29*(7), 413-416.

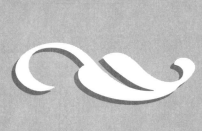

PART IV
THE QUALITATIVE RESEARCH PROCESS

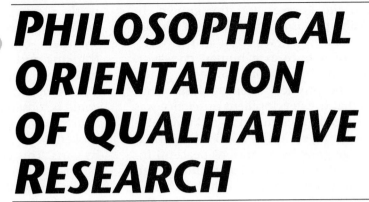

CHAPTER 19

PHILOSOPHICAL ORIENTATION OF QUALITATIVE RESEARCH

GERI L. DICKSON

Is the cosmos defined in terms of particles or in the terms of forces extending throughout space in fields? Are particles or fields the basic unit of all objects in the universe? For physicists the answer, which is critical to their research, depends on their scientific perspective. Do they subscribe to the basic assumptions and concepts of Newton or to those of Leibniz?

In the eighteenth century this metaphysical disagreement in physics created strains and tensions that are still noticeable in contemporary science. Isaac Newton's fundamental belief was in particles, that is, the atom and universal gravitation. Gottfried Leibniz believed that ordinary observable objects were not divisible into parts, but were the manifestation of underlying collections of force, that is, energy fields (Gale, 1979). These fundamental beliefs about the nature of physics not only colored and directed the experiments scientists conducted, they also shaped the knowledge gleaned from those experiments. This historical scenario illustrates how scientific discoveries are defined by a scientist's perspective.

Just as important today is the fact that the basic assumptions of research help to determine its questions, its methods, and the outcomes of knowledge. Any research is more than a method or methods; it is a system of inquiry based on a philosophical perspective, often called a world view. In this chapter the philosophical bases of nursing research are discussed to distinguish the differences between the underlying philosophical assumptions of research using qualitative or quantitative methods. The nature, applications, evaluation, and some issues surrounding research using qualitative methods also are addressed in this chapter.

HISTORICAL OVERVIEW: FROM A QUANTITATIVE TO A QUALITATIVE PERSPECTIVE

During the mid-twentieth century questions were raised in the scientific world about the philosophical bases of science, particularly the long-held belief in a value-free objective science created by distance

411

between the knower and the known. In 1970 Kuhn published his history of physics and introduced a new picture of the development of science as a human endeavor. Studying the history of knowledge generated in the physical sciences, Kuhn concluded that the development of science was not the steady accumulation of knowledge usually portrayed in the textbooks. Rather, knowledge grew by a series of peaceful interludes, called normal science, interrupted by intellectually violent revolutions when one conceptual world view was replaced by another. To illustrate this view of science, Kuhn originated the concept of paradigm, a unique view of the world that prescribes the nature and direction of science within the discipline. Any specific scientific community consists of people who function within a particular paradigm of knowledge (Kuhn, 1970).

Each specific paradigm gives rise to certain basic beliefs about what constitutes reality, about what counts as knowledge and creates a particular concept of the topic of study. These basic beliefs are not tested but serve as the starting point of the research. The basic beliefs are the assumptions of the paradigm. They provide a foundation—philosophical, theoretical, instrumental, and methodological—for the research and enable the researcher to see and interpret the world from one perspective rather than from another (Morgan, 1983). The beliefs of the paradigm structure the research questions to be asked and eliminate other questions. However, when the beliefs about reality change, the rules of the old paradigm no longer "fit," and the paradigm may be altered or abandoned entirely.

THE TRADITIONAL VIEW:
A QUANTITATIVE PERSPECTIVE

Research methods that arise from the traditional view of research in nursing have a quantitative perspective and rely on a world view consistent with beliefs of an empirical/analytical paradigm. Early in the twentieth century the dominant way of thinking and reasoning about science was based on objective data—the empirical. Valid empirical knowledge was that which could be observed with all the senses. To be analytic, the knowledge of the whole was broken down and known from the study of its parts. This view of science was advanced as detached from ethical and moral issues.

The roots of this world view of science began in the sixteenth century, when science was established as a separate and unique branch of knowledge, different from the prevailing paradigm of religion and ethics. During the eighteenth-century intellectual period known as the Enlightenment, this empiric form of knowledge was fostered and became known as the empirical/analytical paradigm of knowledge. This form of science often is referred to as positivism and in its most rigid form as logical positivism.

Certain beliefs or assumptions provide the foundation for the empirical/analytical approach to science, particularly assumptions about reality, theory, objectivity, control, causation, observation, prediction, and measurement (Allen, Benner, & Diekelman, 1986; Dickson, 1993). Cook (1983), a recognized expert in quantitative research, described these assumptions as "built on the supposition that an external world of objects exists, that these objects are lawfully interrelated and that the relationships are mediated by a real force in objects that is called causation" (p. 78). These beliefs naturally support the need for objectivity to give credibility to the scientist, for he or she is able to stand at a distance and through empirical study derive knowledge; "the knower can be completely differentiated from the known" (Allen, et al., 1986, p. 25).

This representation of science stresses

not only its general and systematic character but also its quantitative and experimental features. The advent of experimental and quasi-experimental studies (Campbell & Stanley, 1963) contributed the means to make the study of people the same as the study of the organisms of the natural sciences. Within this scientific paradigm, variables are distinct and analytically separate parts of an interacting system in which variables are presumed to be measurable independently of one another. Measuring and quantifying phenomena as distinct and analytically separate allows for statistical analysis with inferences about the whole drawn from these analyses of the parts. This approach is at the heart of quantitative modes of inquiry.

A DIFFERING VIEW: A QUALITATIVE PERSPECTIVE

To understand the emergence and use of qualitative methods, it is important to appreciate how and why they were developed in nursing. Modern nursing generally is accepted as beginning with the work of Florence Nightingale in the mid-nineteenth century. Because she had a substantial education and background in statistics and was a prolific writer, Nightingale is considered the first nurse researcher. By using statistics and her detailed pie-shaped graphs, Nightingale was able to demonstrate that nursing care made a difference in the lives of the sick and wounded British soldiers in the Crimea. When the Nightingale model of nursing and education came to the United States, nurses devoted their energies to education, licensure, and improving the life of their patients/clients.

Gradually, as these issues were resolved, nurses began to conduct research and to search for a means of reporting it. As a result the first nursing research journal, *Nursing Research,* began publishing in 1952. In the 1970s other research journals were established, but *Nursing Research* continues to be a major resource in the dissemination of nursing knowledge.

As nurses began to conduct clinical research, professional leaders strongly encouraged nurses to engage in science-based practice. At the same time nursing grand theories were being developed that were based on a philosophical position of wholeness. The focus of nursing moved away from the traditional disease/medical one and toward the person, and nurses cared for the person in all aspects, not just the physical body. Careful study and analysis of the empirical/analytical scientific paradigm and the holistic philosophy of nursing reveal basic incongruities, paradoxes, and conflicting ideologies. Although the assumptions of the empirical/analytical paradigm call for a reduction of the whole to a study of its parts, the nursing core philosophy is one of caring for the patient in all dimensions, not just the biomedical. By the 1980s the nursing literature began to reflect questions about these incongruities (Munhall, 1982; Tinkle & Beaton, 1983).

Munhall (1989) has described this reflective era of nursing science as an "interpretive turn," in which some nurse researchers began to think of nursing as a human science, different from the natural or social sciences. An increased interest and exploration of research methods appropriate for a human science based on the wholeness of the individual accompanied the "interpretive turn." "These research methods, although highly differentiated, have been grouped together and called qualitative to contrast them conceptually with the quantitative" (Munhall, 1989, p. 20). The philosophical underpinnings of these qualitative methods are based in a rejection of a cause-and-effect model, the experimental method, and a philosophical base of "universal laws" that is devoid of any sociohistorical context.

The next hurdle came in establishing a new paradigm. Although many of today's nurse researchers hold advanced research degrees in nursing, many of the earlier nurse researchers were educated in disciplines that used the scientific method based on the empirical/analytical paradigm. However, during the 1960s some nurses were exposed to a variety of methodologies more holistic than those found in the traditional paradigm. Approaches to knowledge such as those found in anthropology and the Chicago school of sociology were encountered by nurses.

Thus as the twentieth century wore on, the time was ripe for the development of a competing paradigm of science—one consistent with a core nursing philosophy of wholeness. Subsequently, qualitative research methods in nursing were formed. These scientific methods are suited to the everyday nursing practice of collecting subjective, qualitative data, as well as quantitative data, about clients. Qualitative data allow nurses to explore such phenomena as empathy, caring, suffering, restlessness, and hope, which are not easily segmented and measured.

A basic assumption underlying qualitative methods is the belief that people choose their reality by assigning meaning to the objective world (Benoliel, 1984; Tesch, 1990). Thus there can be multiple realities, not just one world with universal laws. Attempting to move beyond the individuals as a sum of the parts, the perceptions and experiences of individuals are valued, and their experiences are situated within a historical and social context. Terminology that has developed from this qualitative paradigmatic view of science includes *holistic, naturalistic, organismic, process-oriented, the lived experience, open system,* and *dynamic reality.* As such, the scientific paradigm that supports qualitative research methods offers a world view of

science that is congruent with nursing's larger world view of the discipline (Munhall & Oiler, 1986).

Benoliel (1984), instrumental in fostering the development of qualitative methods in nursing, identified qualitative approaches to science as "modes of systematic inquiry concerned with understanding human beings and the nature of their transactions with themselves and with their surroundings" (1984, p. 3). New paradigms require new lenses to view research, as well as new ways to conduct and to evaluate the process of research.

The development of new qualitative approaches to research in nursing may not constitute a paradigm shift, but it certainly has added a new paradigm to the research endeavor. Nursing's complex clinical problems require methods arising from more than one paradigm to answer the research questions that nurses have about people.

❧ THE NATURE OF QUALITATIVE RESEARCH

The human science paradigm from which qualitative methods arise is sometimes called a symbolic interactionist paradigm, because some methods historically have arisen from this philosophical view. The notion of a symbolic interactionist paradigm arise from sociology, whereby the belief is held that people negotiate their reality in interactions with others. To give a nursing perspective to this paradigm a better choice for naming the nursing scientific paradigm is the humanistic/holistic paradigm.

CHARACTERISTICS OF METHODS FROM THE HUMANISTIC/HOLISTIC PARADIGM

Although the methods of qualitative research in nursing may vary, they all share the following: (1) a world view that assumes multiple realities created by people, (2) a value placed on the perceptions and experiences of people, and (3) a recognition of the unique context from which the experience arises. Additionally, the focus of analysis in qualitative research is on words rather than on numbers. However, it is important to remember that it is not a technical question of whether to use statistics or words that drives one's choice of methods, but rather a decision based on one's beliefs about science and the formation of a research question.

Munhall & Oiler (1986) identified qualitative methods as legitimate aspects of the realm of science that lead to knowledge about people and their worlds. Although sometimes a research program of a particular phenomenon may begin with a qualitative study, no hierarchy of value of methods is implied in the choice. Most qualitative researchers do not hold the belief, sometimes expressed, that qualitative research may only be helpful as a preliminary step to developing quantitative information, but quantitative methods are preferred (Allen, et al., 1986). The selection of methods is most often based on answers to the question, "What do you wish to know?" and "What is your world view of reality?" Qualitative methods lead to knowledge generation and are scientific.

Qualitative research gained a degree of credibility when it became a subject heading in 1988 in the *Cumulative Index of Nursing and Allied Health Literature*. There qualitative studies are defined as "the non-numerical organization and interpretation of observations for the purpose of discovering important underlying dimensions and patterns of relationships" (*Cumulative Index*, 1988, p. 657). This definition emphasizes the aim of qualitative research, which is to discover meaning and understanding, rather than to verify truth or predict outcomes as in quantitative research. Al-

though qualitative researchers may count words or occurrences and report frequencies and characteristics of participants, inferential statistical analyses are not generally used.

Research *with* people, rather than *on* people, is a goal. In fact, experiential, collaborative research is frequently conducted. Research problems that are important, complex, and not amenable to "technical rationality" fit well with a qualitative approach. For example, phenomena responsive to qualitative study and that have been studied by nurses include the understanding of body experiences by healthy and chronically ill adults (Price, 1993), the patient's perceptions of suffering in a nursing home (Starck, 1992), the nurse's use of intuition (Agan, 1987), the meaning of empathetic nursing (Zderad, 1969), and living with an incurable disease (Meisenhelder & LaCharite, 1989).

Research from this perspective is conducted where the people are living and often is referred to as field research. This allows nurse researchers to get a picture of a phenomenon from the unique perspective of the patient/client. Some people call this type of research "naturalistic inquiry" (Lincoln & Guba, 1985).

Because the data are words or texts placed in the context of the particular research problem, the primary instrument of data gathering becomes the researchers themselves, rather than a questionnaire or a pencil-and-paper test. The research process is a human experience in which the researcher, instead of a computer, analyzes and collects the data. Interpretation of the data in both paradigms is a human endeavor; in the quantitative mode the researcher interprets the statistics, and in qualitative research the researcher interprets the meaning of the words.

A basic belief of the humanistic/holistic paradigm is that realities cannot be studied independently from their context, nor can they be separated into parts for study. The context, both social and historic, of each research problem is important. As Lincoln and Guba (1985) point out, a fundamental assumption is that "the very act of observation influences what is seen, and so the research interaction should take place with the entity-in-context for the fullest understanding" (p. 39). Understanding, based on the particulars of the contextual values, illustrates that the whole *is* greater than the sum of the parts.

A primarily inductive approach to data and theory building is generally used, rather than the hypo-deductive approach that begins with a theoretical perspective and hypotheses predicting the outcomes. In the inductive approach the data are allowed to "speak for themselves," and the analysis process progresses from the generalities of the data to the specific results of the study. This inductive process is more likely to identify the multiple realities found in the data and is able to identify the mutually shared influences that interact with the context.

DATA COLLECTION AND ANALYSIS

Consistent with the scientific paradigm and resultant methods, sample size is based on a nonprobabilistic approach. In fact, the use of the word "sample" implies that the subjects are representative of some larger population and does not clearly describe the participants in a qualitative study. The numbers of people studied is neither based on a belief in a normal distribution within a population, nor does it require a randomized or representative sample to produce the most reliable results. Inferential statistics are not used, and therefore calculating the sample size based on the power of the statistic is not required. Because the context is critical, each study's sample is based

on the number and type of participants necessary to gather as much information as possible about the topic, including all of the various ramifications and constructions (Lincoln & Guba, 1985).

With qualitative methods the number of participants selected for study is done with a purpose in mind. The idea of purposive or theoretical sampling is based on a belief that it increases the range of data exposed, "as well as the likelihood that the full array of multiple realities will be uncovered" (Lincoln & Guba, 1985, p. 40). Because data collection and beginning analysis are carried on simultaneously, it is possible to ensure maximum variation by choosing purposively differing experiences of the phenomenon. Although readers of qualitative research may identify with the findings, it is not the goal to make generalizations about the larger population based on probability and statistical inference from the research sample.

As the first data in a qualitative study are collected through interview or observation, they are analyzed and form the basis for further collection of data. The data collection continues until no new information is forthcoming. Therefore the number of participants is not determined in the proposal stage, but participants are added until saturation occurs. Because of their more active role in the research process, the people who are studied often are called informants, respondents, or participants rather than subjects.

✑ THE PURPOSES OF QUALITATIVE APPLICATIONS

In all kinds of research the purpose or the problem under study sets the direction for the research question, the type of research, and the analysis to be used. Knafl and

Howard (1984) in a landmark article identified four distinct purposes of qualitative research that can be linked clearly to the methods employed. They suggested that qualitative studies are designed to (1) describe a phenomenon, (2) sensitize others to the experience of a phenomenon, (3) develop research instruments, or (4) create a theoretical explanatory model. Others generally have suggested that qualitative approaches can be used to explore and describe as well as to discover and explain (Wilson, 1992).

Each purpose may require a slightly different qualitative approach to answer the questions posed by the researcher. Qualitative methods are a family of ways to collect and analyze phenomena of interest and include such techniques as grounded theory, phenomenology, hermeneutics, ethnography, case studies, and historical approaches. Broadly speaking, critical theory and feminist studies that use textual analysis are also qualitative studies. Sometimes a researcher may combine methods by using words as data along with a blended method of analysis, for example, combining ethnographic and phenomenologic methods. In addition, a study may have more than one purpose, which makes it difficult to use mutually exclusive categories for instruction. However, the purpose of the study, the research question, and the methods must be consistent with one another. The following examples of studies demonstrate research problems in which various qualitative methods have been used for different purposes. Some may fit into more than one category, but these examples give a good sense of when and how qualitative methods may be used.

TO GAIN A DIFFERENT PERSPECTIVE

One appropriate use of qualitative methods is to gain a new and different perspective when the existing quantitative methods do not capture the phenomenon under study. A classic example can be found in the work of J. Quint (later, Benoliel, 1966; 1967), who described the unique patient perspective of what it meant to be dying and what it meant to have a mastectomy.

The focus in Quint's (1963; 1967) qualitative research was different from that found in traditional studies. For example, in a study of women who had mastectomies, Quint (1967) reported that she was not concerned with mastectomy as a treatment procedure, but rather "with mastectomy as a significant personal event which initiated a series of reactions and actions, not only within and by the women themselves, but also within and by their personal associates and the personnel who staffed the hospital and clinic" (p. 111). Quint (1963) described these reactions and actions to mastectomy by identifying several categories of responses. They were Shock of the Unexpected, A Personal Social Loss, The Incision, The Uncertain Future, The Fear of Death, The Doctor, Is Any Woman Immune?, and Nurses' Reactions. These descriptive categories matched her purpose of describing the experience of a mastectomy from the point of view of the woman experiencing the surgery. Quint had studied with the grounded theorists, Glaser and Strauss, and was one of the first nurses to report studies in which she used qualitative methods.

Other more recent nursing studies that used qualitative methods to understand previously studied phenomena from a different perspective include those of Bowers (1987) and Dickson (1990). Bowers looked at intergenerational caregiving from the perspective of the persons involved in caring for their elderly parents. Bowers challenged the traditional empirical/analytical way of approaching this subject in which data are operationally defined variables that force conceptualization and analysis into discrete either/or categories. Instead, she used a qualitative approach to explore the meaning and to gain understanding of the experience of caregiving without violating the integrity or significance of the subjects' experiences by making them fit into the researcher's conceptualization of caregiving. This approach led to Bowers identifying a previously "hidden" aspect of care: protecting the elder's personhood by maintaining a reciprocal relationship between the caregiver and the elder in which the care of the elder was not the focus. This need for protection of the elder's self-esteem had a powerful influence on caregiving decisions, even if it resulted in withholding the most efficacious medical or physical care.

Dickson (1990), while attending to historical and social factors, studied experiences of the menopausal transition of midlife women. The traditional biomedical view of menopause today is one of a hormone-deficiency disease. Because the biomedical view is based on a linear, causal model of science and supports a view of women as hormone and reproductive systems, the scientific concept of menopause as a hormone-deficiency disease is logical. Hence, symptoms can be identified and measured; hormones can be prescribed to relieve the symptoms.

In contrast, Dickson (1990) approached the experiences of menopause within the context of women's lives beginning with a historical and social context. Using a qualitative textual analysis of the biomedical literature, she found that since the late 1880s the concept of menopause in the biomedical literature has changed from that of menopause as "a moral fault," to "involutional melancholia," to the current "hormone-deficiency disease." Using a post-structuralist interpretive framework, she compared the concepts of menopause found in the literature with those of contemporary women she interviewed. Although the women had expectations of experiences of menopause similar to that in the biomedical literature, they also had experiences that reflected a distinctly female point of view. In addition, Dickson (1990) made the following observations: the women encountered a variety of menopausal experiences; their experiences were often not acknowledged by physicians; women rarely talked to those close to them about their experiences; and women report experiencing life as the "other" or second, but not equal, sex.

Another example in which recent qualitative research has shed new light on nursing education is the work of Diekelmann (1992). She conducted interviews with nursing students and their teachers to analyze their words describing the experience of testing within the context of learning and teaching nursing. Diekelmann identified issues that may be used as the basis for further research or to help the discipline develop changes in educational practices.

TO DESCRIBE AREAS IN WHICH NOT MUCH IS KNOWN

Other studies use qualitative methods when they rely on in-depth descriptions of experiences about which little is known. For example, Wilson's work (1977) with schizophrenic patients resulted in a theory of "infracontrolling," which explained how social order was maintained in a milieu of espoused freedom. The study of life in an experimental community for mentally ill persons was an area about which little was known.

Another and more recent example is the work of Heidt (1990), who studied the experience of therapeutic touch with seven nurses and seven patients. Although few in number, previous studies of therapeutic touch had used experimental methods to test the effects of therapeutic touch on patients with specific health problems. Heidt used a qualitative approach, grounded theory, to study the experiences of the nurses who gave and the patients who received therapeutic touch. From the analysis of interviews and participants' observation, Heidt developed a theory explaining the process of therapeutic touch. The core variable in the process of therapeutic touch for nurses and patients in the study was opening to the flow of universal life energy. Three subcategories of opening were identified along with three themes describing the experience in each of the three subcategories.

Another example is the work of Aroian (1992), who developed the concept of social support as it was evidenced in Polish immigrants. She used an ethnographic approach to do a content analysis of immigrant interviews and field notes. The results of her study were used to develop preliminary guidelines for health care professionals and policy makers to decide when formal support may be needed to supplement the immigrants' natural networks.

A pioneer in using ethnographic methods in nursing research is Leininger (1966; 1984; 1991). She has been studying caring in various cultures since the 1960s. In a 1984 study she looked at the care and health values, beliefs, and practices of two subcultures in the southern United States: rural African-Americans and Anglo-Americans. Because specific interventions can be developed from the study, the results of her research are particularly helpful to nurses and may help the community as a whole maintain favorable health care practices.

Watson (1988) also studied caring using qualitative methods. Her method choice was phenomenology, which seeks the meaning or the "essence" of the experience. The reporting of such research can be very creative. After studying loss and caring experiences in the Aborigine community in the outback of Australia, Watson was moved to write a poetic expression of her findings (pp. 94-100).

Rather (1992) found little research available about the perceptions of registered nurses (RNs) returning to school to obtain a baccalaureate degree. Other researchers had looked at selected aspects of the return to school experience, but only one was found to explore the whole experience in the context of an RN's previous educational experiences. That research approached the study of RN students from the perspective of professional resocialization.

Instead, the goal of Rather's research was to understand the everyday experience as it was lived by the returning RN student. She interviewed 15 RN students about their perceptions and experiences of returning to school. She used a qualitative method called hermeneutics to interpret the students' interviews. The interviews, as in most qualitative methods, were tape recorded and transcribed to a written text for analysis. Rather identified common meanings and relational themes across the texts of the students. From these, Rather developed what is called "constitutive patterns" that express relationships between themes. She reported on the major finding of her research, which was the constitutive pattern of "Nursing as a Way of Thinking." It was important to the students to look at nursing as a thinking process rather than as merely gaining information. As a result, teaching methods used with traditional undergraduate students fail to facilitate the returning RN students' learning. A suggestion that came from the texts of the students' interviews was the idea of the teacher as consultant or coparticipant, rather than as an informer of nursing facts.

Another area in which little is known is that of the significant others of murder victims. Cowles (1988) conducted a grounded theory study of 12 survivors of murder victims. From her study she developed a substantive theory of personal world expansion. This presents a beginning understanding of the experience of grieving after such a trauma by the analysis of the actual reports of families and friends.

TO SENSITIZE HEALTH CARE WORKERS AND OTHERS

Qualitative methods also can be used in studies to sensitize health care providers to particular experiences of persons requiring nursing care. A classic qualitative study with this purpose is the work of Fagerhaugh and Strauss (1977) regarding pain management. Fagerhaugh and Strauss used the grounded theory method in a field study in several clinics and hospitals to observe, interview, and generally study who got pain medication and why they received it. From the study they developed a substantive theory about pain interactions. The theoretical constructs that emerged from the study were assessing, legitimizing, and relieving pain. These were placed in the context of organizational setting, political processes, and the disease-oriented ideology of the hospitals. The results of this study were used to sensitize health care workers to their role in the dynamics of pain management.

Another area in which greater sensitivity is a concern is that of schizophrenics living in the community. The schizophrenic adult often appears normal, but is unable to hold a job and develop independence. Therefore for some individuals the need for parenting continues. In a qualitative study of parents continuing to care for adult schizophrenic children, Chesla (1991) found that parents coping with the extreme breakdowns in expectations for their children and themselves had to find new meanings and practices to continue their parenting. She identified four distinct forms of parents' caring practices: "engaged care, conflicted care, managed care, and distanced care" (p. 454). An additional outcome of this work was that the family behavioral patterns of these four forms of caring were identified. As a result the study findings may help nurses and others understand and assist with nursing strategies for families to engage in satisfying parenting of a seriously mentally ill offspring.

Some contemporary problems demand new sensitivity and understanding. A study by Gregory and Longman (1992) about the suffering of mothers whose sons had died from AIDS gives a poignant message about suffering. This study allows nurses to understand the daily struggle of living with AIDS and how each mother "was faced with the intrapersonal and socially constructed metaphors and meanings of AIDS" (p. 353).

TO DEVELOP A RESEARCH INSTRUMENT

Quantitative study often presupposes qualitative study of a phenomenon, even if it is a study of the literature. A research program may be developed that begins with interviews and observations of potential subjects in the field and moves on to test hypotheses in a quantitative way. A classic example of this approach is found in the work of Kramer (1968; 1969) and the experiences of baccalaureate graduates in their first hospital jobs. Her studies began with direct observation in "natural" settings where she interviewed various participants. From the field study "propositions and hypotheses emerged which were subsequently tested" (Kramer, 1969, p. 198). Based on the testing of the propositions and hypotheses, Kramer developed an instrument to measure the nurses' responses to their first hospital job. From that data Kramer went on to generate the theory, Reality Shock, about new graduates' first experiences in the workplace. She proposed a bicultural approach (combining the school and the hospital culture) to resolving the tensions between what the new graduate learns in nursing school and what is experienced in the hospital.

Another example of qualitative work used as a basis for instrument development is the work of Miller (1985; 1988) and the concept of hope. A qualitative research study of the perspectives of hope of 59 persons who were survivors of a critical illness contributed to understanding the key elements of hope. From their responses and the literature, the instrument—The Miller Hope Scale—was constructed. Miller continues to work on this concept.

TO CREATE A THEORETICAL EXPLANATORY MODEL

In a study of couples and infertility Blenner (1990) identified a theoretical model to explain the process of coming to grips with infertility. Blenner explored the perceptions of 25 couples as they underwent infertility assessment and treatment. Using a grounded theory method, she developed a substantive theory about each couple's passage through infertility treatment. A substantive theory identifies a core psychosocial process from which to develop a model to explain what is happening. Blenner identified three concepts and eight stages that couples go through when dealing with infertility. These processes are helpful in planning nursing interventions with couples experiencing infertility.

In a study of women facing breast cancer surgery, Pierce (1993) describes the decision-making process and provides the empirical grounding from which to generate a theoretical framework for more structured research. Forty-eight women who were confronted with making the decision about treatment choices, lumpectomy (followed by adjuvant therapy) or mastectomy, were interviewed after diagnosis but before treatment. The interviews were tape recorded and transcribed to textual data. The narrative materials were sorted and coded according to the constant comparative method of analysis of grounded theorists Glaser and Strauss (1967). Based on five indicators of decision-making behavior, three styles of decision makers were identified: deferrer, delayer, and deliberator. Nurses may use this knowledge of decision making "in understanding the decision behavior of patients confronting health care choices" (p. 17).

TO DESCRIBE THE EVERYDAY EXPERIENCES

Most recently, increasing numbers of phenomenological studies have begun to appear in nursing journals. These studies look at the everyday experiences of persons who are or who may become patients/clients of nurses. The lived experience of the phenomenon is studied by the researcher from the perception of the patient/client. Prior to these studies not much was known from the experience of the patient/client about such topics as postpartum depression (Beck, 1992), the "inner strength" of women (Rose, 1990), and the human quality of nurses as persons (Taylor, 1992). In addition, nurse theorists Rosemary Parse (1990) and Margaret Newman (1992) are developing phenomenological qualitative methods that are consistent with their theories.

A review of nursing journals reveals that qualitative studies in nursing are increasing

Table 19-1
Examples of Qualitative Research by Primary Purpose

Purpose	Author	Title	Publication
To gain a different perspective	Quint (1967)	The case for theories generated from empirical data.	*Nursing Research*
	Bowers (1987)	Intergenerational caregiving: Adult caregivers and their aging parents.	*Advances in Nursing Science*
	Dickson (1990)	A feminist poststructuralist analysis of the knowledge of menopause.	*Advances in Nursing Science*
To describe areas in which not much is known	Wilson (1977)	Limiting intrusion—Social control of outsiders in a healing community.	*Nursing Research*
	Heidt (1990)	Openness: A qualitative analysis of nurses' and patients' experience of therapeutic touch.	*IMAGE*
	Aroian (1992)	Sources of social support and conflict for Polish immigrants.	*Qualitative Health Research*
	Leininger (1984)	Southern rural black and white American lifeways with focus on care and health phenomena.	*Care: The essence of nursing and health* (pp. 133-159).
	Watson (1988)	*Nursing: Human science and human care.*	(Book)
	Cowles (1988)	Personal world expansion for the survivors of murder victims.	*Western Journal of Nursing Research*
	Rather (1992)	"Nursing as a way of thinking"—Heideggerian hermeneutical analysis of the lived experience of the returning RN.	*Research in Nursing and Health*
To sensitize health care workers	Fagerhaugh and Strauss (1977)	*The politics of pain management.*	(Book)
	Chesla (1991)	Parents' caring practice with schizophrenic offspring.	*Qualitative Health Research*
	Gregory and Longman (1992)	Mothers' suffering: Sons who died of AIDS.	*Qualitative Health Research*
To develop a research instrument	Kramer (1968)	Role models, role conceptions, and role deprivation.	*Nursing Research*
	Miller (1985)	Inspiring hope.	*American Journal of Nursing*
	Miller and Powers (1988)	Development of an instrument to measure hope.	*Nursing Research*

Table 19-1—cont'd
Examples of Qualitative Research by Primary Purpose

Purpose	Author	Title	Publication
To create a theoretical explanatory model	Blenner (1990)	Passage through infertility treatment: A stage theory.	*IMAGE*
	Pierce (1993)	Deciding on breast cancer treatment: A description of decision behavior.	*Nursing Research*
To describe everyday experiences	Rose (1990)	Psychologic health of women: A phenomenological study of women's inner strength.	*Advances in Nursing Science*
	Beck (1992)	The lived experience of post-partum depression: A phenomenological study	*Nursing Research*

in number. An interdisciplinary journal with a nurse-researcher editor, *Qualitative Health Research,* is devoted to health research using qualitative methods. Table 19-1 summarizes the range of studies used as examples in each of the categories of purposes of nursing research: to gain a different perspective, to describe areas in which not much is known, to sensitize others, to develop a research instrument, to create a theoretical explanatory model, and to describe an everyday phenomenon from the participant's perspective. Most of nursing's research journals are represented in this table, but a review of the recent literature shows that *Advances in Nursing Science, IMAGE: Journal of Nursing Scholarship,* and *Qualitative Health Research* publish most of the nursing qualitative studies. Because of a page-length restriction on manuscripts in most journals and the bulk of textual data generated in qualitative research, sometimes a book-length report is better suited than a journal article. A prime example is the qualitative study done by Benner (1984) of nurses and their practices. Her phenomenological study became the well-read book *From Novice to Expert* (1984).

METHODOLOGICAL ASSUMPTIONS IN QUALITATIVE RESEARCH

The various methods of qualitative research arise from the same basic philosophical orientation of the research paradigm. The methods, however, can be considered a family of methods with each having a somewhat different set of assumptions accompanying the method of analysis. The methodological assumptions might be compared to those of the different methods in quantitative research, such as experimental or quasi-experimental studies, correlational methods, and multivariate analysis. Each has a somewhat different set of assumptions underlying the method of analysis, but arises from the larger empirical/analytical paradigm.

Some of the research methods, such as grounded theory or phenomenology, call for the researcher to suspend any prior theoretical commitments or at least to make explicit and put aside assumptions about the phenomenon under study. Nevertheless, these two methods do not require the researcher to remain uninformed about the relevant scholarship in the area nor to ignore the theoretical orientation of the discipline of the researcher (Sandelowski, 1993). Certain assumptions inherent in nursing will shape the researcher's thinking in regard to the phenomenon under study. These disciplinary assumptions should be consistent with the method of inquiry. For example, in nursing the core philosophical view is that of the wholeness of the person as client of the nurse, and research should not try to fragment the wholeness.

In addition, a researcher may use a particular nursing theorist as a basis for a study, and that theory will provide a direction for data collection and interpretation. However, nursing theorists are not the focus of discussion here. Refer to nursing books devoted to theorists and their theories for such a discussion.

Information regarding the designs of qualitative studies can be found in Chapter 20, but the assumptions and use of particular qualitative methods most frequently found in the nursing literature will be discussed here: grounded theory, phenomenology, hermeneutics, ethnography and ethnoscience, and case study.

GROUNDED THEORY

In grounded theory the goal is to conduct empirically grounded research on a particular topic that will lead to a theory about the topic of study based on the participant observations and interviews of the researcher and participants. The data are words, that is, the texts of the interviews and the researcher's log of observations. Analysis of the words is done concurrently with the collection of data. In fact, the analysis of data provides the direction for further sampling to occur. Often, the direction of the research develops as the study is under way, and this is sometimes called an emergent design.

In their work on pain management, Fagerhaugh and Strauss (1977) explained how that research evolved out of previous research on the care of the terminally ill in hospitals. This earlier work provided the beginnings of a substantive theory or a theoretical perspective about pain management. The earlier work led to a number of hypotheses about assessing, legitimizing, and relieving pain that were qualified in the new work on pain management. One goal was to extend a previous line of theorizing. Another goal "was the practical application of this research, for effective theory should have both immediate and long-range applicability" (p. 305). The short-range goal was the sensitization of health care workers, and the long-range one was to develop further hypotheses regarding pain management.

A current example of a grounded-theory nursing study is the work of Sohier (1993). Her study explicated the grieving process in the parents of gay men dying from AIDS. Interviews were conducted with gay men and their biological parents. Participant observation occurred during support groups for parents and sons. Sohier described the evolutionary process in the emerging theory, the major conceptual categories, and the concept indicators confirming the major concepts. The major conceptual category was "Gaining Awareness." The conceptual indicators were Suspicioning, Challenging, and Confronting. Positive, neutral, and negative strategies used by the parents were identified. The parents who were able to develop a satisfactory solution to the moral questions surrounding homosexuality were able to achieve a meaningful closure with their gay sons. Only five out of 54 parents were able to achieve this meaningful closure: filial reconstruction.

PHENOMENOLOGY

Phenomenology is both a philosophy and a method. As a method it is the study of phenomena, the appearance of things

(Cohen, 1987). The focus of study is on the practical world of the "lived experience," from the perception of the person experiencing it. The subject matter of phenomenology, with the goal of describing and understanding, is on human responses such as pain or courage to such experiences as cancer or perinatal loss. An assumption is made that people know and can talk about their experiences and the meaning of those experiences in their lives.

History usually credits German philosophers Husserl (1859-1938) and Heidegger (1889-1976) with being the originators of the movement. The philosophical roots have varied over time, even within the lives of the originators between their earlier and later works. The development of phenomenology grew out of critique of the science-based realism, objectivity, and overwhelming focus on the empirical in the empirical/analytical kind of science. Phenomenology developed out of a concern for the experience and its meaning for people rather than the measurement of behavior and determination of the laws of science.

The German philosophers had an impact on French philosophers who continued in the phenomenological tradition. Breaking with the positivists, the phenomenologists remained interested in studying meaning and existence. Two French philosophers, Sartre and Merleau-Ponty, played major roles in the development of phenomenology. The focus of phenomenology became the person, a being-in-time, in his or her world. A branch of psychology began to use this philosophy in practice. In clinical practice they began seeing patients as they really are and knowing them in their own reality (Cohen, 1987). Nurse theorists, particularly Paterson and Zderad (1976) and Watson (1979; 1988), espouse values consistent with existential phenomenology. These values include viewing the person as a human evolving, as a person in a particular important context, at a particular time, and with an identifiable interaction between researcher and researchee.

Several phenomenologists have developed methods that nurses have used. For example, nurse researchers have found useful the phenomenological methods of Giorgi (1970), Colaizzi (1978), and van Manen (1990). Giorgi and Colaizzi, in particular, have been used by a number of nurses. Some examples of Giorgi's phenomenology in nursing studies include Rose's (1990) study of women's inner strength, a study of the experience of caring by Forrest (1989), a study of the drive to be thinner by Santopinto (1989), and of living with addiction by Banonis (1989). The work on the experience of postpartum depression by Beck (1992) and the following study by Price (1993) are examples using Colaizzi's method.

Van Manen's work has been used as the phenomenological basis for studies about women in an anthology edited by Munhall (1994). Twelve nurse researchers studied the everyday world of women at various stages in life. Mothercare, abuse, menopause, anger, and chronic illness are some of the experiences seen through the eyes of women.

Price (1993) explored the understanding and meaning that healthy and chronically ill adults have about their body experiences. This study provides clinical significance for nursing because it revealed not only the existence of symptoms but also of a body as a whole

> that is inherently understood, always ready-to-hand, and that forms the basis of personal body explanation. Such, in turn, determines the range and type of possibilities for health maintenance or restoration and what the individual sees as "me." (p. 50)

This concept of body listening and body awareness is considered by nurses to establish care plans that address the possibilities individuals hold for themselves. A method closely related, philosophically, to phenomenology is that of hermeneutics.

HERMENEUTICS

Through the work of Martin Heidegger (1889-1976) in the phenomenological movement, hermeneutics moved into a position central to European philosophy. It too is based on a view of science as a human science. Hermeneutics are based on the interpretation of a text. It can be such written texts as the Bible or in modern times the interviews of a nurse researcher. It is an interpretive method and moves beyond knowing to really understanding a phenomenon.

There are different philosophical positions that rely on the interpretation of texts called hermeneutics. Many nurse researchers have done studies using Heideggerian hermeneutics. The most well known of these is the work of Benner (1984) and her model of nursing practice, *From Novice to Expert.* She observed and listened to nurses at all levels of experience tell their stories of nursing. From these she developed exemplars and paradigm cases to illustrate each of the five levels a nurse goes through in becoming proficient in practice, according to the Dreyfus and Dreyfus model of skill acquisition. In addition, she created seven domains of practice from the data. These domains recognize the knowledge embedded in nursing practice.

A somewhat different perspective on hermeneutics is that of critical hermeneutics. This arises from the continental style of critical theory that has as its goal to uncover hidden practices that may oppress people (Allen, 1985). A critical hermeneutic study of the language used to describe, explain, and interpret the concept of nursing

process in introductory nursing texts was conducted by Hiraki (1992). She used a theoretical framework that combined the hermeneutics of Ricoeur (1983) and the critical social theory of Habermas (1971). This was helpful in making explicit the "cultural and political meanings hidden in the taken-for-granted metaphors used to describe the nature of nursing care and what constitutes nursing knowledge for beginning nursing students" (p. 1). Hiraki concluded that the language in the textbooks portrayed a technical, rational view of nursing care. Educators may find these results helpful in planning curricula that focus on the professional development of nursing practice.

ETHNOGRAPHY AND ETHNOSCIENCE

Ethnography is a qualitative method that uses participant observation and interviews of key and general informants as the source of the data. The focus of ethnography is the social and cultural world of a particular group of people. It grew out of anthropology and the study of culture, usually in cultures foreign to one's own. According to Spradley (1980), the central aim of ethnography is to describe a way of life different from the native point of view. A belief underlying ethnography is that the behavior of people can only be understood within the cultural context in which it occurs (Omery, 1988). This differs from phenomenology, which focuses on the meaning of the experience rather than on the role of culture in shaping the experience.

Ethnoscience is the systematic study of nursing and phenomena of interest to nurses that was developed by Leininger (1985). In this instance the culture is that of nursing in hospitals or other settings, wherever nursing is practiced. An example of an ethnoscience study is the work of Gates (1991) in a study of dying cancer patients. She conducted interviews with general informants such as nurses, other care providers, family members, and visitors, as well as with the key informants, the patients who had been diagnosed with terminal illness. Field notes based on observations also were included in the data. The data were studied and analyzed following Leininger's three phases of reviewing, coding, and classifying data to develop descriptors and patterns of care and cure from the descriptors. These patterns of care and cure are helpful to nurses in caring for dying patients.

Another ethnoscience study from a cultural point of view was done by Nikkonen (1992) with psychiatric patients in Finland. Although observation provided data, the patients and members of the staff also were interviewed. Over time four stages of caring for the group of patients were identified from the data: formation, reformation, fragmentation, and reintegration. These stages related to the changes observed in the ward during the time of the study, which occurred over a span of 11 years, 1977 to 1988. A stable and mature staff was identified as an important factor in the patients' recovery.

CASE STUDY

The case study method is not a new use of research. In fact, some of the most durable and influential theories have been developed through the use of case studies of patients, namely, the theories of Freud and Piaget. Both used the case study method with a small number of people from whom they developed their theories of ego development and child learning.

The qualitative case study comes from a holistic perspective. "That is, investigators use a case study design in order to gain an in-depth understanding of the situation and its meaning for those involved" (Merriam, 1988, p. xii). The general philosophical underpinnings of the qualitative paradigm with the focus on meaning in context is the methodological assumption of the case study method.

An example of a nursing qualitative case study is the work of Yuen (1991). The primary concern of the researcher was the effect of the hospital learning milieu on the first-year graduates' awareness of the need for ongoing education. Four case studies were conducted in four different clinical settings. Each area in the clinical setting was observed for a total of 4 hours a week with particular reference to the first-year nurse graduate's learning behavior. For nurses to develop a concept of lifelong learning, the investigator found that (1) there must be a well-planned learning program, and (2) there must be a supportive clinical learning environment. Good programs without support of the unit managers did not succeed in fostering learning. Also, if nurses are to develop a desire to continue to learn, they must have the freedom to test or apply significant new knowledge in their work situations.

✎ EVALUATION OF QUALITATIVE STUDIES

The assumptions underlying the humanistic/holistic research paradigm are different. The research questions and methods of qualitative research are different from those found in the empirical/analytical paradigm. It follows then that the evaluation measures should also be different. Although evaluation is a focus of Chapter 23, there are some general, helpful guidelines that are gaining acceptance in evaluating qualitative studies. These are summarized in the box.

PHILOSOPHICAL AND METHODOLOGICAL CONSISTENCY

The first thing to consider when evaluating qualitative studies is whether philosophical

---

EVALUATING QUALITATIVE STUDIES

1. Are the philosophical and methodological assumptions of the study congruent with each other?
2. Are the results of the study credible?
3. Can the results of the study be transferred to another context? Does the descriptive data contain enough detail to allow for this?
4. Are the researcher decisions documented sufficiently?
5. Was the study conducted in an ethical manner?

---

and methodological assumptions of the study are congruent. This means that the assumptions underlying the research must be consistent with those of the humanistic/holistic paradigm, and the method and its assumptions must be consistent with what the researcher wants to know. The philosophical paradigmatic assumptions include a belief in multiple realities, the importance of the context of a phenomenon, a noncausal model, the experiences of people, and analysis based on words rather than numbers. In addition, the assumptions of the method selected should be consistent with the research questions. For example, if a researcher is looking for an explanatory model of a particular phenomenon, a grounded-theory study would be appropriate. If the goal is to understand the experience of living with pain from the perception of a person with chronic back pain, a phenomenological study would be the right choice.

The traditional forms of evaluating validity and reliability do not apply in qualitative research. The threats to internal and external validity (Campbell & Stanley, 1963), which lie at the heart of quantitative evaluation, do not apply here. Yet means of evaluating qualitative studies have been identified that are different from the techniques used to evaluate experimentally designed or correlational studies.

TRUSTWORTHINESS

In qualitative research the idea of validity and reliability that has gained the most acceptance among all researchers is the concept of trustworthiness developed by Lincoln and Guba (1985). Rodgers and Cowles (1993), qualitative nurse researchers who incorporate and build on Lincoln and Guba's ideas, recently wrote about the use of documentation in allowing for evaluation of qualitative studies.

The concept of trustworthiness includes credibility, transferability, dependability, and confirmability (Lincoln & Guba, 1985). In dealing with credibility the goal is to increase the possibility that the research will produce credible results. Lincoln and Guba suggest that one way to enhance credibility is through prolonged engagement in the field or with the participants in the research. Prolonged engagement also leads to the identification of contextual factors that might impinge on the phenomenon under study (Lincoln & Guba, 1985). Another technique, member checks, also increases the credibility of a study. This process involves checking with or getting feedback from the participants to ensure that the researcher has captured their words and their meaning by "playing back" to them the interpretations of the data. Agreement by the participants validates the researcher's interpretation. If the participants do not agree, the researcher must make the necessary changes or supply logical justification for the interpretation of the data.

Transferability is the ability of others to use your results; that is, the results can transfer to another context. One way to build this process is to have a rich, "thick" description of the phenomenon. This means that not just any descriptive data will do, but the data should provide for the widest possible range of information for inclusion in the thick description (Lincoln & Guba, 1985). The specifics of what constitutes a rich, thick description have not been fully identified by Lincoln and Guba, but purposive sampling continues until no new information is obtained. At that time, with careful analysis, a description of considerable depth and breadth should be possible.

The specifics of dependability, although referring to the dependability of the inquiry, are not well spelled out by Lincoln and Guba (1985). Some suggestions include having at least two researchers who can examine the process and the product of the research. However, it is suggested that dependability and confirmability may occur simultaneously. Confirmability is described as the process of developing an audit trail of the researcher's decisions. This allows others to observe the rationale for choosing participants, for interpreting the data, and how the issue of trustworthiness was addressed. To greatly enhance the research, particularly with novice researchers, an experienced qualitative researcher may examine the data, notes, and log of the researcher to validate the decisions.

DOCUMENTATION OF THE RESEARCHER DECISIONS

Rodgers and Cowles (1993) outline how to document researcher decisions and conduct an audit. They cite four areas (contextual, methodological, analytical, and personal) in which documentation will provide the data for completing an audit. The first is contextual documentation, which relates to the field and to the field notes of the researchers. Second is the documentation of all of the methodological decisions made throughout the study. The process of keeping memo notes related to the researcher's decisions as the study progresses is important for the dependability of the study.

The next source of documentation is the analytic notes, which are kept during the process of "sorting, categorizing, and comparing data and in conceptualizing patterns that emerge as the data are examined and coded" (Rodgers & Cowles, 1993, p. 222). The analytic notes reflect the researcher's thought processes in making analytic decisions. The last source of documentation is a personal log. The log is based on the researcher's reflection on collecting and analyzing data, as well as developing self-awareness of any personal biases and strategies for maintaining "neutrality" (Lincoln & Guba, 1985). Rodgers and Cowles also suggest that the log can be used as a means of catharsis, that is, to discharge feelings and recount difficulties encountered as a result of intense engagement in the research process.

These recommendations are the beginnings of a new means of evaluating qualitative studies. Researchers need to pay attention to finding a system that works for them to provide documentation for all of the above areas. It is important to write as soon as possible after each event and not rely on memory to record later. Rodgers and Cowles (1993) point out that "the more descriptive, detailed, and candid the notes are, the more they enhance the rigor of the study" (p. 225). That is what trustworthiness of qualitative studies is all about—enhancing the rigor of the study.

⟡ SOME ISSUES IN QUALITATIVE RESEARCH

Research in nursing is a relatively new venture, dating back to the mid-twentieth century. Qualitative research is a still younger enterprise with articles appearing in nursing journals since the late 1960s. Most of the research methods used now have been borrowed from other disciplines. As attempts are made to develop a method that captures the holistic focus of nursing—and that is unique to nursing—debates about the emerging qualitative methods are found in the literature. Several issues related to conducting studies of this design will be identified and discussed here.

REVIEW OF THE LITERATURE

An area often debated by nurse researchers is the use of the literature in qualitative research. However, there is agreement that the type of tight literature review that supports and defines the variables of choice, as done when using quantitative methods, is not done when conducting qualitative research. Some qualitative researchers believe that a literature review should be done first to provide justification for the study and to place it in context. Others think a comprehensive review of related literature is necessary to produce a scholarly document. Another point of view often shared is that after the study is completed the findings of a study should be examined in relation to the existing literature of the topic of study (Burns, 1989).

Some of the grounded theorists, such as Glaser (1978), recommend that the literature not be reviewed prior to entering the field as it may mislead or distract the researcher. Using this approach, the review of the literature is done after the findings of the study have been generated—this is the substantive theory. Then the theory

can be placed within the context of the literature and what is known about the topic.

The literature approach most often supported by qualitative researchers is to examine the relevant literature and to selectively use this work. The literature often is carefully "examined for explicit and implicit assumptions, for biases in measurement and unsubstantiated conclusions" (Field & Morse, 1985, p. 35). Generally, the literature review in a qualitative study supports the study and provides the rationale for the choice of method in studying the phenomenon. Besides providing the prevailing view of the phenomenon under study, the literature provides the historical and social context of the study.

In addition, after the study is completed, Burns (1989) suggests the findings should be situated in relation to the existing body of knowledge about the topic of study. The implications for nursing practice and further research are generated from the examination and discussion of the results of the study in comparison with other knowledge found in the literature.

METHODOLOGICAL TRIANGULATION

Researchers in nursing often debate the issue of whether one can combine methods from a paradigm that supports qualitative research with quantitative methods from an empirical/analytical paradigm. Using different methods in one study is called triangulation of methods. The purists insist that because the underlying world views are different, the methods cannot be mixed (Allen, et al., 1986; Powers, 1987). Others state that different methods may be mixed, or triangulated, in the same study to fully explicate the topic studied (Duffy, 1987; Haase & Myers, 1988).

Whichever view the researcher subscribes to, it is important to acknowledge that each method arises from a particular conviction about research and knowledge generation. And further that each method can stand alone and has its own place in nursing inquiry. Each method has merit if the researcher has conscientiously selected a given design to answer an appropriate research question.

However, it must be noted that the addition of a few open-ended questions on an instrument designed to measure a topic of interest does not constitute a qualitative study. Nor does hastily adding a questionnaire to the interview contribute to an empirical/analytical stance. It is important that the substance and form of the chosen research method or methods be philosophically and methodologically congruent.

ETHICAL CONSIDERATIONS

People whose "realities" are the focus of qualitative research through observation and/or interviews need to be informed of the study and its purpose as do subjects in quantitative research. Institutional review boards (IRBs) of hospitals, universities, or other agencies involved will need to approve of the research project. Sometimes, in the event the study involves patients in more than one agency, each IRB must approve the study. If the participants are not part of an agency, approval is necessary from the IRB of the agency of the researcher. Often, as Munhall (1988) has pointed out, because qualitative research is conducted in an ever-changing field, obtaining participant consent may be an ongoing process. This means that the researcher continually assesses the effects of the involvement in the field and renegotiates the consent. "Continually informing and asking permission establishes the needed trust to go on further in an ethical manner" (p. 157).

Other ethical concerns include the selection of the phenomenon to study. How will the study affect the people and/or organization being studied? Because of the very nature of qualitative research, the influence of each study on the people involved is carefully considered.

Participant observation plays a role in data collection in both ethnography and grounded-theory studies. The people being observed need to be aware that they are part of a study and have the same right to refuse as other participants in research.

Gaining access to the area of study and becoming a participant-observer allows for a certain degree of trust to develop. Occasionally, an informant, after trust is developed, may share a "secret" with the researcher (Field & Morse, 1985). Permission should be clarified to include such pieces of data in the study. If permission is denied, the information cannot be included and must be discarded.

In becoming a part of the environment while conducting research in the "field," qualitative researchers may encounter situations that other researchers do not. During the planning stage of the study the appropriate response in such situations should be thought out. The observation of unethical or illegal behavior may occur. For example, if a researcher studying the experience of being an AIDS patient in a dedicated AIDS unit witnesses unethical treatment by the staff, how should the researcher respond? According to Munhall (1988), nurse researchers "are morally obliged from the therapeutic [nursing] imperative to report such violations" (p. 158). In addition, illegal behaviors of the patients, such as abusing illegal substances, may occur. Again the investigator should have a procedure for handling such events and should anticipate how this may influence the trust between researcher and participant.

Qualitative researchers have an obligation to maintain the privacy and confidentiality of the participants. How the findings of the study will be used needs to be communicated to the participants at the onset of the study. The circumstances of the research, such as settings and names, are changed to ensure confidentiality of the institutions and/or participants. Qualitative researchers also bear the responsibility to accurately and faithfully describe the experiences of others. Including the participants as part of the member checks of the studies will help to ensure the trustworthiness of the results.

As more and more nurse researchers become involved in studies of a qualitative nature, the different ethical considerations of qualitative methods will become more commonplace. Perhaps, then, additional guidelines for qualitative research will emerge that take the unique perspective of that research into consideration. The complex problems of nurses and their clients require a variety of methods to provide for a science-based practice.

SUMMARY

- Members of a scientific community share a particular world view of science called a paradigm, and a specific scientific community is made up of people who share the same paradigm.
- The assumptions of the paradigm— philosophical, theoretical, instrumental, and methodological—afford a foundation for research and allow the researcher to see and interpret the world from one perspective rather than from another.
- An "interpretive turn" has been identified in recent nursing research in which some nurse researchers began to think of nursing as a human science, different from the natural or social sciences.

- The philosophical underpinnings of qualitative methods are based in a rejection of a cause-and-effect model, the experimental method, and a philosophical base of universal laws that do not account for the sociohistorical context of human experience.
- The scientific paradigm in nursing that relies on qualitative methods for analysis of data is the humanistic/holistic paradigm. The assumptions of this paradigm are congruent with the holistic philosophy of nursing practice.
- Qualitative methods are legitimate members of science, and they lead to knowledge about people and their worlds.
- The aim of research using qualitative methods is to discover meaning and understanding, rather than to verify truth or predict outcomes.
- Because data are words or texts placed in the context of the particular research problem, the primary instrument of data gathering is the researcher.
- Because the context is critical, each study's sample is based on the number and type of participants necessary to gather as much information as possible about the topic, including all of the possible ramifications and constructions.
- In qualitative research, the data collection and analysis are carried on simultaneously and interactively.
- The purposes of qualitative applications are to describe a human phenomenon from a different perspective or, when little is known, to sensitize others to the experience of a human phenomenon, as a basis for instrument development, to create a theoretical explanatory model, or to describe and interpret the meaning of everyday human experiences.
- Qualitative methods are a family of ways to collect and analyze phenomena of in-

terest and include grounded theory, phenomenology, hermeneutics, ethnography, case studies, historical, and feminist methods.

- Because the assumptions underlying the humanistic/holistic research paradigm are different, so are the evaluation measures.
- The assumptions of the given paradigm, the research method, the investigator's theoretical perspective, and the research questions must all be consistent with each other.
- In qualitative research, the concept of validity and reliability that has gained the most acceptance among qualitative researchers is trustworthiness as developed by Lincoln and Guba.
- The concept of trustworthiness includes credibility, transferability, dependability, and confirmability.
- Four areas of documentation are necessary to establish the confirmability of a study through an audit trail. They are contextual, methodological, analytical, and personal documentation.
- The use of the review of the literature, methodological triangulation, and the considerations of ethical research are all concerns of the qualitative nurse researcher.

FACILITATING CRITICAL THINKING

Nursing has a relatively short history in conducting research. Most early research studies were based in an empirical/analytical paradigm using quantitative methods. As the focus of nursing practice evolved from a medical, task-oriented focus to one based on people and their wholeness, a need arose for a different kind of research based on a different scientific paradigm. Hence, nurse researchers began to conduct studies that moved away from a cause-and-effect model to one that focused on the experiences of people and patients. Answer the following questions using a critical thinking process:

1. Compare and contrast five differences between the philosophical assumptions of the empirical/analytical paradigm and the humanistic/holistic paradigm presented in this chapter.
2. One's belief about science provides the philosophical basis for conducting research and provides the support for the research question and purpose. For example, if one wants to look at the experience of breast cancer from the perspective of the women undergoing the disease and its treatment, qualitative methods are a good fit. The findings of such studies as those completed by Quint (1963), Bowers (1987), and Dickson (1990) are reported differently from quantitative studies. Contrast the differences between those reported in the above studies and the possible outcomes of a quantitative study of women and breast cancer.
3. Reflect on your clinical practice and identify a research problem or question for which qualitative methods may provide an answer. Using the characteristics of qualitative methods, describe how the study might be presented.
4. From a recent nursing research journal, select an article of research in which a qualitative research method was used. Identify the philosophical assumptions underlying the research. Are the assumptions clearly identified? Or are they implicit in the method?
5. In the article selected for question 4, did the authors consider the credibility of the research? Did they describe the trustworthiness of the research? How did they describe it?

References

SUBSTANTIVE

AGAN, R. D. (1987). Intuitive knowing as a dimension of nursing. *Advances in Nursing Science, 10*(1), 49-62.

AROIAN, K. J. (1992). Sources of social support and conflict for Polish immigrants. *Qualitative Health Research, 2*(2), 178-207.

BANONIS, B. C. (1989). The lived experience of recovering from addiction: A phenomenological study. *Nursing Science Quarterly, 2*(1), 37-43.

BECK, C. (1992). The lived experience of postpartum depression: A phenomenological study. *Nursing Research, 41*(3), 166-170.

BENNER, P. (1984). *From novice to expert.* Menlo Park, CA: Addison-Wesley.

BLENNER, J. L. (1990). Passage through infertility treatment: A stage theory. *IMAGE: Journal of Nursing Scholarship, 22*(3), 153-158.

BOWERS, B. J. (1987). Intergenerational caregiving: Adult caregivers and their aging parents. *Advances in Nursing Science, 9*(2) 20-31.

CHESLA, C. A. (1991). Parents' caring practice with schizophrenic offspring. *Qualitative Health Research, 1*(4), 446-468.

COWLES, K. B. (1988). Personal world expansion for the survivors of murder victims. *Western Journal of Nursing Research, 10,* 687-699.

DICKSON, G. L. (1990). A feminist poststructuralist analysis of the knowledge of menopause. *Advances in Nursing Science, 12*(3), 15-31.

DIEKELMANN, N. L. (1992). Learning-as-testing: A Heideggerian hermeneutical analysis of the lived experiences of students and teachers in nursing. *Advances in Nursing Science, 14*(3), 72-83.

FAGERHAUGH, S., & STRAUSS, A. (1977). *The politics of pain management.* Menlo Park, CA: Addison-Wesley.

FORREST, D. (1989). The experience of caring. *Journal of Advanced Nursing, 14,* 815-823.

GATES, M. F. (1991). Culture care theory for study of dying patients in hospital and hospice context. In M. M. Leininger (Ed.), *Culture care diversity and universality: A theory of nursing.* New York: National League for Nursing.

GREGORY, D., & LONGMAN, A. (1992). Mothers' suffering: Sons who died of AIDS. *Qualitative Health Research, 2*(3), 334-357.

HEIDT, P. R. (1990). Openness: A qualitative analysis of nurses' and patients' experience of therapeutic touch. *IMAGE: Journal of Nursing Scholarship, 22*(3), 180-186.

HIRAKI, A. (1992). Tradition, rationality, and power in introductory nursing textbooks: A critical hermeneutics study. *Advances in Nursing Science, 14*(3), 1-12.

KRAMER, M. (1968). Role models, role conceptions, and role deprivation. *Nursing Research, 17*(2), 115-120.

KRAMER, M. (1969). Collegiate graduate nurses in medical center hospitals: Mutual challenge or duel. *Nursing Research, 18*(3), 196-210.

LEININGER, M. (1984). Southern rural black and white American lifeways with focus on care and health phenomena. In M. M. Leininger (Ed.), *Care: The essence of nursing and health.* Thorofare, NJ: Slack.

LEININGER, M. M. (Ed.). (1985). *Qualitative research methods in nursing.* Orlando: Grune & Stratton.

LEININGER, M. M. (Ed.). (1991). *Culture care diversity and universality: A theory of nursing.* New York: National League for Nursing.

MEISENHELDER, J. B., & LACHARITE, C. (1989). Fear of contagion: The public response to AIDS. *IMAGE: Journal of Nursing Scholarship, 21,* 7-9.

MILLER, J. F. (1985). Inspiring hope. *American Journal of Nursing, 85,* 22-28.

MILLER, J. F., & POWERS, M. J. (1988). Development of an instrument to measure hope. *Nursing Research, 37,* 6-9.

MUNHALL, P. L. (Ed.). (1994). *In women's experience.* New York: National League for Nursing.

NIKKONEN, M. (1992). Caring in the preparation of long-term psychiatric patients for non-institutional care: Ethnonursing study. *Journal of Advanced Nursing, 17,* 1088-1094.

PIERCE, P. F. (1993). Deciding on breast cancer treatment: A description of decision behavior. *Nursing Research, 42,* 22-27.

PRICE, M. J. (1993). Exploration of body listening: Health and physical self-awareness in chronic illness. *Advances in Nursing Science, 15*(4), 37-52.

RATHER, M. L. (1992). "Nursing as a way of thinking"—Heideggerian hermeneutical analysis of the lived experience of the returning RN. *Research in Nursing and Health, 15,* 47-55.

ROSE, J. (1990). Psychologic health of women: A phenomenological study of women's inner strength. *Advances in Nursing Science, 12*(2), 56-70.

SANDELOWSKI, M., HOLDITCH-DAVIS, D., & HARRIS, B. G. (1990). Living the life: Explanation of infertility. *Sociology of Health and Illness, 12,* 195-215.

SANTOPINTO, M. (1989). The relentless drive to be ever thinner: A study using the phenomenological method. *Nursing Science Quarterly, 2*(1), 29-36.

SOPHIER, R. (1993). Filial reconstruction: A theory of development through adversity. *Qualitative Health Research, 3,* 465-492.

STARCK, P. L. (1992). The management of suffering in a nursing home: An ethnographic study. In P. L. Starck, & J. P. McGovern (Eds.), *The hidden dimension of illness: Human suffering.* New York: National League for Nursing.

TAYLOR, B. J. (1992). Relieving pain through ordinariness in nursing: A phenomenologic account of a comforting nurse-patient encounter. *Advances in Nursing Science, 15*(1), 33-43.

WILSON, H. S. (1977). Limiting intrusion—Social control of outsiders in a healing community: An illustration of qualitative comparative analysis. *Nursing Research, 26,* 103-111.

YUEN, F. (1991). Case study of learning milieux: The modifying effect of the workplace. *Journal of Advanced Nursing, 16,* 1290-1295.

CONCEPTUAL

ALLEN, D. (1985). Nursing research and social control: Alternative models of science that emphasize understanding and emancipation. *IMAGE: Journal of Nursing Scholarship, 17*(2), 58-64.

ALLEN, D., BENNER, P., & DIEKELMANN, N. L. (1986). Three paradigms for nursing research: Methodological implications. In P. L. Chinn (Ed.), *Nursing research methodology.* Rockville, MD: Aspen.

HAASE J. E., & MYERS, S. T. (1988). Reconciling paradigm assumptions of qualitative and quantitative research. *Western Journal of Nursing Research, 10*(2), 128-137.

HABERMAS, J. (1971). *Knowledge and human interests.* Boston: Beacon Hill.

MUNHALL, P. L. (1989). Philosophical ponderings on qualitative research methods in nursing. *Nursing Science Quarterly, 2*(1), 20-28.

NEWMAN, M. A. (1992). Prevailing paradigms in nursing. *Nursing Outlook, 40*(1), 10-13.

POWERS, B. A. (1987). Taking sides: A response to Goodwin and Goodwin. *Nursing Research, 36,* 122-126.

WATSON, J. (1979). *The philosophy and science of caring.* Boston: Little, Brown.

WATSON, J. (1988). *Nursing: Human science and human care.* New York: National League for Nursing.

ZDERAD, L. T. (1969). Empathetic nursing: Realization of a human capacity. *Nursing Clinical of North America, 4,* 655-662.

METHODOLOGICAL

BENOLIEL, J. Q. (1984). Advancing nursing science: Qualitative approaches. *Western Journal of Nursing Research, 6*(3), 1-8.

BURNS, N. (1989). Standards for qualitative research. *Nursing Science Quarterly, 2*(1), 44-52.

CAMPBELL, D. T., & STANLEY, J. C. (1963). *Experimental and quasi-experimental designs for research.* Chicago: Rand McNally College Publishing Company.

COHEN, M. Z. (1987). A historical overview of the phenomenological movement. *IMAGE: Journal of Nursing Scholarship, 19,* 331-334.

COLAIZZI, P. (1978). Psychological research as a phenomenologist views it. In R. Valle & M. King (Eds.), *Existential phenomenological alternatives for psychology.* New York: Oxford University Press.

COOK, T. D. (1983). Quasi-experimentation: Its ontology, epistemology, and methodology. In G. Morgan (Ed.), *Beyond method: Strategies for social research.* Beverly Hills, CA: Sage.

Duffy, M. E. (1987). Methodological triangulation: A vehicle for merging quantitative and qualitative research methods. *IMAGE: Journal of Nursing Scholarship, 19,* 130-133.

Field, P. A., & Morse, J. M. (1985). *Nursing research: The application of qualitative approaches.* Rockville, MD: Aspen.

Giorgi, J. A. (1970). *Psychology as a human science: A phenomenologically based approach.* New York: Harper & Row.

Glaser, B. (1978). *Theoretical sensitivity.* Mill Valley, CA: The Sociology Press.

Glaser, B. G., & Strauss, A. L. (1967). *The discovery of grounded theory.* Chicago: Aldine Publishing.

Knafl, K. A., & Howard, M. J. (1984). Interpreting, reporting, and evaluating qualitative research. *Research in Nursing and Health, 7*(1), 17-24.

Lincoln, Y. S., & Guba, E. G. (1985). *Naturalistic inquiry.* Beverly Hills, CA: Sage.

Merriam, S. B. (1988). *Case study research in education: A qualitative approach.* San Francisco: Jossey-Bass.

Morgan, G. (1983). Research strategies: Modes of engagement. In G. Morgan (Ed.), *Beyond method.* Beverly Hills, CA: Sage.

Morse, J. (1992). The power of induction. (Editorial). *Qualitative Health Research, 2,* 3-6.

Munhall, P. L. (1988). Ethical considerations in qualitative research. *Western Journal of Nursing Research, 10*(2), 150-162.

Munhall, P. L., & Oiler, C. J. (1986). Language and nursing research. In P. L. Munhall, & C. J. Oiler (Eds.), *Nursing research: A qualitative perspective.* Norwalk, CT: Appleton-Century-Crofts.

Omery, N. (1988). Ethnography. In B. Sarter (Ed.), *Paths to knowledge.* New York: National League for Nursing.

Parse, R. R. (1990). Parse's research methodology with an illustration of the lived experience of hope. *Nursing Science Quarterly, 3*(1), 9-17.

Ricoeur, P. (1983). Hermeneutics and the human sciences. (J. Thompson, Trans.). London: Cambridge University Press.

Rodgers, B. L., & Cowles, K. V. (1993). The qualitative research audit trail: A complex collection of documentation. *Research in Nursing and Health, 16,* 219-226.

Sandelowski, M. (1993). Theory unmasked: The uses and guises of theory in qualitative research. *Research in Nursing and Health, 16,* 213-218.

Spradley, J. (1980). *Participant observation.* New York: Holt, Rinehart, and Winston.

Tesch, R. (1990). *Qualitative research: Analysis types and software tools.* New York: The Falmer Press.

van Manen, M. (1990). *Researching lived experiences.* New York: State University of New York.

Wilson, H. S. (1992). *Research in Nursing* (2nd ed.). Redwood City, CA: Addison-Wesley.

Historical

Cumulative index to nursing and allied health literature. (1988). Glendale, CA: Author.

Dickson, G. L. (1993). The unintended consequences of a male professional ideology on the development of nursing education. *Advances in Nursing Science, 15*(3), 67-83.

Gale, G. (1979). *Theory of science.* New York: McGraw-Hill.

Kuhn, T. S. (1970). *The structure of scientific revolutions* (2nd ed.). Chicago: University of Chicago Press.

Leininger, M. (1966). *Convergence and divergence of human behavior: An ethnopsychological comparative study of two Gadsup villages in the Eastern Highlands of New Guinea.* Unpublished doctoral dissertation, University of Washington.

Munhall, P. (1982). Nursing philosophy and nursing research: In apposition or opposition? *Nursing Research, 32*(3), 176-181.

Paterson, J. G., & Zderad, L. T. (1976). *Humanistic nursing.* New York: Wiley.

Quint, J. C. (1963). The impact of mastectomy. *American Journal of Nursing, 63*(11), 88-92.

Quint, J. C. (1967). The case for theories generated from empirical data. *Nursing Research, 16*(2), 109-114.

Tinkle, M., & Beaton, J. (1983). Toward a new view of science: Implications for nursing research. *Advances in Nursing Science, 5*(2), 27-36.

CHAPTER 20

QUALITATIVE DESIGNS

INEZ TUCK

There is an increase in the number of homeless persons in the United States. These persons have health care needs, yet health care providers are unsure what these needs are. Epidemiologic data available indicate that homeless persons experience health care problems that are related to their living conditions; for example, nutritional deficits, infestations such as scabies, and wounds from injuries are often evident in this population. However, do these health problems represent the health care issues that nursing professionals see as significant, or are these reported as significant by homeless persons? Homeless persons may not seek care for these health problems. Unstructured interviewing of homeless persons about their health problems and their perceptions of barriers to health care would provide an insider's or emic perspective.

Likewise, premenstrual syndrome (PMS) has been discussed in the literature as a common health problem for women. The condition has been described in terms of a medical diagnosis with recommended treatment. The experience of PMS as described by women is not clearly understood. Asking women to clearly explicate their experiences with PMS or to interpret their view of this phenomenon through the visual arts has not been done.

Qualitative research approaches can provide for in-depth understanding of this phenomenon. Qualitative designs can be used to study these two case illustrations and many other unexplored phenomena, which can provide context and information lacking in studies that are only quantitative in nature. This chapter describes the most frequently used qualitative designs.

The qualitative research process will be described in Chapter 21. One important aspect of the overall research process is the selection of a design appropriate to the problem or the phenomenon of interest. Similar to quantitative research, there are many options for qualitative designs, all offering divergent perspectives of a phenomenon. An understanding of each of these is necessary to make an informed decision regarding the appropriateness of the design for a particular study.

STEPS IN CHOOSING A QUALITATIVE DESIGN

1. Identify a philosophical perspective of qualitative research that is compatible with your world view.
2. Clearly define the phenomenon of interest.
3. Identify the research problem.
4. Pose the research question if appropriate, or clarify the purpose of the study. Word these in a manner consistent with the theoretical underpinning.
5. Using a step-by-step conceptual analysis, determine the best method to study the phenomenon. Choose from alternative methods.
6. Assess your familiarity with the design.

   Enhance your knowledge as appropriate.
7. State the resources available, including time, money, previous research experience, availability of site to study the phenomenon, subjects, consultation, and support.
8. Write the proposal or methodology section of the human subjects' approval form. Obtain feedback regarding the design.
9. Determine the feasibility of conducting the study using the proposed design.
10. After careful assessment of steps 1 to 9, alter the research design as indicated.

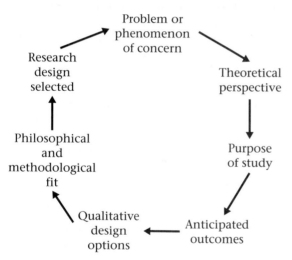

Figure 20-1. Selecting a qualitative design.

The theoretical underpinnings of phenomenology differ from those of ethnography, historical analysis, or grounded theory. While theoretical orientation is a major consideration when deciding a qualitative research design, it is not the only consideration. The selection of a qualitative design not only requires understanding the question to be answered or a sense of the nature of the phenomena to be explored, but the design requires a "fit" with the investigator's own philosophical orientation. Other considerations for the selection of the design are discussed in greater depth in the accompanying box. The steps in choosing a qualitative design are shown in Figure 20-1 and summarized in the box.

When conducting research the investigator starts with a clinical issue of concern, intuitively knowing about the topic or research question. An initial literature review of the problem or concern elucidates the theoretical underpinnings. The literature review also illustrates what is known about a phenomenon and places research findings in their theoretical context.

The transition from intuition, observation, or curiosity of the investigator to exploring topics found in the literature helps the investigator clarify the purpose and anticipated outcomes of the study. Once clarity of purpose is achieved, the investigator begins to consider the options for qualitative designs. In many cases the theoretical perspective has shaped what is written or known about the concern. For example, the clinical skill of contracting comes from the psychological perspective of behaviorism. Understanding patient encounters related to contracts, noncompliance, or behavioral interventions is grounded in the assumptions of behaviorism. When reviewing the options for a research design, the investigator would explore the congruence between the concept or problem as commonly mentioned in the literature and the theoretical underpinnings of the qualitative design.

The investigator reviews the design options and the implications of each method for anticipated outcomes. A particular design will "make sense" to the investigator. There will be a fit between the individual's world view and preference for a design, the supporting literature about the concern, and the assumptions of the qualitative method. These steps are the conceptual phase of the research process. The selection of the research design comes after introspection and reflection on the merits of each type.

❧ THEORETICAL FRAMEWORKS

Quantitative research methods come from the positivist paradigm and an empirical method. The world is viewed as orderly, where phenomena exist in objective reality and can be measured and operationalized. Reality is conceptualized as two-dimensional and can be explained by cause-and-effect relationships. This "way of knowing" is wholly deductive and results in reductionism and compartmentalization. The emphasis is on objectivism and observing truth as a singular objective reality.

On the other hand, qualitative approaches are consistent with the paradigm of idealism. In this paradigm subjective reality of the lived experience is explored. This view of the world complements the nursing reality where empathy, holism, humanism, and intuition are valued. Science as a rational knowledge has a narrow definition that excludes the subjective experience. However, qualitative research offers a unified view of objective and subjective realities and better describes the complexity of lived experiences.

SYMBOLIC INTERACTIONISM

The philosophical foundations of qualitative research were developed in the disciplines of the social sciences: psychology, history, sociology, and anthropology. Symbolic interactionism explains human behavior in terms of meanings and embodies perceptions of the situation. This confluence of meaning and context is the theoretical underpinning of ethnography and grounded theory and is closely linked to phenomenology (Chenitz & Swanson, 1986). Blumer (1969), usually associated with the development of the theoretical framework, stated that "human beings act toward things on the basis of meanings that the things have for them." People conceptually develop symbols that have meaning and interact on the basis of these symbols. "Meaning is then derived out of the social interaction. Meanings are handled in and modified through an interpretive process" (p. 2).

PHENOMENOLOGY

Phenomenology first appeared in the work of Franz Brentano in the nineteenth century and was later developed by Edmund Husserl (1965; 1977). Martin Heidegger (1962) refined the field by combining existentialism with phenomenology. Preeminent French and German philosophers such as Gabriel Marcel (1971), Maurice Merleau-Ponty (1964; 1977), and Jean Paul Sartre (1966) continued the work in this area. Other noted scholars who have written on the subject include Alfred Schultz (1967) and Paul Ricoeur (1973).

Readings in phenomenology are theoretical, span several decades, and require careful deliberation. Phenomenology is concerned with essences and conscious experiences of the world. The individual is viewed as having a stock of knowledge that is used to make sense of the world and to guide his or her own actions. Meaning is constructed in ongoing relations between people as they interact and share an experience. Phenomenology uncovers the meaning of an experience as humanly expressed.

Phenomenology has been incorporated into nursing conceptual frameworks. For example, Paterson and Zderad's (1976) theory of humanistic nursing is developed out of existential phenomenology. The view of nursing in this conceptual framework is to struggle with patients through the peak experiences related to health and suffering. Nursing is concerned with the quality of a person's living or dying. The nurse's offered presence to a client indicates understanding of the meaning of the experience to the extent that one's self can be a gift.

⚬ QUALITATIVE DESIGNS

The research design is an overall plan for answering the research questions and includes the strategies for gathering data. A wide variety of qualitative designs exists

Table 20-1
Selected Qualitative Research Methods

	Phenomenology	**Ethnography**	**Descriptive Studies**
Conceptual origin	Existential phenomenology, psychology emphasis	Social sciences,* anthropology emphasis	Social sciences*
Methodological goal	Understanding of phenomenon	Understanding of phenomenon in cultural context	Description or exploration of phenomenon
Data collection methods	Interviews, written descriptions	Participant observations, interviews, and document retrieval	Interviews, surveys
Role of researcher in data analysis	Intuits, analyzes, describes, validates the subjects' descriptions	Immerses, observes, clarifies and verifies (cultural context)	Collects, analyzes, and interprets
Outcome	Essence of phenomenon, essential definition of structure of phenomenon	Cultural report, case illustration	Narrative report, case illustration

*Social sciences: The traditional disciplines of psychology, sociology, history, anthropology, political science, and economics.

(see Table 20-1). Each offers the researcher a perspective that allows description or exploration of a phenomenon or an opportunity for the development of a substantive theory regarding the phenomenon.

PHENOMENOLOGY

Phenomenology as a method of inquiry comes out of phenomenological philosophical works of Husserl, Merleau-Ponty, and others. There are varying perspectives to understanding the human experience through analysis of the participants' descriptions. The goal is to understand the basic structure of phenomena as humanly experienced by analyzing the verbal explanations of the experiences from the perspective of participants (Parse et al., 1985). The participant's perception of the experience is the focus of phenomenology.

Phenomenology is concerned with investigating questions related to the lived experiences of patients and their families. Nurse researchers such as Munhall and Oiler (1986), Omery (1983), and Watson (1988) have described phenomenology and offer clarification of epistemological (method and ground of patients' knowledge) issues. The approach allowed them to interpret and understand the clients' experiences. Munhall and Oiler (1986) stated that the aim of phenomenology is to "describe the experience rather than define, categorize, explain or interpret it" (p. 81). This view is contradictory to the method of phenomenology if description is thought of as only a restatement of the experience in a narrative report.

Reduction of data does occur in phenomenology; however, it is actually "a

Historical Studies	Grounded Theory	Case Studies	Aesthetic Inquiry
Social sciences,* history emphasis	Social sciences,* symbolic interactionism, sociology emphasis	Social sciences*	Social sciences,* history and art emphasis
Interpretation of phenomenon over time	A theory describing or explaining phenomenology	In-depth description or exploration of single or multiple cases	Visual representation of phenomenon
Document retrieval and interviews	Interviews, observations, and participant observations	Interviews, observations, and document retrieval	Photographs, video, computer image, and artwork
Collects, analyzes and interprets (historical context)	Immerses, observes, compares, conceptualizes, and validates	Collects, observes, describes, and explores	Analyzes, interprets content and context
Biography, case study, historic report	Substantive or formal theory	Case description	Photographic essay, case illustration

---

PHENOMENOLOGICAL METHOD—SPIEGELBERG (1976)

1. Investigate the particular phenomenon.
2. Investigate general essences.
3. Apprehend the essential relationships among essences.
4. Watch modes of appearing.
5. Watch the constitution of the phenomenon in consciousness.
6. Suspend belief in the existence of the phenomenon.
7. Interpret meaning of the phenomenon.

Summary: The researcher uses intuition, analysis, and description while dwelling on the clients' descriptions. Intuiting is coming to know the uniqueness; analyzing is exploring the distinguishing characteristics and relationships to other phenomena to understand the structure; and describing is affirming the connections. Eidetic intuiting occurs when moving from the particular to general essences, and the internal relationship between essences is examined to understand the nature of general essences. Watching modes of appearing means looking at how the phenomena present themselves and take shape in the consciousness. Bracketing is the process of setting aside or detaching the meaning of the phenomena or any presuppositions or personal beliefs. Finally, interpretation is the attempt to identify the "sense" of the phenomena. Inferences are made, and the researcher makes intuitive leaps to understand the concealed meaning.

PHENOMENOLOGICAL METHOD—VAN KAAM (1969)

Modification consistent with Spiegelberg
1. Elicit descriptive expressions.
2. Identify common elements.
3. Eliminate those expressions not related to the phenomenon.
4. Formulate a hypothetical definition of the phenomenon.
5. Apply the hypothetical definition to the original descriptions.
6. Identify the structural definitions.

Summary: Dwells on the descriptions by intuiting, analyzing, and describing as noted by Spiegelberg. Secondly, the common elements are named. These common elements are implicitly or explicitly stated in the majority of the descriptions and are compatible with them all. The common elements are then synthesized into a definition. Independent judges are used for verification.

---

methodological process that is designed to lift these secondary sense-making operations from experience in order to better understand it" (p. 81). Through this reductionistic process, fuller awareness of the experience is gained. There are no prior views (hypotheses) to test or verify; previous knowledge is bracketed or set aside, and the review of literature is preferably completed after the data have yielded the essential structure of the phenomenon.

Method

There are four methods for data analysis recommended for phenomenological studies. Van Kaam (1969), Giorgi (1970), Spiegelberg (1976), and Colaizzi (1978) each developed an approach that can guide

PHENOMENOLOGICAL METHOD—GIORGI (1970)

1. Dwell on the description.
2. Return to the subjects for elaboration on ambiguous areas of description.
3. Identify the natural meaning units for each subject.
4. Identify the themes.
5. Identify the focal meanings.
6. Synthesize the situated structural description.
7. Synthesize the general structural description.
8. Share the structure with other researchers for confirmation or criticism.

Summary: The researcher dwells on the descriptions and forms questions. He returns to the subjects for elaboration. Scenes are identified, and the unit of meaning is determined. The focal meaning is crystallized into themes. Finally, a meaning for all subjects is developed.

PHENOMENOLOGICAL METHOD—COLAIZZI (1978)

1. Read all descriptions to acquire a feeling for them.
2. Extract phrases or sentences that directly pertain to the phenomenon.
3. Formulate the meaning of each significant statement.
4. Organize the aggregate formulated meanings into clusters of themes.
   a. Validate these clusters with the original descriptions.
   b. Note discrepancies; some themes may be contradictory or unrelated; proceed with the conviction that what is inexplicable may be existentially real and valid.
5. Integrate the results in an exhaustive description.
6. Formulate an exhaustive description that is unequivocally a statement of the essential structure of the phenomenon.
7. Return to the subjects to validate the descriptions formulated.

Summary: The descriptions or protocols are read so that phrases or sentences can be extracted. Repetitive statements are eliminated. The meanings inherent in these significant statements are spelled out. The formulated meaning should illuminate the statements and be connected to the protocols. These formulated meanings are grouped into themes that are validated in the original protocols. This back-and-forth process ensures that the themes reflect the meanings and that all are accepted as real without preconceived views of what is real. An exhaustive description is written and validated with the subject.

the researcher in understanding the client's experience. A brief overview of the steps for each of these procedures is outlined in the boxes on pages 442 and 443 (Parse et al., 1985; Munhall, & Oiler, 1986). Again, to ensure adequate understanding of the approach prior to its use, the reader is referred to the original sources for full elaboration. This author outlines a method for data analysis in nursing that involves the use of

---

PHENOMENOLOGICAL METHOD—TUCK

1. Participate in a "bracketing" interview by responding to the research question as if a study participant.
2. Analyze the bracket interview to determine biases and presuppositions.
3. Gather an understanding of the phenomenon by interviewing participants.
4. Dwell on descriptions after reading to acquire a feeling for the data.
5. Read the protocol out loud to the research group to further dwell on the descriptions.
6. Identify meaning units (phrases, sentences, or paragraphs of text) that have significance for the phenomenon.

7. Formulate meanings into themes, theme clusters, and categories that describe the essence of the phenomenon for each protocol.
8. Synthesize the essence of the phenomenon from all participants.
9. Present meanings as description of the structure of the phenomenon to a research group for review.
10. Allow verification of meanings, essences, and structures by the research group.
11. Integrate the essential description of the structure of the phenomenon in narrative form or diagrammatic representation.

---

research groups. The process is described in the box above .

Examples

There are several excellent examples of phenomenological studies in nursing research. Riemen (1986), cited in Munhall and Oiler, studied caring interactions in nurse-patient relationships and offers a useful example of how Colaizzi's procedural steps can be followed. Another example is this author's use of Colaizzi's approach in developing an exhaustive description of caregiving in families with a chronically mentally ill family member.

GROUNDED THEORY

Grounded theory examines the social context of human interaction. Glaser and Strauss developed grounded theory as they studied the experiences of dying patients (Munhall & Oiler, 1986). These two sociologists were the products of different theoretical backgrounds. Strauss came from the Chicago School and was heavily influenced

by symbolic interactionism and the works of W. I. Thomas, G. H. Mead, and Herbert Blumer. Glaser, from a more quantitative theoretical perspective, developed an appreciation for well-thought-out, systematic methods for coding and generating theory; thus the influence of symbolic interactionism on the understanding of one's social reality.

Since 1967 these authors and their associates have written four books describing grounded theory. These primary sources describe the theoretical underpinnings of grounded theory, the qualitative method, and the data collection and analytic processes. The more recent publication by Strauss and Corbin (1990) offers a "how to" approach. The book outlines the steps to guide qualitative analysis in grounded theory. The reader is referred to this publication as a good foundational reference source for understanding grounded theory methodology.

Grounded theory is a qualitative research method that has a systematic procedure for deriving a theory about a phenomenon. The grounded theory approach identifies concepts and the relationship between these concepts in an inductive manner. The researcher returns to the data frequently during the study, revises research questions, and seeks out additional or missing data. This process of comparative analysis continues throughout data collection and allows for provisional testing of the theory. This method is used when there exists minimal knowledge about a phenomenon or when a new perspective is required.

Jeanne Quint Benoliel, a nurse researcher, worked collaboratively with Glaser and Strauss and was one of the earliest nurses to use the methodology. In 1967 she published her work entitled "The Nurse and the Dying Patient," in which she used an inductive process to derive a general theory from a specific patient situation (Munhall & Oiler, 1986). Later, Hutchinson (1986) described how nurses in neonatal intensive care units created meaning for themselves and how the absence of such meaning resulted in staff burnout.

Hutchinson (1986) classified grounded theories as formal and substantive. Formal theories are those that are conceptual in nature, while substantive theories are specific, circumscribed, and limited to a situation. The initial work with dying patients was formal and later circumscribed for specific patient populations as substantive theory. Hutchinson (1986), Glaser and Strauss (1967), Strauss and Corbin (1990) described the terms associated with grounded theory, including constant comparison, memoing, theoretical sampling, bracketing, sorting, basic social psychological process (BSP), saturation, and theoretical sensitivity. The reader is referred to these sources for further description of these key terms.

As indicated, theoretical sensitivity is associated with grounded theory. Strauss and Corbin (1990) describe this term in a chapter in their book and Glaser (1978) has written a book about it. Theoretical sensitivity refers to the researcher's awareness of the subtleties of meaning of data. Theoretical sensitivity comes from having familiarity with the literature, professional and personal experiences, and the analytic process. For instance, interest in a research problem often is peaked by a professional or personal experience. The nursing observation that the elderly cling to small personal objects in nursing homes may be associated with detachment or the types of memories retained. The personal experience of caring for a chronically ill family member may sensitize a potential investigator to seek the deeper meaning of observed phenomena and thereby develop grounded theory.

A question frequently asked is how to use the existing literature in a grounded theory approach. In grounded theory, the literature stimulates theoretical understanding by providing or suggesting concepts that may have been found to be related to the phenomenon under study. The literature does not define the study as in quantitative research but can guide the researcher or facilitate one's thinking. An open mind about the data allows concepts from the literature to be used if they are indeed relevant or evident in the data. The grounded theory researcher develops theory but does not test an existing one. It is assumed that there is no preconceived answer to the research questions. However, in some instances existing theory is supported by the emerging grounded theory and may be incorporated as content seems to fit or make sense. In addition to supporting theoretical sensitivity, uses of literature in grounded theory include stimulating research questions and theoretical sampling or validating the theory when writing the findings. Strauss and Corbin (1990) give detailed descriptions of how to appropriately address these issues.

Method

The grounded theory method, as in ethnography, begins in the naturalistic setting and follows the procedures of field research. Unlike ethnography, however, grounded theory does not seek to understand culture and cultural processes; rather, reality is perceived as a social construct. The investigator in grounded theory immerses herself or himself in a social environment. Observations are made about the structure and patterns noted there. Interactions are studied through interviews and observations made in the field. The method is executed in the field over a protracted length of time. The biases that can be inherent in the participant-observer role are mediated by the length of the fieldwork and the propensity of respondents in the environment to continue to exist or function in their natural environment in a natural way.

Document analysis of organizational charts and policies, patient records, and other sources of data provide additional perspectives for illuminating the social phenomenon. The numerous sources of data complicate analysis, but allow for depth in the theory generated. Multiple methods or triangulation adds to the validity of the data. The use of various data sources is thought to increase the rigor of the study.

Data are collected by tape recorders or written as field notes. Data are prepared for analysis by coding, writing memos, and diagramming. The first step is coding the data by marking or highlighting significant incidents or observations found in the text. The facts or incidents then are abstracted into concepts and are written in the margins of the transcribed interviews or fieldnotes. The fact or incident now has a code and an associated theoretical note. Initially it may not be clear what these codes mean or if they will all be relevant to the emerging theory, because the data analysis process is more extensive than early efforts to form opinions. Recoding of data occurs frequently and is usually a substantial and developmental process for the research.

Memos are researcher's notes that indicate the stage of the analytic process, the conceptualization of ideas, and the thinking process that illustrates the relationship between codes. They are written for the benefit of the researcher and become the basis for writing the theory. Memos should be dated, titled, cross-referenced, and filed. Often a computer file can facilitate the cataloging of memos. Memos are compared and linked into categories. The process continues until the primary category or central core of meaning is found. Diagrams are often used as a visual representation of the categories and the way they are linked. These diagrams are often continuously revised until the developing theory is fully conceptualized. Chenitz and Swanson (1986) provide excellent examples of the data analysis process and have generated many such diagrams.

Through inductive and deductive conceptualization of the text, the central core of meaning and relationships are established. This is followed by the evaluation of "fit," that is, the relevance of those relationships and the extent of their interconnections. The data are constantly re-analyzed to determine the need for additional sampling. Sampling continues until saturation of codes occurs. Saturation or completeness of all levels of codes occurs when no "new" information is available and all data fit into the existing categories. Theoretical sampling includes all persons who have information that is relevant to the phenomenon of concern. However, varied codes may be derived from the diverse sample. The constant comparative method of data analysis is coding and analyzing the data for common patterns within the sample. An incident is compared with another incident, category with category, and construct with construct across all observations.

The final step is sorting through the codes to determine the core variable or basic social psychological process (BSP). The core variable emerges naturally in the process and explains the social process related to the phenomena. Data collection continues until the core variable emerges. A coherent, workable whole integrates the major ideas. The literature is used at this point to support the emergent theory. Developing the theory requires constant reevaluation and examination to assure validity, utility, and comprehension.

Glaser and Strauss (1967) reported a set of criteria for evaluation of grounded theories. A theory must have a "fit" with the situation or explain or predict relevance to the core variable. The theory should be modifiable to other settings, have density, and reflect integration into a tight theoretical framework that has depth. Premature closure of theory would indicate the lack of density. The grounded theory generated would be inclusive of the core variable, but would not reflect all the variation in the data. Having developed a dense theory is one of the true measures of successful work. It is a process where data are compared or contrasted repeatedly over time through the constant comparative technique. Finally, the theory that emerges is relevant for the population studied.

Examples

Nurse researchers who possess creativity and conceptual thinking can use the grounded theory method to develop middle-range, substantive theories to apply to nursing practice. Chenitz and Swanson (1986) described Wilson's study on the treatment of the mentally ill in the community and Hutchinson's study of the environment in the neonatal ICU as two studies indicative of analysis centering around a social process. Chenitz's study of dying in the nursing home is an example of linking a substantive theory to a formal one. More recent examples of grounded theory are the study of the bereavement experience in caregivers by Jones and Martinson (1992) and Burke et al. (1991). Jones used the grounded theory methodology of Strauss to analyze interviews of 13 caregivers. According to this methodology, concepts are derived from the indicators (events, actions, or words) found in the data (Strauss, 1987). The conceptualization of a two-stage pattern of bereavement resulted from the study. Burke et al. (1991) developed the mid-range theory of hazardous secrets and "reluctantly taking charge" from the responses of parents of chronically ill children.

ETHNOGRAPHY

Ethnography is a qualitative method that collects, describes, and analyzes the ways in which people categorize the meaning of their world in a cultural context. It includes knowing how people shape and interpret their experiences in a cultural context. Although there are differences in experiences across cultural groups, all groups assign meaning to their experiences and such meaning shapes their social behavior. Germain (1986) stated that ethnography is a factual description and analysis

---

KEY POINTS OF THE ETHNOGRAPHIC METHOD

1. Data gathering occurs in a naturalistic setting.
2. The native or emic view is critical.
3. The etic view is acknowledged.
4. Participants observation and interviewing are the main data collection techniques.
5. Interpretations are made and inferences are drawn.
6. There are suggested methods for data analysis.

---

of aspects of the way of life of a particular culture or subcultural group (p. 147). Leininger (1984) stated that ethnography documents, describes, and analyzes physical, cultural, social, and environmental features as those factors influencing peoples' patterns. The goal of ethnography is to discover the cultural knowledge people use to organize their behaviors and interpret their experiences (Spradley, 1979).

The ethnographic researcher becomes involved in the culture by living in the setting or environment for an extensive period of fieldwork. Ethnography is done in the context of the culture and results in a detailed description of that culture. Culture is a system of knowledge used by participants to interpret experience and generate behavior. Language expressed by key informants is the guide to establishing the meaning or interpretation essential for constructing cultural knowledge by the researcher. Through the essential methods of participant observation and intensive interviewing of members of the subculture, the researcher learns from informants the meaning they attach to activities, events, behaviors, knowledge, artifacts, rituals, and other aspects of their life-style (Germain, 1986, p. 147).

The ethnographer looks for connections, patterns, themes, or relationships that have meaning for the people in the culture. The themes include shared knowledge, norms, values, belief systems, language, role behaviors, or patterns of interaction. Ethnography contributes to descriptive and explanatory theories of culture. Ethnoscience ethnography yields taxonomic analysis of particular domains. Ethnohistory combines the use of historic sources with theoretical abstractions to provide a complete understanding of culture.

Method

Spradley (1979; 1980), Agar (1986), and Werner and Schoepfle (1987) described in detail the complex process of ethnography. However, a discussion of the intricacies of their data analysis process is beyond the scope of this chapter. Persons intent on conducting ethnographies are encouraged to read these noteworthy sources for further elaboration of the method.

The method of ethnography has been established in the field of anthropology and used by other social scientists. Nurse anthropologists first used the method in nursing research. Now the method is not associated with a particular educational background as much as it is now considered a research design available to any interested nurse researcher.

As a first step in such a study, the investigator enters the field with some general questions about the culture. The culture may be defined as subcultures, ethnic and racial groups, institutions, or community settings such as homeless shelters. The definition of culture is stated in the research questions. A study's target, such as the laboring experiences of the Hopi Indians, establishes the parameters of who will be studied and where the study will take place.

Secondly, the conceptual literature is reviewed to provide the framework for examining the culture. Background information guides the approach to the culture. The investigator is cautioned not to have predetermined biases about the culture or the questions to be asked. Access to site is negotiated with persons significant to the culture. There is often a spokesperson or leader who will give consent. Once established, however, informed consent is not assumed, but is continually obtained. Key informants are the source of data about the culture. The names of persons who become key informants will emerge as the investigator interacts in the field.

The length of time spent in the field is determined by the research question, the complexity of the subculture, the time required for building relationships with the informants, the access to data, and the seasonal or cyclic variations of the subculture (Munhall & Oiler, 1986, p. 152). Fieldwork is both an art and a craft, and the interpretation of data can take a lifetime (Werner & Schoepfle, 1987, p. 16). When no new data emerge, data saturation is met and fieldwork ends.

Germain (1986) described three phases of fieldwork. The initial phase is defined as a period of general observation to obtain a broad view of the culture and to write descriptive accounts of what is observed in the culture, the characteristics of the people, and the environment. Trust and rapport are established with members of the cultural group. The second phase has more focused questions or working hypotheses. Participant observations and interviews are done to answer research questions. Collection of data and data analyses occur simultaneously in a dialectical process. In the final phase, saturation of data is recognized, disengagement occurs, termination of relationships is planned, and the ethnographer leaves the field.

The two methods of data collection are participant observations and interviews. Participant observation refers to the technique in which the investigator is submerged in the culture under study. There is a range of behavior in this role. Field and personal notes are written as the investigator interacts with the culture. Subtleties of human interaction are noted through observations and are recorded. There is researcher involvement in this design, and the interaction between researcher and informants becomes a source of data. The ethnographer brings the "self" to the environment. Notes related to stress, anxiety, and discomfort experienced by the ethnographer can be recorded as an added dimension to the data analysis.

The second data gathering technique, interviewing, may be formal and structured or informal and flexible. Attempts are made to obtain the emic (internal) view from members of the subculture. Patterns or domains are elucidated in the data. Broader cultural patterns emerge and are reported as findings of the research project.

Several other data sources may be used in an ethnographic study. These sources include documents, life histories, films, photographs, and artifacts. Extensive field notes are written about these data sources to describe the observations made. At this point in the data collection process, no interpretations are made by the ethnographer.

After the ethnographer has spent time in the field, he or she begins the process of data analysis. Ethnographers use qualitative content analysis to derive patterns and themes from the data. Categories are extracted from the data by comparing, contrasting, analyzing, and synthesizing (Munhall & Oiler, 1986). Spradley (1979) describes a process in which content from interviews is ordered into domains of meanings and taxonomies are derived. These taxonomies are the emic view of the culture, whereas the researcher derives cultural themes that are the researcher's view (etic) of the whole culture. The unit of analysis (the linguistic expressions) are the domains of meaning.

Agar (1986) discussed the unit of analysis as segments, a subcategory of a larger unit known as strips. Agar described the process of taking words and behaviors and linking and sorting them into patterns, thus developing a coherent sense of the culture. These strips are organized into schema. Agar described the data that seem foreign or different as "breakdowns." Breakdowns occur when there are different traditions from the emic and etic perspectives. These breakdowns must be resolved before understanding is possible. Exploring additional observations found in other segments makes these differences appear similar. As segments become similar, coherence is achieved. Resolution is the process by which segments are understood in view of other segments. Each segment is then considered in a larger context of the strips and schema. Through an expanding process, larger units emerge as schema are derived that make sense of the cultural knowledge and fit the meaning expressed by the informants. Inferences are drawn and are the basis on which schema are derived. Linkages are made and relationships are established between strips. Schema are connected to overriding theoretical schema.

The smaller units of analyses present the emic perspective, while the inferences drawn involve the ethnographer's understandings. To ensure that the ethnographer has considered all possibilities when drawing inferences, Agar suggested looking for examples of anticoherence, the examination of those pieces of the puzzle that do not seem to relate to others previously reviewed. This activity leads to comprehension. Comprehension occurs when the researcher determines if one strip can be used to "comprehend" another. Validation by asking informants is another way to verify coherence in the meaning of data. Coherence is the goal that allows for comprehension. Agar provides excellent examples of this process in his monograph.

As data are analyzed, it is important to recognize the role of the ethnographer in the research process. The cultural background of the ethnographer may well influence the interpretations and meanings associated with the behaviors found in the culture. Ethnographers bring certain traditions of their own into the field. For instance, the views of Western culture have basic assumptions that differ from those found in many other cultures. The cultural influence of the ethnographer is evident in instances of secondary analyses of previously conducted ethnographic studies; different ethnographies emerge when other researchers interpret the findings. Secondly, it is noteworthy that cultures are not static, as is often discovered when a given ethnographer revisits a previously studied culture.

The findings of an ethnography are reported in a narrative form. Reliability is achieved by critiquing the sources and the consistency of responses across informants.

Ethnography is neither a subjective nor objective report but is considered an interpretive one mediating the two.

Aamodt (1991, p. 45) succinctly describes six steps of ethnography. They are:

1. Observe the cultural scene identified in the questions.
2. Develop beginning ethnographic questions.
3. Gather linguistic samples from actors in the social scene of study.
4. Identify culturally relevant domains of meaning.
5. Develop structural questions.
6. Elicit structure for a taxonomy of domains of meaning.

Spindler and Spindler (1970) stated the following criteria for a good ethnography: (1) the observations are contextualized in the naturalistic setting, and any judgments made about what is significant are deferred until the orienting phase of field study is complete; (2) observations are prolonged, repeated, and focused on obtaining the native view of reality; (3) knowledge is elicited from the informant, and any data gathering instruments are generated in situ; (4) the presence of the ethnographer in the study is acknowledged and does not presuppose any responses; and (5) the emic point of view is important for the transcultural perspective.

Examples
Ethnography as a research design has been used by nurse anthropologists to study health beliefs and practices. More recently the method has been used to study the phenomenon of caring by Leininger (1984) and others. Gates (1991), in a study of the caring environments of an oncology and hospice unit, spent 6 months doing field-work in each site. She collected data "in order to discover the universal and diverse patterns which influenced care provided to dying persons" (p. 3). Her methods included unstructured interviews and participant observations. She combined the approaches of ethnography and ethnonursing in her study when determining beliefs and practices about nursing care.

Ethnography combines the use of historic sources with theoretical abstractions to provide a complete understanding of culture. Few ethnohistoric studies have been done in nursing. However, recently, Villarruel (1992) used ethnohistory to study pain in the ancient Aztec and Mayan civilizations. Sources for data analysis were selected on the basis of availability, accuracy, and credibility and included eyewitness accounts, myths, previous ethnographies, archaeology, art, and art history. Thematic and pattern analysis resulted in six categories of beliefs related to pain.

Cognitive anthropology is a method in which themes are found within the data and then are related to cognitive principles. These statements are believed by the participants and accepted as true and valid. For example, one belief that may be identified in a culture is that men are deemed superior to women. Participants share this opinion, and cultural behaviors are ascribed according to the belief. Exploring these belief statements and related principles is the goal of cognitive anthropology.

HISTORICAL RESEARCH
Krampitz (1981) stated that "historiography is the science and art of reconstructing the past from a critical review of documents, artifacts, literature, and accounts of eyewitnesses or participants in the event" (p. 54). Historical research is not the mere reporting of historical facts or description

of past events, but requires interpretation to gain an understanding of the event and demonstrate its relevance to contemporary issues.

Historical researchers cannot alter the data that they gather in surveys or interviews. The data for historical analysis exist as defined by others in a previous period of time and were interpreted and recorded as deemed appropriate for the time. Historical researchers use a myriad of data sources during a historical study.

Historiography is a retrospective approach in which generalizations are drawn only after corroborating and supporting data are found. Hypotheses are supported or refuted by the careful analysis of existing documents and personal accounts. The quality of the study is related to the quality of the archival retrieval of primary sources. Primary, as well as secondary, sources are often used, and the validity and reliability of the sources are crucial to the levels of generalizations that can be generated as findings of the study.

Method

The initial step in historical studies, as in other designs, is the clear identification of the problem and the purpose of the study. The historical analysis is a deliberate and painstaking process. It is imperative that the topic be interesting and challenging to maintain the commitment of the researcher to the project over time. Equally important is the definition of the parameters of the study. The amount of time available to conduct the study, the time frame and era of available data, and the population to be studied are crucial decisions. Identifying where primary sources are located, the type and quantity of sources, and their accessibility will determine the feasibility and depth of the project. Gaining access to materials in the public do-

main may be easier and more fruitful, but also more time-consuming than obtaining access to private collections. Resources available, including the time necessary to complete the study, will ultimately influence the quality of the research results.

After the decision is made to conduct a historical study, specific research questions are written and hypotheses explicitly stated. Failure to limit the scope of the investigation is one of the major pitfalls of new researchers. A comprehensive review of literature will indicate what has been done previously in the subject area. The literature will usually also provide background on how to design the study.

Once the basic decision making has occurred, three additional steps are required to complete the historical approach: (1) the gathering of data, (2) the criticism of data, and (3) the synthesis of data (Christy, 1975; Robnett, 1986). Austin (1958) adds a fourth step, the writing of the research report. These final steps can be instituted only after the initial step of problem delineation is complete.

Gathering the Data. To accomplish the second step, data may be gathered from a number of locations such as libraries, historical societies, museums, and archives. The historical study usually requires an intensive search, and the investigator becomes an amateur detective in following every clue to its source. As one searches through various repositories, the investigator must decide which ones are representative of a phenomenon and which may contain obscure information.

Next primary and secondary sources are identified. Primary sources include original records and documents directly related to the topic. Eyewitness accounts, testimonials, photographs, and artifacts that attest to the event are also primary sources. Official records are considered broadly as including diaries, books, media accounts, minutes, proceedings, laws and legislative actions, letters, autobiographies and memoirs, pamphlets, periodicals, and source books. Documents, as defined by Austin (1958), may be written or unwritten sources, official or unofficial sources, and private or public sources. Secondary sources are second-generation data reported by someone who has secondhand knowledge of the incident or event and is commonly referred to as "hearsay."

Statements found in documents are not presumed to be facts, but must undergo a process of analysis. A statement is nothing more than what someone said about a matter, and there are many reasons why statements may not be wholly or even partially true. Factors that influence "truth" include cultural biases or prejudices, investment or interest in the event, motives for writing the document, political or social climate, cultural or societal values of the time of the document, and control of the media (print, audio, or video). Materials published for propaganda have to be interpreted in view of prevailing social/political forces of the time. An understanding of the era or the environmental context is necessary in determining truth.

The critical evaluation of the content and the source of documents accounts for the categories assigned. The technique of data triangulation or the use of multiple data sources is helpful here. For instance, an eyewitness account by a participant of an event and its corroboration by a newspaper account the next day (two primary sources) are reviewed, and the results indicate that the statement is fact. When corroborating evidence is found for information in primary and secondary sources, the statements are deemed "true"; statements are "probably true" when from one primary source with limited contrary evidence or when a modest disagreement is encountered. "Possible facts" rely on secondary or tertiary documents or exist in those instances where there are contradictory findings. These distinctions in categories, which seem arbitrary when described, are essential when writing the findings.

Copious research notes are encouraged, particularly in documenting the location and condition of sources and the methods used to obtain access. Since documents usually provide leads to other sources, it is important that clear notes be kept and sufficient information obtained to relocate the referenced document. Complete citations of sources are required for any scholarly dissemination of the findings of the study because others may want to retrieve documents for future studies. It is also helpful to record notes about the authors of a document. Historical researchers should employ a system for indexing materials that will facilitate data interpretation and preparation of the research report.

Critical Analysis of Data. Initially, careful review of each document from an investigative perspective is encouraged. Is the document authentic? Is it confined to the time frame studied? Is the incident or event of the study clearly described or made relevant? What is the source of the document? Where is it stored? Does a reputable site house the document? The answers to these questions can ensure external criticism. Experts such as museum curators or historians may be used to further verify the authenticity of documents.

The historical methodology includes the use of internal and external criticism as an attempt to evaluate historical data. External criticism establishes the validity of documents, while internal criticism determines their reliability. Each document must be scrutinized in view of its authenticity and trustworthiness. Examination of original documents should include when, who, where, and under what circumstances the documents were written. In addition, it is vital to determine the credibility of the facility where the document is stored and whether the document has been analyzed by other historians. Techniques such as handwriting analysis and testing of paper and ink for chemical composition and age are sophisticated methods of assuring the authenticity of documents. These are examples of methods to achieve external criticism.

On the other hand, internal criticism is more difficult to achieve. Internal criticism refers to the credibility of the source, that is, the writer, reporter, or publisher. A critical review of the document is required in view of potential biases and inaccuracies in recording or reporting. Determining the biases inherent in the original document is made easier when examined in context. At the same time it is important not to eschew one's own biases in the study by the selection, organization, and interpretation of materials (Krampitz, 1981, p. 56).

Internal criticism is a phase of positive criticism in which the document is read without introducing the investigator's biased interpretations (Christy, 1975). Austin (1958) stated that positive internal criticism directs the researcher to decide the real contextual meaning as compared with the literal one. Negative criticism requires the investigator to disbelieve the data until the credibility is confirmed by other sources.

After sufficient sources are obtained and authenticated, the researcher begins the arduous task of sifting through the documents to reconstruct past events. Although this activity is lengthy and intense, the process can be stimulating and interesting. Images of a puzzle emerge as small pieces of information begin to reflect a larger pattern. Varying documents and personal accounts illuminate the emerging descriptions. Clarification of information and elucidation of meaning define the data analysis process. Data analysis offers refinement of the research questions and frequently leads to other sources of data. Further analyses may suggest previously unknown material and may significantly alter the actual definition of the problem. However, the researcher's familiarity with the topic and prior substantial review of the literature should limit findings to true serendipitous ones.

Data analysis in historical methodology is a process of synthesis and reflection. Shafer (1980) stated that analysis is the systematic attempt to learn about a phenomenon by looking at elements that result in preliminary conclusions. In this context, working hypotheses will not bias interpretation if they are plausible ideas about causes or relationships. However, these tentative hypotheses can be discarded at need. As a result, relationships are established between events, the reconstruction is as accurate as can be achieved from the available data, and the interpretations made are free of bias. The description of the event, an understanding of how the event occurred, and its relationships with other events in the past and present are reflected in a narrative discussion when the historical researcher makes distinctions between major and minor events.

Synthesis of Data. The synthesis actually occurs through the writing process. The findings are reported in the research report in a well-developed style that is interesting and stimulating for the reader. Spieske (1953) stated that the exposition or narrative of historical research must tell not only what happened but why and how it happened. By establishing relationships and making interpretations, the researcher must strive to show that the subject was part of a development or a process. "Continuity he stresses, but causation he does not oversimplify" (p. 37).

Shafer (1980) stated that final synthesis involves interpretation by finding causal relations, assertions of value judgment, and emphasis. Devoting a specific portion of the written account to a particular subject arrangement, grouping the evidence in chronological or topical order, and making fact-based inferences fill in the gaps or supply connections. Preparing the results of a historical investigation is actually a creative process. However, the greater the number of inferences, the greater the likelihood of a research error. Shafer described five categories of synthesis ranging from the literal and real meaning to relevance, the highest level (p. 195).

Writing the Final Report. The final step, writing the formal research report, is the recording of the knowledge gained through the research process, finding meaning in the facts assembled. The best way to proceed is to simply begin to write. This process can be approached in a number of ways, but until the investigator begins to pull the findings together, it seems a formidable task. "The writing of history is a science and an art. As a science, it is a synthesis of verified facts into a readable and understandable account. It involves the processes of documentation, organization, and interpretation. As an art, history must be well written so that its chief purpose may be realized, namely, the extension of knowledge of past events" (Austin, 1958, p. 9).

Skills of the Historical Researcher
Historical research is time consuming, and one must have a keen interest in history and be comfortable with an involvement with objects rather than people. The historical researcher must be able to capture the essence of a person by simply reading their materials. Other necessary skills are an excitement for the reconstructive process and the ability to integrate data from various sources. Patience as a virtue is required of a historical researcher. There is a constant need to search for new materials in unfamiliar sites. Original materials are often housed in secured facilities that require appropriate identification and fees to obtain access. There is typically a lack of funding for this type of research, although available funds are increasing for qualitative studies.

Church (1987) stated that the study of history represents the potential of a unity and continuity in one's identity. An intelligent appreciation of the emergence and evolution of an identified group is fundamental to that group's status as a profession (p. 275). Absence of appreciation for the past can account for the difficulty in developing nursing as a profession. Other professional groups have had a clear understanding of the contributions of the past and of the ways in which future destiny is shaped. It is critical that nursing embrace historical research approaches for continued professional development.

Examples
Historical research provides insight into the profession and the issues that have been significant to its development over time. Austin (1958) proposed six areas for historical research in nursing: (1) biographies of nursing leaders, (2) histories of organizations and professional associations, (3) factors that influence the field, (4) ideas reflected in the philosophy of science in nursing, (5) editing or annotating writings, and (6) compiling and authenticating documents. These areas have been previously researched in nursing. Noted works include the biographies of Lillian Wald (Duffus,

1938; Daniels, 1989) and Florence Nightingale (Woodham-Smith, 1951; Barritt, 1975).

Recently, nursing researchers have begun to generate historical data through oral histories. Interviews with significant nursing leaders provide data about an event in the recent past for analysis as a primary or secondary source and become a data source for studies in the future. An example is the history of African-American nurses described in the book *The Path We Tread* by Mary Elizabeth Carnegie (1986).

Groups of nurses or individuals have been studied in a historical context, such as nurses in the Civil War. Nurses can trace historical research to the early years of the profession's development. Lavinia Dock, Isabel Stewart, and Adelaide Nutting (Dock & Stewart, 1938; Nutting & Dock, 1907-1912) represent this era and are considered the first nurse historians. Another historical researcher, Olga Church, wrote the history of psychiatric nursing, a unique contribution to that specialty practice area.

Sources of nursing data are found in numerous archives such as the ones located at Vanderbilt University and the University of Iowa. Several professional organizations, such as the Heritage Commission of Sigma Theta Tau and the American Nurses' Association, have archival capability. Records and minutes of state boards of nursing are available for historical studies as well.

CASE STUDY METHOD

Case study as a research strategy includes single and multiple case designs and may be descriptive, exploratory, explanatory, or causal. Yin's (1989) monograph is an excellent reference for studying the case study research design in depth. Case studies have been used in a variety of ways. They have been used in nursing and other disciplines as a way of teaching course content. As a

teaching tool, case studies are designed to promote discussion and debate. In other instances case studies are used as a method for evaluating practice. Cases are written to demonstrate continuity and holism in mental health and community health practice. Recently case studies have been utilized by nurses as a research method. It is this use of case studies that will be discussed in this section.

Yin (1989) stated that "the case study allows an investigation to retain the holistic and meaningful characteristics of real-life events—such as individual life cycles, organizational and managerial processes, neighborhood change, international relations, and the maturation of industries" (p. 14). This description covers the potential range of ways in which the case study approach might be used in nursing. As the health care industry evolves, there are opportunities to examine changes in institutional policies and practices. Professional organizations have changed in keeping with the larger societal changes, and those changes could be well documented in case studies. Case studies of patients may be helpful in understanding the implications of these changes on nursing practice.

Method

One of the strengths of the case study approach is the depth of the case descriptions or explorations as they are written. The cases provide sufficient details for the reader to grasp the idiosyncrasies of the phenomenon. However, quantitative cases are often criticized for their lack of objectivity and generalizability. These disadvantages are more often associated with quantitative methods. The researcher must evaluate the quality of case studies in view of the goals of the study. The aim of a qualitative case study is to offer a perspective of the situation. Qualitative case studies are to be evaluated on the ability of the case to illustrate or describe the corresponding phenomenon.

Example

The most widely recognized case study is Whyte's 1943 study entitled "Street Corner Society." This classic study described the single case of an American subculture. Case studies in nursing are often examples of rare or unusual cases such as the breastfeeding experience of a mother with a radical mastectomy.

DESCRIPTIVE METHOD

The descriptive method is a general term that can refer to qualitative case studies or to detailed descriptions of phenomena. Parse et al. (1985) described the descriptive method as similar to descriptive quantitative approaches in that questions are specified, the conceptual framework identified, and the study design fleshed out, including the sampling plan. In this method data gathering may be done by interviews, observations, or open-ended questionnaires. The data are content analyzed and reported in narrative form. Usually there is a specified method for conducting the content analysis.

PHOTOGRAPHY AND AESTHETIC INQUIRY

Photography and aesthetic inquiry is a relatively new qualitative method in nursing. Photographs can provide an excellent source of data in three ways. The first is the analysis of existing photographs. This process is similar to that used in document analysis in historical research. It is important that the researcher places the photos in the context of the time and place in which they were taken. Questions related to the motivation or intent of the photographer, the purpose of the work, and the nature of the content are to be considered.

Verification and authentication of photographs have methodological significance as in historical studies.

Recently the camera has become a research tool for data collection; more recently video and computer-generated images have evolved as sources. Images can be captured with details that otherwise would be unnoticed or forgotten. Often mundane aspects of life can be recorded electronically or by time-lapse photography. The camera facilitates the researcher's objective recollection of visual data. Taylor and Bogdan (1984) described studies by Ryave and Schenkein (the art of walking) and Whyte (description of life in small parks and plazas) as early examples of use of this technology. A study by Ziller and Smith (1977) illustrated how photography can be used to elicit the perspective of the subject. Ziller and Lewis (1981) gave cameras to subjects and asked them to take pictures of who they thought they were. A study by Higgins and Highley (1986) is another example of the use of the camera and photography in research.

Another method using photography involves the researcher taking photos to depict a phenomenon. Photographic essays are a specific example of how situations can be documented by the researcher. This author depicted caring experiences in a photographic essay.

There are other methods using photography or visual media. In photo-interviewing, for instance, subjects are given a photo or asked to take a photo and share the meaning with the researchers. The interviewing schedule directs the responses of the subject regarding the photograph and illuminates meaning.

An example of such an inquiry is a doctoral student's study of premenstrual syndrome (PMS) at the University of Tennessee. Her dissertation research is studying the PMS experience from the perspective of the client by asking her to take photographs of herself on a PMS and a non-PMS day. The investigator proposes that these two sets of photos are different and that the subject can adequately portray these differing experiences in photography. A method of photo disclosure has emerged from this study (Bultemeier, 1993).

Method

Highley and Ferentz (1988) examined the history of aesthetic inquiry and credited John Collier with writing the first text on visual research in anthropological fieldwork. His work, published in 1986, promoted photography in academic and research settings. Highley and Ferentz (1988) further described the 1942 work of Margaret Mead, "Balinese Character," as a classic in this area.

In their discussion of the aesthetic inquiry method, Highley and Ferentz described access and consent as two issues of concern. First, the investigator must obtain blanket access to subjects from an agency and then individual consent from each subject photographed. Clear descriptions of how the photos will be used, where and how they will be disseminated, and ways in which anonymity will be protected are to be included in consent forms.

Two methods for conducting aesthetic inquiry as outlined by Highley and Ferentz are the agency survey and the case study. The agency survey is the sampling of the services of a particular agency that allows the researcher to examine the superstructure. The focus of this type of inquiry is on the service rather than on individuals. The second approach, case studies, examines one situation over an extended period of time. A variety of activities are documented so that all the images present a view of the case. Planning and intuition are useful in deciding the appropriate photos to take to illustrate the case. Collaborative decision making between the investigator and the subject is useful when planning representative photos. Scripting, which is a predetermined list of photos to be obtained, requires prior knowledge of the case.

Data analysis is accomplished through content analysis with emphasis on themes and patterns and sequences of images. In the analyses one photograph rarely stands alone, while a series of photos are more often the unit of analysis. Highley and Ferentz provide an in-depth review of the process of content analysis in their chapter. Briefly, they describe the process of content analysis in four stages. First, the investigator examines the contact sheets as raw data. Second, patterns and themes are identified among the photos. Third, working proofs of 5 × 7 enlargements are analyzed, and themes are further refined. Finally, high-quality prints are placed in sequence emphasizing aesthetic appeal. These prints become the finished product to be disseminated as project findings.

✑ EVALUATING THE QUALITATIVE DESIGN

The choice of research design is critical to the outcome of the study in that the findings are shaped by its design. Marshall and Rossman (1989) stated that the researcher is to explicate the logical and compelling connection between the research question and the choice of methods (p. 46). They suggest the careful matching of the purposes of the study, research questions, research strategies (design), and possible data collection techniques.

An evaluation process is suggested to en-

EVALUATION OF QUALITATIVE DESIGNS

1. Is the phenomenon being studied best understood from a qualitative perspective?
2. Are the theoretical underpinnings of the design understood? Are the assumptions underlying the qualitative design fully described and met by the method?
3. Are the steps in the methodology followed as suggested by published, experienced researchers (mentors, advisors, research consultants)?
4. Are data collected and analyzed appropriately according to the design?
5. Do findings of the research study reflect the outcome proposed by the approach (e.g., a substantive or formal theory is the result of grounded theory design)?

sure that all the underlying assumptions are met and that the design methodology is followed. Questions pertinent to the evaluation of the design are outlined in the box.

Qualitative designs are compatible with the values espoused in nursing. Concepts associated with the qualitative method are holism, naturalistic setting, perception, subjective or lived experiences, interactions, communication, and patterns. By using qualitative designs, nursing research can overcome the limitations of strictly empirical science and can study the phenomena of caring, dying, presencing, touching, and empathy, or situations such as becoming a mother or entering menopause. Only then can our research findings from such studies contribute to the theory base of our applied discipline.

SUMMARY

- Qualitative designs are essential for the development of nursing science in that all nursing phenomena cannot be understood from one perspective.
- It is through the combined efforts of researchers using qualitative and quantitative methods that discovery and verification can take place.

- The valuing of the "science of knowing" is equally shared by qualitative and quantitative researchers who contribute to the body of nursing knowledge.
- Quantitative and qualitative research approaches are complementary and reflect what is known about a phenomenon. Limited knowledge offers opportunities for discovery in qualitative approaches, while verification and validation occurs with hypothesis testing.
- Qualitative research strategies include participant observations, interviews, document analysis, and life histories. These strategies are used in the various research designs and are not necessarily a defining characteristic.
- As found in quantitative strategies, each qualitative method is structured by principles, rules, and certain steps for implementation.
- The various qualitative approaches are best distinguished by their underlying theoretical framework, the wording of the research question, and the methods of data collection and analysis.
- The process of selecting a research design is a nonlinear process and reflects considerable thoughtful consideration and planning.

FACILITATING CRITICAL THINKING

The following clinical situations are areas of concern for nursing practice. To best understand these experiences, the nurse researcher may want to first consider a qualitative research method. What qualitative designs would be most appropriate to answer questions about these phenomena? Read through the situations and propose two possible approaches for each.

CLINICAL SITUATION 1

Breastfeeding is a way to provide passive immunity to newborn infants, enhance mother-infant bonding, and provide nutrition in a cost-effective manner. Even with these significant outcomes, some women choose not to breastfeed. What are reasons women choose to breastfeed their infants? What nursing interventions would facilitate mothers choosing this option more frequently? What type of social support networks facilitate breastfeeding as an option?

CLINICAL SITUATION 2

Menopause is viewed by the medical community as a negative period in the lives of women that requires medical intervention to cope effectively. Others describe menopause as a major life event that focuses on the psychophysiological symptoms and their impact on the woman's relationship with significant others. How do the members of the nursing profession respond to menopause? What type of care is available to menopausal women? What views of menopause treatment are supported by nurses in their practice? Which research approach would allow women to define their experience with menopause?

CLINICAL SITUATION 3

Little is known about the experience of caring for family members who suffer from a chronic mental illness. As a consequence, there are few nursing interventions that support these caretaking activities. Families often receive assistance from community support groups when they are in crisis instead of preventively by professional nurses. What is the family's experience of caregiving? How does the lack of nurses' understanding of the family caregiving experience influence the quality of psychiatric/mental health nursing care to the patient and family?

References
SUBSTANTIVE

BARRITT, E. R. (1975). *Florence Nightingale: Her wit and wisdom.* New York: McGraw-Hill.

BENOLIEL, J. Q. (1967). *The nurse and the dying patient.* New York: Macmillan.

BURKE, S. O., ET AL. (1991). Hazardous secrets and reluctantly taking charge: Parenting a child with repeated hospitalizations. *IMAGE: Journal of Nursing Scholarship, 23*(1), 39-45.

CARNEGIE, M. E. (1986). *The path we tread: Blacks in nursing, 1854-1984.* New York: J.B. Lippincott.

CORBIN, J. (1987). Women's perception and management of a pregnancy complicated by chronic illness. *Health Care for Women International, 84,* 317-337.

DANIELS, D. (1989). *Always a sister: The feminism of Lillian Wald.* New York: Feminist Press at the City University of New York.

DOCK, L., & STEWART, I. (1938). *A short history of nursing, from the earliest times to the present day.* New York: G. P. Putnam.

DUFFUS, R. L. (1938). *Lillian Wald: Neighbor and crusader.* New York: Macmillan.

GATES, M. F. (1991). Transcultural comparisons of hospital and hospice as caring environments for dying patients. *Journal of Transcultural Nursing, 2*(2), 3-15.

HIGGINS, S., & HIGHLEY, B. (1986). The camera as a tool: Photo interview of mothers of infants with congestive heart failure. *Children's Health Care, 15*(2), 119-122.

JONES, P. S., & MARTINSON, I. M. (1992). The experience of bereavement in caregivers of family members with Alzheimer's disease. *IMAGE: Journal of Nursing Scholarship, 24*(3), 172-176.

NUTTING, M., & DOCK, L. (1907-1912). *A history of nursing: The evolution of nursing systems from the earliest times to the foundation of the first English and American training schools for nurses* (Vols. 1-4). New York: G. P. Putnam.

RIEMEN, D. J. (1986). The essential structure of a caring interaction: Doing phenomenology. In P. L. Munhall & C. J. Oiler (Eds.), *Nursing research: A qualitative perspective*. Norwalk, CT: Appleton-Century-Crofts.

VILLARRUEL, A. M., & ORTIZ DE MONTELLANO, B. (1992). Culture and pain: A Mesoamerican perspective. *Advances in Nursing Science, 15*(1), 21-32.

WILSON, H. S. (1982). *Deinstitutionalized residential care for the mentally disordered: The sorteria house approach*. New York: Grune & Stratton.

WOODMAN-SMITH, C. (1951). *Florence Nightingale*. New York: McGraw-Hill.

CONCEPTUAL

AAMODT, A. M. (1991). Ethnography and epistemology: Generating nursing knowledge. In J. M. Morse (Ed.), *Qualitative nursing research: A contemporary dialogue*. Newbury Park, CA: Sage.

CHURCH, O. M. (1987). Historiography in nursing research. *Western Journal of Nursing Research, 9*(2), 275-279.

GERMAIN, C. (1986). Ethnography: The method. In P. L. Munhall, & C. J. Oiler (Eds.), *Nursing research: A qualitative perspective*. Norwalk, CT: Appleton-Century-Crofts.

KRAMPITZ, S. D. (1981). Research design: Historical. In S. D. Krampitz & N. Pavlovich (Eds.), *Readings for nursing research*. St. Louis: C.V. Mosby.

LEININGER, M. M. (1984). *Care: The essence of nursing and health*. Thorofare, NJ: C. Slack.

MUNHALL, P. L., & OILER, C. J. (1986). *Nursing research: A qualitative perspective*. Norwalk, CT: Appleton-Century-Crofts.

OMERY, A. (1983). Phenomenology: A method for nursing research. *Advances in Nursing Science, 5*(2), 49-63.

PARSE, R. R., ET AL. (1985). *Nursing research: Qualitative methods*. Bowie, MD: Brady Communications.

PATERSON, J. G., & ZDERAD, L. T. (1976). *Humanistic nursing*. New York: Wiley.

WATSON, J. (1988). *Nursing: Human science and human care. A theory of nursing*. New York: National League of Nursing.

WHYTE, W. F. (1955). *Street corner society*. Chicago: University of Chicago Press.

ZILLER, R. C., & LEWIS, D. (1981). Orientations: Self, social and environmental precepts through auto-photography. *Personality and Social Psychology Bulletin, 7*, 338-343.

ZILLER, R. C., & SMITH, D. E. (1977). A phenomenological utilization of photographs. *Journal of Phenomenological Psychology, 7*, 172-185.

METHODOLOGICAL

AUSTIN, A. L. (1958). The historical method in nursing. *Nursing Research, 7*(1), 4-10.

BULTEMEIER, K. I. (1993). Photographic inquiry of the phenomenon premenstrual syndrome within the Rogerian derived theory of perceived dissonance. Unpublished doctoral dissertation, University of Tennessee, Knoxville, TN.

CHENITZ, W. C., & SWANSON, J. M. (1986). *From practice to grounded theory*. Menlo Park, CA: Addison-Wesley.

CHRISTY, T. E. (1975). The methodology of historical research: A brief introduction. *Nursing Research, 24*(3), 189-192.

COLAIZZI, P. F. (1978). Psychological research as the phenomenologist views it. In R. Valle & M. King (Eds.), *Existential phenomenological alternatives for psychology*. New York: Oxford University Press.

GIORGI, A. (1970). *Psychology as a human science*. New York: Harper & Row.

HIGHLEY, B., & FERENTZ, T. (1988). Aesthetic inquiry. In B. Sarter (Ed.), *Paths to knowledge: Innovative research methods for nursing*. New York: National League for Nursing.

HUTCHINSON, S. (1986). Grounded theory: The method. In P. L. Munhall & C. J. Oiler (Eds.), *Nursing research: A qualitative perspective*. Norwalk, CT: Appleton-Century-Crofts.

Leininger, M. (1985). *Qualitative research methods in nursing.* Orlando, FL: Grune & Stratton.

Marshall, C., & Rossman, G. B. (1989). *Designing qualitative research.* Newbury Park, CA: Sage.

Parse, R. R., & Coyne, A. B. (1985). *Nursing research: Qualitative method.* Bowie, MD: Brady Communications.

Robnett, M. (Fall, 1986). Historical research. *Iowa Nurse,* 2-3.

Shafer, R. J. (1980). *Analysis and synthesis: A guide to historical method.* Homewood, IL: Dorsey.

Spindler G., & Spindler, L. (1970). Fieldwork among the Menomini. In G. Spindler (Ed.), *Being an anthropologist: Fieldwork in eleven cultures.* New York: Holt, Rinehart & Winston.

Strauss, A., & Corbin, J. (1990). *Basics of qualitative research grounded theory. Procedures and techniques.* Newbury Park, CA: Sage.

Taylor, S., & Bogdan, R. (1984). *Introduction to qualitative research methods: The search for meanings.* New York: Wiley.

Yin, R. K. (1989). *Case study research design and methods.* Newbury Park, CA: Sage.

Historical

Agar, M. H. (1986). *Speaking of ethnography.* Newbury Park, CA: Sage.

Blumer, H. (1969). *Symbolic interactionism: Perspective and method.* Englewood Cliffs, NJ: Prentice Hall.

Glaser, B. G. (1978). *Theoretical sensitivity: Advances in the methodology of grounded theory.* Mill Valley, CA: Sociology Press.

Glaser, B. G., & Strauss, A. (1967). *The discovery of grounded theory: Strategies for qualitative research.* Chicago: Aldine.

Heidegger, M. (1962). *Being and time* (J. Macquarrie, & E. Robinson, Trans.). New York: Harper Brothers.

Husserl, E. (1965). *Phenomenology and the crisis of philosophy.* New York: Harper & Row.

Husserl, E. (1977). *Phenomenological psychology* (J. Scanlon, Trans.). The Hague: Martinus Nijhoff.

Marcel, G. (1971). *The philosophy of existence* (R. F. Grabow, Ed. and Trans.). Philadelphia: University of Pennsylvania Press.

Merleau-Ponty, M. (1964). *The primacy of perception* (J. Edie, Trans.). Evanston, IL: Northwestern University Press.

Merleau-Ponty, M. (1965). *Phenomenology of perception* (C. Smith, Trans.). New York: The Humanities Press.

Ricoeur, P. (1973). Hermeneutic method and reflective philosophy. In R. Zaner & D. Ihde (Eds.), *Phenomenology and existentialism.* New York: Capricorn.

Sartre, A. (1966). *The psychology of imagination.* New York: Citadel.

Schultz, A. (1967). *The phenomenology of the social world.* Evanston, IL: Northwestern University Press.

Spiegelberg, H. (1976) On some human uses of phenomenology. In F. J. Smith (Ed.), *Phenomenology in perspective.* The Hague: Martinus Nijhoff.

Spradley, J. P. (1979). *The ethnographic interview.* New York: Holt, Rinehart & Winston.

Spradley, J. P. (1980). *Participant observation.* New York: Holt, Rinehart & Winston.

Strauss, A. L. (1987). *Qualitative analysis for social scientists.* New York: Cambridge University Press.

Van Kaam, A. (1969). *Existential foundations of psychology.* New York: Doubleday.

Werner, O., & Schoepfle, G. M. (1987). *Systematic field-work* (Vols. 1 & 2). Newbury Park, CA: Sage.

CHAPTER 21

THE QUALITATIVE RESEARCH PROCESS

CARLA MARIANO

Nurses are interested in concepts inherent in the human condition. Empathy, pain, hope, suffering, caring, and fear are some of the phenomena that we experience in our everyday lives. Qualitative research methods enable us to explore these concepts as they are perceived and defined by real people; they allow people to speak for themselves, thereby emphasizing the human capacity to know.

⌘ THE NATURE OF THE QUALITATIVE INQUIRY PROCESS

The qualitative research process proceeds in a spiral, looping fashion. It does not handle time linearly. Data gathering and data analysis are integrated and inform each other. The process is compared to the art of sculpting: The researcher continually molds and remolds rather than taking a snapshot. As Mariano (1990) states, "The qualitative approach is interactive; holistic; flexible, dynamic, and evolving; naturalistic; process oriented; primarily inductive;

and descriptive. It has, as its foci, perspectives, meanings, uniqueness, and subjective lived experiences. Its aim is understanding" (p. 354). Munhall and Boyd (1993) offer additional expressions of qualitative research methods as subjective experience, intuition, shared language, lived experience, dynamic reality, patterns, complementarity, and human development (p. 33).

Patton (1990) and Lincoln and Guba (1985) describe the themes of qualitative inquiry in the following way:

- Qualitative inquiry uses the natural setting. It explores real-life situations as they occur naturally. There is no attempt to manipulate or control predetermined variables or conditions. This type of inquiry is open to whatever emerges versus measuring a very limited number of outcome factors.
- Qualitative inquiry uses inductive analysis. It emphasizes exploration and discovery rather than testing or verifying predetermined hypotheses

that are deductively determined. The researcher attempts to discover salient groupings, patterns, themes, and relationships in the data that help one understand the phenomenon under study.

- In qualitative inquiry the researcher examines the totality and the unifying character of what is being studied. The phenomenon is seen as a complex whole in a particular context. Focus is on interdependencies, not cause-and-effect relationships.
- Qualitative inquiry implies qualitative data, that is, detailed, thick descriptions of the situation using the participants' own words, experiences, and perspectives. Data are narrative versus numerical.
- Qualitative inquiry also implies qualitative methods that are most sensitive and adaptable to the multiple realities being uncovered. These methods are discussed further in the sections on data collection and analysis.
- Tacit or intuitive felt knowledge is used in qualitative inquiry to assist the researcher in appreciating the nuances of experiences, interactions, and values.
- The researcher has direct and close contact with the participants, the setting, and the issue under study. The researcher's insights and experiences are integral to inquiry and the analysis.
- The researcher attends to *process* with the assumption that change is constant.
- Qualitative inquiry assumes that each case is unique. This supposition warrants an idiographic interpretation of findings; in other words, data are interpreted based on the particulars of

the case rather than lawlike generalizations.
- Qualitative research attends to social, historical, and temporal context. Findings of these studies are tentatively applied, that is, they may be applicable in diverse situations based on the comparability of other contexts.
- The investigator strives toward empathic neutrality. The researcher is the human instrument. Although maintaining a nonjudgmental position toward whatever appears, she or he includes personal experience and empathic insight as part of the pertinent data.
- Qualitative inquiry necessitates a flexible design. The design emerges as understanding increases. Purposive sampling is used to uncover multiple realities and discover new paths of inquiry as they materialize.

Figure 21-1 displays the process of qualitative inquiry.

ꙮ GETTING STARTED: AIM OF THE STUDY

The aim of the study includes a description of the focus of the inquiry, the research question/problem statement, and the significance of the study.

FOCUS OF THE INQUIRY

Lincoln and Guba (1985) note that "no inquiry, regardless of which paradigm may guide it, can be conducted in the absence of a focus" (p. 226). Determining the focus of an inquiry serves two purposes. First, it "establishes the *boundaries* for a study; it defines the terrain, as it were, that is to be considered the proper territory of the in-

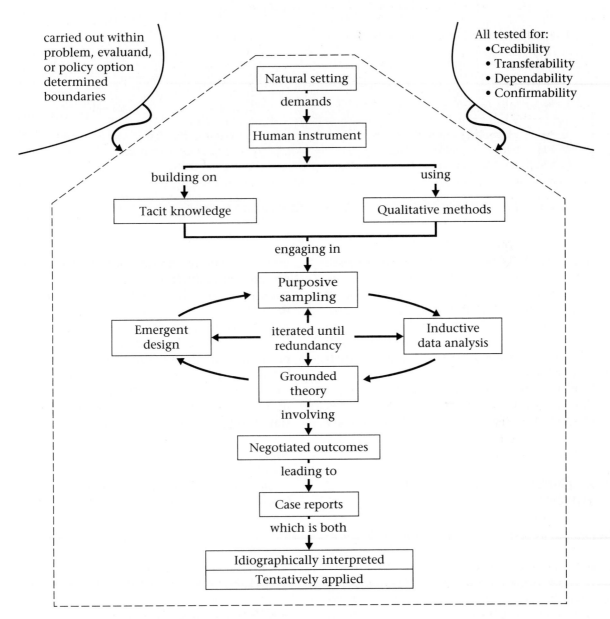

Figure 21-1. The flow of naturalistic inquiry. (Reprinted with permission from Lincoln, Y. S., & Guba, E. G. (1985). *Naturalistic inquiry.* Beverly Hills, CA: Sage, p. 188.)

STEPS IN THE QUALITATIVE RESEARCH PROCESS

1. Determine the aim of the study, and establish:
   a. Focus of the inquiry
   b. Research question/problem statement
   c. Significance of the study
2. Review the literature.
3. Identify the sample.
4. Select a sampling method.
5. Implement the qualitative inquiry.
6. Select data-gathering and -management strategies:
   a. Observation
   b. Interviewing
   c. Data logging
7. Data analysis and interpretation:
   a. Identify a data-analysis technique (thematic analysis; grounded theory development)
   b. Conduct the qualitative data analysis
8. Write the qualitative report.
9. Evaluate the qualitative research process: trustworthiness and ethics

---

quiry" (p. 227). Second, it helps the investigator determine "inclusion–exclusion criteria" for new data that are collected. Not all information collected in a study is relevant, although it may be interesting. Focusing the inquiry assists the researcher in deciding which information to keep and which to eliminate. It is very important to note, however, that as data are collected, the initial research question or problem may change and the focus of the inquiry may shift. That is why qualitative designs are considered emergent designs.

RESEARCH QUESTION/PROBLEM STATEMENT

Qualitative research evolves from a discovery paradigm versus a verification paradigm. It involves learning from those who have actually experienced the phenomenon of interest. The difference between these two paradigms suggests major implications for the type of research question asked or research problem posed. The researcher is not looking for cause-and-effect relationships. Rather, the investigator is exploring how an individual or group experiences a particular phenomenon or creates

meaning. The researcher looks at *what* people are experiencing, *how* they are experiencing it, and how they are *constructing* their reality.

Various sources for researchable questions in the qualitative paradigm include personal and professional experience, the literature, prior research, practical needs, social concerns, or identified priorities for inquiry. Such research questions are not stated in hypothesis form derived from theory; rather, they are broad, open-ended or "open-beginning," context dependent, and people oriented to the human condition.

Open-ended questions allow the inquiry "room to grow." They are asked in the following manner:

- What is the nature of . . . ?
- What is the description of . . . ?
- How do people perceive or experience something?
- What is happening here?

The emphasis of the inquiry is on wholeness and integrity rather than on control and linear relationships. As discussed, defining the research question becomes one of the most important steps in qualitative research as the amount of data gathered can be enormous.

Qualitative research questions are conducive to context. The contexts of both the phenomenon and the researcher are considered. The focus of the inquiry is not the person or event in isolation but the person, event, or phenomenon in its physical, psychosocial, cultural, spiritual, and symbolic milieu. As Lincoln and Guba (1985) state, "naturalistic ontology suggests that realities are wholes that cannot be understood in isolation from their contexts, nor can they be fragmented for separate study of the parts (the whole is more than the sum of the parts)" (p. 39).

The researcher's context is also an important consideration in the development of the research question or focus. The experiences, assumptions, preconceptions, intuitions, and interests of the investigator can influence the entire research process, including what data are collected, how data are collected, how data are analyzed, and what interpretations are proposed (Mariano, 1990). "Inquiries are influenced by *inquirer* values as expressed in the choice of a problem . . . and in the framing, bounding, and focusing of that problem" (Lincoln & Guba, 1985, p. 38).

We all have assumptions, preconceptions, and opinions. However, the qualitative researcher must deal with them both before and during data collection so that she or he does not misinterpret another person's experience. In dealing with assumptions about a particular phenomenon, the investigator: (1) assumes that they are there; (2) draws them out; (3) examines his or her own value stances and judgments; and (4) has his or her work critically evaluated by someone else. This topic will be further discussed under the section on the trustworthiness of a study.

Bracketing is used by qualitative researchers "to meet the ethical dictum of portraying accurately the reality of the phenomenon as it is lived and described by the researcher's informants" (Swanson-Kauffman & Schonwald, 1988, p. 99). This process involves identifying and suspending one's own assumptions, beliefs, culture, attitudes, values, perspectives, and knowledge about the phenomenon under study to "see" and "hear" the experience of another. Unless the researcher explores held beliefs and preconceptions about the phenomenon under study, both data collection and data analysis may become a reflection of the researcher's conception of the event or phenomenon rather than a description of the participant's actual experience.

The qualitative researcher must have a humanistic orientation, "an interest in 'going to the people,' a desire to understand other perspectives, and a willingness to see the researcher/participant relationship as a *partnership*" (Mariano, 1990, p. 356). In discussing the stance of the qualitative researcher, Bogdan and Taylor (1975) note that the researcher is necessarily involved in the participants' lives. The investigator must identify and empathize with participants in order to understand their perspectives. Every person's perspective is viewed as equal to another's. The participants' viewpoints are seen as neither "true nor false, good nor bad. *The researcher seeks not truth and morality, but rather, understanding*" (Bogdan & Taylor, 1975, p. 9).

SIGNIFICANCE OF THE STUDY

In discussing the significance of the study, the researcher demonstrates why it is important to study this particular phenomenon and why it is necessary to utilize a qualitative design. The purpose of qualitative inquiry can be to generate theory or to develop a descriptive base for practice. The researcher discusses the relevance of the inquiry; the contribution of the study to understanding, knowledge, and practice; and the importance of the study to nursing.

Marshall and Rossman (1989) suggest that the significance of the study should answer the following questions:

- Who has an interest in this domain of inquiry?
- What do we already know about the topic?
- What has not been answered adequately in previous research and practice?
- How will this new research add to knowledge, practice, and policy in this area? (p. 31)

REVIEWING THE LITERATURE

In the qualitative paradigm, there are conflicting views on conducting a literature review *before* data collection. One position holds that a preliminary review of the literature should not be conducted as it will unduly bias the researcher in the collection of the data. It may bias observations and questions as the researcher looks to confirm previously held theoretical conceptions. The other position contends that a preliminary review of the literature is valuable for a number of reasons.

Rather than narrowing the investigator's perspective to a preconceived conceptualization of the phenomenon and of how to measure it, a literature review can open the investigator to the complexity of the phenomenon under study. When conducting an ethnography, a literature review also introduces the researcher to the "culture." Knowing something about the people, their language, their norms, often facilitates entrée into and the development of

trust within the group. Most important, a literature review provides additional rationale and credence for conducting the study. It demonstrates that this particular phenomenon has not been studied to date nor has it been investigated in this manner.

The use of a theoretical framework *before* data collection also has opponents and supporters. The qualitative approach is not used to test a theory. Its objective is to develop hypotheses and generate theory. Rather than using an a priori theory, the theory should emerge from the inquiry. On the other hand, the use of a framework is appropriate if the theoretical perspective fits naturalistic axioms. The framework must conform to the philosophical basis from which the researcher approaches the study. Relevant frameworks for qualitative inquiry include phenomenology, culture, symbolic interaction, history, aesthetics, and ethics (see Chapter 19 for further discussion of these theoretical orientations to qualitative research). Patton (1990) also includes ecological psychology (the relationship between human behavior and the environment), chaos theory (the underlying order of disorderly phenomena), hermeneutics (understanding human acts or products through interpretation of meaning and context), and heuristics (development of meaning and knowledge of a significant human experience through personal experience and encounter with the phenomenon) as appropriate theoretical perspectives.

SAMPLING

Qualitative research approaches tend to utilize small samples and emphasize depth versus breadth. The researcher is attempting to obtain understanding through an indepth and detailed exploration of the phenomenon, group, or person. The sample is chosen purposefully rather than randomly or by convenience. Patton (1990) notes that one of the greatest differences between qualitative and quantitative approaches consists in the different logics that underlie sampling methods.

As Patton (1990) states:

> Qualitative inquiry typically focuses in depth on relatively small samples, even single cases (*n* = 1), selected *purposefully*. Quantitative methods typically depend on larger samples selected randomly. . . . The logic and power of probability sampling depends on selecting a truly random and statistically representative sample that will permit confident generalization from the sample to a larger population. . . . The logic and power of purposeful [or selective] sampling lies in selecting information-rich cases for study in depth. Information-rich cases are those from which one can learn a great deal about issues of central importance to the purpose of the research. (p. 169)

THE UNIT OF ANALYSIS

The sample in qualitative research refers to the unit(s) of analysis to be explored. The sample or unit of analysis can be an individual, a group, a culture, an organization or agency, an event or occurrence, a process, or a particular phenomenon that people experience. The researcher must clearly define the unit of analysis as "each unit of analysis [type] implies a different kind of data collection, a different focus for the analysis of data, and a different level at which statements about findings and conclusions would be made" (Patton, 1990, p. 167).

SAMPLING METHODS

The sampling process necessitates an emphasis on both what to sample and how to sample (Kuzel, 1992). "The 'what' to sample may include events, places, persons, ar-

tifacts, activity, and time" (Kuzel, 1992, p. 34). The "how" to sample includes determining which of the various purposive sampling strategies to use. Table 21-1 presents Patton's (1990) summary of the various sampling strategies used in qualitative research.

Theoretical sampling is a method of sampling used to generate grounded theory. In this process

> [the] analyst decides *on analytic grounds* what data to collect next and where to find them. The basic question in theoretical sampling is: *What* groups or subgroups of populations, events, activities (to find varying dimensions, strategies, etc.) does one turn to *next* in data collection. And for *what* theoretical purpose? . . . The process of data collection is *controlled* by the emerging theory. (Strauss, 1987, p. 38)

It is "sampling on the basis of concepts that have proven theoretical relevance to the evolving theory" (Strauss & Corbin, 1990, p. 176).

According to Kuzel (1992), sampling in qualitative research has the following characteristics:

1. The sample design, although preconceived (at least enough to answer the question, Where and with whom do I start?), is flexible and evolves as the study progresses.
2. Sample "units" are selected serially. Who and what comes next? depends on who and what came before.
3. The sample is adjusted continuously or "focused" by the concurrent development of theory.
4. Selection continues to a point of redundancy.
5. Sampling includes a search for negative cases [disconfirming evidence] in order to give developing theory greater breadth and strength (p. 41).

Table 21-1
Sampling Strategies

Type	Purpose
Purposeful Sampling	Selects information-rich cases for in-depth study. Size and specific cases depend on study purpose.
1. Extreme or deviant case sampling	Enables one to learn from highly unusual manifestations of the phenomenon of interest, such as outstanding successes/notable failures, top of the class/dropouts, exotic events, crises.
2. Intensity sampling	Provides information-rich cases that manifest the phenomenon intensely, but not extremely, such as good students/poor students, above average/below average.
3. Maximum variation sampling—purposefully picking a wide range of variation on dimensions of interest	Documents unique or diverse variations that have emerged in adapting to different conditions. Identifies important common patterns that cut across variations.
4. Homogeneous sampling	Focuses, reduces variation, simplifies analysis, facilitates group interviewing.
5. Typical case sampling	Illustrates or highlights what is typical, normal, average.
6. Stratified purposeful sampling	Illustrates characteristics of particular subgroups of interest; facilitates comparisons.
7. Critical case sampling	Permits *logical* generalization and maximum application of information to other cases because if it is true of this one case, it is likely to be true of all other cases.
8. Snowball or chain sampling	Identifies cases of interest from people who know people who know people who know what cases are information-rich, that is, good examples for study, good interview subjects.
9. Criterion sampling	Involves picking all cases that meet some criterion, such as all children abused in a treatment facility. Quality assurance.
10. Theory-based or operational construct sampling	Entails finding manifestations of a theoretical construct of interest so as to elaborate and examine the construct.
11. Confirming and discomfirming cases	Elaborates and deepens initial analysis, seeking exceptions, testing variation.
12. Opportunistic sampling	Involves following new leads during fieldwork, taking advantage of the unexpected, flexibility.
13. Random purposeful sampling (still small sample size)	Adds credibility to sample when potential purposeful sample is larger than one can handle. Reduces judgment within a purposeful category. (Not for generalizations or representativeness.)

Table 21-1—cont'd
Sampling Strategies

Type	Purpose
14. Sampling politically important cases	Attracts attention to the study (or avoids attracting undesired attention by purposefully eliminating from the sample politically sensitive cases).
15. Convenience sampling	Saves time, money, and effort. Poorest rationale; lowest credibility. Yields information-poor cases.
16. Combination or mixed purposeful sampling	Is based on triangulation, flexibility; meets multiple interests and needs.

Reprinted with permission from Patton, M. Q. (1990). *Qualitative evaluation and research methods* (2nd ed., pp. 182-183). Newbury Park: Sage.

The researcher continues to sample individuals, events, situations, and/or settings to the point of redundancy or saturation where no new or disconfirming information or evidence is found.

IMPLEMENTING THE QUALITATIVE INQUIRY

There are five phases in implementing a qualitative inquiry: (1) preliminary fieldwork, (2) gaining entrée and access, (3) focused exploration, (4) leaving the setting or field, and (5) writing the final report (Lincoln & Guba, 1985).

After identifying the focus or the phenomenon of study, the researcher must determine where and from whom information will be collected. In phase 1, it is important to do some background exploration or preliminary fieldwork (informal interviewing and observation) prior to actually adopting the setting for the study. This overview phase allows the researcher to obtain preparatory information and to identify what needs to be followed up on and explored in depth in the actual study.

Qualitative research is conducted in the natural setting, hence, the term *naturalistic inquiry*. In phase 2, the investigator must gain clearance into the setting. This necessitates contacting appropriate individuals at the site of inquiry, gaining permission to carry out the study in the setting, and obtaining consent. If necessary, approval must be received from the agency's Human Subjects Committee or Institutional Review Board.

Some strategies facilitate entry into a setting. Know the access rules. Take advantage of "gatekeepers," hosts or liaisons who can help you gain entrée. Demonstrate how your research can benefit the site. Rehearse beforehand how you will answer questions posed to you regarding the purpose of the study. Be honest about your intentions, but do so in broad and general terms. Cultivate a style that enlists cooperation and demonstrates a genuine interest in the participants' experiences and perceptions. Negotiate early on issues such as publication rights, access to people, documents, and activities, and role expectations of the researcher. Always keep in mind that "entrée is a continuous process of establishing and developing relationships" (Schatzman & Strauss, 1982, p. 22).

Phase 3 of a qualitative study is a "focused exploration" of the phenomenon under study. It is an intense period of data collection, data recording, and preliminary data analysis. This phase is a time of "learning from" the participants and the setting. It can last from weeks to years, as researchers become immersed in "the lives of the people and the situations they wish to study. . . . Prolonged contact in the setting allows them [researchers] to view the dynamics of change and thus see organizations, relationships, and group and individual definitions in process" (Bogdan & Taylor, 1975, p. 5).

In phase 4 of the inquiry, the researcher arranges to leave the field, addressing issues of disengagement and closure. It is not unusual for the researcher to get "hooked" on data collection; however, one must eventually leave the community being studied and return to the community of peers to share findings. The researcher completes data collection when she or he *understands* and no new insights are to be gained. Wilson (1989) offers some guides for leaving the field:

1. Be prepared for some participants to feel abandoned and cheated that the researcher is no longer acutely interested in their life and situation.
2. The length of fieldwork should be clear from the beginning, and withdrawal from the field should be gradual.
3. Any norms for leaving the situation (such as a goodbye party) should be attended to.
4. Commitments made in order to gain entrée, such as presenting the findings or providing the agency or participants with a copy of the final report, must be met.
5. Feelings of guilt and sadness at the ending of fieldwork can be expected,

especially if the relationships with the participants were strong and much trust had been developed.
6. Impersonal explanations (completion of a degree or research grant) are useful in terminating relationships. This eases the process of termination.

The last phase of a qualitative inquiry is the "member check" stage and writing the final report. Although the researcher continually clarifies her or his impressions and beginning interpretations with participants throughout data collection, during the final member check, the "provisional report (case) is taken back to the site and subjected to the scrutiny of the persons who provided information. . . . The task is to obtain confirmation that the report has captured the data as constructed by the informant, or to correct, amend, or extend it, that is, to establish the credibility of the case" (Lincoln & Guba, 1985, p. 236). Then, the final report is written.

✎ DATA GATHERING AND MANAGEMENT

Data for qualitative research studies come from a variety of sources: observations, verbal reports, interviews, documents, photographs, pictures, videotapes, diaries, artifacts, or any combination thereof. Data collection begins with the researcher deciding where and from whom data will be collected. The term *participant* or *informant* rather than *subject* is used in this type of study to illustrate the partner relationship between the researcher and the "knower" of the phenomenon. Informants are defined as knowledgeable persons from within the culture or setting. At the initiation of the study, the researcher often fosters relationships with "key informants" or those who have special knowledge, position, or access to information to which the researcher is not privy.

In qualitative research the investigator is the research instrument. Lincoln and Guba (1985) note that the researcher uses himself or herself as the primary data-gathering instrument because a nonhuman instrument such as a paper-and-pencil questionnaire cannot adjust to or include the multiplicity of realities that the researcher will confront. Only human beings can appreciate, understand, and evaluate meanings that others give to their experiences. In addition, most data gathering instruments are value based; but the human instrument can recognize and consider inherent biases and deal with them accordingly.

Two fundamental techniques are used in gathering data for qualitative studies: observation and interviewing. Supplemental techniques include videotapes, photographs, projective techniques, life history, kinesics (studying body motion communication), open-ended questionnaires, and analysis of various types of documents. As observation and interviewing are most frequently used, they will be described here.

OBSERVATION

Participant observation is a term most frequently used to describe the method of observation used in qualitative research. It is defined by Bogdan and Taylor (1975) as "research characterized by a period of intense social interaction between the researcher and the subjects, in the milieu of the latter. During this period, data are unobtrusively and systematically collected" (p. 5). Spradley (1980) describes the participant observer as an involved "watcher" who is different from an ordinary participant. The ordinary participant engages in

the normal activities required of a particular role in a particular setting. The participant observer not only takes part in the activities but also observes the situation carefully in order to record and analyze what is occurring.

Bogdewic (1992) identifies the focus of participant observation to be on

how the activities and interactions of a setting give meaning to certain behaviors or beliefs. . . . The inhabitants of any organization or group are influenced by assumptions that they take for granted. These assumptions reflect the unique culture of a given organization. Rather than relying on the perceptions of inhabitants, participant observation affords the researcher direct access to these assumptions. (pp. 46-47)

Differences between actual behavior and how people verbalize that behavior become evident. Context as it evolves in everyday life can be examined, and the chain of events that give meaning to a phenomenon can be identified.

Patton (1990, pp. 205-217) outlines five dimensions to describe the variation in approaches to observations. These are described in the box.

Once entrée has been gained and rapport established, what does the participant observer look for? Bogdewic (1992) adapted Goetz and LeCompte's (1984) framework for observation. This includes:

- *Who* is present; what roles they play; how they are characterized; how they became members of this group.
- *What* is going on; how people are behaving; what they are doing and saying; how people are communicating with each other verbally and nonverbally.

DIMENSIONS OF OBSERVATIONAL APPROACHES

1. *Role of the observer:* Full participant observation to partial observation to observation as an outsider or onlooker. Others (Junker, 1960) also discuss the continuum in participant observer roles, from complete participant to participant as observer to observer as participant to complete observer. Wolcott (1988) differentiates between the active participant, the privileged observer, and the limited observer. The style or observation stance that the researcher takes often depends on the research purpose, opportunities in the research setting, and institutional constraints.

2. *Portrayal of the researcher role to others:* Overt observations in which participants know that they are being observed and know who the researcher is; observer role is known by some and not by others;

covert observations in which the participants are unaware that observations are being made or that they are in a research study.

3. *Portrayal of the research purpose to others:* A full explanation of the real purpose of the research/observations to all involved; partial explanations; covert purpose in which no explanations are given to staff or participants; false explanations where staff and/or participants are deceived regarding the purpose of the research.

4. *Duration of the research observations:* A single observation of limited duration (1 hour or 1 day); long-term, multiple observations (months or years).

5. *Focus of the observation:* A narrow focus (a single individual or element of the phenomenon) or a broad focus (a holistic view of the entire phenomenon).

- *When* particular activities occur; what their relationships are to other events; how long certain activities last; what the right timing is for certain activities to occur.
- *Where* particular activities happen; the physical environment's contribution to the occurrence; and the participants's use of space.
- *Why* something is happening; what precipitates or contributes to certain events and interactions; what are the different perspectives on what is happening.
- *How* activities are organized; what rules or norms direct activity and conduct.

Most qualitative researchers would agree that it is important to observe setting (the physical environment), participants' ac-

tions and behaviors, activities (planned and informal), interactions (both dialogue and nonverbal communication), and atmosphere. Also, as Lofland and Lofland (1984, p. 13) note, it is necessary to interweave "looking and listening . . . watching and asking"; therefore, the need for both observation and interviewing during participant observation.

Schatzman and Strauss (1982) and Bogdan and Taylor (1975) offer helpful guidelines for the participant observer role, asserting that the researcher should:

- Become familiar with the layout of the setting, that is, the social, temporal, and spatial maps.
- Take an overview look at things, people, and activities.
- Decide on the vantage points from which to observe, appraising the loca-

tion that will yield the most understanding and varying the positioning—stationary, multiple (changing locations), and mobile (following someone)—as necessary.

- Sample people, places, and events selectively, sampling broadly at first, progressively focusing the observations.
- Choose an unfamiliar setting or one in which the researcher has no professional expertise. In a familiar setting, the researcher shares commonsense assumptions and biases with the participants. The observer may take certain cues for granted, overlook information and perspectives important to the participants, and interpret the data from personal experience. A researcher who is unfamiliar with an area may be more open to discovery and new perspectives about a phenomenon.
- Gather evidence over time. Prolonged engagement allows the researcher to become familiar with and understand the context and culture. It helps the observer to recognize and account for distortions of both the researcher and the participants, and to recognize subtleties of the situation. The researcher has time to "peel away" layers until the real meaning of the phenomenon arises.
- Consider potentially problematic issues before they arise, such as feeling uncomfortable in the setting or in the observer role, being forced into roles other than the researcher role, being told whom to observe in the setting for administrative rather than research purposes, learning the language of the participants or the culture.
- Establish and maintain rapport with-

out imitating the behaviors or the language of the participants. The researcher is there to learn from them, not to become one of them. Dress appropriately in relation to the setting. Although it is important to establish common interests with the participants, relationships should develop slowly. The researcher must become an *unobtrusive* part of the scene, someone whom the participants begin to take for granted and trust. It is important not to disrupt the participants' or the setting's routine. Honesty is imperative, as is reinforcement that participation is voluntary and that all information will remain confidential. The researcher cannot assume that he or she understands everything observed and must play down any aura of expertise by using informal interviewing for continuous validation.

There are some disadvantages to participant observation. This type of data-collection technique can be very costly and time-consuming and often takes as much as 1 to 2 years in the field. The researcher may become overly involved ("going native") with the participants, thereby losing objectivity in reporting and interpreting. There is a heavy reliance on researcher memory to recall events that transpire in the field. Last, the most significant disadvantage can involve ethics, primarily when there is covert observation.

INTERVIEWING

Interviewing in qualitative research takes two forms. The investigator can use informal interviewing during participant observation to clarify what she or he is seeing or to enable the participants to explain or expand on what they are doing. The other form of interviewing is intensive, in-depth interviewing. This has been described as a "conversation with a purpose" (Dexter, 1970; Kahn & Connell, 1957). Interviews allow the investigator to get at people's complex feelings and perceptions. They assist the researcher in uncovering the unanticipated. They also allow the researcher to clarify participant responses and to probe particular statements in more depth.

Interviews should produce interesting and prolific "stories" and narratives. The participant is the knower, the expert, the teacher; the researcher is the learner. A good interview is conducive to openness. The participant feels comfortable and talks freely about his or her ideas, opinions, and feelings. A good interview produces data rich in detail and examples and reveals the participant's viewpoint.

Interviews used in qualitative data collection are different from those used in professional practice. Professional interviews are often closed-ended and focused. Their purpose is to gather information either to develop categorical interpretations (diagnoses) or to substantiate a particular diagnosis:

> In contrast to "structured interviewing" (such as opinion polling), where the goal is to elicit choices between alternative answers to preformed questions on a topic or situation, the intensive interview seeks to discover the informant's experience. . . . The structured interview seeks to determine the frequency of preconceived kinds of things, while the unstructured interview seeks to find out what kinds of things exist in the first place. (Lofland & Lofland, 1984, p. 12)

Interviewing in qualitative research emphasizes listening comprehensively (encouraging participants to tell their whole story in their own language) rather than se-

lectively (Mariano, 1990). As Dobert (1982) notes, "The researcher cannot, like the [practitioner] interviewer, direct the conversation. Indeed, by directing the conversation, the researcher can only uncover patterns predicted in advance" (p. 114). He goes on to say, "The question is not, how do you talk to an informant? But, how do you listen to an informant?" (p. 118).

It is important for the investigator to refrain as much as possible from using questions necessitating only a "yes" or "no" answer. Probe follow-ups can be used to increase detailed exploration: "Tell me more about . . ."; "What did you mean by . . ."; "Can you describe . . ."; "I'm not sure I understand . . . , could you explain it a bit more"; "How did you feel then?" Such probes give the interviewee an opportunity to clarify and expand responses and explicate meaning. They also enhance rapport in that they indicate to the informant that the researcher is truly interested in understanding the participants' experience.

Although questions may change as data are continuously analyzed and different areas become important, it is helpful for the researcher to have an interview guide of five or six broad questions with which to begin. This does not mean that the researcher should *control* the content of the interview, but merely enter into it with some idea of the areas that need to be explored. A funneling approach is most productive with in-depth, unstructured interviewing. This technique begins with very broad, open-ended questions. As the interview continues, or as subsequent interviews are conducted, the questions become more focused and specific.

Spradley (1979) differentiates among three types of questions: descriptive, structural, and contrast. *Descriptive questions* are broad and introductory, and elicit a picture of how people describe their world. These include:

1. Grand-tour questions that endeavor to obtain a detailed account of the interviewee's experience (that is totally directed by the interviewee).
2. Mini-tour questions that investigate smaller aspects of the experience.
3. Example questions in which the investigator asks for a specific example.
4. Experience questions in which the investigator attempts to elicit particular experiences (typical or atypical) that the participant has had with a specific event or setting.
5. native-language questions, which ask for the participants to use their common language (words and phrases).

Structural questions get at how people order, categorize, or structure what they know. They complement descriptive questions. These types of questions are meant to elicit explanations from the participant. They ascertain from the interviewee what things, events, people, and so on are included in a particular domain or are related to one another.

Contrast questions are used to get at the participants' perceptions of differences. They discern what things, people, events, and so on are excluded from a particular domain and how entities differ from one another.

Whenever possible and with the consent of the interviewee, the researcher should tape-record interviews. Interview data should produce voluminous narratives. Even with rapid handwriting, it is almost impossible to remember or write down everything that is said in a conversation. Tape-recording permits the researcher to observe all clues outside of language; to

capture nuances in inflection, speech pattern, and emphasis; to ensure completeness; to review the interview frequently to glean further understandings; to fully attend to the participant, thereby giving the interviewee a sense of importance; and to critique her or his own interviewing style. Additionally, the tape can be given back to the participant following transcription. One must always test the tape-recording equipment prior to each interview to ensure proper functioning. It is disheartening to lose an entire interview because of mechanical failure.

Some principles of sound interviewing should be mentioned. First, rapport must be developed before the researcher deals with sensitive or painful topics. This is achieved by creating an open and safe atmosphere in which the participant *wants* to share his or her story. The following are important ways to establish rapport: maintaining eye contact; paying attention to what the person says, does, thinks, and feels; not interrupting; never assuming (if you are unsure, ask); remaining nonjudgmental (the researcher's intent is to understand, not to evaluate); examining your own style of questioning; and developing a healthy appreciation for silence. It is important to recap frequently and to request elaboration. This facilitates clarity, helps to avoid misinterpretation, and demonstrates that the investigator has heard what was said.

There are some disadvantages to interviewing as a data-collection strategy. In-depth, unstructured interviews are very time-consuming to conduct, transcribe, and analyze. The researcher also can incur great expense if a transcriber is hired to do the tape-recorded transcriptions. The interviewee may expect a direct benefit by participating in the interview session. Finally, the researcher must be proficient in or learn good interview and listening skills.

DATA LOGGING

There are numerous ways to log data in qualitative inquiry. It is helpful to establish three types of records: (1) the data record or the raw data themselves (field notes, interview transcripts), (2) a personal/methodological journal, and (3) an analytical log.

Field Notes

Field notes are detailed recordings of a variety of information collected in the field during a period of observation. Field notes are essential during participant observation as they present a literal account of what occurred in the research setting. The researcher may spend hours at a time observing and interacting with participants. Therefore, the notes should be as comprehensive, complete, and accurate as possible, and they should be written after every observation time. Valuable information can be lost if trusted entirely to memory.

The content of field notes includes both descriptive and reflective notations. The researcher records everything in full detail (thick description) that adds to the understanding of the focus of inquiry. Following are areas that should be described (Bogdan & Biklen, 1982; Spradley, 1980):

- *People:* Physical appearance, clothing, characteristics, mannerisms, style of communicating. The researcher notes characteristics that give insights into how people define themselves or are defined by others.
- *Physical setting:* Physical space, furniture, sounds, objects present, color, smell—everything that captures the "essence" of the setting.
- *Dialogue/interaction:* Conversations among participants and between participants and the observer, gestures, nonverbal communication, speech patterns, tone of voice. This description relays much about intention and meanings.
- *Activities:* Actions that people do individually or together, behaviors observed in carrying out the activities.
- *Events:* Particular happenings that occur in the setting, who was involved, timing of events.
- *Goals:* What the participants are trying to accomplish.
- *Feeling tone:* Emotions felt and expressed, atmosphere.

In addition to describing the above, the researcher records reflections on analysis, method, and the researcher's frame of mind (Bogdan & Biklen, 1982). These notations (Schatzman & Strauss, 1982) can be designated in the field notes as follows:

- *Theoretical notes:* The researcher's beginning interpretations, conjectures, inferences. They are speculations about what is being learned and about emerging patterns and themes.
- *Methodological notes:* Directions to oneself, appraisals of the researcher's approach or style, comments regarding the study design and implementation, and methodological reminders for future plans or points of clarification.
- *Personal notes:* Reflections on the researcher's own feelings, experiences, preconceived ideas, assumptions, and reactions. These reflections assist the researcher in determining his or her effects on the data and the fieldwork experience.

Guidelines for writing field notes are outlined in the box.

GUIDELINES FOR WRITING FIELD NOTES

- Leave the setting when the investigator has observed as much as can be remembered. If the researcher becomes too drained of energy and saturated with too much information, the task of recording may be put off. One hour of observation usually requires 2 to 6 hours of recording. Insufficient recording time results in poor and superficial notes.
- Field notes should be recorded as soon as possible after the observation. Observations are useful only to the extent that they are remembered and transcribed. When using participant observation, discipline is needed to write after *each* observation.
- Descriptive, nonevaluative terms are necessary when describing the setting, the people, the activities/behaviors, and the interactions.
- The observation sessions should not be discussed until they have been recorded. Talking with others about what was seen and heard often influences, and may change, the researcher's recall.
- Write the field notes without editing or critiquing them. Use an organizing framework such as the natural, sequential course of the field observation to chronicle the session.
- An outline of topics and a diagram of the setting often stimulate recall. Line-numbered notes and wide margins for transcriptions enable researcher comments to be made at a later date (this is true for both field notes and transcripts of in-depth interviews). Quotation marks should be used to indicate direct or near exact quotes of the participants.
- Duplicates of the field notes allow copies to be cut up, organized, and reorganized for purposes of analysis.

Personal or Methodological Journals

A personal or methodological journal brings together all the personal and methodological notes taken during the inquiry. It includes the researcher's ideas about the project; the uniqueness of the method; methodological problems and how they were dealt with (such as modifications made during data collection); the researcher's feelings about the study, the participants, the setting; and the researcher's context and frame of mind at the time. This journal often serves as the basis for the methods section of the final writeup of the study.

Analytical Logs

The analytical log is a summary of the theoretical notes, the analytical memos, and the researcher's conceptualizations over the course of the study. It assists the researcher in keeping track of the emerging analytical framework and the actual data relating to it. This document often provides the basis for the findings section of the final report.

⟐ DATA ANALYSIS AND INTERPRETATION

As noted, in qualitative research, data analysis is an ongoing process, and data collection and analysis go hand in hand. The researcher analyzes data that have been collected and in light of that analysis, collects additional data until saturation or redundancy is reached; that is, until no new information is forthcoming from addi-

Quantitative

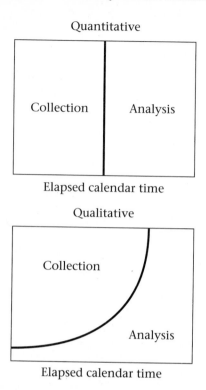

Elapsed calendar time

Figure 21-2. Temporal relations between data collection and analysis. (Redrawn with permission from Lofland, J., & Lofland, L. H. (1984). *Analyzing social settings; A guide to qualitative observation and analysis* (2nd ed.). Belmont, CA: Wadsworth, p. 132.)

tional participants or sources. It is a cyclical and integrative process whose effect can be somewhat likened to a seesaw. However, although the researcher examines themes and develops preliminary hypotheses throughout the progression of the study, "it is during the post-fieldwork stage of the research that he or she concentrates most on the analysis and interpretation of data" (Bogdan & Taylor, 1975, p. 81). Figure 21-2 demonstrates the connection between data collection and analysis in quantitative and qualitative approaches.

Data analysis is the researcher's attempt to *discover* what "all this means." What are the underlying patterns and themes? What is happening here? What is the meaning of this phenomenon? The researcher must scrutinize and examine the data from as many dimensions as possible. The process of data analysis is a putting together. The investigator is endeavoring to abstract meaning, make connections, and develop hypothetical propositions that are based on (grounded in) the data. Like art, it is both creative and interactive. The results of the analysis occur because of the researcher's interaction with the data. However, it is also a scientific process that requires much time, critical thinking, and emotional and intellectual energy. It is *not* merely a projection of what the researcher believes, sees, or feels.

PURPOSES OF ANALYSIS

There are three major purposes of data analysis in qualitative research (Wilson, 1985). The first is to explore and describe. The investigator strives to gain understanding and insight about a particular phenomenon or group of people. What is occurring here? What does something look like? How does something work?

Another purpose of qualitative analysis is to discover and explain. The investigator actively searches the data to discover core patterns and concepts that become the basis for generating hypothetical statements regarding the meaning of the phenomenon under study. The investigator can continue further with this type of analysis by constructing an explanatory scheme, model, or substantively grounded theory that explains a phenomenon under *circumscribed* conditions.

The third purpose of qualitative analysis is to extend an existing theory. Once a theoretical explanation has been developed in one type of situation or circumstance, the investigator may wish to explore whether this theory applies in other contexts or under other conditions. The investigator may also want to extend the theory to a grand or formal theory that illustrates a phenomenon in a multitude of circumstances and cases.

TYPES OF QUALITATIVE ANALYSIS

There are numerous approaches to analyzing qualitative data: content/textual analysis, analytic induction, hermeneutical analysis, aesthetics, matrix analysis, constant comparison, phenomenological analysis, philosophical analysis, quasi-judicial analysis, and reflection, to name but a few. Tesch (1990) identifies at least 26 different approaches to qualitative research, each having a somewhat different analytical focus. She groups analysis into two types: structural analysis and interpretational analysis, which includes theory building and interpretive/descriptive analysis (p. 99). Figure 21-3 provides Tesch's (1990) schemata identifying the four foci of qualitative research with their corresponding analytic techniques.

DOING QUALITATIVE DATA ANALYSIS

Regardless of the analytical approach, interpreting the data to "make meaning" is ultimately the responsibility of the researcher. It must be noted that although there are guidelines and suggestions for qualitative data analysis, there are no hard and fast procedural rules or formulas. "Because each qualitative study is unique, the analytical approach used will be unique. Because qualitative inquiry depends, at every stage, on the skills, training, insights, and capabilities of the researcher, qualitative analysis ultimately depends on the analytical intellect and style of the analyst" (Patton, 1990, p. 372).

There are more qualitative analytical

techniques than this chapter could adequately address, so only two of the more common analysis strategies used in qualitative research will be examined here: thematic analysis and grounded theory development.

Thematic Analysis

The researcher begins the analysis by reading the entire description or log. All the data collected are assembled (such as field notes, transcripts, personal comments, memos) and carefully read through so that the researcher becomes intimately familiar with them. Transcripts of tape-recorded interviews are read while listening to the actual tape recording.

Inductive analysis requires breaking the data into smaller pieces or parts. The researcher starts by tagging or coding meaningful entities in the data. These "meaning units" are labeled by designating in the margin next to the unit what concept or thought that particular unit signifies. These meaning units can either be emic/indigenous or etic/analyst constructed (Patton, 1990). *Emic* labels evolve directly from the data. They are those formulated and expressed by the study participants, the "insider's" views represented in the "insider's" language. *Etic* labels are "outsider" or researcher constructed or drawn from the literature.

After coding several fieldwork logs or interview transcripts, the analyst makes a list of all the substantive labels or codes identified. These are then clustered by similarities and named or categorized. Some of the codes may fit into more than one category. Those that do not fit together should remain separate. Lofland and Lofland (1984) refer to category labels as "thinking units."

Subsequent logs or transcripts should then be analyzed (and previous ones reanalyzed) using the category scheme devel-

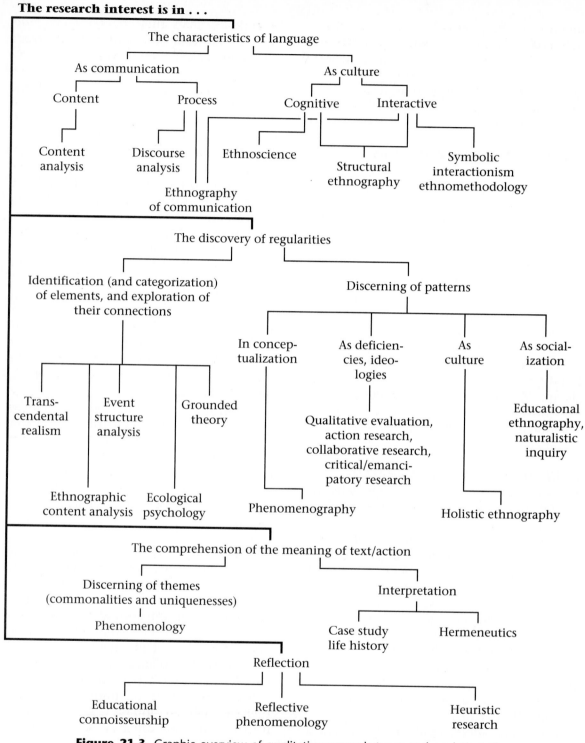

Figure 21-3. Graphic overview of qualitative research types and analytic techniques. (Reprinted with permission from Tesch, R. (1990). *Qualitative research: Analysis types and software tools.* Bristol, PA: The Falmer Press, pp. 72-73.)

oped. In this process, some category labels may change, and subcategories may be developed. It is important that the category labels "fit" the data and that the researcher not force data into categories that do not reflect the actual data. The researcher goes through a process of continually interrogating the data. The researcher has formulated a category when its attributes and characteristics are defined, its boundaries are identified, and it has a name (Schatzman & Strauss, 1982). In addition, the "categories for sorting segments are tentative and preliminary in the beginning: they remain flexible. . . . They are modified accordingly and are refined until a satisfactory system is established. Even then the categories remain flexible working tools, not rigid end products" (Tesch, 1990, p. 96).

Categorical/analytical schemes or concepts can be developed directly from the data, build on the investigator's prior research, or be borrowed from the existing literature. Two such preexisting analytic schemes that are useful for organizing and classifying data are those of Lofland and Lofland (1984) and Bogdan and Biklen (1982). Lofland and Lofland identify the following thinking units, arranged from the microscopic to the macroscopic:

Meanings	Groups
Practices	Organizations
Episodes	Settlements
Encounters	Social worlds
Roles	Life-styles
Relationships	

Bogdan and Biklen present "families" of codes that can be used as coding categories when sorting data:

Setting/context codes
Definition of the situation codes
Perspectives held by subjects
Subjects' ways of thinking about people and objects
Process codes
Activity codes
Event codes
Strategy codes
Relationship and social structure codes
Methods codes

Using the organizing scheme, the data are clustered under established category headings. This can be done manually by cutting up the log or transcript and filing data segments according to the category heading. For this reason, it is imperative that there be duplicates made of the various data sources such as field notes or transcripts. In addition, a number of computer software packages assist the researcher in organizing, filing, and managing data. The reader is referred to Tesch (1990) for descriptions of qualitative analysis computer programs.

After the data are sorted into categories and filed, the researcher reflects on what these clusters mean. The focus is on noting regularities in the data. The researcher can identify patterns or themes reflecting each participant's personal view, develop a personal story for each participant, and then compare all the personal profiles for similarities and differences. Or the researcher can identify general themes or patterns instead of focusing on a personal narrative for each individual.

As patterns, themes, and hypothetical explanations become apparent, the researcher evaluates the plausibility of his or her interpretations and "tests" them against the data. Verbatim narrative from the field notes or interview transcripts are incorporated to link the researcher's conceptualizations with the raw data, and negative cases, disconfirming instances, or alternative explanations are explored. The "researcher must engage in the critical act of challenging the very pattern that seems so apparent" (Marshall & Rossman, 1989, p. 119). This process continues until a comprehensive description and a general pattern of interrelated relationships evolve that can be illustrated and supported by the data. The researcher also validates the findings with the help of the participants themselves ("member checking").

Throughout the inquiry, the investigator writes analytical memos and may use diagrams. Diagrams are "graphic representations or visual images of the relationships between concepts" (Strauss & Corbin, 1990, p. 198). Analytical memos are notations (a sentence, a paragraph, or pages) of the researcher's ideas regarding how data, codes, and categories are related. "Analytic memos can be thought of as conversations with oneself about what has occurred in the research process, what has been learned, the insights this provides, and the leads this suggests for future action" (Ely, Anzul, Fieldman, Garner, & Steinmetz, 1991, p. 80). These memos are invaluable both methodologically and in advancing the analysis. They assist the researcher in speculating, reflecting, conceptualizing, and integrating. Analytical memos and diagrams "help you gain analytical distance from materials. They assist your movement away from the data to abstract thinking, then in returning to the data to ground these abstractions in reality" (Strauss & Corbin, 1990, p. 199). Memos and diagrams evolve and become more conceptual, growing in "complexity, density, clarity, and accuracy as the research and analysis progress. The later memos and diagrams may negate, amend, support, extend, and clarify earlier ones" (Strauss & Corbin, 1990, p. 198). Analytical memos should be written whenever the researcher has a hunch, an idea, an understanding, or a "wondering" about content or process. Each memo should be dated, referenced regarding the evidence (observation or transcript) from which it was obtained, have a heading, and include short quotes or phrases from the actual data. The writing should be unconstrained, and most important, conceptual in nature.

Grounded Theory Development
Grounded theory as a qualitative research method has been described in Chapter 20. The analytical procedures used in the development of grounded theory are an extension of those presented in thematic analysis. The analyst uses *open coding* (tagging data to capture "what is going on"), *selective coding* (clustering codes to create categories), and *theoretical coding* (developing propositions and actively validating proposed relationships in the data) (Wilson, 1985). Using theoretical sampling, the investigator looks for variation and situations that exhibit new category characteristics. Saturation of categories occurs when completeness of all categories is achieved. That is, no new data regarding the categories are discovered.

Strauss (1987) and Strauss and Corbin (1990) present a paradigm model for developing sets of relationships in grounded theory. This paradigm incorporates denoting the phenomenon (the central event, happening); the causal conditions (events or incidents leading to the occurrence of the phenomenon); context (specific properties of, or circumstances surrounding, the phenomenon); conditions (qualifiers under which a phenomenon occurs); actions/interactions (strategies or tactics directed at managing, handling, carrying out, or responding to a phenomenon); and consequences (results, outcomes, or effects of a phenomenon).

Through constant comparison, the researcher generates theoretical constructs and forms a theory. "There is a constant effort to integrate the loosely integrated categories into more generalized ones and to link the categories" (Fagerhaugh, 1986, p. 136). Analytical memos are written, analyzed, reanalyzed, and sorted to reach higher levels of abstraction. There is a continuous search for structure. The researcher compares incident with incident, incident with category, category with category, and construct with construct until a conclusive integrative scheme or core process is discovered. "This analytic scheme accounts for most of the patterns of behavior in the area under study and integrates and interrelates a dense array of other subcategories and propositions . . . [it is] the main theme, or 'story line,' that explains the problem going on in the data" (Wilson, 1985, p. 421). The generation of the theory occurs around this core category/process.

May (1986) notes that "the findings are the theory itself, i.e., a set of concepts and propositions which link them" (p. 148). The researcher presents the theoretical scheme, portions of actual data that include quotations and observations to support the findings, and a discussion of the relationship of the theory to existing knowledge.

ELEMENTS AND PROCESSES OF QUALITATIVE ANALYSIS

Generic elements are common to both strategies of analysis. Data analysis and data collection occur simultaneously and inform each other. The analysis is systematic (but not inflexible) and comprehensive. The investigator divides the data into smaller units for analysis and then reintegrates them into a conceptual whole. The product of these analyses is a higher-order synthesis. As Tesch (1990) states, "The final goal is the emergence of a larger, consolidated picture" (p. 97).

Interpretation is required. Interpretation involves "attaching significance to what was found, offering explanations, drawing conclusions, extrapolating lessons, making inferences, building linkages, attaching meanings, imposing order, and dealing with rival explanations, disconfirming cases, and data irregularities as part of testing the viability of an interpretation" (Patton, 1990, p. 423). Schlechty and Noblit (1982) describe the purpose of interpretation as: (1) making the obvious obvious, (2) making the obvious dubious, and (3) making the hidden obvious.

In this type of analysis, there is an "interpenetration of data and analysis" (Lofland & Lofland, 1984, p. 146), or a balance between the interpretations made and the descriptive evidence that serve as the basis for the interpretations. Conclusions and analyses are directly supported (grounded in) description, evidence from documents, and direct quotations, and the researcher distinguishes between evidence and inference.

In analyzing qualitative data, the researcher uses three dominant processes (Mariano, 1993): reflection, comparison, and creativity. *Reflection* is both personal and data oriented. Personal reflection was discussed with regard to assumptions and bracketing. Data-bound reflection necessitates contemplating, dialoguing with, and critically appraising the data. Through this approach the investigator develops clarity of meaning and advances the descriptive evidence to a more abstract and conceptual plane.

Comparison is used in almost all phases of the analysis. The qualitative researcher is continually attempting to uncover conceptual similarities and differences in the data. Whether the researcher is developing themes and patterns to describe or explain an individual experience or comparing themes and patterns across individual cases or sites, association and contrast are the analytical processes used.

Creativity is the hallmark of qualitative analysis. There is no one "right way" to make meaning. Whatever the analytical approach, the researcher, through a blend of critical thinking and creative insight, must make sense of the data. Using metaphor, analogy, and imagery can often facilitate the genesis of this type of "creative scholarship." Creative thinking can be nurtured if the researcher is open, generates options, diverges before converging, uses numerous stimuli, makes linkages, zig-zags, trusts him- or herself, and works and plays at being creative (Patton, 1990).

Strauss and Corbin (1990) also include theoretical sensitivity as a much-needed quality:

> Theoretical sensitivity refers to the attribute of having insight, the ability to give meaning to data, the capacity to understand, and capability to separate the pertinent from that which isn't. All this is done in conceptual rather than concrete terms. It is theoretical sensitivity that allows one to develop a theory that is grounded, conceptually dense, and well integrated. (p. 42)

This sensitivity is developed through professional and personal background and experiences, as well as through familiarity with the technical literature. It also is obtained during the implementation of the research study by constant interactions with the data. Strauss and Corbin suggest that researchers continually step back and ask whether what is believed to have been observed fits the data; preserve a skeptical attitude and repeatedly check out emerging hunches and hypotheses with the actual data; and carefully follow good research procedures. They end their discussion of theoretical sensitivity by quoting Rapport and Wright (1964, pp. 130-131): "But chance is never the predominant factor in discovery. The beginning scientist who hopes by luck to emulate Lavoisier or Faraday, or even lesser scientists is directed to Pasteur's famous statement that 'chance favors only the prepared mind'" (p. 46).

✎ WRITING THE QUALITATIVE REPORT

Qualitative reports are often book-length narratives. Again, there are no standardized procedures for creating this narrative. The researcher must become engrossed in a process of composing and often artistry. "Probably not much more can be said than that the usual principles of good composition—the writing of understandable prose—apply" (Guba & Lincoln, 1982, p. 375). Bogdan and Biklen (1982) note that when writing up a qualitative study, the researcher engages in a form of translation: "You take what you have heard and seen and put it down on paper so that it makes sense to your readers as it made sense to you. . . . You must also convince the reader of the accuracy of your views" (p. 176). That is to say, the researcher's generalizations and interpretations are grounded in the actual descriptions or quotations from the participants.

The researcher needs to identify the audience for the report. Different audiences may have different concerns and interests in the phenomenon. Therefore the report may demand distinct emphases, specifics, writing style, and even length. In addition to innovative reporting of qualitative inquiry (photographs, videotapes), there are various types of written reports. Ely et al. (1991) define these as follows:

- The case report, "or a story over time about a bounded system such as one

> ### ELEMENTS OF A QUALITATIVE RESEARCH REPORT
>
> - An explication of the problem or question
> - A detailed summary of the context/setting
> - The nature and number of participants and/or settings
> - The time and length of the study
> - The researcher–participant relationship
> - A complete picture of the processes and transactions in the setting that are relevant to the focus of the study
> - A detailed description of the methodology, including an exact reporting of the data-collection procedures and -analysis methods used in the study, the investiga-
>
> tor's credentials, assumptions and biases regarding the phenomenon under study, and an accurate account of the steps taken to ensure the quality and trustworthiness of the inquiry
> - A full discussion of the results of the study or "lessons to be learned." Findings are supported with illustrative examples from the data such as quotations, descriptions, and other appropriate evidence. The findings are compared and contrasted with existing literature and other theoretical perspectives on the phenomenon.

person, one event, or one institution that was the focus of study, in order to illuminate important findings about that person or about the entire broader social unit." (p. 173)
- Composites or vignettes describing findings that pertain to a group rather than any one individual.
- Depictions of "critical incidents" that explicate meaning about the phenomenon under study.
- Presentations that demonstrate a single picture of a phenomenon in its entirety or the phenomenon in its various phases over time.
- Portrayals of contrasts and variance.

The following elements (see the box) should be included in the content of a qualitative research report (Bogdan & Taylor, 1975; Lincoln & Guba, 1985):

The write-up of the inquiry should be fashioned in an engaging style, captivating the audience and enticing them to read more. This requires an investigator who possesses a certain "passion" about the study and strongly desires to share the find-

ings of the inquiry. It also requires an interesting and articulate writing style.

✎ EVALUATING THE QUALITATIVE RESEARCH PROCESS

A number of criteria are used to assess the value of qualitative research studies. These include criteria for establishing the trustworthiness of the study (Lincoln & Guba, 1985; Sandelowski, 1986) and criteria for evaluating the quality of the work (Burns, 1989); Cohen and Knafl (1993) provide an overview of the various frameworks published by nursing researchers for evaluating qualitative research studies.

TRUSTWORTHINESS

To achieve trustworthiness four objectives must be attained: credibility, transferability, dependability, and confirmability. *Credibility* ensures that the researcher has developed plausible interpretations and conclusions. Credibility meets the criteria of validity as described by Goetz and LeCompte (1984): "Validity is concerned

EVALUATING THE QUALITATIVE RESEARCH PROCESS

- Is it credible?
- Are findings transferable?
- Is it dependable?
- Are findings confirmable?
- Are descriptions vivid?
- Are analyses precise?

- Are there theoretical connections?
- Does the work have authenticity, integrity, intellectual vigor, utility?
- Is it aesthetic?
- Is it ethical?

with the accuracy of scientific findings. Establishing validity requires (1) determining the extent to which conclusions effectively represent empirical reality and (2) assessing whether constructs devised by researchers represent or measure the categories of human experience that occur" (p. 210).

Techniques used to achieve credibility include remaining in the field over a long period; triangulating data sources (using a variety of sources in data gathering); peer debriefing (in which the researcher exposes him- or herself to a disinterested peer who probes the researcher's biases, explores meanings, and clarifies the bases for particular interpretations); negative case analysis (searching for and accounting for disconfirming evidence); and having the participants review, validate, and verify the researcher's interpretations and conclusions (member checking). This is done to ensure that the facts have not been misconstrued.

Transferability allows someone other than the researcher to determine whether the findings of the study are applicable in another context or setting. This is accomplished by providing a detailed data base and thick description (a description that enumerates everything that another would need to know to comprehend the researcher's conclusions).

Dependability enables someone else logically to follow the process and procedures that the researcher used in the study. It is

achieved by using an auditor (a person who inspects the inquiry process and determines it to be authentic).

Confirmability guarantees that the findings, conclusions, and recommendations are supported by the data and that there is an internal agreement between the investigator's interpretations and the actual evidence. This also is accomplished by incorporating an audit procedure in the study.

Burns (1989) suggests additional standards for superior qualitative research. These are descriptive vividness; methodological congruence (consisting of precision in documentation and procedure and strict adherence to ethics and auditability); analytical preciseness; theoretical connectedness; and heuristic relevance (which consists of intuitive recognition, relationship to existing knowledge, and applicability).

Garman and Pinanida in their graduate course entitled *Disciplined Inquiry Introduction to Qualitative Research* at the University of Pittsburg use six "qualities" to guide the evaluation of qualitative work:

1. *Verity* (does the work ring true, and is it intellectually honest and authentic?)
2. *Integrity* (is the work structurally sound, and is the research rationale logical and appropriate within a paradigm?)
3. *Rigor* (is there depth of intellect vs. simplistic, superficial reasoning?)
4. *Utility* (is the work useful, professionally

relevant, and does it make a contribution to the discipline?)

5. *Vitality* (is the work meaningful, providing a sense of vibrancy and discovery, and do metaphors and images communicate forcefully?)

6. *Aesthetics* (is the work enriching; does it touch the spirit and give others insight into some universal part of themselves?)

ETHICS

Ethical issues emerge in every phase of the qualitative research process. Ely et al. (1991) note that struggling to be faithful to another's viewpoint, to maintain confidentiality, and to be trustworthy are all endeavors to be ethical. The authors note that ethical considerations are "present from the beginning and are woven throughout every step of the methodology" (p. 218).

The qualitative researcher must attend to potential ethical dilemmas when data collection involves participant observation or when interviewing includes sensitive topics. Anonymity and confidentiality must be ensured as participants may be sharing intimate details of their lives. The investigator might also have to deal with expectations that participants or gatekeepers may have of the researcher in the field, raising the question of "whether or not the researcher should intervene as a 'therapeutic agent' in specific situations or report to an authority certain incidents observed [or communicated] during the course of the fieldwork" (Mariano, 1990, p. 357). Qualitative inquiry necessitates a continuous exploration of one's own values and ethical orientations.

SUMMARY

- Qualitative inquiry is naturalistic, holistic, inductive, and emergent.
- Research questions are open-ended and context dependent.
- In qualitative inquiry, there are contrary

views regarding conducting a literature review and using a theoretical framework *prior* to data collection.

- Qualitative research uses small samples and purposeful sampling strategies.
- Phases of qualitative inquiry include preliminary fieldwork, gaining entry, focused exploration, closure, and member checking.
- Data collection and analysis occur simultaneously.
- Primary data-gathering techniques in qualitative research are participant observation and in-depth interviewing.
- Data logs include (1) field notes and interview transcripts, (2) personal/methodological journals, and (3) analytic logs.
- There are a variety of qualitative analytic techniques.
- Thematic analysis and grounded theory development require interpretation, interpenetration of descriptive data and analysis, reflection, comparison, and creativity.
- Qualitative research reports are lengthy narratives.
- Criteria for trustworthiness of qualitative inquiry include credibility, transferability, dependability, and confirmability.
- Ethical issues emerge in every phase of the qualitative research process.

FACILITATING CRITICAL THINKING

1. You are interested in exploring the experience of hope in women with breast cancer. From a qualitative research perspective:
   a. How would you phrase the research question?
   b. What assumptions do you have regarding this topic?
   c. How would you select participants for the study?
   d. What techniques would you use to collect the data?

e. What approach would you implement in analyzing the data?

f. How would you disseminate your findings to others?

g. What ethical issues might you have to consider?

h. What measures would you take to ensure the trustworthiness of the study?

2. Select a qualitative research article from a referenced journal. Evaluate the research using criteria presented in each step of the qualitative research process.

References

SUBSTANTIVE

LEININGER, M. (Ed.). (1985). *Qualitative research methods in nursing.* Orlando, FL: Grune & Stratton.

MORSE, J. (Ed.). (1992). *Qualitative health research.* Newbury Park, CA: Sage.

MUNHALL, P., & BOYD, C. O. (1993). *Nursing research: A qualitative perspective.* New York: National League for Nursing Press.

CONCEPTUAL

BOGDAN, R. C., & BIKLEN, S. K. (1982). *Qualitative research for education: An introduction to theory and methods.* Boston: Allyn & Bacon.

BOGDAN, R., & TAYLOR, S. (1975). *Introduction to qualitative research methods: A phenomenological approach to the social sciences.* New York: Wiley.

BURNS, N. (1989). Standards for qualitative research. *Nursing Science Quarterly, 2*(1), 44-52.

COHEN, M., & KNAFL, K. (1993). Evaluating qualitative research. In P. Munhall & C. O. Boyd (Eds.), *Nursing research: A qualitative perspective* (2nd ed.). New York: National League for Nursing Press.

DENZIN, N., & LINCOLN, Y. (Eds.). (1994). *Handbook of qualitative research.* Thousand Oaks, CA: Sage.

DOBERT, M. (1982). *Ethnographic research: Theory and application for modern schools and societies.* New York: Praeger.

GARMAN, N., & PIANTANIDA, M. (1986). *Disciplined inquiry. Introduction to qualitative research.* Graduate course at the University of Pittsburgh.

GOETZ, J., & LeCOMPTE, M. (1984). *Ethnography and qualitative design in educational research.* Orlando, FL: Academic Press.

GUBA, E. G., & LINCOLN, Y. S. (1982). *Effective evaluation* (2nd ed.). San Francisco: Jossey-Bass.

JUNKER, B. (1960). *Fieldwork: An introduction to the social sciences.* Chicago: University of Chicago Press.

LINCOLN, Y. S., & GUBA, E. G. (1985). *Naturalistic inquiry.* Beverly Hills, CA: Sage.

MARIANO, C. (1990). Qualitative research: Instructional strategies and curricular considerations. *Nursing & Health Care, 11*(7), 354-359.

MARIANO, C. (1993). Case study: The method. In P. Munhall & C. O. Boyd (Eds.), *Nursing research: A qualitative perspective* (2nd ed.). New York: National League for Nursing Press.

MORSE, J. (Ed.). (1991). *Qualitative nursing research: A contemporary dialogue* (rev. ed.). Newbury Park, CA: Sage.

MUNHALL, P., & BOYD, C. O. (1993). *Nursing research: A qualitative perspective.* New York: National League for Nursing Press.

PATTON, M. Q. (1990). *Qualitative evaluation and research methods* (2nd ed.). Newbury Park, CA: Sage.

POWERS, B. A., & KNAPP, T. R. (1990). *A dictionary of nursing theory and research.* Newbury Park, CA: Sage.

RAPPORT, S., & WRIGHT, W. (Eds.). (1964). *Science: Methods in meaning.* New York: Washington Square Press.

SANDELOWSKI, M. (1986). The problem of rigor in qualitative research. *Advances in Nursing Science, 8*(3), 27-37.

SARTER, B. (1988). *Paths to knowledge: Innovative research methods for nursing.* New York: National League for Nursing.

SCHLECHTY, P., & NOBLIT, G. (1982). Some uses of sociological theory in educational evaluation. In R. Corwin (Ed.), *Policy research.* Greenwich, CT: JAI Press.

STRAUSS, A. L., & CORBIN, J. (1990). *Basics of qualitative research: Grounded theory procedures and techniques.* Newbury Park, CA: Sage.

SWANSON-KAUFFMAN, K., & SCHONWALD, E. (1988). Phenomenology. In B. Sarter (Ed.), *Paths to knowledge: Innovative research methods for nursing.* New York: National League for Nursing.

WILSON, H. (1989). *Research in nursing* (2nd ed.). Menlo Park, CA: Addison-Wesley.

WOLCOTT, H. (1988). Ethnographic research in education. In R. Jaeger (Ed.), *Complementary methods for research in education.* Washington, DC: American Educational Research Association.

METHODOLOGICAL

BOGDAN, R. C., & BIKLEN, S. K. (1982). *Qualitative research for education: An introduction to theory and methods.* Boston: Allyn & Bacon.

BOGDAN, R., & TAYLOR, S. (1975). *Introduction to qualitative research methods: A phenomenological approach to the social sciences.* New York: Wiley.

BOGDEWIC, S. (1992). Participant observation. In B. Crabtree & W. Miller (Eds.), *Doing qualitative research.* Newbury Park, CA: Sage.

CHENITZ, W. C., & SWANSON, J. (Eds.). (1986). *From practice to grounded theory: Qualitative research in nursing.* Menlo Park, CA: Addison-Wesley.

CRABTREE, B., & MILLER, W. (Eds.). (1992). *Doing qualitative research.* Newbury Park, CA: Sage.

DENZIN, N. K. (1989). *Interpretive interactionism.* Newbury Park, CA: Sage.

DEXTER, L. (1970). *Elite and specialized interviewing.* New York: Basic Books.

DOBERT, M. (1982). *Ethnographic research: Theory and application for modern schools and societies.* New York: Praeger.

ELY, M., ANZUL, M., FRIEDMAN, T., GARNER, D., & STEINMETZ, A. (1991). *Doing qualitative research: Circles within circles.* New York: The Falmer Press.

FAGERHAUGH, S. (1986). Analyzing data for social process. In W. C. Chenitz & J. Swanson (Eds.), *From practice to grounded theory.* Menlo Park, CA: Addison-Wesley.

FIELD, P., & MORSE, J. (1985). *Nursing research: The application of qualitative approaches.* Rockville, MD: Aspen.

HYCNER, R. H. (1985). Some guidelines for the phenomenological analysis of interview data. *Human Studies, 8,* 279-303.

KAHN, R., & CONNELL, C. (1957). *The dynamics of interviewing.* New York: Wiley.

KUZEL, A. (1992). Sampling in qualitative inquiry. In B. Crabtree & W. Miller (Eds.), *Doing qualitative research.* Newbury Park, CA: Sage.

LOFLAND, J., & LOFLAND, L. H. (1984). *Analyzing social settings: A guide to qualitative observation and analysis* (2nd ed.). Belmont, CA: Wadsworth.

MARIANO, C. (1993). Case study: The method. In P. Munhall & C. O. Boyd (Eds.), *Nursing research: A qualitative perspective* (2nd ed.). New York: National League for Nursing Press.

MARSHALL, C., & ROSSMAN, G. (1989). *Designing qualitative research.* Newbury Park, CA: Sage.

MAY, K. (1986). Writing and evaluating the grounded theory research report. In W. C. Chenitz & J. Swanson (Eds.), *From practice to grounded theory.* Menlo Park, CA: Addison-Wesley.

MILES, M. B., & HUBERMAN, A. M. (1984). *Qualitative data analysis: A sourcebook of new methods.* Beverly Hills, CA: Sage.

SCHATZMAN, L., & STRAUSS, A. (1982). *Field research: Strategies for a natural sociology* (2nd ed.). Englewood Cliffs, NJ: Prentice-Hall.

SPRADLEY, J. (1979). *The ethnographic interview.* New York: Holt, Rinehart & Winston.

SPRADLEY, J. (1980). *Participant observation.* New York: Holt, Rinehart & Winston.

STRAUSS, A. L. (1987). *Qualitative analysis for social scientists.* New York: Cambridge University Press.

STRAUSS, A. L., & CORBIN, J. (1990). *Basics of qualitative research: Grounded theory procedures and techniques.* Newbury Park, CA: Sage.

TESCH, R. (1990). *Qualitative research: Analysis types and software tools.* Bristol, PA: The Falmer Press.

WILSON, H. (1985). *Research in nursing.* Menlo Park, CA: Addison-Wesley.

HISTORICAL

GLASER, B., & STRAUSS, A. (1967). *The discovery of grounded theory: Strategies for qualitative research.* Chicago: Aldine.

LEININGER, M. (Ed.). (1985). *Qualitative research methods in nursing.* Orlando, FL: Grune & Stratton.

SCHATZMAN, L., & STRAUSS, A. (1982). *Field research: Strategies for a natural sociology* (2nd ed.). Englewood Cliffs, NJ: Prentice-Hall.

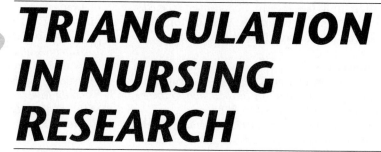

CHAPTER 22

TRIANGULATION IN NURSING RESEARCH

KATHLEEN A. KNAFL • AGATHA GALLO

A faculty member, a graduate student in pediatric nursing, and the student's clinical preceptor at a home health care agency are discussing the student's experiences working with a family that is caring for a ventilator-dependent child in their home. Based on her observations of interactions between the child's parents and the home health care nurses, the student has numerous questions about the respective roles of the parents and the nurses. She has noted that misunderstandings frequently arise over who is responsible for certain aspects of the child's care and that the nurses and parents sometimes are critical of one another's interactions with the child. During the course of their conversation, the student, faculty member, and preceptor begin exploring the possibility of initiating a research project to explore more fully the nature of interactions between home health care nurses and parents and to identify factors that contribute to a positive working relationship. They identify multiple questions they would like to address: How are decisions made about the child's care? To

what extent do family members and nurses work together or separately in providing care to the child? How satisfied are family members with the nursing care their child is receiving? What variables influence the quality of the relationship between the nurses and the parents? How well are parents adapting to this unique parenting situation? As they talk about the plans for their project, they soon realize that no single instrument or data collection approach will address all the questions of interest.

On the one hand, some of the types of data they envision collecting would be qualitative interviews or field note narratives; other data would be quantitative scores. Their questions about the interactions between family members and nurses lend themselves to direct observation of the caregiving situation. Questions about satisfaction with care would have to be addressed through either a questionnaire or an interview with the parents. On the other hand, questions about parental adaptation could be addressed through standardized quantitative measures. In addition to identifying different types of data that could answer their research questions, the three realize that to have a more nearly complete understanding of the relationships between the nurses and the parents they would need to obtain data directly from both groups as multiple sources of data. Moreover, they speculate that mothers and fathers might have different views of their situation and they discuss the possibility of conducting separate interviews and obtaining separate measures of adaptation from each parent. They also realize that as potential collaborators on a study each of them brings a unique perspective to the situation. Even in preliminary conversations they have raised rather different substantive and theoretical questions about their subject matter, and they would like to preserve these unique points of view in their research. Although they realize they probably will have to narrow the scope of the project, they are convinced that their research will provide a more valid, complete understanding of the subject matter if they continue with their plans to use multiple data collection methods and to obtain data from multiple sources. After further discussion, they decide to use both qualitative and quantitative data collection techniques in their study and to gather data from home health care nurses, mothers, and fathers. In planning and carrying out their research, they will be applying principles of triangulation.

In recent years there has been a growing interest among nurse researchers in qualitative research methods. This interest is reflected in a growing recognition of the contributions of qualitative approaches to nursing science. Numerous nursing methods texts devoted to qualitative methods are now available (Chenitz & Swanson, 1986; Field & Morse, 1985; Leininger, 1985; Munhall & Oiler 1986; Strauss & Corbin,

1990). More important, major qualitative studies such as Corbin and Strauss's (1988) work on chronic illness and Swanson's (1991) work on caring have demonstrated the need for qualitative approaches to address some of the most salient research questions facing nursing. In conjunction with a growing interest in qualitative methods there has been a growing number of attempts to combine quantitative and qualitative methods in a single study, an approach often referred to as triangulation. For example, the authors' research on family response to a child's chronic illness has combined data from a variety of standardized quantitative measures of individual and family functioning with interview data (Knafl, Breitmayer, Gallo, & Zoeller, 1987). This chapter presents an overview of approaches to triangulation and a discussion of differing views of the merits and appropriate uses of triangulation. Examples from the authors' own research serve as highlights throughout.

❧ OVERVIEW OF QUALITATIVE RESEARCH

Qualitative research encompasses a family of research approaches such as grounded theory, phenomenology, and ethnography, which are characterized by overlapping, but not identical, goals and techniques. Speaking to the broad spectrum of qualitative approaches, Strauss and Corbin (1990) said:

> By the term qualitative research we mean any kind of research that produces findings not arrived at by statistical procedures or other means of quantification. It can refer to research about persons' lives, stories, behavior, but also about organizational functioning, social movements, or interactional relationships. (p. 17)

Authors differ regarding how they classify qualitative approaches, and even within the discipline of nursing considerable variation exists. For example, Chenitz and Swanson (1986) identified five different approaches; Field and Morse (1985) identified eight; Leininger (1985) identified seven; and Munhall and Oiler (1986) identified five. Taken together, these authors identified a total of 13 different qualitative approaches. In spite of considerable variation among authors, all agreed that ethnography, grounded theory, and phenomenology are members of the "qualitative family." These three major approaches are used to address different kinds of research questions.

Ethnographic researchers study their subject matter from a cultural perspective. They are interested in such things as the shared norms and values of a particular group. Ethnographic studies can be particularly useful in revealing important differences between the values and health beliefs of providers and those of diverse cultural groups. For example, Anderson (1986) analyzed the experiences of Chinese immigrant families with children with chronic illness and found that Chinese parents' views of their parenting role were inconsistent with providers' expectations that they would participate fully in the child's treatment regimen. Her discussion provides important insights into how to include parents whose beliefs differ from those of the dominant culture into the decision-making processes that influence their lives.

In contrast to ethnographic research, the purpose of grounded theory studies is to conceptualize a process that people use to deal with a problematic aspect of their lives. In grounded theory the conceptualization is inductively derived from the data. Francis (1992) used this approach in her study of homeless mothers. Based on interviews with eight women, she identified and developed the process theme of a "Search for Connections" to conceptualize how homeless mothers managed their experience.

Qualitative researchers who use a phenomenological approach focus on the perceived experiences of the individual. As such, phenomenology provides a valuable approach for understanding intangible experiences such as pain, hope, and loneliness. Beck's (1992) study of postpartum depression is an excellent example of a phenomenological study. Beck used phenomenological interviewing and data analysis techniques to describe the essential structure of the lived experience of postpartum depression. This essential structure was comprised of 11 thematic clusters that were derived inductively from the interview data.

Although these three approaches serve somewhat different purposes, they typically use similar approaches to data collection, a situation that sometimes confuses persons not familiar with qualitative research. Qualitative approaches rely on data collection techniques such as intensive interviewing and participant observation, which produce narrative as opposed to numerical data.

Because of their reliance on narrative data, qualitative researchers have devised various techniques for systematically managing and analyzing data sets that typically are comprised of interview transcripts, field notes, and/or memos. A rudimentary understanding of these techniques is necessary to understand how qualitative and quantitative data can be combined in a single study. Tesch (1990) has provided an overview of both major differences and commonalities in forms of qualitative analysis. Among the important commonalities she noted are the reliance on comparison, the use of categorization to organize the textual data, the concurrent or cyclic nature of data collection and analysis, and a final product that reflects some higher level of synthesis. This synthesis may take the form of a thematic description or a more abstract conceptualization.

In recent years a number of excellent texts have been published that are specifically devoted to qualitative data analysis. While some present fairly generic descriptions of qualitative analysis (Miles & Huberman, 1984; Patton, 1990), others focus on specific qualitative approaches such as grounded theory (Strauss, 1987) or present a discussion of analytic techniques specifically geared to different qualitative approaches (Tesch, 1990). Another fairly recent development has been the emergence of software programs specifically designed to assist in qualitative data processing and analysis. The previously mentioned book by Tesch (1990) provides an excellent overview of these programs.

Although brief, this introduction is meant to provide a basis for understanding how qualitative and quantitative data can be combined in a single study. As previously noted, the use of qualitative and quantitative approaches or techniques in a single study often is labeled triangulation.

ꙮ *TRIANGULATION*

Knafl and Breitmayer (1991) discussed the origin and development of triangulation. The term was used originally in surveying and navigation to describe the technique for using two known points to plot the location of an unknown third point. The term was introduced into the social sciences by Campbell (1956), who used it metaphorically to refer to the use of multiple measures to assess a single construct.

Campbell (1956) described the approach, saying,

> In several instances in the present study, there has been achieved what might be called methodological triangulation, in that several different methodological approaches have been employed to get at the same variable, psychologically conceived. . . . The process is one of mutual confirmation among the various approaches. (pp. 73-74)

As initially conceived, triangulation entailed employing multiple measures to investigate a single concept. A key aspect of this view of triangulation is that multiple measures be chosen to counterbalance the threats to validity identified in each. The reasoning behind this approach is that an investigator can be more confident in the study results if they have been confirmed using multiple measures. Thus the original purpose of triangulation was to confirm one's findings.

For example, the authors' ongoing study of family response to childhood chronic illness has compared results from the Feetham Family Functioning Survey (FFFS) (Roberts & Feetham, 1982) with results from open-ended interviews for consistency with regard to parents' views of family life. In so doing the authors expected to find that parents whose FFFS scores indicated a high level of satisfaction with their family life made comments in their interviews that also were indicative of satisfaction. In making the comparison it was important to recognize the relative strengths and weaknesses of both the FFFS and the interviews. A major strength of the FFFS is that it provides an objective measure of satisfaction with family relationships across three areas of functioning. Because the FFFS is comprised of 21 structured questions with fixed response options, it facilitated comparison across the families in the study and between the results of the authors' research and other studies. On the other hand, the structured format of the FFFS limited the areas of family life addressed. Using this instrument alone, an investigator might fail to obtain data on areas of family life that a respondent thinks are important but that are not included in the FFFS. To offset some of the limitations of the FFFS, the study used open-ended interview questions to obtain data on parents' views of family life. During the interviews the investigators encouraged parents to speak openly about how they viewed their family's response to the child's chronic illness. Unlike the FFFS, the interview did not limit parents to preset areas of response. Rather, the mothers and fathers were free to introduce topics they identified as important and relevant to their experience of having a child with a chronic illness. On the other hand, a weakness of the interview data was its inherent lack of standardization, making it difficult to compare the data across subjects and with results of other studies. This example illustrates the original conceptualization of triangulation as a measurement strategy to increase one's confidence in the measurement of a specific construct. If data from the FFFS and the interviews present a consistent view of subjects' satisfaction with family life, the investigators can be more confident in the validity of our results. The data generated by the two measures are mutually confirming. This approach to triangulation contributes to evaluating the validity of one's measures.

Further development of triangulation by Fielding and Fielding (1986) and Jick (1979) extended the meaning of triangulation to encompass the purpose of completeness as well as confirmation. In using triangulation to achieve completeness investigators employ varying methodological strategies to achieve a more holistic, contextual portrayal of the subject matter.

Using triangulation to achieve completeness is particularly relevant for qualitative researchers, whose purpose often is to understand multiple dimensions of their research topic. For example, family researchers are likely to achieve a more complete understanding of their subject matter by obtaining data from multiple family members, studying the family over time, and using multiple measures of family and individual functioning. As will be discussed in the following sections, various researchers have developed approaches to triangulation that support the purposes of confirmation and completeness.

TYPES OF TRIANGULATION

Denzin (1970; 1989) described different types of triangulation, including investigator, data source, data collection methods, unit of analysis, and theory. He described how using one or more of these types of triangulation in a single study could contribute to the confirmation and completeness of the results.

The following discussion provides a description of the major types of triangulation as identified by Denzin and further explicated in nursing by Mitchell (1986) and Kimchi, Polivka, and Stevenson (1991). Examples of the different types are provided from the authors' study of families with a school-age child with a chronic illness (Knafl et al., 1987).

INVESTIGATOR TRIANGULATION

Investigator triangulation occurs "when multiple observers, interviewers, coders, and analysts, each with expertise and with prominent roles in the study deal with the same raw data" (Mitchell, 1986, p. 20). Kimchi et al. (1991) stated that investigator triangulation has been achieved when each investigator has a major role in the project and the investigators have different areas of expertise that are used to inform the design and implementation of the project. For example, in the situation described at the beginning of the chapter, a faculty member, clinical specialist, and graduate student were discussing the possibility of collaborating on a study of interactions between parents and home care nurses. If these individuals brought unique perspectives and areas of expertise to the research and assumed a major role on the project, this would be an instance of investigator triangulation. The use of investigator triangulation assures that the research question will be considered from varying points of view.

The authors' research provides another example of investigator triangulation. The four-member team represented a wide variety of substantive, methodological, and clinical expertise. Knafl, a sociologist, had considerable experience in qualitative research, and her concept analysis of family management style provided the conceptual underpinnings for the research (Knafl & Deatrick, 1990). Gallo, on the other hand, had a strong background in pediatric nursing and issues surrounding family-centered nursing care. Breitmayer, a child psychiatric nurse with postdoctoral work in child development, had a strong quantitative background and expertise in measuring children's functioning and adaptation. As a public health nurse, Zoeller was particularly knowledgeable about community issues and the linkages between the family and other systems such as school and health care.

The varied backgrounds and areas of expertise of the four-member team were particularly helpful in completing the background section for the research proposal seeking support for the project submitted to the National Institute for Nursing Research. While each team member focused on reading in a particular area of expertise, each also shared and discussed the background extensively as the team developed the overall study design. The diverse backgrounds also were useful in selecting data collection instruments and in analyzing the data. In data analysis, team members focused on specific aspects of the study. Knafl's focus was analyzing the parents' responses to having a child with a chronic illness; Breitmayer's the data from the children with chronic illness; and Gallo's the data from the well siblings. Zoeller's efforts were focused on data related to the family's interactions with health care providers and school officials. Team meetings focused on the discussion and integration of findings from the separate analyses. Given the complexity of the family as an area of study, investigator triangulation contributed to the overall success of the project.

DATA SOURCE TRIANGULATION

According to Denzin (1970; 1989), one can triangulate data sources in terms of time, person, or space. This triangulation strategy directs one to collect data over time, from a variety of persons in a variety of contexts. For example, if an investigator were interested in the experience of being a family caregiver to the frail elderly, he or she might want to interview different family members over time and make arrangements to observe family caregivers in a variety of both public and private settings. The purpose in varying these sources of data would be to validate the consistency of the results over time, place, and/or person (Kimchi et al., 1991).

Gallo, Breitmayer, Knafl, and Zoeller's

(1992) analysis of the response of siblings to a child's chronic illness relied heavily on data source triangulation. Mothers and fathers were interviewed to gain a better understanding of how each parent viewed the effect of illness on the sibling and what parenting strategies each used to help siblings adjust to the illness situation. In regard to different points in time, each participating parent was interviewed separately 12 months apart to understand parents' views related to ongoing interactions with their children. The results of this analysis revealed that overall mothers and fathers agreed in respect to the effect of chronic illness on siblings. While the majority of parents reported few effects of illness on the healthy siblings, 20% described adverse effects. Over the two interview sessions, adverse effects decreased in some siblings but increased in others. Additionally, both mothers and fathers indicated that they used equity in parenting, selective telling about the illness, and a positive approach to the illness situation as strategies to help siblings adjust to the chronic illness. These findings indicated that parents tended to have a shared view of the effect of the chronic illness on the sibling and that this effect varied over time for some siblings.

This example illustrates how collecting data from both parents as data sources over two data collection points provides important information about parents' views about the effect of illness on siblings within the context of the family and how these views are generated out of encounters with their children over time.

METHODOLOGICAL TRIANGULATION

Methodological triangulation refers to the use of different data collection techniques in the same study. The techniques are deliberately selected because their respective strengths and weakness are thought to counterbalance one another. Methodological triangulation often involves the use of relatively unstructured techniques such as intensive interviewing and participant observation in combination with more structured data collection techniques such as standardized questionnaires or observational protocols.

Methodological triangulation was an important aspect of the design of the authors' study. Parents from the authors' study (Knafl et al., 1987) were questioned regarding the extent and meaning of their acceptance of their children's chronic illness. They also completed a standardized instrument, Profile of Mood States (POMS) (McNair, Lorr, & Droppleman, 1981), that measures six specific mood states: depression-dejection, tension-anxiety, anger-hostility, fatigue-activity, confusion-bewilderment, and vigor. A total mood disturbance score that estimates global affective states is derived by summing the six individual scores. Higher total mood disturbance scores indicate greater mood disturbance. As shown in Table 22-1, convergence between statements about acceptance in interviews and total mood scores was clear in the two sets of parents used for this illustration. In parent set 1, parents' statements about acceptance were framed in a positive manner and the parents had low mood-disturbance scores (more than one standard deviation below the group mean). On the other hand, statements about acceptance made by parent set 2 indicated nonacceptance and distress. These parents also had high mood disturbance scores (greater than one standard deviation above the group mean). This example shows how using two independent data collection techniques can confirm parents' view of the experience of having a child with a chronic illness through both

Table 22-1
Example of Triangulation Using Two Data Collection Methods

Parent	Parent Set 1 Statements About Acceptance	Total Mood Score	Parent Set 2 Statements About Nonacceptance	Total Mood Score
Mother	"I think it's a great word. I think it's our philosophy. You can either accept that you have it and go on, or you can let it be a problem for you. I think the goal would be acceptance."	− 13 LOW (More than 1 SD below the mean)	"Acceptance. We have accepted it to an extent. We will never fully accept it because we want it cured. And since we do, we can never fully accept it. I can never see any of us feeling that [ill child] is diabetic for the rest of his life."	140 HIGH (More than 1 SD above the mean)
Father	"I guess you'd say that we accepted it. It's part of [ill child] and who she is. I mean, if your child had a different color hair than everyone else in the family, would you accept that? That's the way we look at diabetes."	−23 LOW (More than 1 SD below the mean)	"Acceptance is a failure term for me. I don't believe in accepting things. If I have absolutely no power to do anything over something, I'd probably shoot myself. One way or another I'm coping and doing something to change things as far as diabetes is concerned. But I don't accept it. I don't think I ever will accept it."	60 HIGH (More than 1 SD above the mean)

a structured instrument and open-ended questioning.

THEORETICAL TRIANGULATION

Theoretical triangulation involves building multiple perspectives and hypotheses into a single study. The hypotheses may be formulated at the outset of the study and formally tested, or they may be working hypotheses that emerge during the course of data collection and analysis and are evaluated in terms of competing explanatory frameworks.

Gallo's analyses of two separate case studies describing family response and adaptation to a child's diabetes provide an example of theoretical triangulation. The family management style model (Knafl & Deatrick, 1990) and the family adaptation model (McCubbin & Patterson, 1983) were the two theories used to understand family response in two families from the larger study on how families define and manage a child's chronic illness (Knafl et al., 1987). The objective of the case study analysis was to determine if both models adequately described how these families responded to a child's chronic illness. In the first case study (Gallo, 1990) a family's experience with childhood diabetes was used to illustrate the three components of the family management style model: family members' definitions of the situation, management behaviors, and sociocultural context. A shared family management style was derived from the descriptions of individual family members. The second case (Gallo, 1991) also illustrated a family's experience with childhood diabetes. It used the family adaptation model, which draws on the following components: perceptions of individual family members, the family's resources, and the family members' coping abilities. Although the models presented different components to describe the family experience of childhood chronic illness, they have similar theoretical underpinnings relating to the broad areas of adaptation and coping. This may be one reason why Gallo found that both models adequately described how these two families adapted to childhood diabetes based on the purpose of the models.

A hypothetical example that uses two theories with different underlying perspectives to interpret data from the authors' study on how families define and manage a child's chronic illness illustrates another application of theoretical triangulation. As described earlier, collection of data for the study was based on the theoretical framework of family management style. Family management style is based on the broader framework of symbolic interactionism, which focuses on how individuals define their situation and the consequences of their definitions for action. To understand the data from a different perspective, feminist theories could also be used to interpret these data. Feminist concepts might show how a woman's experiences of caring for a child with a chronic illness are shaped by her position and relative power in the household and the community.

The examples provided above have the necessary requirements for theoretical triangulation: an available body of data and an understanding of at least two theoretical frameworks to be used to interpret the data (Denzin, 1989). Theoretical triangulation in these illustrations sensitizes the reader to different ways that data can be interpreted to illuminate, disclose, and capture the phenomena at hand (Denzin, 1989).

TRIANGULATION OF UNIT OF ANALYSIS
Triangulation of the unit of analysis entails deliberately varying the analytic focus of the investigation. For example, the investigator studying patient-provider interactions may want to analyze both the nature and quality of the interactions themselves, as well as individuals' perceptions of and response to those interactions. In this example both the interactions and the individuals would be considered the unit of analysis. To use multiple units of analysis, separate analyses must be performed for each analytic unit of interest. In this example the investigator might first analyze the data using the interactions as the unit of analysis and then do a second analysis that addressed individual perceptions.

Triangulation of the unit of analysis in the authors' study entailed analyzing and interpreting the data at both the individual and family unit level. At the individual level attention focused on the individual family members who provided data. For example, one aim of the study was to understand how mothers, fathers, children with chronic illness, and well siblings defined the impact of the illness on family life. Thus for the individual as the analytic unit one analysis considered each mother's response to the question, "In what ways does your child's condition have an effect on your family life?" In comparing all mothers' responses the intent of the analysis was to identify themes that characterized the group. A similar analysis could be undertaken with all the fathers, children with chronic illness, and well siblings in the sample. Having completed such an analysis, it would be possible to compare across these groups of family members, noting similarities and differences in the themes that characterized the group. For example, mothers' comments may focus on the effects of the illness on their usual routine or ability to work outside the home; fathers may focus on the financial impact. Even when making comparisons like these across groups, the *individual* family member is still the unit of analysis, not the family as a whole.

In contrast, when the family is the unit of analysis, all members of a single family are viewed simultaneously. The focus then becomes the configuration of themes formed across family members in the same family and the extent to which these themes are shared or complementary versus discrepant or conflicting. It is possible to consider the comparative impact of the illness within the family unit, as well as similarities and differences in how each member of a particular family defines and manages the situation. At this level of analysis comparisons also occur across all family units. For example, it would be possible to compare family functioning in families where family members hold a shared view of the child's illness with those in which the members have highly discrepant views.

ᴥ MULTIPLE TRIANGULATION

Describing the different types of triangulation, Mitchell (1986) built on Denzin's (1970) work to differentiate between simple and multiple triangulation. She pointed out that a study is triangulated when it uses any *one* type of triangulation and that multiple triangulation occurs when *two or more* types of triangulation are used in the same study. Multiple triangulation is especially useful in studying complex phenomena such as family or organizational behavior where data from multiple methods and sources are needed to provide a relatively complete understanding of the subject matter.

Table 22-2 provides an example of multiple triangulation across data sources and methods. Data on the impact of illness from the authors' study are presented from two data sources (mother and healthy sibling) and two methods of data collection (individual interview and two data collection instruments). The Child Behavior Checklist (CBCL) (Achenbach & Edelbrock, 1983) is based on parental reports and measures behavioral problems as one of its components. Children with scores above 63 on behavioral problems are considered maladjusted based on national norms. The Self-Perception Profile for Children (SPPC) (Harter, 1985) measures children's perception of adequacy in six areas, with Global Self-Worth being one area. The sample mean for Global Self-Worth was 3.11; one standard deviation below the mean was 2.43. Table 22-2 presents data from four mothers and their healthy children from the larger sample. Two mothers rated their healthy children as having behavioral problems, and two mothers rated their healthy child as not having behavioral problems. Mothers' comments from the interviews about the effect of chronic illness on the healthy children confirmed these scores on the CBCL and further explained these behavioral problems within the context of the ill child's chronic illness. In addition, mothers' comments about controllability and/or burden of the illness on themselves provided further explanatory insights into the relationships between impact of illness and well-child behavior

Table 22-2
Example of Triangulating Across Data Sources and Methods

Behavior Problems Ratings of Well Siblings by Mothers	Sibling Scores on Global Self-Worth	Mothers' Comments About Effect of Illness on Well Sibling	Mothers' Comments About Controllability and/or Burden of Illness	Siblings' Comments About Effect of Illness on Self
68 HIGH	1.67 LOW	"She is moody and thinks she doesn't get enough attention."	"He'll never be free of [renal disease] . . . either he'll be on dialysis or be transplanted. I really don't have time for much else."	"We got to do more things before he had kidney disease . . . and now it's just a lot different. Sometimes I get mad and think why do I worry about him, but I do, you know. Everyone does."
64 HIGH	2.16 LOW	"She doesn't say too much about it. I don't know if it's because she doesn't understand or she just passes it off. Grandma babies [the ill child] . . . She's the first grandchild, she is her pick."	"I'm trying to get her to remember [her medication and exercises] on her own. With me being pregnant, things are scattered. I have a lot on my mind . . . sometimes I'm so busy I forget."	"Grandma treats her different. Every time [ill child] needs her back scratched, I want mine scratched, too. But Grandma scratches hers and says, 'You always need your back scratched when she gets hers scratched.' "
38 LOW	4.0 HIGH	"[The sibling] is good about it. He handles it pretty well."	"Treatment has become routine."	"We're not treated any differently, but sometimes [my parents] have to care for him more when he's having an [insulin] reaction. But I don't mind."
30 LOW	3.3 HIGH	"Nothing has changed for her brother."	"Things are pretty much back to normal. I don't devote a lot of time to treating her illness."	"I worry about her when she's having a rough day. Other than that, I hardly think about her. Her asthma doesn't really affect very many things."

EVALUATING THE USE OF TRIANGULATION

1. Do the research questions lend themselves to triangulation? Can both narrative (or qualitative) and numerical (quantitative) data be collected? What are the strengths and limitations of measures used to address research questions?
2. Is(are) the purpose(s) for triangulating clearly defined? Does the study confirm results or provide a more complete understanding of phenomena of interest, or both?
3. What types of triangulation are used in the study design? How were the types determined? Do the types seem appropriate to the purpose for triangulation?
4. How complex is the triangulation approach? Is a single or multiple approach appropriate for the purpose to triangulate?

problems. For example, mothers who rated their well children high on behavioral problems on the CBCL also commented on the burden the illness placed on them. Conversely, mothers who rated the well child low on behavioral problems did not comment on the burden of illness and indicated their ability to control the illness treatment.

Because it seemed from the mothers' interview data that effect of illness on self was related to behavioral problems, the healthy children's comments about effect of illness on self and their scores on Global Self-Worth also were examined. Looking first at the interviews, there was a clear consistency between mothers' and siblings' comments about effect of illness on self. For those siblings who were rated high on behavioral problems by mothers, both the mother's and the sibling's comments in the interviews indicated adverse effects of the illness on the siblings. However, for siblings who were rated low on behavioral problems by mothers, both mother and sibling indicated no adverse effects of the illness.

Also interesting was that siblings' scores on the Global Self-Worth subscale were closely related to their perception of the effect of illness on self and mothers' scores on the CBCL. For example, siblings whose mothers indicated behavioral problems both on the CBCL and in interviews also commented on adverse effects of the illness on themselves and rated themselves low on the Global Self-Worth subscale. This example of multiple triangulation provides an illustration of both the confirmation and completeness functions of triangulation as described by Breitmayer, Ayres, and Knafl (1993).

APPROPRIATE USE OF TRIANGULATION

Regardless of one's goal (confirmation, completeness, or both) and approach to triangulation (single or multiple), it is crucial to delineate one's goals in using a triangulation approach (see box). There is a tendency by some to view triangulation as an inherent good and to assume that use of any type of triangulation automatically will strengthen a study's design. In reality, triangulation contributes to the overall quality of a study only to the extent that it facilitates the achievement of some clearly articulated purpose. The examples highlighted how triangulation can serve both a confirmatory and completeness function, as well as the different ways simple and multiple triangulation strategies can contribute to these purposes.

⚘ OTHER TRIANGULATION FRAMEWORKS

Compared to the considerable literature defining triangulation and debating its relative merits, few authors have presented frameworks or models for carrying out triangulated research beyond describing how triangulation has been achieved in a single project (Connidis, 1983; Hinds & Young, 1987; Knafl & Breitmayer, 1991; Knafl, Pettengill, Bevis, & Kirchhoff, 1988; Swanson-Kauffman, 1986). Notable exceptions are Myers and Haase's (1989) guidelines for integrating quantitative and qualitative approaches and Morse's (1991) delineation of several distinct types of triangulation. In an effort to stimulate innovative research designs and explicate the decision-making processes underlying such designs, Myers and Haase (1989) offered the following guidelines for integrating quantitative and qualitative approaches:

1. The world is viewed from a systems perspective.
2. Understanding is grounded in both objective and subjective data.
3. Study design and analysis build on both atomistic and holistic thinking.
4. Both the investigators and the subjects are considered research participants.
5. Maximally conflicting points of view inform the research.

These guidelines provide a useful framework for structuring creative designs and research teams that emphasize diversity. Myers and Haase based their guidelines on the assumption that nursing practice integrates knowledge from both qualitative and quantitative approaches and that each approach should be valued equally. In addition, they pointed to the importance of identifying commonalities across methods rather than emphasizing differences. The authors contended that the consequences of such designs "may be reflected in more unified investigative approaches, broader questions, different team compositions, and costs and benefits at the personal and organizational levels" (p. 301).

Morse (1991) described four approaches to triangulation based on whether the investigator's theoretical orientation is inductive or deductive and whether the qualitative and quantitative aspects of the study are done sequentially or simultaneously. She maintained that, depending on one's theoretical orientation, either qualitative or quantitative methods will take precedence. According to Morse, if theory is being inductively developed from the data, as is the case in a grounded theory study, qualitative methods will take precedence and quantitative methods will be complementary. On the other hand, if the project is deductive and based on existing theory, quantitative methods will have a predominant role and qualitative methods will be complementary. If both qualitative and quantitative methods are gathered at the same time, simultaneous triangulation is occurring. When data from one method are essential for planning and implementing the other method, sequential triangulation is taking place. An important strength of Morse's (1991) framework is that it forces the investigator to consider the relative importance of the qualitative and quantitative aspects of the study. She argued,

> It is obvious that the qualitative and quantitative aspects of a research project cannot be equally weighted; rather the project

must be either theoretically driven by the qualitative methods incorporating a complementary quantitative component, or theoretically driven by the quantitative methods method, incorporating a complementary qualitative component. (p. 121)

This unequal weighting of the qualitative and quantitative components of the study was evident in the examples from the authors' research. The inductive approach to theory development meant that the qualitative aspect of the study was dominant as reflected in the primary aim of the research to use a grounded theory approach to conceptualize how families define and manage a child's chronic illness. At the same time the inclusion of structured, quantitative measures contributed to a secondary aim of exploring the link between various qualitative defining and managing themes and measures of family unit and individual functioning.

Morse (1991) believed that each method must have a "stand alone" quality and advised that results be blended or combined after the separate analysis of data from the qualitative and quantitative sources. She also pointed out the importance of maintaining rigor in both the qualitative and quantitative aspects of the study by applying appropriate evaluative standards to the qualitative and quantitative aspects of the research.

COMPETING VIEWPOINTS ON TRIANGULATION

In addition to varying conceptions of the nature and purpose of triangulation, there are differing views of the relative merits of triangulation. While some investigators have been extremely enthusiastic about the potential gains from using a triangulated approach, others have argued that the combining of approaches is inappropriate. Taking a positive stance, Goodwin and Goodwin (1984) argued that "many studies could be enhanced considerably if a combined approach were taken" (p. 378). In a similar vein, Sohier (1988) stated, "The utilization of multiple methods in nursing research holds the promise of establishing consistency among the theoretical, research, and practice elements, and has the power to demonstrate the holistic nature of the nursing process" (p. 733). These authors argued that the complexity of many research questions in nursing dictates the need for a triangulated approach.

On the other hand, other authors have argued that triangulation is an inherently illogical and therein inappropriate methodological approach. For example, in responding to Goodwin and Goodwin's (1984) positive stance, Powers (1987) argued,

It is neither realistic or possible to capture the best of both worlds by blending qualitative and quantitative methods to create a new paradigm. Research, at any given phase, is guided by a particular mindset, which is the function of the paradigm. (p. 126)

In general, those researchers arguing against a triangulated approach have focused on philosophical rather than methodological issues, maintaining that qualitative and quantitative approaches reflect distinct, competing paradigms or world views. Because these paradigms encompass incompatible views of reality and the generation of knowledge, they cannot be combined in a single study. In *The Paradigm Dialogue* Guba (1991) provided a detailed discussion of the philosophical underpinnings of different research approaches. Readers interested in these issues are referred to this excellent source.

A third group of authors has taken a

STEPS IN DEVELOPING A PLAN FOR TRIANGULATION

1. Identify research questions of interest.
2. Determine the purpose for triangulating based on research questions.
   a. Confirmation
   b. Completeness
3. Identify the types of triangulation to address research design issues.
   a. Investigator
   b. Data sources

    c. Methods
    d. Unit of analysis
    e. Theories
4. Determine the complexity of the triangulation approach.
   a. Single
   b. Multiple

middle ground by both acknowledging the existence of paradigmatic incompatibilities and deliberately ignoring these in favor of a more pragmatic stance. Patton (1985) maintained,

> Pragmatism can overcome seemingly logical contradictions. . . . I try to emphasize the methods implications of the paradigms debate, not because the competing paradigms can be reduced to contrasting methods, but because methods distinctions are the most concrete and practical manifestations of the larger, more overarching paradigmatic frameworks. (p. 30)

The resolution of the debate regarding the relative merits of triangulation is beyond the scope of this chapter. At the same time it is important to recognize the existence of conflicting viewpoints about the methodological approach and to keep them in mind when evaluating an investigator's rationale for selecting a triangulated or nontriangulated approach. This selection typically is based on the overall purpose of the study, as well as a thoughtful consideration of deeper philosophical and methodological issues.

Like all research endeavors, the combining of qualitative and quantitative methods is a highly purposeful activity that is undertaken to achieve clearly explicated ends. Speaking to the potential contributions of both quantitative and qualitative methods, Morse (1991) stated, "Smart researchers are versatile and have a balanced and extensive repertoire of methods at their disposal" (p. 122). The intent of this chapter has been to provide an overview of the issues involved in combining methods and to introduce the reader to several approaches to combining methods and data. In the end it is important to remember that methods are simply a means to an end. Researchers select a particular approach or combination of approaches in order to achieve the best possible design for addressing research questions of importance to the advancement of nursing science.

SUMMARY
- Qualitative research encompasses several distinct approaches, including phenomenology, grounded theory, and ethnography.
- Triangulation is the use of both quantitative and qualitative approaches in the same study.

- Triangulation can be achieved by using multiple measures to assess a single construct. If the measures yield consistent results, the investigator is more confident in the validity of her or his findings. In such instances triangulation is used for the purposes of *confirming* one's findings.

- Triangulation also can be used to achieve a more complete understanding of the subject matter. When triangulation is used to achieve completeness, different methods contribute to understanding unique aspects of the subject matter.

- Five major types of triangulation are investigator, data source, data collection methods, unit of analysis, and theory.

- Simple triangulation occurs when any one of the five types of triangulation is used in a single study; multiple triangulation entails using two or more types.

- Appropriate use of triangulation requires that the investigator clearly articulate her/his purposes in choosing a triangulated approach.

- In most triangulated studies either the quantitative or the qualitative aspect of the study will be dominant, although both may make important contributions to achieving the study aims.

- There is disagreement in the research community regarding the merit and appropriate use of triangulated research approaches.

FACILITATING CRITICAL THINKING

Your research team is planning to use triangulation to study the effects of quadriplegia on the families of adolescent males who sustained an injury.

1. What might be some research questions that support the use of triangulation?

2. What types of measures could be used to collect data from family members?
3. What are the strengths and limitations of the types of measurement used?
4. How might your study design confirm your results?
5. How might your study design provide a more complete understanding of the effect of quadriplegia on the family?
6. How might you use each of the types of triangulation in your study design?
7. Using information from "6," describe a study design using multiple triangulation.

References

SUBSTANTIVE

ACHENBACH, T., & EDELBROCK, C. (1983). *Manual for the child behavior checklist and revised child behavior profile.* Burlington, VT: Department of Psychiatry, University of Vermont.

ANDERSON, J. (1986). Ethnicity and illness experience: Ideological structures and the health care delivery system. *Social Science and Medicine, 22,* 1277-1283.

BECK, C. (1992). The lived experience of postpartum depression. *Nursing Research, 41,* 166-170.

CORBIN, J., & STRAUSS, A. (1988). *Unending work and care: Managing chronic illness at home.* San Francisco: Jossey-Bass.

FRANCIS, M. (1992). Eight homeless mothers' tales. *IMAGE: The Journal of Nursing Scholarship, 24,* 111-114.

GALLO, A. (1990). Family management style in juvenile diabetes: A case illustration. *Journal of Pediatric Nursing, 5,* 23-32.

GALLO, A. (1991). Family adaptation in childhood chronic illness: A case report. *Journal of Pediatric Nursing, 5,* 78-85.

GALLO, A., BREITMAYER, B., KNAFL, K., & ZOELLER, L. (1992, March). *Parents' role in helping well siblings adjust to childhood chronic illness.* Midwest Nursing Research Society Annual Meeting, Chicago, IL.

HARTER, S. (1985). *Manual for the self-perception profile for children.* Denver, CO: University of Denver.

KNAFL, K., BREITMAYER, B., GALLO, A., & ZOELLER, L. (1987). *How families define and manage a child's chronic illness* (Grant #NR01594). Funded by the National Center for Nursing Research, U.S. Public Health Service.

KNAFL, K., & DEATRICK, J. (1990). Family management style: Concept analysis and refinement. *Journal of Pediatric Nursing, 5,* 23-32.

McCUBBIN, H., & PATTERSON, J. (1983). Family transitions: Adaptation to stress. In H. McCubbin & C. Figley (Eds.), *Stress and the family: Coping with normative transitions* (Vol. 1). New York: Brunner/Mazel.

McNAIR, D. M., LORR, M., & DROPPLEMAN, L. F. (1981). *Profile of mood states.* San Diego, CA: Educational and Industrial Testing Service.

ROBERTS, C., & FEETHAM, S. (1982). Assessing family functioning across three areas of relationships. *Nursing Research, 31,* 1-5.

SWANSON, K. (1991). Empirical development of a middle range theory of caring. *Nursing Research, 40,* 161-166.

CONCEPTUAL

DENZIN, N. (1989). *The research act* (3rd ed.). New York: McGraw-Hill.

FIELDING, N. G., & FIELDING, J. L. (1986). *Linking data.* Beverly Hills, CA: Sage.

GOODWIN, L. D., & GOODWIN, W. L. (1984). Qualitative vs. quantitative research or qualitative and quantitative research? *Nursing Research, 33,* 378-380.

GUBA, E. G. (1991). *The paradigm dialogue.* Newbury Park, CA: Sage.

KNAFL, K., & BREITMAYER, B. (1991). Triangulation in qualitative research: Issues of conceptual clarity and purpose. In J. Morse (Ed.), *Qualitative nursing research: A contemporary dialogue.* Newbury Park, CA: Sage.

MITCHELL, E. S. (1986). Multiple triangulation: A methodology for nursing science. *Advances in Nursing Science, 8*(3), 18-26.

MORSE, J. (1991). Approaches to qualitative-quantitative methodological triangulation. *Nursing Research, 40,* 120-123.

PATTON, M. (1985). Logical incompatibilities and pragmatism. *Evaluation and Program Planning, 8,* 307-308.

POWERS, B. (1987). Taking sides: A response to Goodwin and Goodwin. *Nursing Research, 36,* 122-126.

SOHIER, R. (1988). Multiple triangulation and contemporary nursing research. *Western Journal of Nursing Research, 10,* 732-742.

METHODOLOGICAL

BREITMAYER, B., AYRES, L., & KNAFL, K. (1993). Triangulation in qualitative research: Evaluation of confirmation and completeness purposes. *IMAGE: The Journal of Nursing Scholarship, 25,* 237-243.

CHENITZ, W. C., & SWANSON, J. M. (EDS.). (1986). *From practice to grounded theory: Qualitative research in nursing.* Menlo Park, CA: Addison-Wesley.

CONNIDIS, I. (1983). Integrating qualitative and quantitative methods in survey research on aging: An assessment. *Qualitative Sociology, 6,* 334-352.

FIELD, P. A., & MORSE, J. M. (1985). *Nursing research: The application of qualitative approaches.* Rockville, MD: Aspen.

HINDS, P. S., & YOUNG, K. (1987). A triangulation of methods and paradigms to study nurse-given wellness care. *Nursing Research, 36,* 195-198.

KIMCHI, J., POLIVKA, B., & STEVENSON, J. (1991). Triangulation: Operational definitions. *Nursing Research, 40,* 364-366.

KNAFL, K., PETTENGILL, M., BEVIS, M., & KIRCHHOFF, K. (1988). Blending qualitative and quantitative approaches to instrument development and data collection. *Journal of Professional Nursing, 4,* 30-37.

LEININGER, M. M. (ED.). (1985). *Qualitative research methods in nursing.* Orlando, FL: Grune & Stratton.

MILES, M. B., & HUBERMAN, A. M. (1984). *Qualitative data analysis: A source book of new methods.* Beverly Hills, CA: Sage.

MUNHALL, P. L., & OILER, C. J. (1986). *Nursing research: A qualitative perspective.* Norwalk, CT: Appleton-Century-Crofts.

MYERS, S., & HAASE, J. (1989). Guidelines for integration of quantitative and qualitative approaches. *Nursing Research, 38,* 299-301.

OILER, C. J. (1986). Phenomenology: The method. In P. L. Munhall & C. J. Oiler (Eds.), *Nursing research: A qualitative perspective.* Norwalk, CT: Appleton-Century-Crofts.

PATTON, M. Q. (1990). *Qualitative evaluation and research methods* (2nd ed.). Newbury Park, CA: Sage.

STRAUSS, A. L. (1987). *Qualitative analysis for social scientists.* New York: Cambridge University Press.

STRAUSS, A. L., & CORBIN, J. M. (1990). *Basics of qualitative research: Grounded theory procedures and techniques.* Newbury Park, CA: Sage.

SWANSON-KAUFFMAN, K. M. (1986). A combined qualitative methodology for nursing research. *Advances in Nursing Science, 8*(3), 58-69.

TESCH, R. (1990). *Qualitative research: Analysis types and software tools.* New York: The Falmer Press.

HISTORICAL

CAMPBELL, D. T. (1956). *Leadership and its effects upon the group.* Columbus, OH: The Ohio State University Press.

DENZIN, N. (1970). *The research act: A theoretical introduction to sociological methods.* Chicago: Aldine.

JICK, T. D. (1979). Mixing qualitative and quantitative methods: Triangulation in action. *Administrative Science Quarterly, 24,* 602-611.

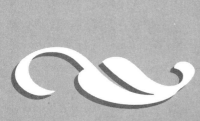

PART V
USING RESEARCH IN PRACTICE

USE OF CRITICAL THINKING IN RESEARCH: THE RESEARCH CRITIQUE

BARBARA RAUDONIS • LAURA A. TALBOT

Before purchasing expensive and durable goods many people frequently read the magazine *Consumer Reports.* Consumers Union, a nonprofit organization, conducts independent, scientific testing of goods and services in order to provide consumers with information and advice. The test results and ratings are published in *Consumer Reports.* Readers refer to these reports because of the rigorous standards, integrity, independence, and no-commercialization policies of the magazine.

Much like the testers in *Consumer Reports,* nurses must develop their critical thinking skills in order to analyze and evaluate research studies. One method to become a critical thinker is the use of the research critique. Critical thinking enables nurses to make informed decisions regarding the implementation of research findings.

CRITICAL THINKING IN RESEARCH

Critical thinking is the art of disciplined reasoning using various tools essential for assessing, integrating, and applying information. Critical thinking provides a framework for practice. Nurses must reason daily through an avalanche of information to be able to use and adapt knowledge in the complex realities of nursing practice.

The use of critical thinking to examine a research study is an important part of developing nursing knowledge. It goes beyond the research findings and conclusions and examines what can be learned from the strengths and weaknesses of a study. By examining previous research, alternate methods and approaches in problem solving can be explored, allowing researchers to learn from other studies and to build on previous research.

At the same time critical thinking enhances the novice researcher's critical and analytical skills in thinking through a research problem. To critically analyze a research study, the reader must have some knowledge of the research process and of the topic being investigated. What better way to learn the research process than to see how an experienced researcher in the

513

field takes didactic material and applies it to a researchable problem.

Critical thinking helps nurses, as consumers of research, distinguish between findings ready to be implemented into practice and those that need replication and further study to ensure quality patient care. Nurses clearly need to examine research findings and conclusions to ascertain what conforms to an acceptable standard of nursing practice and what needs further research. The use of critical thinking is vital in this process.

One method to facilitate critical thinking is the use of the research critique—analyzing and evaluating a research study to ascertain its merit. The function of a research critique is to provide guidelines for a consumer and researcher to learn from the research studies. The process itself provides the following: the development of critical analysis skills; new strategies, techniques, and ideas for further research; establishment and implementation of standards of care; and a systematic way to analyze the study critically. Use of the research critique will enhance conceptual acuity, strengthen intellectual and scientific understanding, and facilitate the use of the research process.

A distinction should be made between the research review and the research critique. In a research review the study is described, focusing on major aspects of the study, then summarizing its major features. One such example is the publication by the American Association of Critical-Care Nurses, *Nursing Scan in Critical Care*. In this publication a reviewer gives a synopsis of a recently published research study, pointing out major characteristics of the study. A commentary follows, highlighting important features of the study. Then the reviewer gives implications for the study's utilization in practice.

The research critique goes beyond this somewhat limited description of a research study. Utilizing specific criteria, the evaluator makes precise and objective judgments about the research study, weighing its strengths and weaknesses. Research critiques are seen in the *Western Journal of Nursing Research*. The research study is presented first by the researcher. A critique by an expert researcher follows, providing constructive comments.

ROLE OF THE RESEARCH CRITIQUE

A critique is meant to be constructive, not punitive. Its purpose is to identify aspects of the study that may provide solutions for immediate problems, improve nursing practice, further a theoretical base, be suggestive of future research, or be deserving of replication.

The person writing a research critique (research critic) has a dual role: to assist the researcher in refining the research study and to assist the consumer of research in the utilization of research findings in nursing practice. As a facilitator, the research critic offers suggestions on how to validate the theoretical framework, refine research design, improve precision of the research instrument, and gain new insight into the overall congruency of the study. As a consumer advisor, the research critic suggests how to apply the research findings in nursing practice and stimulates heightened interest so that new scientific questions are generated for future research.

THE CRITIQUE PROCESS

A general research critique utilizes the techniques of analysis, evaluation, validation, and replication. The first step is analysis—separating the study into parts to better comprehend what the research study is reporting. Each element of the study is examined for strengths and weaknesses.

Next the study is evaluated to assess its overall value or merit. Evaluation uses internal and external standards to make judgments about the study. Internal standards are the evaluation of specific elements within the study such as consistency, accuracy, validity, reliability, precision of measurement, and logical conclusions about the data. External standards are the global evaluation of the study and its clinical contribution in such areas as efficiency, economy, and utility in practice.

The technique of validation weighs the strengths and weaknesses gathered in the analysis stage. The evaluator must determine: (1) whether the strengths of the study outweigh its limitations, or (2) whether the weaknesses of the study invalidate its findings and conclusions. Now the evaluator must exercise judgment in substantiating each conclusion in order to present an objective evaluation. Validation of fact is critical in maintaining an objective stance in the critique process.

The final question is then asked: How can we take what we have learned from this research study and make the next one stronger? Based on the strengths and weaknesses of the study, the evaluator suggests how to capitalize on the strong points and modify the weak aspects of the study. This is how nursing knowledge is built: taking information learned from analysis, evaluation, and validation and going one step further with replication. The recommendations are implemented in a new study. The replicated study is then reevaluated, and the process begins again. Research and critique are an ongoing knowledge-building process.

ELEMENTS EXAMINED IN A RESEARCH CRITIQUE

The evaluator applies critiquing techniques of analysis, evaluation, validation, and replication to the following elements of the research study: conceptual basis, methodology, exposition, substantive contribution, and ethical and legal considerations. To be fair, an evaluator must remember that journal editors have freedom to edit manuscripts according to journal guidelines. Space limitations and journal format are some of the constraints that frequently limit authors' reporting of their entire study.

CONCEPTUAL BASIS

Because the primary purpose of research is to test theory or generate knowledge, it is important that the conceptual basis for the study be appropriate for the type of study being conducted. The research critic must ask the following question: Is there consistency between the theoretical structure of the study and the type of study conducted (see Table 23-1)? For example, exploratory research is used to test or generate explanatory theory. This is the most basic type of research and is used when little is known about the phenomenon to be studied. Concepts tend to be vague and undefined. The characteristics of the phenomenon will be named or classified, and relationships will not be defined.

After examining the overall layout of the study, specific items related to the conceptual basis need to be analyzed and evaluated. They are:

1. Clear identification of the concepts: Are the concepts under study presented clearly in the introduction and easily delineated?
2. Concepts related to the theory: Are the concepts taken from the conceptual/theoretical framework?

Table 23-1

Guidelines for Consistency Among Five Structures for Three Different Types of Studies

	Exploratory	Descriptive	Experimental/ Quasi-Experimental
Theoretical structure:	Conceptual orientation	Conceptual framework	Theoretical framework
	Concepts vague, undefined; no relationships defined	Concepts defined; relationships not defined or relationships between concepts defined but not the direction of characteristics of the relationships	Concepts defined specifically, relationships among concepts defined, characteristics of relationships defined
Research problem:	Research question or statement	Research question or statement	Hypothesis
Design structure:	Ethnomethodology Grounded theory	Quantitatively describe concepts and/or relations	
Data collection methods:	Unstructured techniques Open-ended questions Participant-observation	Structured instruments that have been tested for reliability and validity	Manipulation of independent variable(s), precise measurement of dependent variable(s)
Analysis structure:	Taxonomies Percentages Frequencies	Descriptive statistics	Predictive statistics Probability statistics

Adapted from Hinshaw, A. S. (1978). *Western Journal of Nursing Research, 1*(3), 251, with permission. In Phillips, L. (1986). *A clinician's guide to the critique and utilization of nursing research.* Norwalk, CT: Appleton-Century-Crofts, p. 99.

3. Concepts conceptually and operationally defined: Are the concepts conceptually defined based on the conceptual/theoretical framework? Are the concepts operationally defined using the conceptual/theoretical framework?

4. Use of terms consistent with the theory: Are the terms to describe the concepts consistent with the conceptual/theoretical framework?

5. Reflection of the conceptual/theoretical framework in other aspects of the research study: Are the statement of the problem, study purpose and research question, statement, or hypothesis reflective of the conceptual/theoretical framework?

METHODOLOGY

The methodology section includes the research design, data collection methods, and analysis of variables. The central focus is on this question: Is the methodology appropriate for the solution of the problem? Table 23-1 can assist the critic in examining the consistency between the type of research design and the other components of the study.

The research critic examines the design structure, data collection method, and analysis structure for consistency. In addition, all three should be in logical agreement with the type of study and the theoretical structure. For example, if the research design is experimental, the researcher should use a theoretical framework from which both theoretical structure concepts and relationships are defined. The researcher then formulates a hypothesis in which the independent and dependent variables are identified. The independent variable is manipulated, and the dependent variable is measured. The data are then analyzed using descriptive and/or inferential statistics. This demonstrates the logical flow based on the study type of experimental research.

EXPOSITION

Exposition is an evaluation of the research report for logic, clarity, and consistency among all its components. Most research reports in nursing use the guidelines published in the *Publication Manual of the American Psychological Association* (APA, 1994). The manual provides commonly accepted rules for the preparation of a manuscript and an acceptable method for clear communication. If another guide is used, the writer must be sure that standards of good writing are followed.

To evaluate, the critic examines the writing style to see if there is a logical, orderly presentation of ideas. Continuity in thematic development will clearly demonstrate the relationships between ideas with a smooth transition from one idea to another.

SUBSTANTIVE CONTRIBUTION

A study's substantive contribution is its true contribution to nursing knowledge. The critic first asks the fundamental question: Is the problem studied a *nursing* problem? The researcher should provide evidence of the relationship of the research problem to nursing in the introduction of the study and maintain this theme throughout the research report.

Once a study's basic relevance is established, the critic is ready to determine a study's true substantive contribution to the field. In other words many problems are relevant to nursing but not necessarily substantively noteworthy. Determining the worth of a study means assessing the degree of understanding the research contributes to the phenomenon studied.

In review, to assess substantive contributions, the critic first ascertains whether the researcher discusses the contributions to nursing knowledge in the research report. The critic then determines whether the study contributed what the researcher promised from the information that was provided in the report. Finally, the critic considers the degree to which the study provided new insights and stimulated new avenues of inquiry for the science of nursing.

ETHICAL AND LEGAL CONSIDERATIONS

Ethical and legal considerations focus on the protection of human subjects in a research project. Although laws provide specific guidance in some situations, there are many legal and ethical situations in which there are not firmly established laws or rules. It is the researcher's challenge to design a study to obtain the most valuable information while posing the least possible risk to those participating. The researcher may be caught in an ethical dilemma in which there may be two or more views and means for interpreting a research proposal. Each institution has its own methods of reviewing and interpreting ethical and legal dilemmas. These factors also need to be considered by the research critic when evaluating a study. Chapter 3 discusses these issues in greater depth.

At a minimum a statement in the research report should address human rights issues and the protection of human subjects. Other questions the research critic may want to explore are: How were the subject's rights protected? What method was used to obtain consent? Was enough information given without compromising the study? Was the study approved by an Institutional Review Board?

CRITIQUING QUANTITATIVE AND QUALITATIVE RESEARCH

Whether you are a graduate student or an expert researcher, specific step-by-step guidelines may be helpful in examining the research study. Using a systematic approach to evaluate a study ensures a comprehensive review. The box contains guidelines for critiquing a research report.

GUIDELINES FOR CRITIQUING QUANTITATIVE RESEARCH

When examining quantitative research, the critic examines each major part of the research document: title, statement of the problem, research purpose, theoretical/conceptual basis, review of related literature, hypothesis (research questions), methodology, results, and discussion. As a demonstration, we'll use a quantitative study published by Rentschler (1991) in *IMAGE: Journal of Nursing Scholarship* on factors related to successful breastfeeding. The following section will first present essential elements to examine in each category of a finished study. Next, an excerpt of the Rentschler article will be presented, followed by a critique of the excerpt based on the essential elements.

Title

The title of a study is very important. It can either entice the reader to read the article or turn the reader away. Computer searches frequently rely on key words abstracted from the titles of articles; therefore, titles should reflect the study's variables and method.

The critic evaluates the study title to determine if it is reflective of the hypothesis, suggestive of the research design, and clearly identifies the major variables. Inclu-

---

STEPS IN CRITIQUING A RESEARCH REPORT

1. *Analysis.* Analyze the strengths and weaknesses of each area in a research report:
   a. Conceptual basis
   b. Methodology
   c. Exposition
   d. Substantive contribution
   e. Ethical foundation
2. *Evaluation.* Evaluate the overall merit of each area of the research report:
   a. Conceptual basis
   b. Methodology
   c. Exposition
   d. Substantive contribution
   e. Ethical foundation
3. *Validation*
   a. Do the strengths of the study outweigh the limitations?
   b. Do the weaknesses of the study invalidate the findings and conclusions?
4. *Replication*
   a. Based on this review, how would you conceptualize another study in which you capitalize on the strong points and modify the weak aspects of this study?
   b. How would you envision the resultant critique of this replicated study?

sion of this precise information in the title assists the reader in determining at a glance what the study is examining. It also assists interested readers and other researchers in retrieving specific information when conducting a computer search. Easy access by researchers interested in the topic promotes efficient and effective use of time when retrieval of specific information is vital.

Example. "Correlates of Successful Breastfeeding" is a title from the sample study in *IMAGE: Journal of Nursing Scholarship* (Rentschler, 1991, p. 151).

Critique. The title is brief but explicit and conveys to the reader what the study will be about. The reader can assume from the term *correlates* that the research design will be a correlational study with more than one variable to be measured. The sample is implied by the term *breastfeeding* (that postpartum females will be used).

Statement of the Problem
When critiquing the statement of the problem, the critic should be sure that the statement is telling the reader that (1) a problem exists, (2) there is a need for a research study, and (3) finding a solution is imperative. In addition, the problem needs to be researchable and specific enough to provide guidance for the research design and methodology. From the statement of the problem, the reader should get a sense of the value of the study to nursing and of the intended beneficiaries of the research.

Example. The statement of the problem reads:

> Failure at breastfeeding is not considered serious. But for the unsuccessful mother, failure often produces long-lasting emotional effects (La Leche League International, 1981; Starling, Fergusson, Hor-

wood, & Taylor, 1979; West, 1980). Only about 50 percent of women who attempt to breastfeed do so successfully. The low success rate raises the question: What makes the difference in outcome? (Rentschler, 1991, p. 151)

Critique. This statement of the problem is clear and convincing in its assertion that a problem exists for women attempting to breastfeed. The problem is researchable, significant to nursing practice, and conveys a clear need for resolution. "Successful breastfeeding" and "variables that influence that outcome" are the research variables around which the problem is formulated. The author does not specify the independent variable(s) in the problem statement. Finally, the reader recognizes the obvious beneficiaries of this study—mothers and neonates.

Research Purpose
When examining the research purpose, the overall statement should tell what the researcher hopes to accomplish. It should start with a definitive statement such as: "The purpose of this study is to . . ." What follows is a statement of the study population and a presentation of the relationships among the variables. The critic should examine the statement to be sure that it reflects the problem statement and the type of research design to be used.

Example

> The purpose of this study was to gain a better understanding of the relationship of a pregnant woman's motivation to breastfeed and her knowledge about breastfeeding to success in breastfeeding. (Rentschler, 1991, p. 151)

Critique. The research purpose is clear in stating what the study hopes to accomplish. It has a definitive statement and identifies the study population. The purpose of the study suggests that a potential relationship exists between the variables of motivation, knowledge of breastfeeding, and success in breastfeeding. Because the researcher is examining relationships between variables, the study is a correlational study. Correlational studies seek to describe, predict, or test relationships. When the researcher seeks to predict the value of one variable based on values from another variable, it is a predictive-correlational design. Independent and dependent variables are used in this type of correlational design because the researcher is predicting the dependent variable based on the independent variables.

In this article the independent variables are first presented in the research article's statement of purpose. To make this presentation stronger, the independent variables could be stated earlier, preferably in the title. The purpose is reflective of the problem statement, with the author narrowing the focus by presenting the independent and dependent variables. By indicating that the study is examining "the *relationship* of . . ." the researcher is suggesting that a correlational study will be conducted. The statement "a pregnant woman's motivation to breastfeed and her knowledge about breastfeeding to success in breastfeeding," gives the independent variables of "motivation to breastfeed" and "knowledge about breastfeeding" and the dependent variable of "success in breastfeeding."

Theoretical/Conceptual Basis
The theoretical/conceptual framework identifies and defines the concepts to be studied. The concepts should be evaluated for clarity in statement, understandability, and relevance to the research study. The researcher's presentation of the relationships among the concepts needs to take on a logical, rational flow describing the interrelationships among the phenomena. This flow should move naturally, providing concepts from which the hypotheses can be derived. The level of theory development presented will provide the basis for the type of research design used in the study.

Example. Atkinson's (1964) achievement motivation theory is the theoretical basis for this research study. The Rentschler study (1991) defined Atkinson's three principles:

> The first principle proposes that an individual has greater persistence when the need to succeed is greater than the need to avoid failure. . . . Atkinson's second principle, expectancy of success, is described as what the individual perceives she can accomplish. . . . Atkinson's third principle, the value of incentive, is defined as the perceived benefits to be gained as a result of success at a particular task. (pp. 151-152)

Information theory is based on observations that

> breastfeeding is not instinctual but is a learned behavior (Cadwell, 1981; Grassley & Davis, 1978; Johnson, 1976). Mothers who receive specific information on the advantages and disadvantages of breastfeeding and on the techniques of breastfeeding are more likely to be successful (Cohen, 1980; Ladas, 1970; Sarto, 1963). (Rentschler, 1991, p. 152)

Critique. Achievement motivation theory and information theory are used as the unifying framework for this study. The concepts are clearly stated, easily understandable, and relevant to the research study. The theoretical framework provides clear guidance in conceptualizing the relationships among the concepts of achievement motivation, level of information, and the outcome variable, success in breastfeeding. The level of theory development shows a predictive relationship among the variables in which the independent variables are expected to predict the dependent variable, indicating a predictive-correlational study.

Review of Related Literature

An essential element in the review of the literature involves showing relationships between previous research and the proposed study. This establishes a basis for the research. It is necessary that the written presentation be reflective of an extensive literature review, inclusive of study findings, and not merely provide brief summaries of various articles. Essential works should be presented in a logical and organized fashion. Sources should be current, with classic works included as appropriate. The critic needs to examine the work to be sure that outdated references and studies with irrelevant subject matter are not used and that primary sources are used to the greatest extent possible.

The review of the literature should also relate to the theoretical framework. Background information in the review develops the concepts in the theoretical framework. Previous research studies lend support for the usage of theoretical concepts as research variables in the proposed study. The researcher then concludes with a valid argument on how the present study will build on the theoretical framework and current knowledge base.

Example. Rentschler's review of the literature focuses on the three key concepts: achievement motivation, level of information, and success in breastfeeding.

ACHIEVEMENT MOTIVATION. Motivation has been reported by successful breastfeeding mothers as the basis for their ability to persevere through difficult times (Applebaum, 1975; Cohen, 1980; Ewy & Ewy, 1975; Lawson, 1976; Potter & Klein, 1957; Raphael, 1973). The type and degree of motivation needed for success has not been identified nor has statistical evidence of its influence on success been established. However, successful breastfeeding mothers have been described by Evans, Thigpen, and Hamrick (1969) and Hall (1978) as individuals who are persistent and have high aspirations, which are traits identified in achievers by Atkinson's (1964) achievement motivation theory. (Rentschler, 1991, p. 151)

LEVEL OF INFORMATION. Numerous observers suggest that breastfeeding is not instinctual but is a learning behavior (Cadwell, 1981; Grassley & Davis, 1978; Johnson, 1976). Mothers who receive specific information on the advantages and disadvantages of breastfeeding and the techniques of breastfeeding are more likely to be successful (Cohen, 1980; Ladas, 1970; Sarto, 1963). One proposed mechanism is that providing specific information on a given topic decreases uncertainty (Miller, 1965).

Both Sarto (1963) and Cohen (1980) provided a teaching program for breastfeeding mothers to enhance success in breastfeeding, with the prevention of problems being the focus of the former study and prevention of supplementation with formula that of the other. The programs were offered antepartally and postpartally, respectively. Sarto (1963) reported increased success without statistical evidence, while Cohen provided evidence of a significant difference between those mothers who had been given specific information and those who had not, as to the length of time for which they breastfed.

Studies in which information was not provided, but in which mothers' knowledge of breastfeeding was tested, reported positive correlations between the depth and accuracy of information about breastfeeding and success (Ladas, 1970; Gulick,

1981; Heath, 1977). Mothers with less knowledge of breastfeeding reported experiencing problems related specifically to information they lacked. (Rentschler, 1991, p. 152)

SUCCESS IN BREASTFEEDING. According to the American Academy of Pediatrics (1982), breastfeeding should continue through the first six months of life if optimal benefits to infant and mother are to be attained. In practice, however, most studies have used a duration of only six weeks or less as the criterion for success (Bernard-Bonnin, Stachtchenko, Girard, & Rousseau, 1989; Gulick, 1981; Hall, 1978).

This less stringent criterion is based on studies which report the highest failure rate during the first four to six weeks (Eastham, Smith, Poole, & Neligan, 1976; Samuels, Margen, & Schoen, 1985; Sloper, McKean, & Baum, 1975). The reasons for failure most often cited were mothers' lack of preparation and anticipation for the problems common to the early weeks of breastfeeding. (Rentschler, 1991, p. 152)

Critique. The literature cited by Rentschler provides an ample review with a total of 27 sources referenced in the review of literature. Both historical and contemporary references are used to support the study. The researcher presents a systematic sequencing of sources relevant to the theoretical concepts. Each concept is presented with definitions and an illustration of research support. Conceptual relationships logically unfold, establishing a basis for the proposed research and its variables. The researcher concludes the review with the statement: "In view of the studies cited, it was assumed that the goal-oriented person would seek information about breastfeeding in order to succeed at the task at hand. Therefore, both achievement motivation and level of information about breastfeeding seem to be variables that would explain

successful breastfeeding" (Rentschler, 1991, p. 152). This statement validates the theoretical concepts and lends support for the relationship between the independent and dependent variables.

Hypothesis

The hypothesis should be written clearly and succinctly. Often, the hypothesis will be hidden in the context of the journal article and not obvious to the reader. A statement that asserts "The hypotheses for this study are . . ." takes the guesswork out of deducing the intent of the researcher.

The critic should also consider whether the hypotheses stem from the theoretical framework. Conceptual relationships should make a smooth transition from theoretical concepts to research variables in the hypothesis. This provides the foundation for a research study that is based on theory. To make hypotheses testable, the variables should be operationalized into measurable terms. The critic should examine the research variables to see if they are reflective of the theoretical concepts, stated in measurable terms, and testable.

Example

The hypotheses tested were:
1. There would be a positive relationship between pregnant women's achievement motivation and success in breastfeeding.
2. There should be a positive relationship between pregnant women's level of information about breastfeeding and success in breastfeeding.
3. When taken together the variables of pregnant women's achievement motivation and information about breastfeeding would be better predictors of success in breastfeeding than either one taken alone. (Rentschler, 1991, p. 152)

Critique. The hypotheses were stated clearly and succinctly. Hypotheses 1 and 2 are simple, directional hypotheses. Hypothesis 3 is a complex, nondirectional hypothesis.

The hypotheses are clearly generated from the theoretical framework. There is a smooth transition from the conceptual relationships stated in the theory to the research variables stated in the hypotheses, clearly making this study based on theory.

The researcher operationalized the concepts of motivation and knowledge in the hypothesis. The theoretical concept of knowledge is operationalized to level of information about breastfeeding, and motivation is narrowed to achievement motivation. This focusing establishes that the hypotheses are testable and that they are stated in measurable terms. The researcher clarifies this focusing in the review of the literature. Through a concept analysis, the researcher deduces that "level of information" and "achievement motivation" are sensitive indicators of success in breastfeeding.

Methodology

Methodology includes the research instruments, sample selection, and data collection method. The research instruments measure the variables identified in the hypotheses. The instruments should be congruent with the operational definitions and hypotheses. To ensure that the instruments are measuring the variables they purport to measure, the researcher reports the validity and reliability estimates. The critic now determines if the estimates reported are appropriate values for a valid and reliable instrument based on the reported data. Pilot testing of the instruments makes for a stronger case if a new instrument is used, there has been a change in the target population, items have been added or deleted, and/or reliability estimates are low.

When sampling is examined, a critical factor is the accurate representation of the target population. Sample size and sample selection are two areas that need to be critiqued.

The *sample size* requires a sample large enough to be representative of the study population so as to make generalizations about the target population possible. Statistical methods, such as power analysis, can be used to determine the appropriate sample size and reduce sampling error. Still, sample size means very little if the sample is not representativeness of the population.

Sample selection also addresses the issue of representativeness of the study population. The critic examines how the sample was selected, the method for controlling the variables, and potential sources of sampling bias. Furthermore, the sample selection needs to be reflective of the hypothesis and research design (i.e., an experimental design will have a control and experimental group with subjects randomly assigned).

Data collection methods should be consistent with the research design and appropriate for the solution of the stated problem. If research assistants are used, their training for administration of the instruments should be explained. Included in this section are measures used to protect human subjects. The issues to be discussed are protection from harm, informed consent, confidentiality, and anonymity.

Example

INSTRUMENTS. Achievement motivation was measured by Mehrabian and Bank's (1978) questionnaire Measure of Individual Differences in Achieving Tendency (QMIDAT). The instrument contains 38 items developed from a large pool of items characteristic of most aspects of achieving tendency. The theoretical basis of the instrument is Atkinson's (1964) Achievement Motivation Theory.

Reliability and validity of the 38-item QMIDAT were established on a population of 76 male and 66 female university undergraduates. The Kuder Richardson formula (20) scales were used to obtain a coefficient of .91, providing evidence of internal consistency. Discriminant validity between the achieving tendency measure and the Crowne and Marlowe (1960) social desirability scale was established by a reported correlation of .02. The 38-item QMIDAT was found to correlate ($1 = .14$ $p < .05$) with gender; males had a mean score of 55 ($SD = 34$); females had a mean of 46 ($SD = 36$).

Information about breastfeeding was measured by Gulick's (1981) Information on Breastfeeding Questionnaire (IBQ). It contains 26 items, each with 5 possible responses. The items were construed to reflect information that is available through paperback books and pamphlets, as well as information that may be provided by professionals. A test-retest reliability and Cronbach Alpha reliability coefficient for internal consistency were .87 and .72 respectively.

The Personal Data Inventory (PDI) (Rentschler, 1986) was designed to seek information on those variables cited in the literature as influencing the outcome of breastfeeding experience such as when the decision to breastfeed was made, length of time intended to breastfeed, and demographic information including: age, race, marital status, education level, occupation, and income.

The Breastfeeding Experience Questionnaire (BEQ) (Rentschler, 1986) was used to measure success in breastfeeding. The questionnaire elicited information about factors related to the birth—for example, type of delivery, sex of newborn, birth weight, complications experienced by mother and/or infant—and questions related to breastfeeding, including length of breastfeeding, reasons for weaning, problems encountered, and mother's perceptions of experience. (Rentschler, 1991, p. 152)

SAMPLE. First-time pregnant women who planned to breastfeed ($N = 173$) volunteered to be participants; 15 participants withdrew from the study. Of these 15, four women failed to complete the initial questionnaires, while 11 failed to return the final questionnaire at 6 weeks postpartum. Eight mothers were eliminated as study participants; three experienced infant loss and five decided to bottlefeed. Thus 150 mothers were included in the sample used for testing hypotheses.

The mean age of the participants was 28 years. All were married, most were Caucasian (94 percent). Total family income had a modal range of $31,000 to $40,000. All participants had completed high school; 77 percent had attended college. More than half were salaried professionals or held administrative positions. (Rentschler, 1991, pp. 152-153)

PROCEDURE. Volunteers for the study were sought through prepared childbirth classes. Participants were given a verbal explanation of the purpose of the study and the procedure for collecting data. Individuals' anonymity and confidentiality were assured. During the initial contact, women who were interested and who met the criteria for participating each signed a consent form and completed the PDI data sheet. Arrangements were made then to meet with the participants after their next prepared childbirth class. On the second meeting the subjects completed the QMIDAT and IBQ. The BEQ was mailed to each participant at six weeks postpartum with a request to return the completed form as soon as possible. (Rentschler, 1991, p. 153)

Critique. This researcher pays meticulous attention to the technical and methodological aspects of the study. The independent variables are conceptualized well and operationalized superbly. All four instruments are consistent with the hypotheses. The PDI and BEQ solicited descriptive information about the sample, whereas the QMIDAT and IBQ sought inferential data. The

QMIDAT and IBQ instruments were pretested for validity and reliability. Both instruments were within range for predictive instruments.

The sample was one of convenience that is consistent with a correlational study. The sample size was 150 first-time pregnant women. The researcher does not present a power analysis or justify the appropriateness of the number of participants used. This brings the representativeness of the sample into question. It seems to be skewed toward Caucasian families of high socioeconomic and educational status. This does not seem representative of the proposed target population of pregnant women. If the total sample has completed high school and 77% have attended college, they may already have a high degree of achievement motivation. This may limit the generalizability of these results.

The data collection methods of face-to-face contact at childbirth classes and mailed questionnaires 6 weeks postpartum are consistent with a correlational design. The total dropout rate was 15 with 4 failing to complete the initial questionnaire and 11 failing to mail back the final questionnaire. The researcher had a remarkable return rate on the mailed questionnaire (only 11 failed to return the final questionnaire). Appropriate measures were taken to protect human subjects, including discussions of consent, confidentiality, and anonymity. Based on the information provided in the article, there appears to be no apparent violations of human rights.

Results

When critiquing the results, the critic first considers whether the statistical analysis of the data was appropriate for the research design and hypothesis. Next, the critic evaluates the researcher's relating of the study results to the hypotheses. There should be a discussion of how the results supported or failed to support the hypotheses based on the data analysis. The presentation of data should be clear and concise so that if another researcher wanted to replicate the study he or she could do so. Visual presentations that report statistical results through tables and charts provide volumes of information clearly and concisely.

Example

Of the 150 participants, 107 were successful in breastfeeding; that is, they breastfed for at least six weeks. Of those 43 unsuccessful, more than 50 percent weaned their infants within the first three weeks postpartum. The reasons for weaning reported by these participants varied. The eight categories identified are listed in Table 1. It is worth noting that the two most frequent reasons given for weaning were lack of milk (44 percent) and sore nipples (42 percent).

All three hypotheses were supported. A Point Biserial correlation was used to determine the relationship between success in breastfeeding, a dichotomous variable, and pregnant women's achievement motivation. The results ($rpb = .17$, $p = .018$) indicated a positive relationship between

Table 1
Unsuccessful Breastfeeders' Reasons for Weaning ($N = 43$)

Problem	Frequency	Percentage
Lack of milk	19	44.0
Sore nipples	16	42.0
Baby refused	8	18.6
Baby had colic	4	9.3
Doctor advised	6	14.0
Return to work	13	30.2
Anxious	11	25.6
Maternal problems	7	16.3

pregnant women's achievement motivation and success in breastfeeding. A Point
Biserial correlation was used to determine
the relationship between success in
breastfeeding and pregnant women's level
of information about breastfeeding. The
results (rpb = .32, p = .0001) indicated a
positive relationship. Stepwise Multiple
Regression was used to determine maximum fit of the independent variables, information about breastfeeding and
achievement motivation to the dependent variable, success in breastfeeding. Information about breastfeeding was entered first into the equation because of its
higher correlation with success in breastfeeding; its multiple R was .32 ($F(1.148)$ =
16.828, p = .0001). Achievement motivation entered in step 2, raising the multiple
R to .35($F(2.147)$ = 10.306, p = .0001). Information and achievement motivation
explained 12.3 percent of the variance in
success. These results indicated that
achievement motivation and information
about breastfeeding together are better
predictors of success in breastfeeding than
either one alone. (Rentschler, 1991, p.
153)

Critique. Rentschler presented the study
results in a straightforward and succinct
style. Descriptive statistics were employed
to describe "unsuccessful breastfeeders' reasons for weaning." A table was used to present the eight categories with statistical results. The table was easy to understand. An
error was found in Table 1. The researcher
reports a frequency of 16 sore nipples.
With an N of 43, the percentage should
equal 37.2 and not 42.0.

All three hypotheses were supported,
using the appropriate inferential statistics.
A point biserial correlation is used to determine the relationship between a qualitative
variable and a quantitative variable. Success in breastfeeding, a qualitative variable,
is correlated with the quantitative variable

of pregnant women's achievement motivation. This test of correlation, when a dichotomous variable such as success in
breastfeeding is used, is appropriate for the
level of measurement of the outcome variable.

A regression analysis to test the hypothesis is the method of choice for a predictive
correlation study. A Stepwise Multiple Regression was used to determine the maximum fit of the independent variables,
information about breastfeeding and
achievement motivation, to the dependent
variable. This statistical method was appropriate to predict the strength of each independent variable to the dependent variable.

The researcher related the research results to the hypotheses, stating that the results provided support based on the data
analysis. When closely examined, the results of the point biserial correlation provided a very weak positive relationship between pregnant women's achievement
motivation and success in breastfeeding
(rpb = .17, p = .018). The results of the
point biserial correlation also provided a
weak positive relationship between success
in breastfeeding and pregnant women's
level of information about breastfeeding
(rpb = .32, p = .0001). The stepwise multiple regression reported a higher correlation, indicating that the independent variables are better predictors of success in
breastfeeding when used together versus
separately. There was only one table reporting the statistical results; still, the text was
well written and easy to follow.

Discussion
In the discussion the critic looks to see if
the conclusions and implications presented
come from the study findings; inferences
made should not go beyond the data provided. Conclusions translate the statistical

findings, and implications elaborate on the use of the study findings in practice. Conclusions should be congruent with the stated problem, theoretical framework, and statistical results. Implications for practice, the profession, and nursing science are made.

A discussion of the limitations are presented. The critic must determine whether there is a balance between the contributions made and limitations presented. Based on the limitations, a vital question the critic must answer is: Do the limitations make it impossible to generalize the findings to the target population?

The recommendations for further research should be realistic and meaningful. The financial implications as well as the significance to patient outcomes must be weighed. The proposed recommendations, if implemented in practice, need to be cost- and time-effective and efficient. If not, the justification needs to be discussed before implementation.

Example

Of the 150 participants in this study, 107 were successful, for a success rate of 71 percent. This success rate was higher in comparison to that reported by the national surveys, which at the time was about 60 percent.

The higher success rate observed in this study was most likely related to demographic characteristics of the sample. The participants were generally well educated, relatively affluent, and likely to hold administrative or professional positions. The literature indicates that social class and particularly education level are positively related to the decision to breastfeed (Eckhardt & Henderson, 1984) and to duration (Bacon & Wylie, 1976; Eastham et al., 1976; Gulick, 1981). This seemed to be true in this study, but without knowing

the education level of the women who did not volunteer, a conclusion cannot be drawn.

Beyond the effect homogeneity of the sample may have had on the results of the study, the findings support the premise that women who are knowledgeable about breastfeeding and are high achievers will be successful at breastfeeding.

The need for accurate information about breastfeeding, if success is to be achieved, has been recognized and supported by the findings. The type and number of breastfeeding information sources reported by the participants in this study are interesting and significant for nurses. Books about breastfeeding were mentioned most frequently, followed by friends and female relatives. Mentioned least frequently was advice sought from physicians and nurses. Although statistical analysis was not performed to determine if a particular source of information was related to success, the use of printed information appeared to have the greatest influence.

The relationship between achievement motivation and success in breastfeeding was positive. According to Atkinson's theory, achievement effect or persistence and aspiration level are behavioral indicators of the degree of motivation an individual holds. The need to persevere has been identified by breastfeeding mothers as one of the most important motives for success (Applebaum, 1970; Bacon & Wylie, 1976). In this study, persistence may have been a factor present in those successful mothers who experienced problems and continued to breastfeed in contrast to those who were unsuccessful and weaned. Furthermore, the participants who set a goal for duration of breastfeeding for six weeks or longer were more likely to breastfeed for at least six weeks.

Based on this study's findings it is suggested that the maternal-child nurse provide basic information about feeding choices early in the pregnancy and encourage the women to make a choice (a commitment). Once a decision has been made, the nurse then needs to support the woman's choice by providing specific information and resources relative to the choice. After the woman has given birth, the nurse should be available to reinforce information, to answer specific questions and provide support for the woman as she begins the breastfeeding experience. (Rentschler, 1991, pp. 153-154)

Critique. The researcher initially discusses the major limitation of the study, the homogeneity of the sample. In addition, the sample had a higher success rate than those reported in national surveys. A valid point was made related to the demographic data—this sample was "well educated" and "relatively affluent"—questioning the generalizability of the results. A point was well made in that "the literature indicates that social class and particularly education level are positively related to the decision to breastfeed" (p. 154).

Conclusions made by the researcher are related to the theoretical framework, lending support for Atkinson's theory. Implications made for practice are providing basic information about breastfeeding, answering questions, and encouragement. The researcher does not expand to the profession and nursing science. The overall worth and relevance of this study is important to nursing science and the profession. Making a case would make this section stronger.

The researcher does not provide recommendations for further research. The limitation of homogeneity of the sample would be one area to address in a replication of the study.

CRITIQUING THE QUALITATIVE STUDY: A SPECIAL CHALLENGE
Qualitative (inductive) methodological strategies are gaining acceptance in the discipline of nursing based on the evolving

paradigm shift that has occurred over the past 10 years (Beck, 1993). Nurse scholars, however, continue to struggle with the critical issue of developing criteria for evaluating the rigor of qualitative research. Qualitative and quantitative paradigms are based on different philosophical assumptions, have different goals, use different methods to achieve those goals, and therefore, require separate criteria for evaluation (Leininger, 1993; Lincoln & Guba, 1985).

Morse (1991) and the Editorial Board of *Qualitative Health Research* developed guidelines for reviewing articles reporting qualitative research studies. Their premise is that even the process of evaluating a qualitative study is different from that of an evaluation of a quantitative study. Morse (1991) describes the process as follows:

the reviewer first reads the entire article and then examines the results and discussion sections to assess the significance of the research. Next, the reviewer evaluates the quality of the theory developed and conducts a methodological assessment. Finally, the reviewer considers adherence to ethical standards and compliance with copyright regulations and comments on the writing/editorial study used in the article. (p. 283)

Leininger (1993) believes that those are important questions to ask about qualitative studies but that they do not include specific evaluation criteria. Therefore, she developed six criteria appropriate for analysis of any qualitative research study. Her criteria are: transferability, credibility, meaning-in-context, recurrent patterning, saturation, and confirmability (see Table 23-2 for definitions). Although the six criteria can be used with all qualitative methods, some criteria may be more appropriately developed than others in different studies.

The following section presents an exam-

Table 23-2
Qualitative Criteria and Definitions

Criteria	Definition
Credibility	Refers to the truth as known or experienced by the people being studied
Confirmability	Refers to the repeated direct participatory and documented evidence observed or obtained from primary sources
Meaning-in-context	Refers to data that have become understandable with special referent meanings to the people studied in different or similar environmental contexts
Recurrent patterning	Refers to repeated instances, sequence of events, experiences, or lifeways in different or similar contexts
Saturation	Refers to the "full taking in of occurrences," the researcher has done an exhaustive exploration of whatever phenomenon is being studied
Transferability	Refers to whether particular findings from a qualitative study can be transferred to another similar context or situation and still preserve the particularized meanings, interpretations, and inferences from the completed study

From Leininger, M. (1993). Evaluation criteria and evaluation of qualitative studies. In J. M. Morse (Ed.). *Critical issues in qualitative research methods* (pp. 95-115). Thousand Oaks, CA: Sage.

ple of a critique demonstrating the integration of the broad, process-oriented questions developed by Morse and the specific evaluation criteria developed by Leininger. Criddle's (1993) article entitled "Healing from surgery: A phenomenological study," published in *IMAGE: Journal of Nursing Scholarship,* served as the subject for the critique.

Significance of Research
Example

Healing is a concept central to client care, yet, until recently, it has rarely been explored except in the context of wound healing. Watson (1983) discussed "the dawning of a caring healing consciousness." She said, "More is known about treatment and cure than about healing and human caring processes" (p. 175). Exploration of the concept of caring has begun. More knowledge about the process of healing would complement the study of caring. (Criddle, 1993, p. 208)

A more fundamental exploration of healing might provide a base on which to build further research. Therefore, a phenomenological design was chosen to explore the question: "What is the essence of healing as perceived and experienced by selected individuals who have undergone surgery?" (Criddle, 1993, p. 208)

The experience of healing as perceived by these nine participants was an active process with movement toward achieving balance and wholeness and evolving beyond the place they started before surgery. The data clustered into three substantive themes and one process theme. The substantive themes are: Active Participation, Achieving Balance, and Evolving Beyond. The three main themes all related to a process theme. This theme expressed the dynamic nature of healing and is represented in each of the substantive themes. (Criddle, 1993, p. 209)

This study represents a beginning understanding about the phenomenon of healing. Further exploration is important to assess whether these themes exist in larger populations or in populations with different conditions. Questions such as, "Can one heal while dying?" or "Is it possible to heal with a chronic illness?" are important. Further research could explore whether all the themes described in this study are equally as important as the others. It is not yet known how we can best affect the healing process. Can we help to improve attitudes related to healing, speed up the balance process or ensure a progression to higher levels of functioning? (Criddle, 1993, p. 213)

Critique. The findings of this phenomenological study further the knowledge development of a concept central to providing nursing care to the ill. Although preliminary, a foundation for further investigation is established. New knowledge as well as new questions for further exploration were identified.

CRITERION OF TRANSFERABILITY. This study generated many questions for further investigation of the concept, specifically whether the findings could be transferred to other populations with different conditions. Therefore, this criterion is not completely met, but this is congruent with the design of the study and the state of the knowledge regarding the healing process.

CRITERION OF CREDIBILITY. The data excerpts provide the emic or local perspective of the phenomenon under study: the healing process. These excerpts are "believable" to the reader and support the composite understanding of the process. The standards of trustworthiness, although not described specifically, enhance the credibility of the findings and meet the criterion requirement.

Theoretical Evaluation
Example

The literature related directly to healing is scant and the concept of healing as a phenomenon beyond physical healing is not clearly defined. (Criddle, 1993, p. 208).

A more fundamental exploration of healing might provide a base on which to build further research. Therefore, a phenomenological design was chosen to explore the question: "What is the essence of healing as perceived and experienced by selected individuals who have undergone surgery?" (Criddle, 1993, p. 208)

Active Participation

All participants expressed a specific desire to take conscious control. They thought that they had control and that the success or failure of their healing was at least partially up to them. One participant said, "This really has impacted every part of my life. I don't clean my own house and I can't do what I want to do." Her process of regaining control was long and arduous. She believed control was necessary for healing as she slowly took charge of more and more parts of her life. This was reflected in her statement, "If I resign myself to being helpless and having people care for me, then I can just sit in this bed and rot." (Criddle, 1993, p. 209)

Healing Process

The substantive themes do not have clear boundaries. This overlap is important as an attempt has been made to retain the integrity of the data as a whole. If a phenomenon is unitary, its parts will have independent characteristics and some overlap. For example, Evolving Beyond and Achieving Balance both imply participation on the part of the person healing and therefore relate to the Active Participation theme. The data also are connected by several process subthemes that represent the overall theme, Healing Process. The participants recognized the dynamic nature of healing and attempted to describe what they had experienced related to the process. (Criddle, 1993, p. 211)

Healing as described in this study had some parts that were similar to those described in the existing literature. A sense of being in control was part of the active participatory process for the participants of this study. Healing and control have been linked in prior work. (Criddle, 1993, p. 212)

Critique. The author presented an adequate number of data excerpts that enable the reader to follow the theoretical development of the themes. Integration of the staged process subthemes with the substantive themes resulted in a preliminary description of the healing process. The resultant description attempts to depict the dynamic nature of the process and the relationships between the themes. The data underwent a descriptive level of analysis. The author also clearly integrated the findings of the study with the existing literature.

CRITERION OF MEANING-IN-CONTEXT. In this phenomenological study this criterion is very important and was met. The research question set the context for searching for the essence or meaning of healing to all the participants. The common context was that of a surgical procedure, although there were individual variations in the specific type of procedures. The findings consisted of the common themes through the process of healing. The most common belief was that a positive attitude was necessary for positive healing. If the context were changed, the meaning would also change.

Methodologic Assessment
Example

A more fundamental exploration of healing might provide a base on which to build further research. Therefore, a phenomenological design was chosen to explore the question: "What is the essence of healing as perceived and experienced by selected individuals who have undergone surgery?" A pilot study with two partici-

pants was conducted before the actual study, which included nine participants. All participants had a recent operation from which they were expected to return to their presurgical level of functioning with no disfigurement beyond the incision. No illnesses were expected to be fatal and they had been hospitalized from two to nine days with a variety of surgeries. Two had knee reconstructions, one had a spinal fusion, two had intestinal resections, one had a hip replacement, one had a herniorrhaphy, one had a hysterectomy, and one had an oophorectomy. The participants' ages ranged from 28 to 65 years. Two participants were male and the rest were female. Three participants had significant post-operative complications. (Criddle, 1993, pp. 208-209)

The participants were interviewed one week post hospital discharge and three weeks after the first interview. The questions were initially broad and open-ended with neutral probes to elicit the participant's own experience of healing. Initial questions related to what they thought happened when they healed and what they thought healing was. More specific questions were generated from prior comments of each participant as well as other participants, but only after each participant's own initial description of healing was exhausted. Interviews were transcribed verbatim from audio tape recordings and analyzed using a coding and memo system. These codes and memos were grouped and transformed into a composite understanding of the phenomenon of healing. The participants were contacted again to verify that the researcher's description of healing was what they experienced as the essence of healing. Standards of human subject protection were adhered to, and Lincoln and Guba's (1985) standards of trustworthiness were applied, including a thorough audit by a knowledgeable reviewer who had no prior contact with the study. (Criddle, 1993, p. 209)

Critique. Based on the state of knowledge regarding the concept of healing, a phenomenological design was an appropriate choice. The research question is clearly stated. Although a pilot study was conducted, no information was given related to the changes made based on those initial findings. The type of sample is not described—was it a theoretical or purposeful sample? However, the nine participants were described in aggregate by gender, age, and type of surgery. It is not explicitly stated that the data collection continued until saturation was achieved. However, the participants were recontacted to verify the researcher's interpretation of the data. A general reference to the standards of trustworthiness (Lincoln & Guba, 1985), including an audit, was made. But the particular strategies used to meet the criteria were not addressed.

Although the use of a phenomenological design was clearly stated, identification of a *specific* method was not documented (i.e., was it the method established by Heidegger, Husserl, or others?). The precise method of data analysis was not described either. Although codes and memos were used and transformed to a composite understanding, further description or documentation of the *particular* method, such as Colaizzi's (1978) method of data analysis, van Manen's (1984) methodological outline, or Spiegelberg's (1982) steps of the phenomenological method, would have clarified this issue for the reader. Finally, there was no evaluation of the method used or of any problems encountered.

CRITERION OF RECURRENT PATTERNING. Although essence/meaning is the focus of the study, recurrent patterning was identified in the data using codes and memos in order to finally transform the findings into a composite of understanding the healing process for these participants.

CRITERION OF SATURATION. In this study ful-filling the criterion of saturation is implied, via the design, sample size, multiple interviews, and sequencing of interview questions and probes. It would have helped the critic if saturation had been addressed more explicitly.

CRITERION OF CONFIRMABILITY. This criterion was met when the participants were recontacted for the purpose of verifying the researcher's description of the healing process. No discussion was included that described any discrepancies between the participants' interpretations and that of the researcher.

Adherence to Ethical Standards
Example. "Standards of human subject protection were adhered to" (Criddle, 1993, p. 209).

Critique. Without further elaboration the reader must assume all appropriate measures were taken to protect the participants and that consents were signed.

Writing Style and Clarity
Critique. The article is written in a clear, concise style. The presentation of the findings follows a logical flow and is supported by well-chosen data excerpts.

Summary Statement
Overall, this was a well-developed and well-written research study and report. One strength was the research question's strong influence on the choice of the appropriate qualitative method. In addition, the research study as reported in the article met the qualitative criteria and guidelines for a systematic evaluation.

Primarily, weaknesses were in the identification of specific methods of analysis. Although reporting the findings is the likely priority and journals have page limitations, a few concise phrases or sentences addressing the issue of methods of analysis would have been helpful to the reader.

EVALUATING THE RESEARCH CRITIQUE

1. Did the critic give an objective presentation?
2. Does the critic present both the strengths and weaknesses of the study?
3. Were all the critical components critiqued based on the type of research (i.e., quantitative or qualitative)?
4. Did the critic weigh the strengths and weaknesses of the study?
5. How feasible and essential are the suggestions made by the critic?
6. Does this critique provide new insights and generate more questions for future research?

THE CRITIC'S COMMENTS

Many times a reader will take a critic's comments as the uncontestable truth. The comments and suggestions also need to be examined (see box). The reader of a critique needs to assess how feasible and essential the suggestions made by the research critic in the critique are (Stetler & Marram, 1976). It is good to be idealistic when suggestions are made to the researcher, but if they cannot be carried out, how useful are they? A commonsense approach to a critic's comments is as important as the critique itself.

SUMMARY

- A research critique is a systematic method of critically analyzing and evaluating research. It presents the strengths and weaknesses of a research study, then makes recommendations on how to improve specific elements for utilization and future replication.
- A research review provides a description of a research study. A research critique makes precise and objective judgments about the strengths and weaknesses of a research study.
- A general research critique utilizes the techniques of analysis, evaluation, validation, and replication in the critique process.

- The elements critiqued in all research studies are conceptual basis, methodology, exposition, substantive contribution, and ethical and legal considerations.
- Critiquing quantitative research involves examining each major part of the research process with careful and exact judgments of the title, statement of the problem, research purpose, theoretical/conceptual basis, review of the literature, hypothesis/research questions, methodology, results, and discussion.
- A critique of qualitative research involves an evaluative process that systematically uses specific criteria (see Table 23-2) to assess the significance of the research, its theoretical and methodological development, and the researcher's adherence to the ethical standards.

FACILITATING CRITICAL THINKING

1. As a critic of quantitative research, go to the literature and select a quantitative research article to critique. One example of a quantitative article is Aiden, L., et al. (1993). Nursing practitioner managed care for persons with HIV infection. *IMAGE: Journal of Nursing Scholarship, 25*(3), 172-177.
   a. Examine the title of the research article.

b. Critique the statement of the problem.

c. Comment on the research purpose.

d. Review the theoretical/conceptual basis.

e. Critique the review of the literature.

f. Evaluate the research hypothesis.

g. Critically examine all aspects of the methodology (i.e., instruments, sample, and procedure).

h. Analyze the study results.

i. Examine the study's discussion (i.e., conclusions, limitations, and research recommendations).

j. Is there a good integration of all components of the research study?

2. As a critic of qualitative research, go to the literature and select a qualitative research article to critique. One example of a qualitative article is Morgan, D., & Laing, G. (1991). The diagnosis of Alzheimer's disease: Spouse's perspective. *Qualitative Health Research, 1*(3), 370-387.

a. Evaluate the significance of the research findings.

b. Critique theoretical assessment of the study.

c. Conduct a methodological assessment.

d. Consider the researcher's adherence to ethical standards.

e. Comment on the clarity and presentation of the article.

f. Critique the article, using the six evaluative criteria listed in Table 23-2: credibility, confirmability, meaning-in-context, recurrent patterning, saturation, and transferability.

References

SUBSTANTIVE

CRIDDLE, L. (1993). Healing from surgery: A phenomenological study. *IMAGE: Journal of Nursing Scholarship, 25*(3), 208-213.

RENTSCHLER, D. (1991). Correlates of successful breastfeeding. *IMAGE: Journal of Nursing Scholarship, 23*(3), 151-154.

CONCEPTUAL

ATKINSON, J. W. (1964). *An introduction to motivation.* Princeton: Van Nostrand.

METHODOLOGICAL

AIDEN, L., LAKE, E., SEMAAN, S., LEHMAN, H., O'HARE, P., COLE, S., CUNBAR, D., AND FRANK, I. (1993). Nursing practitioner managed care for persons with HIV infection. *IMAGE: Journal of Nursing Scholarship, 25*(3), 172-177.

AMERICAN PSYCHOLOGICAL ASSOCIATION. (1994). *Publication Manual of the American Psychological Association.* Washington, DC: The Association.

BECK, C. T. (1993). Qualitative research: The evaluation of its credibility, fittingness, and auditability. *Western Journal of Nursing Research, 15*(2), 263-266.

COLAIZZI, P. F. (1978). Psychological research as the phenomenologist views it. In R. Valle & M. King (Eds.), *Existential phenomenological alternatives for psychology* (pp. 48-71). New York: Oxford University Press.

LEININGER, M. (1993). Evaluation criteria and evaluation of qualitative studies. In J. M. Morse (Ed.), *Critical issues in qualitative research methods* (pp. 95-115). Thousand Oaks, CA: Sage.

LINCOLN, Y., & GUBA, E. (1985). *Naturalistic inquiry.* Beverly Hills, CA: Sage.

MORGAN, D., & LAING, G. (1991). The diagnosis of Alzheimer's disease: Spouse's perspective. *Qualitative Health Research, 1*(3), 370-387.

MORSE, J. M. (1991). Editorial: Evaluating qualitative research. *Qualitative Health Research, 1*(3), 283-286.

PHILLIPS, L. (1986). *A clinician's guide to the critique and utilization of nursing research.* Norwalk, CT: Appleton-Century-Crofts.

SPIEGELBERG, H. (1982). *The phenomenological movement: A historical introduction* (3rd ed.). Boston: Martinus-Nijhoff.

VAN MANEN, M. (1984). Practicing phenomenological writing. *Phenomenology and Pedagogy, 2*(1), 36-69.

HISTORICAL

STETLER, C., & MARRAM, G. (1976). Evaluating research findings for applicability in practice. *Nursing Outlook, 26*(9), 559-563.

CHAPTER 24

USING RESEARCH TO IMPROVE NURSING PRACTICE

CAROLYN J. PEPLER

Persons with acquired immunodeficiency syndrome (AIDS) often have complex networks of social support. Awareness of such social support can benefit both nurse and client; this multifaceted concept has been related both directly and indirectly to healthful outcomes (Cohen & Syme, 1985; Stewart, 1989). One group of nurses working with persons with AIDS noted that their clients' support systems changed over time, but sharing this information was difficult because the nurses' observations were vague and anecdotal. Specific information about a particular client's support was often clear to only one nurse, who had been working with the client for a long period. These nurses decided to try to find a better way to collect and record data about their clients' support systems. Their literature review led them to begin testing a combination of a sociogram with a semistructured interview for data collection and recording. With more detailed data, changes in the client's social support system over time are expected to be clearly visible to any health professional working with the client. Thus these nurses are using nursing research to improve their practice.

Amid debates about nursing theories, research methods, and practice modes, there is a consensus among most authors that nursing is a practice discipline. The knowledge nurses seek to attain is knowledge that will ultimately be relevant and practical in nursing. To achieve this end the American Nurses Association created guidelines for the establishment of research not only as the base for practice, but as the norm within practice and education (American Nurses Association, 1989). Similarly, the Canadian Nurses Association has established a goal to develop a "research reality" in nursing (Canadian Nurses Association, 1990). Research is becoming part of the fabric of practice. It provides the basis for many nursing decisions: those that an individual nurse makes about care for a particular client or group of clients, those that administrators make about policies that affect nurses and their practice, and those that nursing teachers and students make about learning. This is the broad goal of research

STEPS IN RESEARCH UTILIZATION

1. Clarifying the problem or clinical question
2. Searching the literature
3. Evaluating scientific merit of the research findings
4. Assessing the clinical merit of the findings, including the feasibility and "fit" of using the findings in a particular setting
5. Testing the use of findings or the innovation
6. Decision making about utilization
7. Implementing a change in practice

utilization that nurses are working to realize.

Research utilization has two major components: the interpretation and use of other people's research findings in practice and the use of rigorous research methods in the process of practice (Crane, 1989; Horsley, 1985; Stetler, 1985). The process of interpreting and using research findings in practice can be described as separate steps. Each step is essential to reach the goal of research-based practice. Although they are generally sequential, each one may lead to clarification or modification of earlier steps. In many ways the steps parallel the research process. The steps, which are expanded on in detail in this chapter, are listed in the box.

The second component of research utilization, the use of research methods in practice, is an integral part of sound clinical, administrative, and educational nursing practice and is essential for quality management. It can be interpreted as "the use of inquiry in nursing, using the methods of science, that is, describing, categorizing, classifying, measuring, relating, quantifying, analyzing, synthesizing, and hypothesis testing" (Canadian Association of University Schools of Nursing, 1986, p. 7). Stetler (1985) explains that "either the overall process can serve as a model for problem solving or individual components can be used independently to facilitate decision making" (p. 42). Research methods may be used separately or in conjunction with the use of research findings. The purpose of the process is what differentiates *doing research* from *using research methods in practice*. The purpose of conducting research is to generate knowledge, whereas the purpose of using research methods in practice is to solve specific problems and to ensure a high level of quality in practice.

This chapter focuses on the first component of research utilization—that is, it will address the broad framework of knowledge utilization, models for transfer of knowledge to practice, achieving the steps to build practice on research findings, strategies to overcome barriers, and criteria for evaluating the use of findings in practice.

KNOWLEDGE UTILIZATION

Havelock (1986) has described six components of the knowledge process: generation, verification, transformation, transfer, reception, and utilization. When the overall process is conceptualized with researchers as generators or producers of knowledge and clinicians as consumers or users without adequate attention to the intervening components, both knowledge generation and utilization may be seriously jeopardized. As will be seen in the models for transfer of knowledge to practice, the role of clinicians in these stages can have long-term effects on the ultimate use of knowledge generated and verified in the conduct of research.

Transformation of knowledge is the process of collecting, summarizing, sorting, translating, altering presentation medium or style, and adapting knowledge for its maximum use. The researcher may be largely responsible for the initial interpretation, organization, and summarizing of the findings of a study, but the use of those findings in practice is enhanced when clinicians are involved in the transformation (Horsley, Crane, Crabtree, & Wood, 1983; King, Barnard, & Hoehn, 1981). For example, Schepp (1991) demonstrated clinical sensitivity in her report on the contribution of different factors to the coping effort of mothers of hospitalized children, but the report is a description of model testing through multiple regression analysis. A clinician who can adapt this information into language that is meaningful for practicing nurses can enhance the usability of the findings. Knowledge of research, statistical analysis, and clinical practice, as well as skills in transforming information, are needed for this process.

The transfer of knowledge is also referred to as the dissemination or diffusion of knowledge. It is the process of communicating research findings from those who produce them to potential users, including other researchers and clinicians. As in any communication process, the message must be in understandable form; that is, it must have been transformed, and it must be available to the recipient. The manner of transfer will be dependent on the researcher's purpose and goal.

Suppose a researcher has studied a clinical intervention to enhance the problem-solving skills of diabetic clients. Details of the statistical analysis of relationships among outcome variables, which is intended as a base for further research, would be appropriate to "send" to researchers as consumers, and a research journal would be an appropriate channel. On the other hand, information about the clinical details of the intervention will be useful knowledge for the clinician, and the researcher should relay this knowledge in a clinical journal to reach many more clinicians.

The reception of knowledge includes the series of processes that go on at the receiver's end. They start with attention and end with agreement or disagreement. Suppose a clinician is thumbing through the journal in which the problem-solving study is reported. "Problem solving" draws his or her attention and is recognized as a topic of interest. The interest may be vague and the article is dismissed. Another clinician may have been trying specifically to help a diabetic client learn to improve problem-solving skills. Here awareness is increased in intensity, because this is something with real relevance to the reader's personal practice. The reader understands the concept and integrates it with what he or she already knows and understands. At this level the clinician is ready to agree or disagree with the intervention and findings in the article. The strength of agreement or disagreement will have an effect on the ultimate utilization, but even if the findings are rejected, the knowledge that someone has studied problem solving in diabetic clients may remain.

Once knowledge has been received, according to Havelock (1986), it is ready to be used. He identifies four types of utilization. The first is *communicative utilization*. This may be the process used by a teacher who passes knowledge on to students. The teacher needs to understand the information rather than simply parroting the ideas, but even reporting findings without complete comprehension is a level of communicative utilization. It may not be successful in terms of actual use. For example, if a head nurse attempts to explain the problem-solving study to staff nurses but is not able to articulate the ideas clearly, it is unlikely that any further utilization will take place. However, another nurse might pick up the ideas and discuss the intervention with a colleague, thereby strengthening the likelihood of its use. Communicative utilization is not an essential step, but it is a very good test of ultimate utilization.

Another type of research use is the process of *confirmation or disconfirmation* that occurs when new knowledge strengthens or weakens a person's current knowledge base. It is improbable that a major change will result from one new piece of knowledge when nothing was previously known about the topic. New research findings are likely to be used when they confirm a nurse's clinical knowledge. The third type is *conceptual utilization*. In the example at the beginning of the chapter the nurses had read about social support and its relationship to health. They had changed the way they thought about the concept as they collected information from clients. They had become more observant of the variations across clients and over time. They were using their new knowledge conceptually. Only when they gained additional knowledge about the measurement of social support and the use of sociograms did they move to *behavioral utilization,* actually changing their practice.

A change in behavior constitutes the final type of utilization. This occurs when an innovation is adopted, with or without adaptation. This is also a complex process that can be facilitated or blocked along the way. For instance, a decision may be made to adopt an innovation at an administrative level, but for many reasons addressed later in this chapter the change is never implemented. If it is implemented sporadically, it never becomes part of the routine of the institution. *Routinization,* also called internalization or institutionalization, is the ultimate form of using new knowledge.

Knowledge utilization is complex and can be difficult. When new knowledge is not immediately put to use, it is not constructive to "blame" researchers for being too obscure or clinicians for being too obtuse. Exploring the process to uncover and overcome barriers is likely to be more productive.

❧ MODELS FOR THE TRANSFER OF KNOWLEDGE TO PRACTICE

Examination of the following models helps to identify potential barriers to the use of knowledge and provides the basis for strategies to overcome them. Crane (1985) described four theoretical models that have evolved in the knowledge utilization process. Several major projects in nursing have used these models: The Western Interstate Commission for Higher Education in Nursing (WICHEN) project (Krueger, Nelson, & Wolanin, 1978); the Nursing Child Assessment Satellite Training (NCAST) projects (Barnard & Hoehn, 1978); the Conduct and Utilization of Nursing Research (CURN) project (Horsley, et al., 1983); and the Orange County Research Utilization in Nursing (OCRUN) project (Donaldson, 1991). Other researchers have been working with clinicians to build and refine more flexible models to bridge the gap between researchers and practicing nurses (Registered Nurses Association of

British Columbia, 1991; Stetler, 1985; Stetler & Marram, 1976).

The most widely used model from a researcher's perspective is the research, development, and diffusion model (Havelock & Havelock, 1973). The research questions arise from the researcher; the research base for innovations is comprehensive; and the results are diffused in the usual research channels, publications, and conference presentations (Figure 24-1). The major limitation of the model is that findings may never reach the majority of clinicians, or they may reach some, but for a variety of reasons are not put into practice. With widespread dissemination following transformation of the information, some clinicians may be able to use the results.

Another model is the social interaction and diffusion model (Havelock & Havelock, 1973; Rogers, 1983). The research questions still originate with the researcher, and the research is extensive, but the diffusion process involves a social system or group process in which ideas are discussed (Figure 24-2). Factors such as group membership, opinion leaders, and informal contact have a significant effect on adoption of innovations. For example,

an informal leader in a clinical journal club can be pivotal in influencing utilization.

A familiar model for clinicians is the problem-solving model (Figure 24-3). In this case the questions start from a problem identified in a clinical setting. From a variety of solutions, one is selected that can be adapted and implemented in the particular situation. The process may include evaluation of the effectiveness of the innovation in solving the problem. If it works, the chances of its being adopted are high. This model's major flaw is that there is no requirement for the solution to be research based. Rigorous evaluation could meet this requirement for sound practice, but once a solution appears to be solving a problem, it may be difficult for clinicians to design a study to question its efficacy.

The fourth model discussed by Crane (1985) is the linkage model developed by Havelock (Havelock & Havelock, 1973). The user system (clinicians) is linked with a knowledge-generating system (researchers), which together identify relevant research questions and find solutions to clinicians' problems (Figure 24-4). Communication systems are built in for clinical questions to become research questions and for the

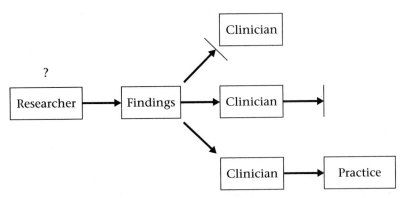

Figure 24-1. The research, development, and diffusion model.

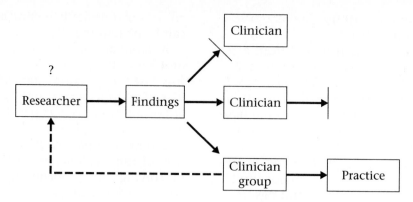

Figure 24-2. The social interaction and diffusion model.

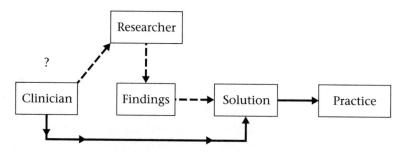

Figure 24-3. The problem-solving model.

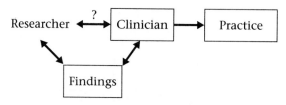

Figure 24-4. The linkage model.

knowledge generated through the research process to be transferred to the clinicians in a usable form. A variation of this model was tested in the CURN project (Horsley, et al., 1983) and is the basis for the current OCRUN project (Donaldson, 1991). In the CURN project clinicians and researchers worked together to identify relevant clinical problems. Research reports of tested interventions addressing these problems were critiqued, and the information was transformed into a clinical protocol that could

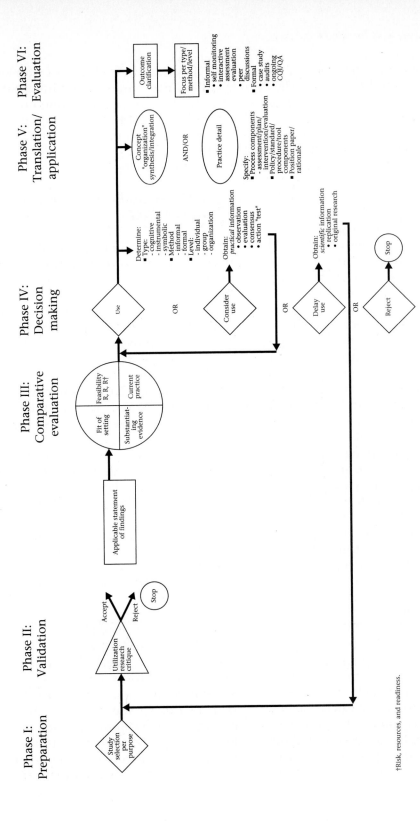

Figure 24-5. The Stetler model for research utilization. (From Stetler, C. B., Refinement of the Stetler/Marram model for application of research findings to practice. *Nursing Outlook* [in press].)

†Risk, resources, and readiness.

be readily understood and implemented by clinicians (Horsley, et al., 1983). The CURN model also calls for a clinical trial of the intervention in the particular setting, decision making regarding the intervention, and planned change in clinical practice.

Stetler and Marram (1976) analyzed the application of research findings from a clinical perspective and developed a model incorporating three phases: validation of the findings, comparative evaluation, and decision making. Stetler (1994) has refined and expanded the model, which now has six phases (Figure 24-5). The first two phases include the preparation, which is a purposeful examination of the reason for the research review, and validation, which is an assessment of the strengths and weaknesses in research reports with a focus on the study's potential applicability. Comparative evaluation assesses the feasibility of using the findings in a given setting, with consideration of factors such as fit, current practice, risks, and potential value of the research. The decision-making phase outlines a number of choices: to use the findings, to consider use, to delay use, or to reject the study. Each decision is considered with attention to all the issues surrounding it. Translation/application is an important new phase in the model to think through the research information into action terms. For example, if the use is to be a cognitive application, similar to Havelock's (1986) conceptual utilization, there is need to think through how a nurse will change the way he or she thinks about a particular issue in practice. The final phase is evaluation of the research utilization, a phase missing in the original model.

The Registered Nurses Association of British Columbia has launched a provincewide program to help nurses understand and use research in their practice. Like the Stetler/Marram model, the process is intended to start with clinicians who identify a clinical issue and seek out information in the literature. It gives direction on when to abandon or continue a project and includes evaluation of the implementation of findings.

✎ PUTTING RESEARCH TO WORK IN PRACTICE

Building nursing practice on research findings is essential for the continued development of nursing as a practice profession (Barnard, 1980; Mercer, 1984), for the self-perception of nurses in practice (Cronenwett, 1987; Fitch, 1992; Goode, et al., 1987), for improved client outcomes (Coyle & Sokop, 1990; Horsley, et al., 1983), and for the efficiency and effectiveness of practice, including cost-effectiveness (Funk, Champagne, Weise, & Tornquist, 1991b; Heater, Becker, & Olson, 1988; Rosswurm, 1992).

It is important to examine the seven steps involved in using research findings in practice that were listed at the beginning of this chapter. Each step involves inquiry and commitment on the part of nurses. All nurses may not have all the skills needed to complete all steps (Kirchhoff, 1991), so cooperative participation of nurses with varying skills is needed. No nurse should be expected to complete all the steps alone.

CLARIFYING THE PROBLEM OR CLINICAL QUESTION

Any change or development in practice must start with an idea or a question— What is going on . . . ? Why is it that . . . ? Is there a better way to . . . ? What if . . . ? As with the development of research questions addressed elsewhere in this textbook, being specific about the issue or the problem will facilitate its resolution. If postoperative patients are unwilling to walk outside their rooms, is the problem one of pain management, preoperative preparation, patient insecurity with cumbersome apparatus, or body image with tubes and other appendages? Which clinical interventions could or should be examined or changed? Which body of literature might be helpful?

Nurses giving direct care clearly need to be involved in clarifying these questions, and discussion at the unit level is essential regardless of whether the issue was identified by clinicians or administrators. Exploring the question with one or two others will usually help to clarify the issue, but focused discussion in a larger group provides an opportunity for input from different perspectives. Some staff may not have observed the phenomenon, some will not see it as a problem, others may have found a personal solution by trial and error, and still others may have made a change in their personal practice as a result of a research report they read.

Ideas may be triggered when nurses attend conferences or browse through the literature. The follow-up to discuss the question with others in the particular setting is important for clarification of the issue and for involvement and commitment of coworkers in addressing the question.

SEARCHING THE LITERATURE

Chapter 7 addresses the literature review as a basis for the conduct of research. The literature is equally important for the use of research in practice because it is the primary source of findings. There are differences in the approach to literature review depending on the purpose. A researcher attempts a comprehensive review of broadly related literature to define the question clearly and to determine gaps that need further study. A clinician looking for ideas related to a particular clinical problem also needs to search the literature thoroughly, but this search may be more focused. Both researchers and clinicians will find the materials they need more efficiently by using electronic search methods. Techniques for using on-line and CD-ROM sources are addressed elsewhere.

The clinician will find that articles on a topic of interest are useful for different purposes. Very often the literature includes opinion articles supporting the observation that an issue is indeed a problem recognized by other nurses. Another type of article is a descriptive report of an intervention or approach used in one setting but not rigorously tested or evaluated. These types of articles will be of interest and may help to define the problem, but they will not serve as the basis for clinicians to build their practice on research.

The research literature reporting on specific studies falls into three broad categories that can be useful for clinicians. These are reports of (1) descriptive studies of the phenomenon, (2) methods to measure a construct or parameter, and (3) tested interventions. A common purpose of the first type of study is to clarify a phenomenon through detailed analysis, either qualitative or quantitative. Studies often provide information on the occurrence of the phenomenon or problem and characteristics of the clients and families. Some examples are family caregivers' descriptions of the impact of cancer pain on the family (Ferrell, Rhiner, Cohen, & Grant, 1991), the level of hope in psychiatric and chemically dependent patients (Holdcraft & Williamson, 1991), the coping effort of mothers of hospitalized children (Schepp, 1991), women's images of being healthy (Woods, Laffrey, Duffy, Lentz, Mitchell, & Taylor, 1988), and factors related to dyspnea in clients with chronic obstructive lung disease (Gift,

Plaut, & Jacox, 1986). This type of literature usually helps nurses expand their perspective of the problem by providing a rich and detailed description of the phenomenon or by identifying correlates. These studies do not offer behavioral strategies for clinicians, but they may provide a base from which to use the findings cognitively to broaden one's thinking about a problem such as pain or about a group of clients such as psychiatric patients. This helps nurses become more particular and more articulate about their observations.

The second category of studies, those addressing measurement methods, can be especially helpful in strengthening observations in direct care and in collecting broad-based data for needs assessments and program planning. Two types of studies are included in this category. The first type focuses on the development of measurement methods or an instrument, for example, a measure of safe sex behavior in adolescents and young adults (Diorio, Parsons, Lehr, Adame, & Carlone, 1992). The purpose of the second type of measurement study is to test instruments used in current practice (e.g., glass and electronic thermometers to measure temperature in full-term babies) (Hunter, 1991), tools for assessing chemotherapy-induced nausea and vomiting (McMillan, Johnston, Tedford, & Harley, 1989), and indirect methods of blood pressure measurement (Rebenson-Piano, Holm, Foreman, & Kirchhoff, 1989). Some instruments are developed and tested for research purposes, and others such as the Braden Scale for Predicting Pressure Sore Risk (Bergstrom, Braden, & Laguzza, 1987) are specifically intended for clinical practice. Many measures that are initially developed for research purposes have potential for use in practice such as measures of social support (Stewart, 1989).

Reports of tested interventions provide a strong base for research utilization. Table 24-1 gives examples of intervention studies in different clinical settings. Studies will vary in terms of specific method, but it is important to search for studies with experi-

Table 24-1
Generic Models for the Transfer of Knowledge to Practice

Model Type	Research Question Source	Research Strength	Transfer Channel	Strengths and Limitations
Research, development, & diffusion	Researcher	+	Research publications Conferences	Strong research Limited access by clinicians
Social interaction & diffusion	Researcher	+	Publications Conferences Journal clubs	Better access, but possibly limited understandability or relevance
Problem solving	Clinician	−	Clinical texts & articles, possibly research articles	Highly relevant, but weak research base
Linkage model	Researcher & clinician	+	Research publications	Highly relevant with strong research base

mental or quasi-experimental designs. Another essential requirement is that studies have been replicated and that there is consistency across replicated studies (see Evaluating Scientific and Clinical Merit). A recent and useful addition to the *Cumulative Index to Nursing and Allied Health Literature* is the heading "Replicated Studies." This is particularly helpful in electronic searches, where subject headings can be combined.

Perhaps the greatest "finds" for a clinician are the critical reviews and metaanalysis reports. One consistent source of review articles is the *Annual Review of Nursing Research,* which provides comprehensive reviews of the research related to a particular nursing phenomenon such as sleep (Shaver & Giblin, 1989) and interpersonal communication between nurses and patients (Garvin & Kennedy, 1990). Both research-focused and clinical journals may include a regular review or "state-of-the-art" section or occasional extensive critiques. These review articles may be broad-based such as an analysis of critical care nursing practice research (VanCott, Tittle, Moody, & Wilson, 1991) and an update on nursing research related to persons with HIV infection (Larson & Ropka, 1991), or they may be specific such as a summary of research on exercise and functional capacity after myocardial infarction (Folta & Metzger, 1989), a critique of prenatal attachment research (Muller, 1992), and a review of children's perspectives of stress and coping (Atkins, 1991).

Metaanalysis is a sophisticated technique of analyzing combined data from related or replicated intervention studies to test the strength of the findings. While clinicians may find the analysis complex, the interpretation of the findings can be highly relevant for practice. Table 24-2 gives examples of metaanalyses pertinent to different areas of practice.

The literature is essential to the development of research-based practice. However, accessibility, understandability, and usability of research reports have been identified as barriers to their actual use. Strategies to

Table 24-2
Examples of Metaanalyses Pertinent to Clinical Practice

Authors/Date	Study Population	Interventions	Outcome Variables
Goode, et al., 1991	Adults & children with peripheral heparin locks	Heparin flush Saline flush	Patency, phlebitis, duration
Hathaway, 1986	Surgical patients	Preoperative instruction	Physiological, psychological, psychophysiological outcomes
Heater, et al., 1988	Patients at all developmental stages	Nursing interventions	Behavioral, knowledge, physiological, psychosocial outcomes
Olson, et al., 1990	Children and parents	Care practices Anxiety reduction techniques Stimulation of premature infants	Behavioral, developmental, physiological, psychosocial outcomes

overcome these barriers are discussed later in this chapter. Another essential step, once articles have been obtained, is the critical appraisal of the research.

EVALUATING THE SCIENTIFIC MERIT OF RESEARCH FINDINGS

Research findings that are to serve as a base for clinical practice must be sound. The developers of the CURN model identified three criteria for determining the validity of research findings: scientific merit, replication, and risk (Haller, Reynolds, & Horsley, 1979). The evaluation of the scientific merit has been discussed in the previous chapter. Replication and risk are criteria that are highly relevant to the clinical usefulness of findings.

Replication may be either an exact or literal replication following the details of the original design, or it may be a construct replication in which a similar hypothesis is tested using a new method or design (Blomquist, 1986; Haller & Reynolds, 1986). The latter helps to establish the validity of the construct across different situations and populations, increasing the generalizability of results. Replications provide the substantiating evidence that research conclusions are sound (Stetler & Marram, 1976). In either form the process is critical for research-based practice because it enhances scientific merit and helps to prevent both type I and type II errors (Haller, et al., 1979). Type I errors, or false positives, are potentially hazardous to clients, so building practice on the basis of one study would be unethical. The rigor with which the criterion of replication is applied is to some extent dependent on the risk factor.

Risk can include both the potential hazard to the client and the potential costs to the organization. In a situation where the risk is small, the findings may be applied more liberally. If an innovation can be safely and cost effectively implemented *and* clinically evaluated, the decision to try it prior to rigorous replication may be appropriate. For example, a study of the effect of offering choices to mildly to moderately demented nursing home residents found that residents made decisions when given the opportunity (Pepler & Koestner, 1992). Participants with the least cognitive ability, whose Folstein Mini Mental Status scores were less than 12, were able to make a choice between alternatives without anxiety, although they were less able to respond to open-ended choices. The intervention is simple, virtually cost free, and the effects can be closely monitored for a careful clinical evaluation.

ASSESSING THE CLINICAL MERIT OF THE RESEARCH FINDINGS

Once these three criteria have been considered, relevance to clinical practice can be evaluated. Appraising clinical merit involves examination of the following:

1. The significance of the problem or phenomenon
2. The relative advantage of the innovation, including costs
3. The fit with the setting
4. The feasibility of the adopting innovation
5. The feasibility of evaluating the innovation (Horsley, et al., 1983)

In determining whether to use an innovation in practice, the clinician will weigh the significance of the problem or phenomenon against the relative advantage of the innovation over current practice. If an innovation relates to a minor or rarely encountered problem or involves a change in which human and financial costs are excessive, the costs of changing current practice may not be worthwhile. The advantages need to be examined in relation to who benefits and how much. A new approach that benefits clients significantly might well be worthy of adoption, even if it costs the nurses in terms of effort or the agency in terms of dollars. Advantages that are visible or tangible are more readily recognized and can be more convincing than those that are abstract or "soft." Fortunately, better measures of variables such as quality of life are becoming available and their significance is more widely recognized. Obviously the ideal innovation is beneficial in terms of client and nursing outcomes and costs less than present practice!

A good "fit" with the organization is another important consideration (Horsley, et al., 1983). This does not imply that an organization cannot change to fit an innovation, but a change that is consistent with the philosophy and policies of an agency is more likely to occur. For example, if the philosophy is one of patient autonomy and collaborative practice among different health professionals, the introduction of patient-controlled analgesia (PCA) is likely to fit with nurses' and physicians' beliefs. PCA is much more liable to be effectively implemented in such a setting than one in which either nurses or physicians believe that patients will take too much analgesia. Other factors in the organization to be considered, as well as philosophy and policy, are the structure, the decision-making processes, and the personnel.

Assessing the feasibility of adopting an innovation involves comparing the needed resources with those available or obtainable. It may be possible to modify either the innovation or the resources within budgetary and other constraints, but sometimes the innovation may have to be rejected for the particular setting despite its clinical merit. For instance, a change calling for a different location of bathrooms may not be possible at a given time, but the research should be considered when renovations are planned. Another aspect of feasibility assessment is the consideration of the complexity, reversibility, and divisibility of the innovation. A new technique or strategy that is relatively straightforward or easily learned may be attainable within limited resources and more readily adopted than one that is complex and involves a major training program for staff. If an innovation can be introduced temporarily and can be readily reversed if it does not have the desired outcomes, staff will be more willing to give it a try. Similarly, if it can be introduced gradually, unit by unit or section by section, it will be less threatening as a major change.

Evaluation of the clinical merit of the findings is as essential as evaluation of the scientific merit. It is a complex process requiring clinical knowledge and skills and a thorough understanding of the particular setting. Part of the assessment of clinical merit includes the necessary step of testing innovations in terms of desired outcomes and costs. The ease with which a new idea or technique can be tested and the costs and political reality of the impact of that testing will have important implications for its clinical merit.

TESTING THE FINDINGS IN PRACTICE

A new approach or idea must be tested in practice before its adoption. This evaluative process should be carried out systematically and rigorously, but the process differs from the conduct of research. Its purpose is to examine the feasibility of using the innovation in a particular setting. It serves as the base for decision making about the adoption of the innovation.

The CURN model for developing research-based practice calls for a clinical trial comparing baseline measures with actual outcomes after the introduction of the innovation (Horsley, et al., 1983). The innovation should be carried out within the scientific limits of the independent variable in the original study, possibly with minor adjustments relevant to the setting. For example, if a trial of positioning of premature neonates were to be conducted, parameters of gestational age, birth age, weight, and diagnosis in the original studies (Fox & Molesky, 1990) would have to be respected, but the particular type of mattress used in the neonatal intensive care unit might be different. The outcomes should include as many as possible of the dependent variables in the research and should be measured with the same instruments when clinically feasible. The use of some research instruments, a laboratory, and direct invasive measures may not be possible. Reliable indirect measures may be used, such as measuring blood pressure with a sphygmomanometer rather than having an intraarterial line.

The trial is planned in detail, including identification of needed resources and costs. It is essential to involve the nursing staff and other health professionals in early discussions and to obtain the necessary sanctions and approval. The staff involved in implementing the innovation will need to learn the technique, and a separate group, independent of those implementing the innovation, will need to learn how to use the dependent measures.

The political reality of the agency or institution may have a significant effect on the trial and needs to be considered. Suppose a long-term care institution is considering the introduction of a no-restraint policy based on the evidence of the potential harm of the use of restraints and the effectiveness of alternative methods of maintaining resident safety (Maciorowski, Munro, Dietrick-Gallagher, McNew, Sheppard-Hinkel, & Wanich, 1988). If the nursing staff is skeptical about the research evidence, the nursing department will have to consider not only the effect of alternative interventions, but also the political outcomes of the process. If the test is carried out on a unit where the staff are perceived by staff on other units to be more enthusiastic or vigilant, a successful outcome may not convince staff on other units. On the other hand, there may be a risk in conducting the test on a unit where the staff are less enthusiastic, as the outcome may not be positive.

Other factors to be appraised when planning a trial are concurrent phenomena and surrounding events. Obvious occurrences such as seasonal changes in staffing or client populations could affect the outcome of a trial, and since health care agencies are rarely static, flexibility and tracking of concurrent events are necessary. A trial may have to be discontinued if there are major changes in the environment.

In the revised Stetler model (Stetler, 1994) a different level of testing can be appropriate. With certain innovations a systematic test in an individual nurse's practice can precede a larger clinical trial, or the change may remain an individual change rather than an institutional one. For instance, based on a study by Rosendahl and Ross (1982), a nurse may decide to examine the purposeful use of specific attending behaviors when interacting with clients. A nurse manager might use data from a review of nurse turnover literature (Cavanagh, 1989) to test a particular strategy with the staff. These individual tests are not merely a matter of trial and error, because the innovation is based on research findings. The type of testing is dependent on the innovation, the research base, and the level of utilization, discussed in the following section.

When a research base is expected to inform policy and lead to a change in practice, the care taken in the evaluation phase can have a significant influence on ultimate use. Systematic evaluation of a new approach or technique not only affects decision making regarding the approach's usefulness, but it also affects attitudes fundamental to successful change.

DECISION MAKING ABOUT UTILIZATION

At the end of an evaluation process, either a formal clinical trial or an individual test, a decision will have to be made about the utilization. The innovation may be adopted, modified, or rejected (Horsley, et al., 1983). The Stetler model (1994) provides other options for use of findings that are cognitive, instrumental, or symbolic types of application (see Fig. 24-5).

The decision is based on the data from the trial or testing period. The first step is a careful consideration of what the data actually represent: How many people (clients, staff) participated? How consistently was the innovation carried out? How consistently were the observations made? It is useful to summarize the data in terms of means, percentages, or frequency distributions. The outcome data are then compared to the predicted outcomes from the research. Is there a difference between the baseline data and the outcomes after the innovation or between the two groups if a comparison group was used? If the difference is in the expected direction and the innovation is satisfactory in terms of feasibility, a decision may be made to adopt the innovation. If there is no difference, or if the difference is the reverse of the expected outcome, the innovation should be reexamined for possible explanations of the outcome. If the trial was consistently carried out and the data are complete, there may have been circumstances in the setting that influenced the results. The innovation may need to be adapted or modified to facilitate its use. It should then be retested

prior to a decision. If no explanations or benefits are found, then the innovation should be rejected as a model for practice. Even new practices with a strong research base may not be beneficial in every setting or with all clients.

A decision to use findings in other ways may result from a rejection or from a smaller scale test. Suppose a strategy to promote urinary continence in a long-term care setting was unsuccessful. A decision might be made to reject the particular strategy but to conduct a thorough evaluation of current practices and continue to search the literature for alternative solutions.

Utilization at a cognitive level can be beneficial for both clients and nurses, especially if the nurse alters his or her thinking purposefully as a result of research findings, rather than in a vague or haphazard way. The details of variables or factors in descriptive or instrument development research can increase the nurse's scope for observations and provide a better foundation for clinical decision making. For example, knowledge of the findings in a correlational study of fatigue in people with breast or lung cancer (Blesch, Paice, Wickham, Harte, Schnoor, & Purl, 1991) could prompt the nurse who is more aware of the client's mood and its effect on fatigue to help the client obtain more rest.

Cognitive use of findings as a base for clinical practice can have an important effect not only on a nurse's personal practice but on the practice of groups of nurses. One neonatal intensive care nurse's careful examination of physiological and behavioral parameters in one infant's 6 months of life and of the related literature led to a new perspective on observations by all staff (Youngkins, 1991). An expanded knowledge base from new research findings enhances nurses' satisfaction with practice and their self-perception (James, Milne, & Firth, 1990).

IMPLEMENTING A CHANGE IN PRACTICE

The principles of change theory are beyond the scope of this chapter, but factors to be considered include communication, involvement and commitment, staff development, and continued monitoring of the process. The process of communication about a proposed research-based change in practice requires thoughtful planning with nursing administrators, staff educators, and staff nurses. Just as the involvement of nurses at all levels enhances the testing of findings described above, it is essential for an effective change process. The first step may be to help administrators understand the rationale for the change without feeling inadequate in their knowledge of research. A face-to-face explanation with the opportunity to have questions answered is likely to gain the strongest support. For explanations to staff nurses, a nurse who was involved in the evaluation trial may be the best person to explain the problem and the proposed change. A researcher or clinician with research preparation may be helpful to explain the research base.

Many changes involve or affect other health care workers, as well as nurses, and explanations need to be appropriately delivered to these groups. Professionals with a knowledge of research will appreciate the reports of the original research. The strength of the research will have a significant effect on the willingness to support a change.

The same factors as those that must be considered in examining clinical merit and designing a trial to test findings, such as complexity of the innovation, measurability of results, costs, and the political reality of the institution, relate to the likelihood of adoption of changes in practice. Innovations with tangible benefits and low costs or effort are likely to be the most readily adopted, but many worthwhile innovations require considerable work to learn and adopt the practice. Resistance to change is a common phenomenon that may be overcome when nurses perceive the problem as relevant to their practice, have an increased understanding of benefits, and believe they are being supported. Time and an opportunity to learn a new approach are needed. Interference with change may result if nurses are expected to make a change for which they are not adequately prepared. A program of gradual or phased change may be most effective.

Once a change has been implemented, the innovation and its outcomes need ongoing monitoring. This may be incorporated into an existing quality improvement program, or it may be specifically planned in the change process. An innovation that was appropriate at one time or with one group of clients may not be useful in different circumstances.

꧁ OVERCOMING BARRIERS TO USE OF RESEARCH IN PRACTICE

Diffusion and adoption of innovations do not happen by osmosis. The invisible wall between researchers and clinicians varies according to conditions. It is essential to allow knowledge to flow in both directions.

BARRIERS TO RESEARCH UTILIZATION

Several nurses have studied the use of research by practicing nurses in general hospitals (Brett, 1987; Coyle & Sokop, 1990; Crane, 1989; Ketefian, 1975; Kirchhoff, 1982) and in community nursing settings (Krueger, 1982; Luker & Kenrick, 1992). Although the quantity, sophistication, and client focus of nursing research have increased over the same time period (Jacobsen & Meninger, 1985; Moody, Wilson, Smyth, Schwartz, Tittle, & Cott, 1988), there are still gaps between the researcher and the practitioner. Brodie (1988) characterized the phenomenon as "voices in distant camps" (p. 320). Nurses have been expressing concerns about the gap for over 30 years (Halpert, 1966; Malone, 1962; Notter, 1973; Roberts, 1967).

Nurses responding to an extensive survey of perceived barriers to the use of research by clinicians reported 28 barriers (Funk, et al., 1991b). These barriers were classified as characteristics of the nurse, the setting, the research, or the presentation of the research. The clinicians perceived the setting as the major contributor to the barriers, accounting for eight of the top 10 barriers (Table 24-3). The quality of the research was less likely to be a barrier, but the

Table 24-3
Rank Ordering of Barriers to Research Utilization, Showing Type of Barrier

Rank Order	Barrier	Type of Barrier*
1	The nurse does not feel she/he has enough authority to change patient care procedures.	Setting
2	There is insufficient time on the job to implement new ideas.	Setting
3	The nurse is unaware of the research.	Nurse
4	Physicians will not cooperate with implementation.	Setting
5	Administration will not allow implementation.	Setting
6	Other staff are not supportive of implementation.	Setting
7	The nurse feels results are not generalizable to own setting.	Setting
8	The facilities are inadequate for implementation.	Setting
9	Statistical analyses are not understandable.	Present
10	The nurse does not have time to read research.	Setting
11	The nurse is isolated from knowledgeable colleagues with whom to discuss the research.	Nurse
12	The relevant literature is not compiled in one place.	Present
13	Implications for practice are not made clear.	Present
14	The nurse does not feel capable of evaluating the quality of the research.	Nurse
15	Research reports/articles are not readily available.	Present
16	The research has not been replicated.	Research
17	The research is not reported clearly and readably.	Present
18	The research is not relevant to the nurse's practice.	Present
19	The nurse feels the benefits of changing practice will be minimal.	Nurse
20	The nurse sees little benefit for self.	Nurse
21	The nurse is uncertain whether to believe the results of the research.	Research
22	The nurse is unwilling to change/try new ideas.	Nurse
23	The literature reports conflicting results.	Research
24	The research has methodological inadequacies.	Research
25	There is not a documented need to change practice.	Nurse
26	The nurse does not see the value of research for practice.	Nurse
27	Research reports/articles are not published fast enough.	Research
28	The conclusions drawn from the research are not justified.	Research

Adapted with permission from Funk, S. G., et al. (1991). Barriers to using research findings in practice: The clinician's perspective. *Applied Nursing Research, 4*(2), 92.
*Present = Presentation.

way the findings were presented was perceived as a great or moderate barrier by more than half the nurses who responded. Characteristics of the nurse, such as being unaware of the research or being isolated from knowledgeable colleagues, were seen as important by the majority of nurses, but only about one third thought nurses' lack of recognition of the value of research was a barrier. This supported the finding in Crane's (1989) study of the use of new knowledge in direct patient care, cognitively or behaviorally, and in generalized use in practice. She found that organizational factors were more influential than individual factors. In an earlier survey by Miller and Messenger (1978) nurses linked problems with the research and the setting as major obstacles.

Goode and her co-workers (1991) added the nursing profession as an organizational system as a source of barriers. Problems include the variations in nurses' educational backgrounds, the diverse contexts in which nurses work, the limited activities related to the identification and prioritizing of clinical problems for study, and the cumbersome knowledge dissemination system. These were also identified in the experiences of six critical care nurses (Newman, Beattie, Harris, Farrar, Simko, & Appel-Hardin, 1989).

FACILITATING TECHNIQUES
Nurses also identified seven facilitators to research utilization (Funk, et al., 1991b). These were:

1. Enhancing administrative support and encouragement
2. Improving availability and accessibility of research reports
3. Increasing advanced education and the nurses' research knowledge base
4. Providing networks and mechanisms for colleague support
5. Conducting more clinically focused, relevant research
6. Increasing time available for reviewing and implementing research findings
7. Improving the understandability of research reports

Administrative support, colleague networks, and time are related to the setting. The accessibility of reports, the nurses' knowledge base, and the relevancy of research may all be influenced by the administration, but the individual nurse and the researchers are also involved. The understandability of the reports is largely in the hands of the researcher, but the journal editors and the readers have a role as well. The profession as a whole can also influence the relevancy of research to practice and the development of research-based practice (International Council of Nurses, 1986).

The Coordinator of Nursing Research in a midwestern children's hospital identified nine themes of research utilization techniques in the literature that reflect the same broad categories (Edwards-Beckett, 1990). She provides examples of techniques that could be implemented by individual nurses, groups, and the organization or profession as a whole (Table 24-4).

Specific strategies to overcome barriers related to the setting, the usability of research, and the nurse's knowledge base are discussed in the following sections. Within each area of potential obstacles, strategies related to the infrastructure, communication, and education are important, but the relative importance varies from area to area.

The Setting
The infrastructure to support research utilization in either a health care agency or an educational institution is critical. Not only

Table 24-4
Examples of Techniques for Relating to Research Utilization Themes as Implemented by an Individual, Group, or Organization/Profession

Themes	Individual	Group	Organization/ Profession
Awareness of current literature	Reads articles on own	Journal club	Designated in job description
Educational technique	Takes research course	Inservices	Utilization taught in nursing programs
Organizational promotion	Participates in traineeships	Policy change based on research	Utilization in philosophy
Supervision of research utilization	Brings articles to proper channels	Committee to promote research	Research department
Resources for research	Provides peer support	Research groups for support	Providing release time
Conduct of research	Identifies problems	Research groups conduct clinical trial	Departmental implementation of study
Dissemination of research findings	Discusses with peers	Inservices	Research symposium
Interactions of clinicians and researchers	Discusses with researchers	Regular research presentations	In-house research and publication
Rewards	Discussion between individuals	Improved unit practice	Improved standards of care

Adapted with permission from Edwards-Beckett, J. (1990). Nursing research utilization techniques. *Journal of Nursing Administration, 20*(11), 26.

does the organizational structure demonstrate the support, but it facilitates the process (Horsley, Crane, & Bingle, 1978; Lawson, 1987; Rosswurm, 1992). The primary requisite is that research utilization be highly valued with an absolute commitment to its promotion. The philosophy and mission statement of the institution and Department of Nursing will clearly identify this position (Baker, 1978; Fitch, 1992; Lawson, 1987; Snyder-Halpern, 1991). Senior nursing administrators in clinical agencies have a key role in facilitating the development of research-based practice in their setting, starting with the creation of a climate of inquiry (Hefferin, Horsley, & Ventura, 1982; Simms, Price, & Pfoutz, 1987). The commitment means en-

couragement to question, openness to change, and recognition for using research. It also means creating the infrastructure and providing the budget to support both the structure and the process of research utilization (Snyder-Halpern, 1991).

Structural elements include (1) positions for nurses whose responsibility includes research; (2) a nursing research committee with a mandate to promote and guide research utilization; and (3) support services, including access to a library and research consultation.

All nurses in an agency may not have the requisite knowledge and skills, so a structure incorporating positions in which nurses are accountable for facilitating research utilization is important (Kirchhoff,

1991). There are two categories of positions whose mandate is focused on research: the clinical nurse researcher (CNR) and the clinical nurse specialist (CNS). The CNR should be a doctorally prepared nurse with research and clinical experience (Hagle, Kirchhoff, Knafl, & Bevis, 1986). Knowledge of statistics, grantsmanship, evaluation research, and administration are assets. The roles are relatively new and may be enacted in different ways, emphasizing either the conduct or facilitation of research (Knafl, Hagle, Bevis, Faux, & Kirchhoff, 1989). Whatever the particular organizational structure, the CNR should possess strong interpersonal skills that are highlighted by patience, flexibility, and approachability. Researchers responding to a Delphi survey characterized the clinical researcher as "a dynamic facilitator" (Snyder-Halpern, 1991, p. 83).

The role of the clinical nurse specialist as a pivotal clinician linking research and practice has been discussed by many authors (Barnard, 1986; Cronenwett, 1986; Hamilton, Vincent, Goode, Moorhouse, Hawker, Worden, & Jones, 1990; Hickey, 1990). CNSs are expected to be master's prepared and to be expert clinicians. The CNS is in an ideal position to assess the system readiness for research utilization, work with the staff to identify clinical problems, and help the staff plan, implement, and evaluate the use of findings that are clinically relevant in a particular area (Cronenwett, 1986; Hickey, 1990). In a study of their practice, CNSs reported that they used research (1) to help staff in complex patient situations such as pain management or treating drug abuse; (2) in the development of broad programs, for instance, programs related to staff orientation or services for persons with AIDS; and (3) in the development of documents for nursing department policies or procedures (Stetler & DiMaggio, 1991).

In any given agency, the nursing research committee's responsibilities may include (1) the promotion and implementation of research utilization, (2) staff development for research, (3) the facilitation of the conduct of research, and (4) the review of proposals from employees or others seeking access to subjects for research projects. The specific mandate will vary, but any agency with a commitment to research will benefit from an active committee.

One 42-bed rural hospital has had a significant international impact on research utilization through the production of a series of videotapes on their committee's structure and activities (Horn Video Productions, 1986). The committee based its process on the CURN project (Horsley, et al., 1983) and used a systems model developed by Conway (1978) to think through utilization projects (Goode, et al., 1987). Feedback and evaluation have been rewarding for all concerned.

In comparison to a small rural hospital, a 1500-bed tertiary care Veterans Administration facility has five research committees, one in each of the major clinical areas (Lawson, 1987). Responsibilities include the review and critique of relevant literature and dissemination of findings, the identification of potential research projects, review of proposals, and recommending speakers for research presentations. Committee chairpersons comprise a central research council, but the decentralized structure allows for participation by nurses from all areas and attention to research activities that are relevant to the particular client group.

A specialty hospital for the care of children has a Nursing Research Utilization Subcommittee currently at work developing a guide to research critique (Van Koot & Laverty, 1992). The Nursing Quality Practice Committee at the same hospital has a mechanism to encourage the production of policies and procedures that are based on research findings.

The research committee also has a significant role in informing researchers about the agency and in facilitating research (Vessey & Campos, 1992). The structure and functions of research committees will vary, but the organizational commitment to research-based practice is essential.

The creation of focused positions and committee structures confirms the administrative resolution to build improved practice on research. It also indicates a commitment to allow the requisite time for research activities. All staff need to be involved at some level: identifying clinical problems, reviewing the literature, testing the innovation, or implementing the new practice. Phillips (1986) identified eight roles for nursing staff as consumers of nursing research. These are "(1) facilitator, (2) advocate, (3) activist, (4) risk-taker, (5) learner/teacher, (6) innovator, (7) negotiator, and (8) collaborator" (p. 70). The particular roles that a nurse assumes will vary according to knowledge, skills, and position, but the expectations for participation in research activities should be clearly identified in job descriptions for all nursing staff. Involvement is important, not only to accomplish the activities, but also to provide a sense of ownership of the process and outcomes (Fitch, 1992; Goode, et al., 1987; Phillips, 1986).

Two additional components of structural support for staff nurses are necessary in the setting: access to library facilities and consultation with researchers. Some facilities may have limited library resources. Subscriptions to a selection of core journals, including broad-based research journals and those with a clinical focus, are a worthwhile investment. Nurses on a particular unit will benefit from shared ownership of a subscription to a clinically relevant research journal. Interlibrary loan with other clinical agencies, universities, or government libraries can be arranged (Goode, et al., 1987) and should be built into process costs for research utilization.

Not all agencies will be able to have a clinical nurse researcher, but it is still essential to create links between researchers and clinicians. Links can be made through consultation with prepared nurses in universities and other agencies. University connections may also serve as the structure for staff education, and there are several strategies that a clinical setting and university may employ (Davies & Drake, 1992; Janken, Dufault, & Yeaw, 1988; Pinch, 1989; Swanson, Easterling, Costa, & Creamer-Bauer, 1990). The focus is on student-staff collaboration in identifying clinical problems and reviewing the literature. Projects may be initiated by either the school or the clinical agency, and the agency may or may not be part of the university. One university in Canada found that all the health care agencies in the geographic area wanted to participate in staff/student projects (Davies & Drake, 1992). The process is immediately advantageous for the staff and the student in terms of learning, accomplishing a practical endeavor, and gaining mutual respect. The clinical agency stands to benefit with both current staff and future graduates.

It is clear that communication among staff nurses, CNSs, administrators, committee members, educators and students, and health professionals is critical. The following section will focus on communication between researchers and clinical staff.

The Usability of Research

The ultimate usability of research is based on the clinical relevance of the research question, the quality of the research, the transformation of the findings into language understandable to clinicians, and the accessibility of the findings to clinicians. Whether the research findings are actually used goes beyond these issues to those factors in the setting discussed above and factors related to the nurse to be addressed later in the chapter.

The linkage model (Figure 24-4) provides one of the best overall frameworks for developing research questions that are clinically relevant. The questions arise from an interactive process between researchers and clinicians. The process does not occur naturally because researchers and clinicians are likely to work in different contexts (Horsley, et al., 1983), and researchers have tended to seek patterns and rationale, while clinicians look for a prescription to deal with a unique clinical situation (Duffy, 1985). The researchers in the linkage model may include CNRs in clinical settings who have direct and regular contact with clinicians, researchers involved in their own clinical practice, and researchers based outside agencies, usually at universities.

One of the key characteristics identified by CNRs as essential to success in their role is the ability to communicate. Both CNRs and clinical nurse executives emphasized the need to be able to work with people, to be down-to-earth, and to be patient, along with the personal qualities needed for research, such as creativity and inquisitiveness (Hagle, et al., 1986). Since these positions are relatively new, time is usually needed initially for informal interactions with staff to discuss the role and involve staff in its development (Fitch, 1992; Knafl, et al., 1989). To contribute to the science of nursing and, also, to maintain credibility and funding as a researcher, the CNR needs to maintain his or her own program of research (Hagle, et al., 1986), but this needs to be balanced with helping others with research.

Researchers based outside the clinical agency and staff in agencies where there is no CNR need to create opportunities for interaction. Researchers often need access to a clinical agency for subjects in their studies. Communication concerning this access can start early in the planning process so that research questions can be directed to produce more relevant answers. Clinicians who have ideas but limited research knowledge may find a researcher through publications such as directories, journals, or conference proceedings or informally through contacts with colleagues and friends (Rempusheski, 1992). Willingness to seek each other out is the first step, but willingness to listen and expand a personal perspective is required for success.

The researcher who is involved in clinical practice, either a university faculty member in practice (Pinch, 1989) or a CNS (Cronenwett, 1986; Hickey, 1990), has direct access to relevant questions, but needs time and consultation to develop them. Clinicians working with such practitioner-researchers will contribute to the research and learn about the process by seeking opportunities to discuss clinical issues.

More formal approaches to the development of critical questions include consensus conferences and formal establishment of research priorities. A consensus conference is an invitational conference that brings together researchers and clinicians with a common focus of interest. The interest may relate to symptom management such as pain control; a group of clients, for example, oncology patients; or a practice concern such as ethical issues. Usually there is a relatively small number of participants so that in-depth discussions can take place and research proposals can begin to be formulated or clear recommendations can be generated for research priorities.

Professional associations, funding agencies, and major consortia are usually responsible for the establishment of research priorities. Hinshaw (1988) reported on the National Nursing Research Agenda, which "encompasses several components: identification of major program areas of study for nursing research, development of program priorities, projection of resources needed to put the program priorities into practice, and specification of an evaluation and update plan for the growth and scientific advances of program areas" (p. 56). Target areas of concern at a national level are identified, such as research on low-birthweight infants, building on the landmark research of Brooten and her colleagues (1986), to focus research and develop a comprehensive body of relevant knowledge for practice. Research questions that begin at the bedside in one clinical agency may become nationally significant.

Transforming research findings into language understandable to clinicians may be done by the researcher or the clinician. A clinician with an understanding of research methods and terminology is in the best position to do this because there is an opportunity for direct interaction with staff and clarification. In a published report, the researcher should identify implications for practice, but sufficient detail for direct use by practitioners can rarely be included. It is important that the limits of generalizability be clearly specified in all reports. The researcher might be aware of how findings might be used in a particular setting, but the readers need to make the interpretation and judgment about use in their own clinical setting. One useful strategy is that of dual publication, with the research details in a research journal and the clinical details in a clinical one. Clinical journals that focus on research such as *Heart and Lung* and *Oncology Nursing Forum* and research journals with a clinical focus such as *Applied Nursing Research* and *Clinical Nursing*

Research have the usability of research findings as a major criterion for publication. A newsletter with research findings interpreted for their application in practice can also be useful.

The ideal situation is for researchers and clinicians to talk to each other about findings. This can happen in either the researcher's or the clinician's setting, but may be most accessible for groups of nurses in the clinical setting. Agencies can invite outside researchers to make presentations in their facilities at relatively low cost, and all researchers who conduct studies in clinical agencies should present their findings to the staff as a whole and particularly to the group of nurses specifically involved. These focused presentations give the best opportunity for discussion of research utilization. Clinicians should be encouraged and supported to attend clinical research conferences and similar meetings and to report to their colleagues shortly after the conference. Universities frequently sponsor research days for presentation of student and faculty projects. Clinicians should be invited and should take advantage of the opportunity to ask questions and discuss the applicability of findings.

Another aspect of accessibility is the clinician's access to published materials. The amount of time a nurse spends reading professional journals and specific research journals correlates with the adoption of innovations in practice (Brett, 1987). The administration is responsible for the infrastructure, the library and its budget; the clinical staff should be responsible for working with the library staff to ensure that the holdings are relevant to their practice. The clinician is also responsible for seeking out the materials. Strategies to get materials to nurses and vice versa include the circulation of a copy of the tables of contents of relevant journals, either by the librarian or a "library representative"; subscription to one or two especially relevant journals on the units; an "article of the week" identified by nurses and made available on the unit; and library time on duty.

While communication between researchers and clinicians is crucial, education for nurses to understand what is being communicated is equally essential. Education includes both formal and informal opportunities to learn. Strategies to increase the nurse's knowledge of research and research-based practice are discussed in the following section.

The Nurse's Knowledge Base

The nurse's knowledge base clearly begins to be developed in the basic educational program, whether at a diploma, associate degree, baccalaureate, or master's level. Students who learn that practice is built on scientific rationale will search for and question the underlying explanation as they practice. They will challenge traditional practices that have become routines and rituals (Walsh & Ford, 1989). Clinical teachers need to help students make purposeful links between the research base and practice. All nursing courses should include some lecture-discussions with researchers who present their research and discuss the applicability of findings. This introduces students to the world of nursing as a research reality with clear connections to real people.

Specific strategies for learning about research and its use in undergraduate programs include experiences for students in the clinical research projects of faculty members (Pinch, 1989), introductory research courses based on a model of research utilization (Larson, 1989; Stetler, 1989), student projects based on staff questions (Davies & Drake, 1992), and student-staff discussions of clinical issues and potential research questions (Janken, et al., 1988; Swanson, et al., 1990). Williams (1987) suggested that students would benefit from structured learning about development of standards of care and practice policies.

Continuing education for practicing nurses is an ongoing need. One program in a tertiary-care hospital has included nurses with varied backgrounds (Pepler, 1992). The course is based on the steps in this chapter built on both the CURN and Stetler models. It is focused on helping learners work through the process with a topic in which they are particularly interested. The pursuit of clinical issues of personal interest has a high level of relevance for each learner. Also, because they come from different clinical areas, they readily enter discussions as experts in their own field and learners about research utilization.

At a more informal level unit-based journal clubs provide the opportunity for social interaction to enhance diffusion of knowledge (see Figure 24-2). Clinicians' discussions of a pertinent research article results in both a greater understanding of the research and brainstorming about its applicability. Journal clubs may be most effective when a series of research papers on a given topic are discussed over a few weeks. This gives the group a broader perspective on the topic and increases their knowledge about findings that are confirmed in replication or about the particular issues with conflicting findings. Interest is boosted and nurses become engrossed when they see findings from several studies fitting together.

Communication strategies are useful such as a unit "inquiry notebook" where nurses jot down ideas and questions—why don't we . . . ? why do we . . . ? what is the best way to . . . ? These start others thinking and enhance discussions when staff get together. Unit-based activities may be linked with quality improvement projects (Ahier, Coghlan, Martin, & Worthen, 1992; Rosswurm, 1992).

Another learning strategy for practicing nurses is involvement in research. Nurses frequently participate in other health care professionals' projects by one or more of the following: notifying the researcher when potential subjects are admitted, carrying out research protocols such as giving experimental drugs, collecting data such as vital signs or specimens, or being subjects themselves in studies of nurses. Nurses need to discuss the research with the researchers, whatever health discipline is involved. Asking questions about how and why the protocol was developed as it was, how the outcome measures are linked to the theory, and how the findings are related to practice will increase the nurse's understanding of the place of research in practice.

The advantages of having a nursing research program in a clinical agency are that nurses are stimulated to question their practice, patient care is improved, and patient care costs can be reduced. However, barriers remain for various reasons. Strategies to overcome these are related to (1) changes in the setting, including philosophy, infrastructure, and support; (2) enhancement of the usability of research in terms of relevance and presentation; and (3) improvement in nurses' knowledge base and understanding of the process of research utilization.

∾ SUCCESSES IN ESTABLISHING A RESEARCH REALITY

A research reality for nursing is a nursing practice environment in which nursing decisions are based on research findings.

Nurses in such an environment have the knowledge base and the autonomy to question their practice, whether in direct care, administration, or education. Practice is built on strategies that have been studied and found to have predictable outcomes. The reality may be a future goal, but fortunately nursing is moving in this direction. The following are examples of successes with applicability in the care of the elderly, new mothers and babies, adults in acute care, children in pain, and in staff support and student learning.

First, patient falls in acute care have many potentially serious consequences for patients and staff. One acute care institution sought to decrease falls by applying relevant interventions found in the nursing research literature (Kilpack, Boehm, Smith, & Mudge, 1991). A group of CNSs explored the literature on falls and developed a list of research-based interventions. Two units with the highest number of falls were selected for a clinical trial. An educational program heightened staff awareness of falls. The literature showed that repeat falls were common, so the CNS worked with nurses who were caring for patients who had had one fall. Nurses selected interventions from the list that were specifically relevant and feasible to be incorporated into the care of that particular patient. Additional interventions were also used. Data from a 1-year trial were compared to the previous year, and falls decreased from 4.7 falls per 1000 patient days to 4.4. This decrease occurred despite an increase in patient acuity and an all-hospital fall rate increase of 3.0 to 3.6 per 1000 patient days. On the basis of the data and the experience the CNSs made major clinical practice recommendations that are being implemented by the Department of Nursing.

Similarly, in a small rural hospital nurses became concerned that new mothers were frustrated with conflicting information on breastfeeding (Goode, et al., 1987). Individual nurses and doctors had their own ideas and good intentions, but the information mothers got was not research based. The Nursing Research Committee reviewed the literature, both the books available to mothers and the research publications. A teaching program was developed with a detailed protocol and teaching record. Follow-up telephone interviews indicated that mothers who had learned about research-based breastfeeding techniques from staff who were consistent in providing information were knowledgeable and believed that the teaching had been helpful. Consistency in teaching helped the mothers learn, and the success of the tested techniques reinforced that learning. The authors concluded that "there is nothing more rewarding than instituting a protocol based upon research that improves patient outcomes" (Goode, et al., 1987, p. 17).

A third project involved the use of the extensive literature on heparin and saline flushes to maintain patency of intermittent peripheral IV access devices and potential cost savings (Goode, Titler, Rakel, Ones, Kleiber, & Small, 1991). In a West Coast university medical center the Nursing Research Utilization Committee evaluated the efficacy of using normal saline rather than heparin (Donaldson, 1991). The review of the literature showed that this technique is scientifically and clinically sound, but the adult medical-surgical and the critical care units were using heparin flushes every 4 to 6 hours and after each use of the intermittent peripheral IV access device. A clinical trial that included a master plan, interdisciplinary communication, and a staff educational program was conducted for 1 month. Data analysis indicated that saline was as effective as heparin in maintaining patency and took less administration time.

In addition, research has demonstrated that saline is less irritating and is compatible with more medications than heparin. The committee concluded that normal saline was the solution of choice, and the nursing administration has approved their recommendation. Approval of the hospital Pharmacy & Therapeutics Committee was pending at the time of publication.

Pain management is a critical aspect of nursing care in any clinical area, but an increased number of requests for consultation related to postoperative pain relief in a children's hospital triggered a research utilization project (Ahier, et al., 1992). The standard practice was the administration of postoperative analgesia by intramuscular injection, which could have a ripple effect on the child's dislike or fear of needles, leading to underreporting or denying of pain and nurses avoiding giving needles because of the child's fear. The investigation revealed that nurses and surgical residents lacked knowledge about pediatric pain assessment, the effect of narcotic analgesia, and the use of PRN analgesics. A review of the literature supported these obstacles to pain management and identified strategies to overcome them. An overall plan was developed by the multidisciplinary team that included the use of the Oucher tool for pain assessment (Beyer & Aradine, 1989) and intermittent or continuous use of intravenous morphine infusion for postoperative pain management. An essential component of the planned change was education for nurses, physicians, and parents, all of whom had misconceptions about children's pain management. The changes were carefully monitored through the quality improvement program, and intramuscular injections have been virtually eliminated.

Improved patient outcomes and lowered costs are not the only advantages to sys-

EVALUATING THE USE OF RESEARCH FINDINGS IN PRACTICE

1. How significant was the clinical problem?
2. How thorough was the literature search?
3. How sound was the research base?
4. How carefully was the innovation tested?
5. How readily was the idea or innovation learned?
6. How widely was it adopted?

tematic research utilization. Staff in a community hospital participated in an inquiry group process to address areas of concern (Parker, Gordon, & Brannon, 1992). Although the overall intent of the program was to involve nurses in research by using a nontraditional approach, opportunities arose for nurses to develop strategies to implement research findings. One identified concern was the need for support mechanisms for nursing staff. The inquiry group reviewed the literature and studied various models of employee assistance programs. They also interviewed representatives from ongoing programs in the area and were able to make well-informed recommendations to the nursing administration for establishing an employee assistance program.

Nursing students can also benefit from a program based on research. Senior students in an articulated associate degree-baccalaureate degree program participated in a course based on Benner's (1984) research on the progression from novice to expert in clinical practice (Carlson, Crawford, & Contrades, 1989). The course included a seminar, a scholarly paper, and clinical experience. Students examined their own progression in clinical expertise and in their ability to relate current research to the clinical situation.

Many examples of research utilization are reported anecdotally. For nurses attempting to start the process, reports of projects using more systematic strategies are useful.

✎ EVALUATING THE USE OF RESEARCH FINDINGS IN PRACTICE

The evaluation of research utilization includes (1) the evaluation of the process related to a specific project, (2) the ongoing evaluation of the implementation of a particular innovation, and (3) the overall assessment of research-based practice in an agency.

Examination of the process may help to identify areas where the mechanisms are weak or need adjusting in a particular setting. Difficulties encountered at any stage in one project may be found in subsequent projects, and obstacles may be discouraging to nurses who are dealing with multiple demands to improve practice. The time taken to evaluate the process may save time, effort, and antagonism in future projects. The questions listed in the box will help to guide the evaluation of the process of a research utilization project.

After an innovation has been tested and implemented, it is essential to continue to monitor its effectiveness and its costs as knowledge increases and other changes occur in the agency. It is hazardous to depend on once-tested nursing interventions because nursing is continuing to develop its knowledge base. For example, structured preoperative teaching has been found to be effective in increasing postoperative activity and reducing postoperative complications (Hathaway, 1986). It is widely used in various forms, but as day surgery and same-day admission for surgery increase, earlier tested techniques need reexamination. There are also many unanswered questions about preoperative preparation that need further study, such as details of timing, format, and patient and family participation. Raising questions about "tested" techniques is as important as questioning traditional practice.

Evaluating clinical practice and identifying problems is a component of quality improvement, that is, using research methods to monitor and improve nursing practice. Watson, Bulechek, and McCloskey (1987) provide a model, the Quality Assurance Model Using Research (QAMUR), for building research utilization into the quality assurance process. It provides a framework for identifying both problems for which there is a research base and problems for which the conduct of research is needed. The major advantage of this model is that research utilization is perceived as part of continuing quality management, rather than the testing of one innovation. It includes the concept of the use of research methods in the practice of nursing, which is one component of research utilization. Hunt (1987) found that the implementation and monitoring of a widespread change in practice needed a systematic approach to research utilization that was provided in the structure of a quality assurance program.

Overall evaluation of research utilization in practice is most effectively done where there is a structure for nursing research, most often a committee whose mandate includes evaluation. Most reports on the development of a structure for nursing research highlight the initial need to increase awareness and educate nurses about the value of research-based practice. They also identify ways to build the research base into practice, such as basing new procedures on research and citing studies in the procedure manual. A research committee may assess the extent to which these are happening.

At the next level the group may examine whether specific strategies to facilitate the process of research utilization are being used. The process can be evaluated through examination of the use of any of the strategies identified above to overcome barriers. Are unit-based groups identifying problems and completing the process of scrutinizing the literature, testing findings, and making changes? If the process is starting, but blocking at some point, what is causing the block? Are there barriers that are still obstructing the process? What further strategies might overcome them?

Evaluation and dissemination of successes will breed more success. Creating opportunities for nurses to report on research utilization activities on their own units will not only prompt them to begin the process and carry it through but can also encourage self-evaluation of the process. Reporting to other nurses can enhance self-esteem and increase the potential for further utilization. While examination of a process can identify problems to be remedied, it can also lead to well-deserved pride that patient care has improved.

SUMMARY

- Research utilization includes the process of building practice on a research base.
- The overall process is one of knowledge dissemination, which includes the generation and validation of knowledge, its transformation and transfer to users, and its interpretation and utilization.
- Research findings become usable knowledge when nurses alter the way they think about a clinical situation; research

findings change behaviors when nurses adopt a new way of practicing.

- The steps in the process of research utilization include:
  1. Clarifying the problem or clinical question
  2. Searching the literature
  3. Evaluating scientific merit of the research findings
  4. Assessing the clinical merit of the findings, including the feasibility and "fit" of using the findings in a particular setting
  5. Testing the use of findings or the innovation
  6. Decision making about utilization
  7. Implementing a change in practice
- Barriers have been identified in the setting, the nurse, the research, and its presentation that can obstruct research utilization at different points.
- Strategies to overcome these barriers include providing a facilitative infrastructure, enhancing communication, and educating nurses.
- Evaluation of research utilization includes examination of the actual process in a particular project, building on going monitoring of a tested innovation into a quality improvement program, and assessing the overall level of research utilization in an agency.

FACILITATING CRITICAL THINKING

1. You are a member of the Nursing Research Utilization Committee in your hospital. The committee has been asked to develop a plan to enhance the dissemination of new knowledge in nursing. What factors will you have to consider in developing your plan?
2. As a head nurse on a surgical unit, you are concerned about the way patients are prepared for surgery when they are admitted on the day of surgery. What strategies would you use to facilitate staff involvement in reviewing the literature related to this problem?
3. You find several studies demonstrating the effectiveness of preadmission preparation and the use of telephone calls between the preparation and the admission. You would like to improve the practice on your unit, but are uncertain about how effective this approach would be for the patients on your unit. How would you test its effectiveness? Whom would you involve in the process?
4. As a community health nurse, you learn that there have been several studies about fatigue in new mothers and fathers. How would you find this information and use it in your practice?

References

SUBSTANTIVE

ABRAHAM, I. L., NEUNDORFER, M. M., & CURRIE, L. J. (1992). Effects of group interventions on cognition and depression in nursing home residents. *Nursing Research, 41*(40), 196-202.

AHIER, J., ET AL. (1992). Children win with improved pain management. *Canadian Nurse, 19*(1), 19-21.

ATKINS, F. D. (1991). Children's perspectives of stress and coping: An integrative review. *Issues in Mental Health Nursing, 12*(2), 171-178.

BENNER, P. (1984). *From novice to expert.* Menlo Park, CA: Addison-Wesley.

BERGSTROM, N., ET AL. (1987). The Braden scale for predicting pressure sore risk. *Nursing Research, 36*(4), 205-210.

BEYER, J., & ARADINE, C. (1989). Patterns of pediatric pain intensity: A methodological investigation of a self-report scale. *Clinical Journal of Pain, 3*, 130-141.

BLESCH, K. S., ET AL. (1991). Correlates of fatigue in people with breast or lung cancer, *Oncology Nursing Forum, 18*(1), 81-87.

BROOTEN, D., ET AL. (1986). A randomized clinical trial of early hospital discharge and home follow-up of very-low-birth-weight infants. *New England Journal of Medicine, 315*(15), 934-939.

CARLSON, L., CRAWFORD, N., & CONTRADES, S. (1989). Nursing student novice to expert: Benner's research applied to education. *Journal of Nursing Education, 4*(28), 188-190.

CAVANAGH, S. J. (1989). Nursing turnover: Literature review and methodological critique, *Journal of Advanced Nursing, 14*(7), 587-596.

COHEN, S., & SYME, S. L. (1985). *Social support and health.* Orlando, FL: Academic Press.

DIORIO, C., ET AL. (1992). Measurement of safe sex behavior in adolescents and young adults. *Nursing Research, 42*(4), 203-208.

DONALDSON, N. E. (Fall 1991). Peripheral saline locks: An alternative to heparin flushes. *The ORCUN Oration.*

FERRELL, B. R., ET AL. (1991). Pain as a metaphor for illness. I. Impact of cancer pain on family caregivers. *Oncology Nursing Forum, 18*(8), 1303-1309.

FOLTA, A., & METZGER, B. L. (1989). Exercise and functional capacity after myocardial infarction. *IMAGE: Journal of Nursing Scholarship, 21*(4), 215-219.

FOX, M. D., & MOLESKY, M. G. (1990). The effects of prone and supine positioning on arterial oxygen pressure. *Neonatal Network, 8*(4), 25-29.

GARVIN, B. J., & KENNEDY, C. W. (1990). Interpersonal communication between nurses and patients. *Annual Review of Nursing Research, 8,* 214-234.

GIFT, A. G., PLAUT, S. M., & JACOX, A. (1986). Psychologic and physiologic factors related to dyspnea in subjects with chronic obstructive pulmonary disease. *Heart and Lung, 15,* 595-601.

GIFT, A. G., MOORE, T., & SOEKEN, K. (1992). Relaxation to reduce dyspnea and anxiety in COPD patients. *Nursing Research, 41*(4), 242-246.

GOODE, C. J., ET AL. (1991). A meta-analysis of effects of heparin flush and saline flush: quality and cost implications. *Nursing Research, 40*(6), 324-330.

HATHAWAY, D. (1986). Effect of preoperative instructions on postoperative outcomes: a meta-analysis. *Nursing Research, 35*(5), 269-275.

HEATER, B. S., BECKER, A. M., & OLSON, R. K. (1988). Nursing interventions and patient outcomes: A meta-analysis of studies. *Nursing Research, 37*(5), 303-307.

HOLDCRAFT, C., & WILLIAMSON, C. (1991). Assessment of hope in psychiatric and chemically dependent patients. *Applied Nursing Research, 4*(3), 129-134.

HUNTER, L. P. (1991). Measurement of axillary temperatures in neonates. *Western Journal of Nursing Research, 13*(3), 324-335.

JAMES, L., MILNE, D., & FIRTH, H. (1990). A systematic comparison of feedback and staff discussion in changing the ward atmosphere. *Journal of Advanced Nursing, 15,* 329-336.

KILPACK, V., ET AL. (1991). Using research-based interventions to decrease patient falls. *Applied Nursing Research, 4*(2), 50-56.

KRAMER, N. A. (1990). Comparison of therapeutic touch and casual touch in stress reduction of hospitalized children. *Pediatric Nursing, 16*(5), 483-485.

LARSON, E., & ROPKA, M. E. (1991). An update on nursing research and HIV infection. *IMAGE: Journal of Nursing Scholarship, 23*(1), 4-12.

MACIOROWSKI, L. F., ET AL. (1988). A review of the patient fall literature. *Journal of Nursing Quality Assurance, 3*(1), 18-27.

MCMILLAN, S. C., ET AL. (1989). Measurement of chemotherapy-induced nausea and vomiting. *Applied Nursing Research, 2*(2), 93-94.

MULLER, M. E. (1992). A critical review of prenatal attachment research. *Scholarly Inquiry in Nursing Practice, 6*(1), 5-22.

OLSON, R. K., HEATER, B. S., & BECKER, A. M. (March/April 1990). A meta-analysis of the effects of nursing interventions on children and parents. *CN, 15,* 105-109.

O'SULLIVAN, A., & JACOBSEN, B. S. (1992). A randomized trial of a health care program for first-time adolescent mothers and their infants. *Nursing Research, 41*(4), 210-215.

PEPLER, C. J., & KOESTNER, J. (1992). Dementia and nursing home residents' response to choice, National Nursing Research Conference, Charlottetown, PEI.

REBENSON-PIANO, M., ET AL. (1989). An evaluation of two indirect methods of blood pressure measurement in ill patients. *Nursing Research, 38*(1), 42-45.

ROSENDAHL, P. P., & ROSS, V. (1982). Does your behavior affect your patient's response? *Journal of Gerontologic Nursing, 8,* 572-575.

SCHEPP, K. G. (1991). Factors influencing the coping effort of mothers of hospitalized children. *Nursing Research, 40*(1), 42-46.

SHAVER, J. L., & GIBLIN, E. C. (1989). Sleep. *Annual Review of Nursing Research, 7,* 71-93.

STEWART, M. J. (1989). Social support intervention studies: a review and prospectus of nursing contributions. *International Journal of Nursing Studies, 26*(2), 93-114.

VANCOTT, M. L., ET AL. (1991). Analysis of a decade of critical care nursing practice research: 1979 to 1988. *Heart and Lung, 20*(4), 394-397.

WALSH, M., & FORD, P. (1989). *Nursing rituals: Research and rational action.* Oxford: Heinemann Professional Publishing.

WOODS, N. F., ET AL. (1988). Being healthy: Women's images. *Advances in Nursing Science, 11*(1), 36-46.

YOUNGKINS, J. M. (1991). The impact of one staff nurse's research. *American Journal of Maternal Child Nursing, 16,* 133-137.

CONCEPTUAL

AMERICAN NURSES ASSOCIATION. (1989). Education for participation in nursing research. Kansas City, MO: ANA Cabinet on Nursing Research.

BRETT, J. L. L. (1987). Use of nursing practice research findings. *Nursing Research, 36*(6), 344-349.

BRODIE, B. (1988). Voices in distant camps: The gap between nursing research and nursing practice. *Journal of Professional Nursing, 4*(5), 320-328.

CANADIAN NURSES ASSOCIATION. (1990). Research imperative for nursing in Canada: The next five years 1990-1995, Ottawa, Canada: The Association.

CANADIAN ASSOCIATION OF UNIVERSITY SCHOOLS OF NURSING. (1986). Accreditation program, Ottawa, Canada: The Association.

COYLE, L. A., & SOKOP, A. G. (1990). Innovation adoption behaviour among nurses. *Nursing Research, 39*(3), 176-180.

CRANE, J. (1985). Research utilization: Theoretical perspectives. *Western Journal of Nursing Research, 7,* 261-268.

CRANE, J. (1989). Factors associated with the use of research-based knowledge in nursing. Doctoral Dissertation, University of Michigan.

FUNK, S. G., ET AL. (1991a). BARRIERS: the barriers to research utilization scale. *Applied Nursing Research, 4*(1), 39-45.

FUNK, S. G., ET AL. (1991b). Barriers to using findings in practice: The clinician's perspective. *Applied Nursing Research, 4*(2), 90-95.

HAVELOCK, R. G. (1986). The knowledge perspective: Definition and scope of a new study domain. In G. M. Beal, W. Dissanayake, & S. Konoshima (Eds.). *Knowledge generation, exchange, and utilization.* Boulder: Westview Press.

HAVELOCK, R. G., & HAVELOCK, M. (1973). Training for change agents, Ann Arbor: Center for Research on Utilization of Scientific Knowledge, Institute for Social Research, The University of Michigan.

HINSHAW, A. S. (1988). The Center for Nursing Research: Challenges and initiatives. *Nursing Outlook, 36*(2), 54-56.

INTERNATIONAL COUNCIL OF NURSES. (1986). ICN position statement—Nursing research, Geneva: author.

JACOBSEN, B. S., & MENINGER, J. C. (1985). The designs and methods of published nursing research: 1956-1983. *Nursing Research, 34,* 306-312.

KRUEGER, J. C. (1982). Using research in practice. A survey of research utilization in community health nursing. *Western Journal of Nursing Research, 4,* 244-248.

LUKER, K. A., & KENRICK, M. (1992). An exploratory study of the sources of influence on the clinical decisions of community nurses. *Journal of Advanced Nursing, 17,* 457-466.

MERCER, R. T. (1984). Nursing research: The bridge to excellence in practice. *IMAGE: Journal of Nursing Scholarship, 16*(2), 47-51.

MOODY, L. E., ET AL. (1988). Analysis of a decade of nursing practice research. *Nursing Research, 37,* 374-379.

REGISTERED NURSES ASSOCIATION OF BRITISH COLUMBIA. (1991). Making a difference: From ritual to research-based practice, Vancouver, BC: author.

ROGERS, E. M. (1983). *Diffusion of innovations* (3rd ed.). New York: The Free Press.

STETLER, C. B. (1985). Research utilization: Defining the concept. *IMAGE: Journal of Nursing Scholarship, 17,* 40-44.

METHODOLOGICAL

BAKER, V. (1978). Nursing administration and research. *Nursing Leadership, 2,* 5-9.

BARNARD, K. E., & HOEHN, R. E. (1978). Nursing child assessment satellite training: Final report, Hyattsville, MD: DHEW, PHS, HRA, Division of Nursing, Contract No. HRA 231-77-002.

BARNARD, K. E. (1986). Research utilization. The clinical role. *American Journal of Maternal Child Nursing, 11,* 224.

BLOMQUIST, K. B. (1986). Replication of research. *Research in Nursing and Health, 9,* 193-194.

CONWAY, M. E. (1978). Clinical research: Instrument for change. *Journal of Nursing Administration, 8*(12), 27-32.

CRONENWETT, L. R. (1986). Research contributions of clinical nurse specialist. *Journal of Nursing Administration, 16*(6), 6-7.

CRONENWETT, L. R. (1987). Research utilization in a practice setting. *Journal of Nursing Administration, 17*(7,8), 9-10.

DAVIES, B., & DRAKE, E. (1992). Student-staff collaborative power for nursing research, *Canadian Nurse, 88*(1), 30-32.

DONALDSON, N. E. (1991). Research utilization in clinical settings: Models and strategies, Nursing research: Global health perspectives, 1991. Los Angeles: International Nursing Research Conference.

DUFFY, M. E. (1985). Strenthening communication signals to build a research-based practice. *Nursing and Health Care, 6*(5), 238-239.

EDWARDS-BECKETT, J. (1990). Nursing research utilization techniques. *Journal of Nursing Administration, 20*(11), 25-30.

FITCH, M. I. (1992). Five years in the life of a nursing research and professional development division. *Canadian Journal of Nursing Administration, 5*(1), 21-27.

GOODE, C. J., ET AL. (1987). Use of research based knowledge in clinical practice. *Journal of Nursing Administration, 17*(12), 11-18.

GOODE, C., ET AL. (1991). *Research utilization: A study guide.* Ida Grove, IO: Horn Video Productions.

HAGLE, M. E., ET AL. (1986). The clinical nurse researcher: New perspectives. *Journal of Professional Nursing, 2*(5), 282-289.

HALLER, K. B., & REYNOLDS, M. A. (1986). Using research in practice: A case for replication in nursing. II. *Western Journal of Nursing Research, 8*(2), 249-252.

HAMILTON, L., ET AL. (September/October 1990). Organizational support of the clinical nurse specialist role. *Canadian Journal of Nursing Administration, 3,* 9-13.

HEFFERIN, E. A., HORSLEY, J. A., & VENTURA, N. R. (1982). Promoting research-based nursing: The administrator's role. *Journal of Nursing Administration, 12*(5), 34-41.

HICKEY, M. (1990). The role of the clinical nurse specialist in the research utilization process. *Clinical Nurse Specialist, 4*(2), 93-96.

HORSLEY, J. (1985). Using research to practice: The current context. *Western Journal of Nursing Research, 7*(1), 135-139.

HORSLEY (1983). *Using research to improve nursing practice: A guide.* New York: Grune & Stratton.

HORN VIDEO PRODUCTIONS. (1986). *Using research in clinical nursing practice.* Ida Grove, Iowa: author.

HUNT, M. (1987). The process of translating research findings into nursing practice. *Journal of Advanced Nursing, 12,* 101-110.

JANKEN, J. K., DUFAULT, M. A., & YEAW, E. M. S. (1988). Research round tables: increasing student/staff nurse awareness of the relevancy of research to practice. *Journal of Professional Nursing, 4*(3), 186-191.

KIRCHHOFF, K. T. (1991). Who is responsible for research utilization? *Heart and Lung, 20*(3), 308-309.

KNAFL, K. A., ET AL. (1987). Clinical nurse researchers: strategies for success. *Journal of Nursing Administration, 17*(10), 27-31.

KNAFL, K. A., ET AL. (1989). How researchers and administrators view the role of the clinical nurse researcher. *Western Journal of Nursing Research, 11*(5), 583-592.

LARSON, E. (1989). Using the CURN project to teach research utilization in a Baccalaureate program. *Western Journal of Nursing Research, 11*(5), 593-599.

LAWSON, L. (1987). Developing a research structure within the nursing department. *Journal of Nursing Administration, 17*(11).

NEWMAN, L. S., ET AL. (1989). Application of research in clinical practice. *Dimensions of Critical Care Nursing, 8*(6), 364-366.

PARKER, M. E., GORDON, S. C., & BRANNON, P. T. (1992). Involving nursing staff in research, a non-traditional approach. *Journal of Nursing Administration, 22*(4), 58-63.

PEPLER, C. J. (1992). Fostering change through education. *Canadian Nurse, 88*(1), 25-27.

PHILLIPS, L. R. F. (1986). *A clinician's guide to the critique and utilization of nursing research.* Norwalk, CN: Appleton-Century-Crofts.

PINCH, W. J. (1989). Integrating research into practice. *Nursing Education, 13*(3), 30-33.

REMPUSHESKI, V. F. (1992). A researcher as resource, mentor, and preceptor. *Applied Nursing Research, 5*(2), 105-107.

ROSSWURM, M. A. (1992). A research-based practice model in a hospital setting. *Journal of Nursing Administration, 22*(3), 57-60.

SIMMS, L. M., PRICE, S. A., & PFOUTZ, S. K. (1987). Creating the research climate: A key responsibility for nurse executives. *Nursing Economics, 5*(4), 174-179.

SNYDER-HALPERN, R. (1991). Attributes of service-based nursing research programs useful for decision-making. *Nursing Administration Quarterly, 15*(4), 82-84.

STETLER, C. B. (1989). A strategy for teaching research use. *Nursing Education, 13*(3), 17-21.

STETLER, C. B., & DiMAGGIO, G. (1991). Research utilization among clinical nurse specialists. *Clinical Nurse Specialist, 5*(3), 151-155.

SWANSON, J. M., ET AL. (1990). Student-staff collaboration in identifying nursing problems and reviewing the literature. *Western Journal of Nursing Research, 12*(2), 262-265.

SWANSON, J. M., ET AL. (1992). Program efforts for creating a research environment in a clinical setting. *Western Journal of Nursing Research, 14*(2), 241-245.

VAN KOOT, B., & LAVERTY, P. (1992). A research foundation for policies and procedures. *Canadian Nurse, 88*(1), 39-41.

VESSEY, J. A., & CAMPOS, R. G. (1992). The role of nursing research committees. *Nursing Research, 41*(4), 247-249.

WATSON, C. A., BULECHEK, G. M., & McCLOSKEY, J. C. (1987). QAMUR: A quality assurance model using research. *Journal of Nursing Quality Assurance, 2*(1), 21-27.

WILLIAMS, C. (1987). Research utilization: Preparing graduates for responsibilities in development unit policy. *Journal of Professional Nursing, 3*, 264.

HISTORICAL

BARNARD, K. E. (1980). Knowledge for practice: Direction for the future. *Nursing Research, 29*(4), 208-212.

HALPERT, H. P. (1966). Communication as a basic tool in promoting utilization of research findings. *Community Mental Health Journal, 2*, 231-236.

HALLER, K. B., REYNOLDS, M. A., & HORSLEY, J. A. (1979). Developing research-based innovation protocols: Process, criteria, and issues. *Research in Nursing and Health, 2*, 45-51.

HORSLEY, J. A., CRANE, J., & BINGLE, J. D. (July 1978). Research utilization as organizational process. *Journal of Nursing Administration, 8*(7), 4-6.

KETEFIAN, S. (1975). Application of selected nursing findings into nursing practice: A pilot study. *Nursing Research, 24*, 89-92.

KING, D., BARNARD, K. E., & HOEHN, R. (1981). Dissemination the results of nursing research. *Nursing Outlook, 29*(3), 164-169.

KIRCHOFF, K. T. (1982). A diffusion survey of coronary precautions. *Nursing Research, 31*(4), 196-201.

KRUEGER, J. C., NELSON, A. H., & WOLANIN, M. O. (1978). Development, collaboration and utilization. *Nursing Research.*

MALONE, M. F. (Spring 1962). Research communication. *Nursing Forum, 1*, 56-59.

MILLER, J. R., & MESSENGER, S. R. (1978). Obstacles to applying nursing research findings. *American Journal of Nursing, 78*(4), 632-634.

NOTTER, L. E. (1973). Twelve years and sixty editorials later. *Nursing Research, 22*, 387.

ROBERTS I. (1967). Dissemination and use of research reports. *International Journal of Nursing, 14*, 43-45.

STETLER, C. B. (1994). Refinement of the Stetler/Marram model for application of research findings to practice. *Nursing Outlook, 42*(1), 15-25.

STETLER, C. H., & MARRAM, G. (1976). Evaluating research findings for applicability in practice. *Nursing Outlook, 24*(9), 559-563.

PART VI

CONDUCTING NURSING RESEARCH

CHAPTER 25

WRITING A RESEARCH PROPOSAL

AUDREY G. GIFT

Whereas previous chapters have focused on developing a research plan, this chapter focuses on communicating that plan to others in the research proposal.

❧ PURPOSE OF THE PROPOSAL

The proposal is written for a variety of reasons with slight differences in what is expected for each situation.

CRITIQUE BY PEERS

Critique of the proposal can be helpful in making the research easier to understand, improving the research design, or simply clarifying points that were unclear in the written proposal. Critique enhances the learning experience when the research is part of the requirements for an academic degree, but it is also desirable in other situations. Arrangements for critique are negotiated with those who would be most likely to help improve the study.

HUMAN SUBJECT REVIEW

If the research involves human subjects, it is essential that a proposal be written so that a federally regulated Internal Review Board (IRB) can decide if the research procedures will pose any undue risk to the subjects. A separate section on human subject guidelines is required. The process for obtaining informed consent is particularly important.

A description of the study subjects is necessary. If vulnerable subjects, such as unconscious or confused patients, are to be included, the proposal should explain why this is essential and how their rights will be protected. The proposal should indicate that subjects will not be pressured to be in the study, will not be discriminated against if they decide not to participate, will have

571

the opportunity to withdraw from the study if they should decide to do so, and will have the risks and benefits explained to them. The procedures section must indicate exactly what will be done to each subject in the study, when it will be done, and how long it will take. This section should also indicate how consent will be obtained.

The proposal is often accompanied by other forms specifically designed by the IRB to let them know who the person responsible for the study (the principal investigator or the faculty advisor for a student) is and the type of human subjects review desired (exempt, expedited, or full review). When the study is approved, a form or letter indicating that human subject assurances have been given must be received by the principal investigator before data collection can begin.

INSTITUTION BASED RESEARCH COMMITTEE

Before one can gain access to subjects in an institution, that agency's own research committee will review the research proposal to determine the impact of the study on the institution. The proposal should include the following: the site within the institution of the study, the specific criteria and procedures to be used to determine subject eligibility and exclusion, the exact research procedures, the amount of time required of each subject (patient or staff), and assurances that human subject guidelines will be followed. It is essential to plan the study in a manner that will minimize the impact of the research on the routines in the institution.

SUBMISSION FOR FUNDING

A proposal may be written to solicit possible funding. In this situation it is essential to communicate very clearly how the research idea matches the goals of the funding organization. If the funding agency has published guidelines regarding the type of research they will fund, budget limits for their studies, or other requirements for funding, these must be strictly adhered to in writing the proposal. A budget and a justification for the items on the budget are required as well.

PROPOSALS AS CONTRACT

The proposal forms a contract indicating exactly what is to be done. This is especially true when it is written as part of an academic degree or when it has been accepted for funding. There are to be no substantive changes in the contract except when written special permission has been requested by the investigator and accepted by the whole academic committee or the funding agency (Locke, Spirduso, & Silverman, 1987). The terms of the contract are not to be altered by a unilateral decision.

✺ WRITING STYLE

All research proposals, regardless of the intended audience, are to be written in scientific style. They are to be succinct and clearly written in an orderly, logical manner. This is especially true when writing a grant. Funding agencies often impose page limitations that must be strictly followed. Redundancy, wordiness, and embellishments should be avoided. The first draft of the manuscript should be set aside and reread later with the intent of eliminating as many words as possible and of improving the flow of ideas.

One exception to being succinct is the requirement that sexist language be avoided. For instance, the use of "man" or "he" as inclusive terms can be misleading in scientific studies. The writer is required to be specific about the gender being discussed. Also stereotyping, such as using the term "mothering" when nurturing or parenting is discussed, conveys unsupported or biased connotations about roles and should be avoided. The *Publication Manual of the American Psychological Association* (4th ed., 1994) gives examples of how to avoid sexist language.

In addition, care should be taken to use the correct verb tense for each section of the manuscript. The literature review section should be in the past tense (e.g., "Jones showed . . .") or the present perfect tense (e.g., "Researchers have shown . . ."). The methods section is a description of the research that will be done; therefore, it should be written in the future tense (e.g., "Subjects will be asked to . . .").

The proposal should look attractive. A word processor allows for easy correction of errors and facilitates revisions. The pages should be numbered the document printed using an easy-to-read type. This attention to detail will put the reviewer in a favorable frame of mind when reading the proposal.

✍ PROPOSAL DEVELOPMENT PROCESS

Even though it is customary to present a discussion of a research proposal in the order in which the sections are presented in the final document, that is rarely the order in which they are actually written. Therefore, this chapter will be organized to reflect the research study development process. Once the sections are written, they are arranged to follow the recommended order for submission of the proposal and must be read to ensure that information is presented in a logical order. Selecting someone to review the proposal and critique it is essential. At the end of this chapter the order of the sections for the final document will be discussed.

GETTING STARTED: DECIDING ON THE QUESTION

Initial focus should be on the research question or questions. This will guide the rest of the proposal. The studies to be included in the review of the literature, the design, and statistics are selected to address the research questions. The questions may need to be modified as the research study develops more fully, but the main focus should not be lost in these changes.

The formulation of these questions cannot be done in isolation but, rather, is based on knowledge of previous work in the area and of the clinical situation of interest. By knowing the body of knowledge already developed, the researcher is able to identify a conceptual framework and the variables related to it. Questions can then be derived to test this framework, expand it, or test its application with a new population. When little information is available on the topic as it relates to the population of interest, one should explore the literature available on the phenomenon with other related populations. If the researcher does not already have this in-depth understanding of the content area, this step in the planning may require a thorough review of current literature, direct consultation with content and methodological consultants, or interactions with the subject group. This stage is often very time-consuming, especially for the first study done by a novice researcher, but the amount of time needed will usually decrease with each related study. It is essential that the study be accurately conceptualized so as to contribute to the scientific knowledge in the field. This step is, therefore, extremely important (Hill (Part 1), 1988a).

Research questions may be stated in the form of questions or as hypotheses. For hypotheses, sufficient information must be available to make a tentative prediction about the relationship between variables. Otherwise, the exact form is a matter of personal preference or the preference of the student's committee. If the proposal is written for an academic degree or for a funding agency, the guidelines may indicate a preference. Research questions or hypotheses should be clearly stated, include the study variables, be realistic, measurable, and worded in a manner that will match or be consistent with the research design and chosen statistics.

SIGNIFICANCE OF THE STUDY

Once the questions have been formulated, an introduction to the study needs to be written. This section will precede the research questions in the document and will indicate to the reader why the study questions matter. The introduction answers the crucial "so what" question. It indicates to the reader why it is important to know the answers to the research questions (Gordon, 1989). This section might include the incidence of the problem to be researched, information about the devastating effect of not dealing with the problem, or any other information indicating the importance of studying this problem. The length of this section will vary according to the target group for the proposal but is generally rather short.

BACKGROUND FOR THE STUDY/ REVIEW OF THE LITERATURE

The focus of the review of the literature section is to place the present study in the context of previous research. It is especially important to indicate the strengths and weaknesses of prior research. The investigator can outline how the proposed research will improve on previous studies. It might take the information one step further, use more sophisticated methods or measures, have a stronger design, examine a new population of subjects, have a broader focus, or in some other way make a unique contribution to nursing knowledge. At the end of the review, the reader should have a clear idea of how this study fits within the present literature and of the variables to be included. The goal of this review is conceptually to set the stage for the study. This is often different from previous academic assignments and may be difficult for the writer at first.

The conceptual framework used to guide the study is presented just before or after the review of the literature. If a framework that has been used in studying this problem in the past would help the reader by guiding the review of literature, then it should be presented *before* the review of the literature. If, on the other hand, the framework is derived from the review of the literature, it would be best presented at the end of the review of literature. The conceptual framework indicates how the variables of the study are related to one another and can be used to predict or hypothesize the study findings. It provides the investigator with focus and direction in planning the study and interpreting the results.

METHODS SECTION

The methods section of the proposal consists of several subdivisions. These can vary with different studies, but generally they include the research design, sample, measurement instruments, procedures, and plan for analysis. If different treatments are being tested, a section in which they are described must also be included. This section usually precedes the procedure section. Each subdivision of this section will be discussed in detail.

The Research Design

The ideal research design is the one that will best answer the question being asked. Some researchers describe experimental designs as ideal; however, it is not necessarily the best method for all research questions. The design should be chosen to answer the research questions (Hill, Part 2, 1988b). The description of the design usually comes at the beginning of the methods section of the proposal and may be described in one sentence or may require several paragraphs. Often a quantitative design can be described by simply naming the design or using brief diagrams that represent observations (O) and treatments (X) (see Chapter 12). Time intervals can also be included. Such figures can quickly convey the design and eliminate lengthy descriptions of sequences and intervals. For a qualitative study, the research procedures to be followed are indicated.

Possible threats to internal, external, construct, and statistical conclusion validity are to be addressed in the proposal. Although the methods section is the appropriate place to address these threats, each one may fit best within a different subsection of the methods section. Those threats to validity that are eliminated or most affected by the study design should be described in the design section. Others may be best addressed during the description of the sampling technique, the measures, the procedures, or the analysis. The methodological choices made to minimize the validity threats should be made explicit in the text.

Selecting the Setting

Formulating the research design cannot be done in isolation from the setting in which it is to be carried out. It may not be possible to carry out the ideal design in the chosen setting. Feasibility must be assessed early in the research process. It is critical that the investigator consult personnel in the clinical setting to formulate a plan that will minimize disturbance in the clinical routine. In some institutions, such as hospitals, patient care is a priority over academic concerns. Access to patients or staff may be refused if the study interferes with

---

EXAMPLE OF DESIGN SECTION

This is an experimental design with subjects randomly assigned to a treatment or control group. To prevent the threat of compensatory equalization of treatment, treatment and control subjects will be cared for by nurses on different floors. Thus the nurses caring for the control subjects will not be taught the treatments and will not have access to the equipment. This will also prevent the threats of resentful demoralization and compensatory rivalry of control subjects, who will be unaware of the treatments being administered to the other subjects. To ensure that randomization eliminated selection threats, the treatment and control groups will be compared on demographics and on the premeasures.

---

care or is time-consuming for patients or staff. Also, if the study is expected to have an impact on care given by a health care provider, the details of the study design and protocol need to be discussed with health care providers and administrators early in the planning stage. It is helpful to work with personnel at all levels within the organization to identify sources of support and to prevent potential roadblocks.

Some institutions are not sophisticated about nursing research and federal guidelines regarding research. As a result, they may impose needless restrictions on a nurse conducting research. For example, a hospital may require that before any patient can be asked to participate in a nursing study the physician caring for that patient must give permission for the patient to be approached. Although it would be appropriate to add this extra step for a study interfering with the medical management of the patient, it is not necessary in every study. Federal guidelines for protection of human subjects require consent of the individual who will be studied. Only when people are declared incompetent to make such decisions for themselves is a guardian required for the consent. If needless restrictions are imposed on a study, a nurse re-

searcher would be wise to consider another institution in which to conduct research.

Special events that may be planned to occur in the target institution can also distort the study findings. An example would be a health fair to screen and educate clinic patients about hypertension just before a study of patient knowledge of hypertension is to be implemented. Another example would be a pay raise for nurses just before a study questionnaire is administered to determine nurse job satisfaction. Such events distort the generalizability of the study findings and should be avoided if at all possible. Requesting a delay of the event until after the completion of data collection or selecting a different research site are strategies for dealing with such problems.

The researcher needs to verify the availability of potential subjects in the chosen setting and determine the likelihood of subjects being available at the time of data collection. If too few subjects are available, the researcher will want to rethink the study or select a different site. This is especially important if the study is to involve patients admitted to the hospital in a cyclical or seasonal pattern.

The courtesy of keeping personnel in the institution informed of the study during

---

EXAMPLE OF SAMPLE SECTION

A convenience sample will be obtained from all adult patients admitted to a large metropolitan medical center with a diagnosis meeting the American Thoracic Society (1987) definition of Chronic Obstructive Pulmonary Disease and experiencing dyspnea at the time of admission. Those who have an additional medical diagnosis that might interfere with their sensory perception (such as diabetic neuropathy) or a diagnosis (such as cancer or AIDS) that might involve extreme emotional disturbances will not be included. A history of psychiatric problems and inability to understand English are additional exclusion criteria.

Power Analysis. The effect size was found in preliminary studies to range from 1.08 to .625. Considering the smallest effect size, a sample size of 20 in each group would be needed to achieve 80% power.

---

the planning and approval stages should not be ignored. Before the study is to begin, the best method for informing staff and professional personnel in the institution about the study should be decided. There should be a clear understanding of responsibilities of all personnel.

The Sample

The sample to be included in the study, the site, and sampling plan need to be described in such a way that the reviewer can judge the adequacy of the technique. All criteria used to screen potential subjects for inclusion and exclusion from the study should be specifically stated. Factors used to describe potential subjects often include their medical diagnosis, age group, cognitive functioning, ability to understand English, and the like.

The sampling method needs to be identified. If a convenience sample is to be used, this should be made clear. The entire population may not be identifiable, making simple random sampling impossible. The best sampling technique will depend on the research question. The investigator must consider the relative importance of internal versus external validity for the study. There is no single best sampling technique for all studies. (See Chapter 13 for more detail.)

The ideal sample size should be indicated in the proposal by including a power analysis, a procedure for estimating sample size requirements. Investigators breaking new ground must first conduct a pilot study to obtain the information needed for a power analysis, such as the means, standard deviations, and, if possible, the expected difference between groups.

Measurement

In this section of the proposal all the instruments and data collection forms used in the study are described. It is critical that the researcher be very familiar with all such instruments before using them in a study. Copies of instruments and permission for use should be obtained far in advance of proposing a study and included in the proposal's appendix. Likewise, working with a physiological instrument or practicing the procedures for analyzing a biological sample will help the researcher determine the usefulness of the measure for the particular study being planned.

The description of the instrument should start by indicating which variable it is designed to measure. The theoretical definition of the variable as it is to be used in the study, the construct used to devise the instrument, and a connection between the theoretical and operational definition of the variable need to be clarified here. A full description of the measure should then be given. For example, if it is a paper-and-pencil test, the length of the instrument, type of questions asked, the range and type of scale used for obtaining answers, the full range of possible scores for the instrument, the reading level, the time expected for subjects to complete the survey, and the scoring procedure are to be included in this description.

The type of reliability and validity established for the instrument and the method by which it was done need to be specified and references given for additional information. Types of reliability checks to be included in the conduct of the study should be specified. Internal consistency, such as calculation of a Cronbach's alpha for items on the scale, and stability of the measure, such as the use of test-retest reliability, are the most frequently used methods for establishing reliability of instruments within a study. If multiple data collectors are involved, it is essential to establish and maintain interrater reliability through training and retraining.

Some research designs allow concurrent comparisons of instruments and the establishment of an instrument's validity within the study. This is essential if the instrument does not already have well-established validity.

Scoring techniques for the instrument should be described. This helps communicate the level of measurement each instrument represents. These methods should be known early in the formulation of the study. Instruments that require skilled professionals or specialized equipment to administer or to score may be too expensive for the unfunded researcher. The time required for scoring is helpful information

when planning a time frame for completion of the study.

For clinical or physiological measures it is important to identify the exact instrument used to measure the variable, the manufacturer of the instrument, the calibration procedures to be applied, and the exact protocol to be used when obtaining the measure. Information about the precision and accuracy of the instrument are usually available from the manufacturer.

If a biologic specimen is required in the study, the collection procedures, handling procedures, and the assay or technique for specimen analysis need to be fully described. The specificity and sensitivity of the assay or technique are to be stated. In some circumstances these can only be run in specific national laboratories, and it is sufficient to state the name of the laboratory and their protocol.

Treatments

If the study is one in which different groups of subjects are to receive an experimental treatment or test, the precise technique or treatment needs to be indicated in the proposal (Tornquist & Funk, 1990). If more than one treatment is provided or a control (nontreatment) group is used, the investigator should describe each group and treatment separately. The length of the treatment as well as the setting in which it will be provided should be stated for each group.

Procedures

Once the design and measures have been determined, the flow of events in the execution of the study are fairly easy to anticipate. The procedures section of the proposal states exactly what is to be done to the subjects in the study, including all measures taken and treatments given. It begins with a description of where and how subjects will be identified for inclusion in

EXAMPLE OF MEASUREMENT SECTION

Anxiety will be assessed using the Spielberger Anxiety Inventory, which is a self-report scale designed to measure both state (SSAI) and trait (STAI) anxiety. State anxiety is a transitory emotional state or condition that is characterized by subjective, consciously perceived feelings of tension and apprehension as well as heightened autonomic nervous system activity that may vary in intensity and fluctuate over time. Trait anxiety is a personality trait regarding the tendency to perceive stressful situations as dangerous or threatening. The inventory consists of two scales of 20 statements each, one asking the subject to indicate how he or she feels at the moment (for the state anxiety scale) and how he or she usually feels (for the trait anxiety scale) on a range from 1 to 4, "not at all" to "very much so." It is designed for a fifth-grade reading ability. The scales are balanced for acquiescence set with 10 items reversed on each scale. It requires approximately 10 minutes to administer it the first time. The inventory, commonly used in the written form, can also be administered in the narrative mode, as will be done in this study (Spielberger, Gorsuch, Lushene, Vagg, & Jacobs, 1983). The state anxiety scale has been shown to be sensitive to changes in dyspnea intensity in COPD patients (Gift, Plaut, & Jacox, 1986).

Reliability was established using two methods, stability and internal consistency. The test-retest correlations for the scales range from .32 to .54 for the state scale, reflecting the transitory nature of that scale, and .73 to .86 for the more stable trait scale. Internal consistency, using Cronbach's alpha, was found to be .83 and .92 for the state and trait scales, respectively. Construct validity for the state scale was established by demonstrating significantly higher scores in an anxiety-producing situation than in a more relaxed situation. The Inventory has also been shown to correlate with other measures of anxiety (Spielberger et al., 1983).

Scoring is done on each scale by weighing each item from 1 to 4, with 4 always indicating higher anxiety regardless of the wording of the item. The weights for each item are then totaled for the subject's score on each scale (Spielberger et al., 1983). In the present study the validity of the scale will be determined by comparing the state anxiety scores to scores on the anxiety subscale of the Brief Symptom Inventory (BSI). A Cronbach's alpha will be determined for reliability of both scales.

EXAMPLE OF TREATMENT SECTION

Group A: Treatment Group. The teaching of relaxation techniques will be done at the patient's bedside by the research assistant. Teaching will be done in a standardized manner with subjects placed in a comfortable position and asked to listen to a prerecorded tape teaching them progressive relaxation techniques according to the procedure recommended by Bernstein and Borkovec (1973) for tension release in 16 muscle groups. The achievement of relaxation will be determined by measuring peripheral skin temperature, heart rate, and respiratory rate. Preliminary studies indicate that relaxation is achieved when subjects are able to elevate their skin temperature by at least 2 degrees, decrease their heart rate by at least three beats per minute, and decrease their respiratory rate by at least two breaths per minute during relaxation. The relaxation tape runs for 30 minutes.

Group B: Control Group. Subjects entered into the control group will be cared for by the medical and nursing staff on a separate unit without being taught relaxation techniques for dyspnea reduction.

EXAMPLE OF PROCEDURES SECTION

As soon as possible after admission to the hospital, subjects will be approached by a research assistant, provided information about the study, and asked to sign a written consent. All those willing to participate will have their medical records reviewed for demographic information and health history. All subjects will be asked to indicate the intensity of their dyspnea (VADS), to complete the Spielberger State Anxiety Inventory (SSAI), and the Brief Symptom Inventory (BSI).

Subjects will then be randomly assigned to treatment or control group with those assigned to the treatment group admitted to the treatment unit. The treatment group will receive relaxation instruction as indicated. Afterward they will complete the VADS, SSAI, and BSI. Those assigned to the control group will be admitted to a control unit and asked to complete the VADS, SSAI, and BSI minutes after being admitted to the unit.

EXAMPLE OF ANALYSIS SECTION

To address specific aim 1 and 2, the treatment group will be compared to the control group using a 2×2 repeated measures ANOVA (2 group x pre- vs. post treatment). An alpha level of .01 will be used.

---

the study and how consent will be obtained. Then each measure and procedure is listed in order of sequence. A description of the data collectors and place and time of the measurements and/or treatments must also be included. If the data collectors are to be blinded (purposefully unaware) to the group assignment of subjects when they collect the data, this needs to be indicated. The future tense is used in writing the procedures section.

Analysis
In this section the researcher indicates the data analysis procedure or procedures to be used to answer each separate research question. It is clearest to repeat each research question and list the analysis technique and level of statistical significance to be used to answer it (Fuller, et al., 1991). This is helpful even though one analysis technique may be used to answer several questions.

REVISING THE PROPOSAL

The proposal writing process is one of constant building and improvement. Once the first draft of the proposal has been written as clearly and accurately as possible, it should be reviewed and critiqued by others (see box on p. 581). Reviewers should have clinical and/or research expertise and be willing to participate. These may be faculty or peers or other investigators who deal with the same subject population or specialty under investigation. Experts who can strengthen the proposal are the most valuable. The time spent in reviewing and improving the proposal early in the process will result in a stronger study.

It is often frustrating for novice researchers to realize that when one part of the proposal is changed, there are ramifications for other parts of the proposal. Using a word processor has become a necessity because of the many revisions commonly required. Periodically during the development stage, the proposal needs to be read through from beginning to end for consistency. For example, when a measurement instrument is changed, the procedures section would need to be revised to include the new measure and delete reference to the old one. Changing research questions requires even more extensive changes in the rest of the proposal.

SEQUENCE OF SECTIONS IN THE PROPOSAL

The order in which the various sections of the proposal are to appear is determined by the agency for whom the proposal is being written. The format recommended by the American Psychological Association (APA, 1994) is as follows:

Title page
Abstract
Significance of the study
Study background/literature review
Methods section
    Design
    Sample
    Measures
    Procedures
    Analysis
References
Appendices

If the proposal is written for a funding institution, a budget and budget justification will be required and will usually precede the study. A timeline, if included, will usually follow the budget pages. Biographic sketches of key personnel, other sources of support, a description of the resources, and environment for research are required sections in federal funding proposals and usually follow the timeline and precede the body of the proposal. If a section indicating previous work of the principal investigator is required, it will usually be presented after the background of the study.

It is important for investigators to be aware of any specific agency or university guidelines that may be required for sections of the proposal and the exact order in which they are presented. Some agencies will not review proposals that do not follow their specific proposal guidelines, regardless of the quality or merit of the study.

TITLE PAGE
The title for the study should indicate the topic, the study design, variables of interest, and the population studied. It often will serve as a guide for key words used to index the work in the library. The recom-

EXAMPLE OF AN ABSTRACT

This is the first known nursing intervention study aimed at relieving the distressing symptom of dyspnea in inpatients with chronic obstructive pulmonary disease (COPD). An experimental design is used to test the effectiveness of progressive relaxation techniques in the reduction of dyspnea. Forty COPD subjects admitted to a local medical center will be randomly assigned to treatment or control groups. Subject records will be reviewed for demographics and health history. All subjects will rate the intensity of their dyspnea (VADS) and complete the Spielberger State Anxiety Inventory (SSAI) and the Brief Symptom Inventory (BSI). Those assigned to the treatment group will be taught relaxation techniques using a taped message lasting 30 minutes. Afterward they will again be asked to complete the VADS, SSAI, and BSI. Control subjects will receive routine care and complete measures identical to the treatment subjects', 30 minutes after the first measures. A 2 × 2 analysis of variance (ANOVA) with one repeated measure will be used to analyze the data.

Key Words: Dyspnea, relaxation, COPD, Anxiety

REDUCING DYSPNEA USING TAPED RELAXATION

TECHNIQUES IN THOSE WITH COPD

BY

AUDREY G. GIFT, RN, PhD, FAAN.

ASSOCIATE PROFESSOR

UNIVERSITY OF PENNSYLVANIA

SCHOOL OF NURSING

PHILADELPHIA, PA

RUNNING HEAD: Relaxation for dyspnea relief

Figure 25-1. Example of a title page.

mended length of titles is 12 to 15 words. Some agencies will require the title to fit within the number of characters allocated for titles on their computer data base. An example is a limit of 56 characters, including spaces. This allows few words and makes brevity essential.

The title page will also include the author's name and affiliation. Some will request that the author indicate key words for characterizing the proposal and perhaps a running head, which is an abbreviated title to appear at the head of each page. The *Publication Manual of the American Psychological Association* restricts running heads to a maximum of 50 characters, counting letters, punctuation, and spaces between words. An example is shown in Figure 25-1.

Funding agencies and some universities require their own form to be used as the first page of the document instead of the title page. This allows them to have the information they require in a familiar format.

THE ABSTRACT

The abstract is a brief but comprehensive presentation of the research proposal. It is usually the last section to be written, even though it is usually the first page of the submitted proposal. It is the first section read by reviewers and funding agencies—and often the only section they read. This brief statement must communicate to the reader

	Jan	Feb	Mar	Apr	May	June
Principal investigator						
Hire personnel	X	X				
Recruit subjects			X			
Train personnel			X			
Supervise personnel				X	X	X
Write research report						X
Research assistant						
Administer treatment			X			
Collect data			X	X		
Enter data into computer					X	X
Analyze data						X

Figure 25-2. Example of a timeline.

the essential parts of the proposal and should follow the same order of presentation as the proposal itself. It is essential that the abstract be as clear as possible. Often abstracts are restricted to a limited number of words, usually 100 to 150. If so, this will be specified in the guidelines for the proposal, but abstracts are rarely longer than one typed page. Abstracts should include only material discussed in the body of the proposal. Abbreviations and references should not be used. The active, rather than the passive, voice is used in the abstract.

TIME SCHEDULE

It is important for the researcher to estimate how long the research project will take to complete. A timeline will also indicate who will be doing what at each stage of the research process. This is very helpful to investigators allocating resources, hiring staff, and planning a budget for the research project. It also allows the grant reviewer to know exactly what the researcher intends to do at each phase of the research. It should, of course, be only a summary of what the researcher has already indicated in the proposal but formatted in a specific timeline.

The format for a timeline can vary. It may list dates by which each activity should be completed or begin and end, which is easily done with a chart or diagram. It is common to use weeks or months across the top of the page with personnel and the activities listed along the left-hand column. An X under the date next to the activity would indicate when it was to be performed. This indicates what each person will be doing at each time and can give the reader an idea of simultaneous activities. An example of a timeline is shown in Figure 25-2.

The personnel required to carry out the

EXAMPLES OF REFERENCES FROM TWO MANUALS

1. A reference list written according to the *Publication Manual of the American Psychological Association, 4th ed.* (APA, 1994) would have all references listed in alphabetical order using the following format:

Moore, T., & Soeken, K. (1992). Relaxation to reduce dyspnea and anxiety in COPD patients. *Nursing Research, 41,* 242-246.

2. A reference list written according to the *American Medical Association Manual of Style* (AMA, 1989) would have references numbered and listed in the order in which they appear in the text. References would have the following format:

1. Moore T, Soeken K. Relaxation to reduce dyspnea and anxiety in COPD patients. Nursing Research 1992;41:242-246.

---

study should be obvious from the description of the research. Time to hire personnel, order equipment, orient staff, collect data, and carry out other research procedures needs to be estimated. To construct a timeline, specific information is required about the potential availability of subjects, refusal rate projections, and for a longitudinal study, the expected mortality rate. These data are necessary to build a feasible estimate of the time required for data collection. The data-scoring, -entry, and -analysis phases must also be estimated.

The timeline is also used during the planning phase as a basis for preparing the budget for a funded study. Personnel positions are described, as are their activities; the percentage of time they require to complete tasks can then be estimated. The timeline also indicates why the study is judged to take the time indicated. Once the project is under way, the timeline can be used as a guide to project progress.

REFERENCES

The reference section lists all the journal articles or other sources of information cited in the text. The specific manual of style recommended by the institution for whom the proposal is being prepared should be

followed for the list of references and the format of citations in the text. If no manual of style is stipulated, one should be chosen by the researcher and the form for citations and references followed. The box outlines two common styles.

APPENDIX

The appendix is the section in which all supporting documents are contained, such as data collection tools and accompanying letters of permission to use. Many funding agencies and universities require letters of agreement from agencies indicating the willingness of the institution to cooperate with the study. If instruments are copyrighted, or if their circulation is restricted, a few sample items may be reproduced.

GRANT WRITING

When a proposal is written for a funding agency, additional sections frequently need to be added to the proposal. It is essential that the researcher use these sections to indicate how the research study being proposed meets the funding objectives of the agency. In addition, extra sections are added to the proposal to enable the funding agency to evaluate the competence of the researcher, merit of other members of the research team, resources in the research environment, and the appropriateness of the proposed budget.

BIOGRAPHIC SKETCH

The biographic sketch displays the competence of the principal investigator (PI), the individual responsible for carrying out the research. It is vital that this biographic sketch indicate the experience of the PI with the research being proposed, the population to be studied, the instruments to be used, or any other experience that will contribute to the success of the research. A publication track record, particularly publications of earlier, related research, indicates that the PI is likely to publish the findings of the study.

Biographic sketches are also usually required for coinvestigators and consultants. These other research team members especially matter if the PI is not an experienced researcher. It is important to communicate to reviewers how team members will contribute and how as a group they present all the skills needed to carry out the research.

OTHER SUPPORT

Funding allocated to the principal investigator and other key personnel on the grant is listed. The source of the support, the percentage of time committed to that project, the dates of the project, and costs that indicate the size of the project are to be included. Any overlap between other funded projects and the proposed one should be discussed.

PRELIMINARY STUDIES

This section describes all previous studies conducted by the research team that relate to the present study. The purpose of the section is to indicate the competency and

experience of the research team beyond the biographic sketches. Both published and unpublished studies by the investigator(s) should be included in this section. A suggested format is to indicate the aim of each preliminary study, the research methods, and the findings.

Pilot testing done for the proposed study is explained in this section. Pilot testing helps predict the expected findings of the study and provides data to indicate that the proposed study will produce the expected results. The researcher also demonstrates that subjects and other resources are available for the study.

RESOURCES

This section describes the environment in which the study is to be carried out. Available facilities, such as computer access, consultation services, and library facilities should be described in detail. The commitment of the institution to the research should be clarified here. Space and equipment allocated for the research indicate to the funding agent the agency's level of commitment.

Consortium arrangements with facilities such as clinics or hospitals may be described in this section or in a separately labeled section. Letters of support from these agencies are to be included in the appendix.

BUDGET

When the proposal is written as a grant to obtain research funding, it is necessary to include a budget. A budget consists of a listing of the money required to carry out the research proposal and a justification for how that money will be used. This is done to allow the funding agency to decide whether the project is worth the expense. Funding agencies typically have a budget range for the studies they fund. It is wise to ensure that the project is within that range. This information is obtained by contacting the funding agency and asking about previously funded studies.

It is very important to anticipate exactly what research costs will be. Should the research grant be awarded, the study must be carried out within the budgeted amount. Experience dictates that costs are always greater than expected, so the researcher should make every effort to estimate the cost of the research accurately. Each budget category should be examined separately, and the real cost should be estimated as closely as possible. When appropriate, a cost-of-living increase to salaries and some purchased goods should be added and indicated in the budget justification section (Krathwohl, 1988).

The first step in preparing a budget is to read the guidelines provided by the funding agency carefully. Often funding agencies divide costs into categories specified in the guidelines. The actual budget may be written on a form specifically designed by the agency; it should be accompanied by the budget justification. Agencies differ in the types of items or services they will fund. Some will not allow computers to be purchased, some have limits on salaries, consultant fees, and the like. It is essential that the researcher adhere to these guidelines. It is also important to note how much flexibility the agency will allow in moving funds from one budget category to another after the grant is awarded. If there is little flexibility, it becomes vital that much care be given to determine appropriate costs in each category. Categories commonly used for budget preparation are the following.

Personnel
This first category includes all individuals considered necessary to conduct the re-

search. For most nursing research, this is the largest budget category. Referring to the timeline for the study will help determine who will be needed, the amount of effort required, and the length of time they will be needed. The name of the person (if known), the title indicating his or her responsibilities, the percentage of time to be devoted to the project, and salary and fringe benefits are commonly required in the budget.

The budget justification section is usually a separate section, but rather than writing it after the whole budget has been developed, it is easier to write it as each category of the budget is thought out. For personnel, each person is listed on the justification form along with a description of exactly what he or she is expected to do. The evaluators will be judging whether the appropriate number and type of personnel needed to complete the research have been included.

Consultants
An important part of personnel included on a grant consists of the consultant(s). Because they are only available for a short time during the study, they are usually listed separately from personnel. They tend to be included on an hourly or daily basis with a set fee for that amount of time. The fee is determined by the consultant and should be negotiated when they are invited to participate in the study. It is imperative that the researcher contact consultants during the planning stage of the study before they are listed on a grant. Most will want to see a copy of the grant beforehand to evaluate its scientific merit and decide whether they wish to participate. If you need help from them to improve the scientific merit of the proposal, ask for that early in the planning stage.

The budget justification for the consultant(s) should include a brief description of their credentials to indicate what they will contribute to the quality of the study.

Equipment

Equipment refers to those items that are permanent or may be used again after the project has been completed. Some funding agencies will allow the equipment to remain with the research institution at the completion of the project, and others collect the equipment so that it may be used by other researchers. This is usually specified at the time the grant is awarded. List each type of equipment separately, indicating the manufacturer and its cost. The budget justification section for equipment should indicate how each item will be used and by whom.

Supplies

Supplies are consumable goods, such as office supplies, clinical materials, or tests. It is almost impossible to be certain about the exact costs and quantities of these items, but a reasonable estimate must be included.

Travel

This is sometimes subdivided into local, national, and on rare occasions, international travel. List first the travel needs inherent in the research design, such as costs for home visits if they are required. Travel for consultants needs to be included, and often so does travel to present research findings. It is best to include a breakdown of those costs with airfare, hotel costs, meals, and such listed. Consult the guidelines provided by the funding agency to determine if there is a limit for travel costs.

Patient Care Costs

This includes any costs incurred by patients treated in either an outpatient or inpatient facility. The health care institution determines these costs. If subjects are paid for their participation in the research study, include these costs here. Rationale for the costs are included in the budget justification.

Other Expenses

This section includes all expenses not included in other categories. Costs for computer time, postage, publication, library fees, copying, and telephone service are items commonly included in this category. Justification for each item in this category is required.

Indirect Costs

Large granting agencies will pay research institutions for the overhead costs of maintaining the institution. If these costs are allowed, they will help finance such things as the bookkeeping office, purchasing department, library, and general building and ground maintenance. The allowance for these costs in the budget will be specified in the guidelines for the research award.

Second Year of Funding

When a research project lasts more than 1 year, the researcher is expected to specify the costs anticipated for the second year of funding. This budget will be considerably less detailed than the first-year budget. Items continue to be listed in their categories but are usually not itemized within the category. Justification focuses on reasons for changes from the first to the second year. Any expected percentage increase in items, such as salaries, should be included.

REVIEW OF THE BUDGET

The business or administrative office in the institution that will receive the funds must approve the budget well ahead of the deadline for submission of the grant. Changes are often made, more information may be required, and typically the forms have to be retyped.

FUNDING SOURCES

Funding for research can come from a variety of sources. These sources can be categorized as being within the institution itself (internal sources) or from outside the institution (external sources). Only external sources will be discussed here. The most important factor to consider when selecting a source for funding is the institution's mission or funding objectives. Each organization targets certain research topics for funding and will not fund projects outside of that area. Communication with the funding source to determine their funding goals, the titles of previously funded projects, and the budget amounts they routinely award is essential (Strickland, et al., 1987).

Nursing Organizations

Nursing organizations, such as Sigma Theta Tau, The American Association of Critical Care Nurses, and the Oncology Nurses Society, have research programs that allow them to fund small research projects. Information packets contain guidelines indicating the focus of their particular research interests, what to include in a proposal, submission deadlines, and funding amounts.

Businesses and Corporations

If a research proposal involves the testing of a particular piece of equipment or of a commercially available product, the researcher should explore the possibility of obtaining funding from the company that produces the product. Although the dollar amounts of research awards from these sources are often small, many will fund the research and/or supply their products for the study.

Nongovernmental Agencies

Nongovernmental agencies, which include organizations such as the American Heart Association, American Cancer Society, and American Lung Association, have a focus for their research effort. Their area of research interest is usually obvious by the title of the organization. They may, however, focus on a particular problem of interest to them. It is helpful to know of such priorities ahead of time. They also usually have funding initiatives for a particular level of researcher, such as funding for only beginning researchers or for only those with an established research program. Funding success will be determined by how well the project and researcher meet the guidelines.

Foundations

A number of foundations fund research (Beard, 1985). A foundation is a nongovernmental, nonprofit organization with its own funds. Often these are from an individual, family, or corporation. A foundation usually has programs managed by its directors and trustees and is established to maintain or aid charitable, religious, educational, social, or other activities serving the common good. It may provide financial assistance to other nonprofit organizations. Foundations from which nurses have received funding include The Robert Wood Johnson Foundation, American Nurses Foundation, and the W. K. Kellogg Foundation.

Consult a directory to obtain information about foundations. One such directory is *The Foundation Directory,* which lists over 7000 foundations. Librarians can assist in locating other, similar listings of funding opportunities. Directories can be used to locate a foundation interested in funding research that matches your area of interest (Kemp, 1991). Examine the current goals and objectives of these institutions for their research priorities.

It is important also to know the budget amounts on grants funded by each foundation. Foundations tend to award research proposals at a specific time of the year. It is important to meet the funding deadlines as some foundations change their funding priorities annually, and a proposal delayed for a year may no longer fall within their priorities.

Federal Institutions

Research funding comes through the Public Health Service, specifically the National Institutes of Health. The Institutes are organized around substantive areas of research from which nurse researchers are eligible for funding (Cowan, 1992). The research interests of nurses, however, make them more likely to seek funding from the National Institute of Nursing Research and such institutes as the National Institute on Aging, National Institute of Mental Health, and the National Institute of Child Health and Human Development. The Agency for Health Care Policy and Research (AHCPR) is another possible source of funding. Federal funding for research is highly competitive.

The Public Health Service published *Healthy People 2000* in 1990, focusing on health promotion and disease prevention. This document provides a guideline for research funding priorities for most federal funding agencies. In addition, each government funding unit publishes information about its particular research goals. It would be wise to examine these before beginning a study. The *NIH Guide for Grants and Contracts* is published to announce scientific initiatives and changes in focus for grants

and contract activities of the National Institutes of Health.

EXPECTATIONS OF THOSE WHO FUND RESEARCH

Agencies require periodic reports of the progress of the research, often annually. Reports generally need to include what has been done, the number of subjects admitted to the study, any problems encountered, findings to date if they are known, and a projected schedule of activities for the next reporting period.

Funding agencies expect the research to be published, and most expect to have the agency listed as the funding source. The agency may also expect the researchers to attend annual meetings or make presentations regarding their research. Assuming that the research results are favorable to the agency, it may take an active role in publicizing the project findings. Requests to notify the local newspaper, report on the project in its trade journal, or use the researcher's name in its publications are not uncommon.

SUMMARY

- The purpose of the research proposal determines the sections to be included and the amount of attention to be given to each.
- Research proposals are to be written in a scientific style using nonsexist, inclusive language.
- Sections of the proposal do not have to be written in the order in which they will appear in the submitted document.
- The research questions or hypotheses provide the focus for the whole proposal.
- The introductory part of the proposal indicates why it is important to know the answers to the questions being posed in

the research. This is usually labeled "Introduction" or "Significance of the Study." The second part, the "Background" or "Literature Review," places the present study in the context of previous work and provides the scientific rationale or the framework for variables included in the study.

- The methods part of the proposal consists of several sections.
  The design is described first.
  The sample to be included in the study and the techniques to be used to obtain the sample need to be described in the second section.
  All research instruments to be used in the study and their reliability and validity data are listed in the measures section.
  The procedures section consists of a description of all procedures used to obtain the research data.
  The last section of the methods part of the proposal specifies the techniques to be used for data analysis. How these methods will answer the research questions should be made clear.
- Critique by experts and subsequent revisions of the research proposal are important to improve the quality.
- All proposals need a title page, abstract, and reference list.
- It is helpful for the reviewer to have a time schedule for the research to refer to while reading the proposal.
- When a proposal is written to obtain funding, additional sections such as biographical sketches, preliminary studies, resources to support research, and a budget are needed.
- Budget categories include personnel, consultants, equipment, supplies, travel, patient care, other costs, and indirect costs. Justification of items in each budget category is required.

- Funding sources include nursing organizations, businesses and corporations, nongovernmental agencies, private foundations, benefactors, and the federal government.
- The proposal should be written in a manner that addresses the objectives of the target audience or funding agency.

FACILITATING CRITICAL THINKING

Obtain and review a research proposal. Consider the following questions in your review:

1. Does the proposal communicate the importance of the research?
2. Is the proposal clear and specific with logical consistency among the sections?
3. If there is a budget, is it appropriate with adequate resources identified to complete the research?
4. Does the proposal meet the funding agency's goals?
5. Does the proposal have scientific merit?
6. Are there adequate facilities for the research to be carried out?

References

SUBSTANTIVE

NAYLOR, M. D. (1990). Special feature, an example of a research grant application: Comprehensive discharge planning for the elderly. *Research in Nursing & Health, 13*, 327-347.

CONCEPTUAL

AMERICAN MEDICAL ASSOCIATION. (1989). *The American Medical Association manual of style* (8th ed.). Baltimore: Williams & Wilkins.

AMERICAN PSYCHOLOGICAL ASSOCIATION. (1994). *Publication manual of the American Psychological Association* (4th ed.). Washington, DC: The Association.

GORDON, A. L. (1989). Ingredients of a successful grant application to the National Institutes of Health. *Journal of Orthopaedic Research, 7*, 139-141.

METHODOLOGICAL

BEARD, M. T. (1985). Foundations: Finding the right funding source. *CNR: Newsletter for the American Nurses Association, Council of Nurse Researchers, 12*(1), 1-3.

COWAN, M. J. (1992). Facts about the National Center for Nursing Research. *Cardiovascular Nursing, 28*(2), 9-14.

FULLER, E. O., HASSELMEYER, E. G., HUNTER, J. C., ABDELLAH, F. G., & HINSHAW, A. S. (1991). Summary statements of the NIH nursing research grant applications. *Nursing Research, 40,* 346-351.

HILL, M. N. (1988a). Writing a research proposal: The first step in conducting research, Part 1. *Cardiovascular Nursing, 24,* 1-4.

HILL, M. N. (1988b). Writing a research proposal: The first step in conducting research, Part 2. *Cardiovascular Nursing, 24,* 7-11.

KEMP, C. (1991). A practical approach to writing successful grant proposals. *Nurse Practitioner, 16*(11), 51-56.

KRATHWOHL, D. R. (1988). *How to prepare a research proposal* (3rd ed.). Syracuse: Syracuse University Press.

LOCKE, L. F., SPIRDUSO, W. W., & SILVERMAN, S. J. (1987). *Proposals that work: A guide to planning dissertations and grant proposals that work* (2nd ed.). Newbury Park, CA: Sage.

STRICKLAND, O. L., BURGESS, A. W., OBERST, M. T., & KIM, H. S. (1987). Private sector support of nursing research. *Nursing Research, 36,* 253-256.

SULTZ, H. A., & SHERWIN, F. S. (1981). *Grant writing for health professionals.* Boston: Little, Brown.

TORNQUIST, E. M., & FUNK, S. G. (1990). How to write a research grant proposal. *IMAGE: Journal of Nursing Scholarship, 22,* 44-51.

CHAPTER 26

USING COMPUTERS IN THE RESEARCH PROCESS

BARBARA S. THOMAS

The history of science contains many examples of new avenues of research opened by developments in technology, including microscopes, x-rays, and computer technology. Computer technology has changed our everyday lives: the ways we communicate, travel, and manage our finances, for example. Changes in health care delivery affect all professionals, including nurses. Research, both basic and applied, has been changed forever through the development of increasingly powerful computers.

This chapter introduces students to the use of computer technology in nursing research. An overview of computer hardware and software is followed by descriptions and illustrations of computer applications that deal directly with very important components of the research process: *the literature review, data collection,* and *data analysis.* The last of these, data analysis, is no doubt most familiar to students because computers have had the most impact on this phase of research in all fields. The speed with which computers can process words and numbers has taken the drudgery out of an-

alyzing data! Further, computers have enabled investigators to address increasingly complex and sophisticated problems. Studies that would have been prohibitive in terms of time and labor before computers are now commonplace.

An example from a survey study illustrates the efficiency of computers in analyzing research data. In investigating high school students' use of alcohol and other drugs (AOD) and adverse consequences experienced from AOD use, data were collected from over 1000 students. A 60-item questionnaire was used to collect information about sociodemographic variables, risk factors, AOD use, and adverse consequences. Using optical scanning, data were entered into a computer file in a few minutes at a cost of about $30. In a single analysis, new variables, *use scores* (the sum of eight items), and *adverse consequences scores* (the sum of 12 items) were computed for each subject (1000+); frequency distributions and descriptive statistics were produced for each of the 60 items and the two new computed scores; and 200 tables were

593

produced from cross-classifying the 20 use and consequences items with the 10 sociodemographic variables. Chi Squares and their significance levels were also computed for each of these 200 tables. This entire job was completed in just *14 seconds of computer time*. The output consisted of 125 pages at a cost of $3.21 for computing and printing.

Imagine the time and effort needed for these tasks without computers! The simplest task, computation of the use and adverse consequences scores for over 1000 subjects, would require more than 30 hours, assuming that each set of scores could be calculated in only 2 minutes! All of the other computations are much more labor-intensive than the mere calculation of the two scores.

Computing often appears more complex than it really is because of the special terms and acronyms associated with it. Every specialty has its own vocabulary, and computing is no exception. The box on pages 595 and 596 provides a glossary of very basic computer jargon and acronyms. Refer to it as needed as you read this chapter.

COMPUTER SYSTEMS: AN OVERVIEW

A computer system consists of the computer and various configurations of additional electronic equipment functioning together as a unit. The system is also called *hardware*. In addition to the computer itself, a typical system consists of an input device such as a keyboard to allow an investigator to put information such as data and computer programs (the applications or *software*) into the computer, a central processing unit (CPU) and storage devices, and an output device such as a monitor or printer to allow the computer to report results to the investigator. Figure 26-1 illustrates these basic components.

TYPES OF COMPUTERS

Computers can be classified in three major ways according to (1) what they do, (2) their size, and (3) their configuration (the type of CPU and operating systems installed). The first classification system, function, refers to the differences between analog and digital computers. Analog computers, common in research laboratories, measure changing values of a variable continuously. In acute care settings analog computers function as patient monitors. Digital computers accept and process data (represented as zeros or ones) according to coded instructions provided in the computer program. This chapter deals primarily with digital computers because they are the type that nurses use to analyze their research data. It should be recognized, however, that analog-to-digital systems are common data sources for some kinds of nursing studies.

Size as a way of classifying computers is not as important as it once was. The term *mainframe* has been reserved traditionally for the largest computers, *minicomputers* for medium-sized computers, and *microcomputers* for the smallest computers. Distinctions based on power of the CPU and size of the memory were once clear-cut, and differences among the categories were substantial. However, some microcomputers now have processing power and memory comparable to early mainframes and minicomputers, and distinctions between minicomputers and mainframes are becoming even more blurred. The notion of large, medium, and small is still valid, but it is somewhat more useful to think of mainframes and minicomputers as *time-sharing machines* and microcomputers as *personal computers* (PCs). Many people can use a time-sharing computer at the same time, while personal computers are used by individuals.

The very large time-sharing computers,

THE LANGUAGE OF COMPUTING: TERMS AND ACRONYMS

AI—Artificial intelligence; human intelligence mimicked by computers.

batch processing—The execution of an entire program from a single input.

bug—A mistake in a computer program or job stream.

CPU—Central processing unit; controls and performs all arithmetic and logical operations.

CRT—Cathode ray tube; monitor for visual display of input/output.

code—Representation of information in symbolic form.

data—Information.

data base—Software for organizing information in different fields in a computer-readable form.

downloading—The process of files transfer from a time-sharing computer to a PC (or to any remote system).

error message—A printed notation of an error detected by the computer usually found during execution of the program in data analysis.

execute—Complete a computer program from input to produce output.

expert system—A computer program based on human (expert) decision making for computer-based problem solving.

field—Any unit in a computer file for storing the values of a variable (e.g., age of each subject would be entered in a single field).

file—A collection of logically related fields treated as a unit (e.g., a data set).

fixed field format—Coding variables into a computer file with each variable assigned to the same field (columns) throughout the data set.

floppy disk—A magnetic disk used as a computer memory device (usually $5\frac{1}{4}''$ or $3\frac{1}{2}''$).

free field format—Coding variable in the same sequence for all subjects with no regard for the fields each occupies; delimiters are used between each variable.

hard copy—Computer input or output printed on paper or some other permanent medium such as microfiche.

hard disk—A random-access mass-storage device that is resident in the computer—either PCs or time-sharing.

hardware—The physical components of a computer system.

indexing program—Software for creating indexes of text stored according to keywords or codes that allow rapid searches of the file.

input—Information and commands entered into a computer system.

input device—Designated data or programs entered into a computer system.

interactive—A process of computing whereby a user's input produces immediate responses from the computer.

JCL—Job control language; statements used in time-sharing computers to identify valid users; to specify resources, files needed for processing, and CPU time; and to separate one job from another; usually the first input in a job submitted to a time-sharing computer.

job stream—Input consisting of job control statements, program control statements, and data.

keyboard—Most common input device; resembles a typewriter except that special function keys are important parts of keyboards.

leading zeros—Zeros that precede a number to ensure that the value conforms to its assigned field, e.g., 0253 for 253 in a four-digit field.

library—A stored collection of programs, routines, and subroutines that are accessible from a computer system's memory.

light pen—A hand-held stylus that can translate light on a screen into an electronic signal transmitted to the computer.

load—To enter data or other input; to transfer stored information from an auxiliary storage device to a computer's main memory.

Continued.

THE LANGUAGE OF COMPUTING: TERMS AND ACRONYMS— cont'd

log on—To access a time-sharing computer by entering required information such as identification numbers and passwords.

mainframe computer—The largest computers; capable of serving many users simultaneously; usually found in large universities or businesses.

Mb—Abbreviation for megabit.

MB—Abbreviation for megabyte.

microcomputer—A personal computer (PC) having only one microprocessor.

microprocessor—A tiny but increasingly powerful chip containing electronic circuitry to perform logical, arithmetic, and controlling functions for computers.

minicomputer—Medium-sized time-sharing computer system; usually found in universities and medium-sized businesses.

modem—A device for communicating between computers using modulated telephone signals for the transfer of digital computer signals.

monitor—The screen of a PC or computer terminal.

motherboard—The circuitry that connects the various components of the computer system (input, output, storage).

mouse—A small input device that is moved across a flat surface to control the position of the cursor on the screen.

network—A system of connected PCs or terminals and peripherals that allows users to share software and peripherals.

OCR—Optical character recognition; input device based on optical scanning.

OS—Operating system; a collection of system programs that controls the overall operation of the computer system.

output—The results of a job; information produced.

output device—Any medium for producing results of a computer job as displayed, printed, or graphic information.

peripheral—Any device connected to and controlled by a computer.

processor—A device that can perform operations on data.

program—A set of commands that defines a job to be executed by a central processor.

RAM—Random access memory; active information storage used while the computer system is being used; RAM is lost when the computer is turned off.

ROM—Read only memory; information stored on special memory chips that can be read; no data can be added to ROM.

SAVE—An important command that enables a user to preserve the data or program created at a session for later retrieval.

search—A command that allows a user to locate coded information in certain types of software such as word processors, data bases, and indexing programs.

software—Instructions for computers.

statistical package program—Instructions for performing statistical analyses.

time-sharing—A computer system capable of handling multiple jobs.

upload—Transfering files from a PC or other remote system to a central system (usually a time-sharing computer).

built to serve many users simultaneously, are commonly owned by universities, corporations (including hospitals), and research institutions. Their cost makes them prohibitive for individuals or small companies.

Since many users have access to a time-sharing computer, there have to be provisions for identifying individuals as valid users. In general, *logging in* requires entry of identification numbers and passwords to ensure that unauthorized individuals do

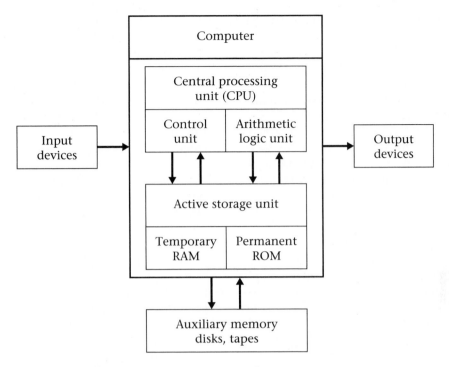

Figure 26-1. Components of a computer system.

not gain access to computer files. In many instances there are different levels of access within a single system. For example, in a Hospital Information System's (HIS) patient data base, physicians' and nurses' information needs differ from those of the pharmacy or accounting staff. Different codes are assigned to provide different levels of access, generally on a *need-to-know* basis.

Similar situations arise in academic situations. Investigators need to know that they alone have control over access to their research accounts. Thus they are assured that their intellectual property rights are protected, that the participants' anonymity and confidentiality are protected, and that pranksters cannot tamper with or destroy valuable data or other files. Faculty who teach computing generally need access to

their students' files for various reasons, often to place data sets or problems in students' files, negating the need for individual students to engage in data entry. Also problems on the computer can be assigned and checked, troubleshooting is facilitated, and messages can be relayed so that students will receive them as soon as they log on. However, students do not normally have access to their instructors' files, although the instructor can set up the class account for such access. *Security* is an important consideration in the use of time-sharing computers.

Cost is also important. Since computing costs money, the costs of creating and maintaining files, performing computations, and producing output need to be charged to the user. Thus the expenses incurred by a nurse investigator working on a grant-supported project are charged to that grant account. Universities, colleges, and departments include computing costs in their annual budgets. Within the department, different accounts are established for different users such as for classes, faculty research, and students' projects.

Identification numbers and passwords serve a third purpose. In addition to security and costs, a user's output must be separated from that of other users. Thus use of identification numbers and passwords is required to allow the user to specify type, location, and labeling of output.

Microcomputers, by contrast, are personal computers. They may be fairly large desktop units, portable laptops, superportable notebooks, or even handheld devices. Although microcomputers can be linked in networks to share software, each microcomputer functions as a single user machine, hence the label *personal computer.*

Configuration refers to a computer's type of microprocessor and operating system (OS), which can be thought of as its control tower. The microprocessor consists of the electronic circuits that are needed to translate instructions and data into machine-readable form. The following discussion focuses only on personal computers, but different configurations in time-sharing computers pose parallel concerns. Intel's 486 microprocessor is more powerful than its 386, which is in turn more powerful than its 286. Improved microprocessors have appeared in rapid succession, contributing to difficulties in keeping current about computer technology. The operating system is simply a set of programs (coded instructions) that manages all operations, including storage, use of software, and translation of data.

Among microcomputers, the individuality of these components is illustrated by the fact that software created for one type of operating system generally has been useless on another. For example, the operating systems of the Apple II series and the Apple MacIntosh series differ, making software for the two types of microcomputers incompatible even though they are both manufactured by Apple. By contrast, IBM microcomputers have been imitated to create IBM-compatible microcomputers (IBM clones); these have been and continue to be built and marketed by many companies. Since their operating systems are compatible, many software applications for all of these systems are compatible. However, many applications require a certain level of microprocessor or specific internal configurations to support special features such as graphics, animation, or sound recognition. Math coprocessors are needed to run statistical programs.

New technology has changed this compatibility issue, however. Until recently a word processing program for an Apple MacIntosh microcomputer could not be used on either an Apple IIc or on an IBM or IBM-compatible microcomputer. Their operating systems were not compatible. The use of coprocessors and certain types of interface technology (more simply, "conversion programs") appears to have solved this problem. However, just as IBM advocates and MAC advocates have neither disappeared nor joined forces, nor can it be inferred that compatibility problems have disappeared entirely.

COMPONENTS OF A COMPUTER SYSTEM

Figure 26-1 represents the components of a computer system—the hardware—as an input device, an information processing unit, and an output device. This is a simplified representation of highly complex technology. However, it is sufficient for our purposes. Investigators in any field need a basic understanding of computer capabilities, but knowledge of the intricacies of computer hardware or the skill to write a computer program are not needed for effective use of the technology. One does not need detailed knowledge about an automobile's engine or the skill of an automobile mechanic to drive a car. However, knowing how computers operate in a general way is necessary to use the technology efficiently and to work with consultants on special problems.

Input Devices

The first input devices were keypunch machines. Although these are virtually obsolete today, it was easier in many ways for novices to understand and learn how to process data when their computing jobs consisted of a deck of keypunched cards in a specific sequence than it is now with nothing concrete to illustrate the task.

In the 1960s and early 1970s computer input consisted of a deck of cards that were coded for both data and commands. Special thin cardboard cards consisting of 80 vertical columns of numbers were fed one at a time into a keypunch machine. Using a keyboard similar to that of a typewriter, cards were punched at various points along the 80 vertical columns to represent numbers, letters, and punctuation marks. Since the cards contained only numbers, a system of multiple punches was used to represent letters and punctuation marks. The deck of cards was then placed in a precise sequence to be read into the computer by a card reader. As you might guess, the first cards indicated that the person submitting the job was a valid user by an identification number and usually a password.

What are some of the input devices available today? The most common consists of a keyboard attached to either a microcomputer or a computer terminal. In addition to normal typewriter keys, a special numeric keypad speeds up data entry consisting solely of numbers. Function keys, also unique to computer keyboards, are usually labeled F1, F2, and F3 on to F12 or even F24. These keys are programmable, meaning that they can be used to perform functions or commands normally requiring many keystrokes; they are shortcut keys. Finally, the keyboard has utility keys, another form of shortcut key. The arrow keys allow the user to move quickly from any part of the screen to any other part. Other utility keys such as ESC, CTRL, and ALT are used alone or in combination with another key or keys to perform special technical jobs. For example, CTRL-ALT-DEL will restart an IBM or IBM-compatible computer and delete whatever is on the screen. The computer's manual explains the use of special keys. In addition, most software applications, such as word processing programs, designate special tasks for the function and utility keys. The mechanics of using the keyboard approach do not differ a whole lot from earlier use of keypunch machines. The critical difference is that data or commands are entered directly into computer files that can be stored, manipulated, and used with statistical package programs.

Electronic scanners are widely used to read information by scanning a printed page. Probably the most familiar types are the bar code readers in many of today's supermarkets. Also, is there a student who has never taken a test using an answer sheet with instructions to use a number two pencil? Testing services commonly score such tests using optical scanners. Along with the scanning, programs are included for scoring items, for producing scale and subscale scores, for performing item analyses, and for producing test statistics, such as split-half reliabilities and Cronbach's alpha.

As noted earlier, analog computers measure variables continuously and are used in acute care settings as patient monitors. These analog computers can be connected to digital computers so that they function as input devices. The input consists of the values of the variables being monitored. Two other tools commonly used in clinical settings are also input devices: light pens and touch screens. In allowing users to make choices using these devices, input in the form of commands is transmitted very quickly. Devices like these, which require virtually no computer skills, are called user-friendly.

Two additional input devices merit mention. One is the mouse, a user-friendly way of entering commands. The mouse is a small boxlike device that when moved across a flat surface causes a cursor on the screen to move among choices of a menu. The menu is usually displayed in graphic form or in a combination of graphics and text. When the desired selection is reached, a button on the mouse is clicked and the command is executed. Second, voice recognition is now a means of input. Such input has been possible for several years but has not, at this writing, become cost-effective for research applications. However, a notion of the potential power of voice recognition can be gained by considering its use on telephone calling cards. In areas where Touch-Tone telephones are not available or simply as an alternative, a caller can read his or her number into the telephone. Security can be built in so that another person's voice will be recognized as invalid!

Nurse researchers also need to know about files transfer programs. Data or commands entered in one computer can be transferred to another. When the transfer is from a microcomputer to a time-sharing computer, the operation is called uploading. Transferring data or instructions from a time-sharing computer to a microcomputer is called downloading.

To illustrate both, consider two situations. In one a nurse who lives some distance from a time-sharing computer has a personal computer (PC), but for various reasons (such as insufficient memory capacity) this PC cannot be used for the required statistical analyses. The nurse may enter the data into a PC file, save it on a diskette, and upload the file to the distant time-sharing computer for analysis. One alternative would be to go to the time-sharing computing facility, and after establishing an account and obtaining an ID and password, upload the data using files transfer software. These data could then be analyzed using the more powerful statistical package programs available on the time-sharing computer.

Another alternative involves the use of a special device, a modem. A modem can link the nurse's PC to the time-sharing computer via telephone lines. In essence, the electronic computer signals are translated into telephone tones, transported over telephone lines, and then changed back into binary electronic signals. Through the modem, an investigator can access a time-sharing computer as if she or he were using a terminal connected to it. The costs include the usual computing costs of the time-sharing computer, the electricity used by the PC, and the telephone charges. On college and university campuses, having PCs as terminals for the time-sharing computers is common, and generally fiber optic technology is used rather than modems.

The second hypothetical situation occurs when a nurse uses a time-sharing computer for both data entry and analysis. This is most common in completing a thesis or dissertation or when working on a special project such as faculty research. At the end of the project there is no need to maintain the data sets or job streams on the time-sharing computer's disk. However, they need to be preserved for possible future secondary analyses or for checking results at some future time. The data sets and job streams may be downloaded to tape, to a PC hard drive, or to a floppy diskette. (Note: Granting agencies often require investigators to retain data sets for a specified term such as 3 years.) The nurse researcher does not need to know the intricacies of *how* these operations are accomplished, but it is essential that there be awareness of these options.

Central Processing Unit

As depicted in Figure 26-1, the heart of a computer system is the information processing unit. Its unique component is the central processing unit (CPU), consisting of a microprocessor to transform information into machine-usable form, two types of memory circuits, and the motherboard, where connections among the different components of the system are made.

The two types of memory circuits are RAM (random access memory) and ROM (read only memory). During a data processing job, information such as data and commands are entered using one of the input devices described above. The CPU stores these data temporarily and maps the location of each segment of information entered. Thus access and retrieval of this information is very fast, hence the term *random access*. By contrast, if many data entries were stored on a tape recorder, one would have to go through the tape to find the desired segment of information, a time-

consuming process. Generally, RAM storage disappears when the computer is turned off. For this reason, investigators store their data files and programs on secondary storage devices such as hard drives or floppy diskettes for future use.

The other type of resident memory, ROM, provides for manufacturers' instructions for vital operations in using the computer. Erasing or writing over these instructions would produce disastrous results, hence the term *read only memory*.

The motherboard refers to the component that contains the circuitry for the microprocessor's link to input, output, and optional devices. Add-on options include the math coprocessor mentioned above plus many others such as color graphics, a modem, and a mouse.

The terminology used throughout this discussion of hardware is most suitable, but not unique, for PCs. For example, all computers have CPUs and internal storage units, RAM and ROM. All use secondary storage devices. However, in some cases the terminology for mainframes and minicomputers differs somewhat. For example, in time-sharing computers, there is generally an array of CPUs using several operating systems, and the *motherboard* is generally called the *backplane*. It is essential that the investigator understand the concepts of input and electronic processing and use ROM for essential instructions and RAM (temporary memory) for a current job and to obtain useful output. Using secondary storage devices to create retrievable files for data sets or job streams is necessary for continued work on a project.

Output Devices

Although a variety of output devices are available, the two most important to nurse researchers, video monitors and printers, will be given the most attention. The most common monitors today, those of desktop PCs, are cathode ray tubes (CRTs). Technically, they are the same as the picture tube of a television set. From one perspective, the CRT can be considered part of the input device system since the characters typed on a keyboard are displayed on the CRT as they are entered. As an output device, monitors display results of the information processing completed by the computer. They are available in either black-and-white or color versions and can display numbers, letters, symbols, or graphics, depending on the options that have been installed in the motherboard. The resolution of monitors varies greatly with high-resolution, noninterlaced color monitors at the high end of the cost range.

Although the CRT is still the most common output device, other options have been developed as the size of computer systems has been reduced. In addition to desktops, PCs are also available in portable, laptop, and notebook computers. (Handheld computers are also available, but are not generally used for a full range of statistical analyses at this time.) Liquid crystal or plasma screens, which are smaller and can produce better resolution for this reduced size than cathode ray tube technology, have been adopted for these small PCs.

Printers are the second most common output device. Generally, data entry and preliminary data analysis such as production of histograms and frequency distributions can proceed with input displayed only on the monitor. The investigator can scan the data for errors or outliers and inspect distributions to see if transformations or nonparametric approaches may be needed. However, when statistical analyses are performed to describe the sample or to answer research questions, hard copy is generally needed. In many cases the researcher needs a printer capable of producing graphics as well as text. Although daisy wheel printers were popular earlier, they cannot be used for graphics, making today's most popular options (in order of increasing cost) dot matrix, ink jet, and laser printers. Dot matrix printers use small pins in their printheads; these pins form characters by hitting an inked ribbon. The number of pins determines the quality of the output. Those with fewer than 24 pins produce rather low-quality print; the print is perfectly acceptable for output from statistical analyses but is inadequate for manuscripts or graphics. Those with print heads using 24 or more pins retain the advantage of low cost while offering the user speed plus fairly high-quality print and graphic capabilities.

The next step up is the ink-jet printer. As the name implies, tiny drops of ink are deposited on paper to form dots that in turn form characters. The quality of the print approaches that of more expensive laser printers, but they are slower and generally have fewer optional features than laser printers.

The technology of the laser printer is based on depositing toner in dots on special paper that is electrically charged and then heated. Laser printers vary in the dot density produced, but all of them print characters of very high quality and give the user remarkable flexibility in printing both graphics and text on the same page in complex layouts.

Selection of a printer for a PC depends on whether the PC or a time-sharing computer is used for statistical analyses. If the PC is used for statistical analyses as well as word processing, high speed and low quality are appropriate for the output, but quality must be adequate for preparing a research report and for producing graphics. A 24-pin dot matrix or low-cost ink-jet printer would furnish adequate speed and quality at the lowest cost. On the other hand, researchers who use time-sharing computers and receive printed output as part of the job can select a personal printer for its word processing and graphics capabilities rather than its speed. The high-end ink-jet and laser printers may be judged worth the extra cost because of the superior quality of reports prepared using them.

Additional output devices include plotters, magnetic disks, magnetic tape, and voice synthesizers. When graphics are to be produced directly from the output of a computer, plotters are useful. When storage of the output is a major concern, magnetic disks or tapes are appropriate. To date, voice synthesizers have little or no applicability to research applications.

SOFTWARE

The computer system described above has the potential to perform vast numbers of operations, but can do nothing without instructions written in a language it can understand. Software is a catchall term to refer to the intelligence behind the computer system, that is, coded instructions known as computer programs. A person who develops software is a programmer. Instructions to be understood by the computer must be written in a programming language such as FORTRAN, BASIC, PL-1, or COBOL, which is converted into machine language.

Software may be designed to direct the activities performed by the components of the system. The most well known of these utility programs are the disk operating systems (DOS) programs. Other programs, designed to perform specific tasks, are called applications programs. Examples of these include word processing, spreadsheets, database, and statistical programs. The emphasis in this chapter is on statistical programs.

THE USE OF COMPUTERS IN RESEARCH

LITERATURE REVIEW

As noted before, a comprehensive literature review is essential for seeing what has been done in an area of interest, in locating gaps or inconsistencies that merit study, for defining concepts both conceptually and operationally, and for ideas that will facilitate development of workable research designs. Reinventing wheels is not productive if a research question has been answered definitively; nor is it sensible to develop a data collection instrument if one of established validity and reliability is available.

Computer technology has eased literature reviews enormously. First, there are electronic card catalogs. Computer searching is much faster than hand searching. In addition, with a PC, a modem, and appropriate software, a library's holdings can be searched from your home or office at any time. In addition to locating pertinent references, you can generally learn the book's location and whether the book is available.

The literature search need not be limited to books or to local holdings. A modem can be used for off-site searches for journal articles and even newspaper articles from various data bases. Of course, the capabilities vary with the resources available at the library, but even small libraries have electronic card catalogs and access to some data bases. Working with the librarian to identify useful data bases and procedures for using them effectively saves a lot of time. Procedures are available for broadening a search or narrowing it. For example, *neonate* or *infant* can be used to pick up articles indexed by either term. The connecting word *and* can be used to limit a search to sources containing two or more terms, for example, both *child* and *abuse*.

Data base searching has become much more user-friendly and less costly in recent years so that investigators can perform their own literature searches at minimal expense. In most cases the search will provide the number of entries found ("hits") before bringing them to an active file for scanning or printing. Thus if 2756 entries are reported, an investigator might choose to limit the search, not only by key words but also by years to bring the costs down, at least for the initial search.

CD-ROM technology consists of a CD-ROM player, a CD-ROM disk, and a computer. CD-ROM disks (not unlike compact disks) store vast data bases; currently, a single disk can store the equivalent of 1440 Mb (megabyte) hard drives (Hall & Marshall, 1992). The user selects an appropriate disk and simply enters key words for the search. The appropriate references are brought to the active file (the computer screen where they can be reviewed), printed as hard copy, or copied onto a floppy disk. Such a search requires minutes, compared with a "hand search," which might require several days.

Word processors and data base systems can be used to record notes and label them with codes regarding the nature of their usefulness. In reality you are indexing your notes for speedy retrieval. For example, all references that contain ways of collecting data on relevant variables can be given a single code in a word processor or indexing program or placed in a specific data base field. As the search proceeds it is simple to retrieve all such references and make some decisions about usefulness for the current study.

DATA COLLECTION

Most experienced investigators are accustomed to viewing the data collection process as a necessary preliminary step to the use of computers for analyzing their data. Data are collected from physiologic or psychologic measures, patients' charts, observation, interviews, questionnaires, Q sorts, and the like. These data are then coded for data entry and subsequent analysis using computer technology. This tradition should be questioned, however, at the planning stage of a study.

The availability of powerful notebook computers makes it possible for the investigator to enter data directly into a computer file, saving time and money and eliminating or reducing the errors that might occur when transposing chart information into codes and codes into data files. Consider first a retrospective study using patients' charts as the data source. Instead of tediously recording information on forms for later transfer to a data file, the investigator can use the notebook (or laptop or even portable) computer at the site, recording the information in word processing or data base software for direct use in computer-based analyses. The only preliminary work involved is designation of variables and the order in which their values will be recorded. This same approach can be used for any study based on existing records.

Prospective studies are candidates for computer-based data collection as well. In many situations it is feasible to have participants enter their own data following clear, simple directions for using a carefully constructed electronic questionnaire. Specially designed software can be developed or existing data collection programs can be purchased and customized for each study.

Examples of this sort of software, the capabilities of each, the cost, and the source are published yearly in a reference publication called *DATA SOURCES*. Although it is designed for business applications, the section "Research and Survey Analysis," identifies a number of programs that are useful for data collection and even analysis in nursing studies. The programs differ considerably in power, flexibility, user-friendliness, and cost. Such programs can be used to facilitate the process for either interviews or questionnaires. Since computer technology is changing so rapidly, this sort of information must be updated regularly.

Consider first the telephone interview. Computer-assisted telephone interviewing (CATI) is simple to conduct with a multipurpose program like Sawtooth Software's *C12* package (DATA SOURCES, 1994). The computer can dial the telephone number (e.g., from a list or randomly generated numbers having the same first three digits), pause to let the investigator introduce herself or himself, explain the purpose of the study and obtain consent for participation. At this point the computer program prompts the interviewer to enter an identification code for this subject and begin collecting data. Preselected logic instructions are used to bring questions to the screen in a specified or random order. For closed-ended questions, the options are also displayed, allowing the investigator to enter the respondent's choice directly into a file for future analysis. For example, a question such as the following may appear on the screen:

*Do you have any preschool-aged children in
   your home?*
(1) YES
(2) NO

The investigator reads the question and options. If the interviewee responds *yes*, the investigator presses the number 1, and these data are recorded in a predetermined space in the data record. Moreover, this software can be programmed to branch to additional questions about preschool children when a *yes* response is given, while a *no* skips these questions and directs the interview in another direction.

For open-ended questions, protocols adopted in advance dictate whether the exact response or a shortened version is to be entered. The investigator and research assistants follow these protocols to enter the response.

Naturally, this same technology can be used for person-to-person interviewing or for questionnaires in which the research subjects enter their own responses. For questionnaires, Sawtooth Software's program *C13 System for Advanced Computer Interviewing* (V 1.0) for PC-MS/DOS systems writes and administers computer-aided questionnaires. When a computer poses the questions and stores the answers, an interview becomes a questionnaire! A novel feature is that it can handle open-ended responses, as well as single or multiple responses.

Voice recognition software would be nice for an interview. Creative Research Systems has a program called *Voice Capture Module* as part of its larger package, *Survey System* (V 5.0), that records voices of subjects interviewed onto disk and integrates them into research presentations. The interview can be face-to-face or by telephone. It is voice activated to allow for unlimited comment length.

The advantages of using software for data collection include (1) elimination of paper-and-pencil interview forms that must be coded and entered into a computer file, (2) standardization of the interview process so that all interviewers follow the same sequence of questions and branching, (3) elimination of errors in data entry since the fields for each response are predetermined and transcription from a form to a computer file has been eliminated, and (4) elimination of the high costs of transcribing audiotapes from interviews.

Note that as with any other approach the data collection instrument and procedures should be pretested. Moreover, normal protocols for assuring that ethical issues have been properly reviewed are needed.

DATA ANALYSIS

The Process

Using computers for data analysis involves a series of decisions. These include choices among methods of preliminary analyses (e.g., to examine distributions of variables, to identify errors or outliers), mode and coding guide for data entry, selection of statistical computations, selection of alpha levels, and choices in the use of statistical package programs, output options, and so forth. This section of the chapter is designed to assist students in making these choices. Although many decisions are dictated by such factors as the research questions posed and the level of data to be analyzed, many other decisions allow investigators to make choices among equally valid options. In this section guidelines for recognizing and implementing required approaches and for making appropriate selections from optional procedures are discussed.

Software for Statistical Analyses

Probably the first nurses to use statistical programs for analysis of their research data used programs developed at the university they were attending. For example, by the early 1960s at the University of Iowa an entire library of statistical programs had been developed by professors in various departments such as psychology and computer science and by the computing center staff. Although procedures for accessing the mainframe were consistent, the many differences in program control among these programs made their use for a variety of analyses rather difficult. At that time a bestseller on campus was a manual of directions for using the most popular programs; in addition to instructions for input, illustrations of typical output were also included (Snider & Thomas, 1971).

Statistical package programs became commercially available about the same time. The "Big Three," Biomedical Data Processing (BMDP) (introduced in 1961), Statistical Analysis System (SAS) (introduced in 1966), and Statistical Package for the Social Sciences (SPSS) (introduced in 1970) dominated the market. Each was available initially only for time-sharing computers. (Microcomputers did not yet exist!) Other packages are also available, such as IMSL (International Mathematical and Statistical Library), a package of more than 900 mathematical and statistical FORTRAN subroutines that is especially useful for scientific, mathematical, and statistical applications.

For the early microcomputers statistical applications software was very limited because this hardware had neither the power nor the memory to handle much data or complex computations. Computing and output were limited and slow. As microcomputer technology improved, applications software was developed to handle more data and perform more operations.

Although it is possible to buy single-purpose programs (e.g., for analysis of variance or questionnaire analyses), most microcomputer programs are multipurpose programs, and many include graphics capabilities as well. The "Big Three" have versions for MS/DOS, WINDOWS, Apple MAC, and OS-2 platforms.

Preparing Data for Analysis

Before data can be processed by computer-based programs, preliminary work must be completed. Data are the raw material on which the computer software works and must be error-free and machine readable.

The investigator must make decisions about the computer programs to be used *before* preparing the data for analyses. Whether the study involves qualitative data, quantitative data, or both, protocols are needed to ensure that

1. Raw data must be treated as confidential information and should be stored in locked files.
2. All members of the research team are trained in relation to data management protocols adopted to ensure that confidentiality is not breached.
3. Identification codes are set up according to the size of the sample.
4. Data are scanned for obvious errors; resolution of errors must be consistent.
5. Data are scanned for missing information; subjects whose answers are too incomplete to be useful are eliminated.

Although all of these items are self-explanatory, illustrations for the last two might be helpful. As a first example, in a questionnaire item, subjects are asked to check the answer that indicates their *highest* educational attainment. A subject checks BSN and MA. It's fairly simple to ignore the BSN, but the person doing the data entry must know what to do. Instructions to enter only the highest are unnecessary if the investigator is entering the data, but this is often not the case. It is the investigator's responsibility to devise a sound coding guide so that a novice can deal with problems in the data correctly. Obviously, the data must be scanned to identify these problem areas.

Sometimes the situation is more complex. Suppose that answer sheets designed for optical scanning have been used for a questionnaire. Subjects were instructed to select from among four options: Strongly agree (1), Agree (2), Disagree (3), and Strongly disagree (4). An individual has marked various items with 1s, 2s, 3s, 4s, and a few 5s. Do you eliminate this subject from the sample because the "5" responses are obvious errors? Or do you assume that the 5s were meant to be 4s?

When data collection tools such as questionnaires are incomplete, the decision concerning use of the data is usually based on the relevance of the missing data to specific research questions or hypotheses. If the completed portion is useful for a question or hypothesis, it may be retained for that analysis, with missing data codes used to eliminate the subject from other analyses. If the completed portion is not useful for even one segment of the study, the investigator will no doubt make the decision to eliminate that subject, and not waste data entry effort on useless information.

Quantitative Data. In preparing quantitative data for statistical analyses, one needs to look ahead to consider the statistical package to be used and the tests to be run. Plans for analysis should generally include description of the sample, analyses needed to answer research questions or test research hypotheses, and analyses needed to support the credibility of the study.

Each of the Big Three mentioned earlier will perform a wide variety of analyses. In addition, there are a number of packages available commercially for single-task or multifunction uses.

The first task is to scan the raw data for missing, illegible, or meaningless entries. Since every variable must be coded into numbers for every subject, decisions about missing data codes are needed. The decision about missing data codes is related to the statistical software to be used. For example, MINITAB will not accept a blank for missing data; use of asterisks is recommended. With any statistical package, care should be exercised in choosing to use zeros as missing data codes. Many programs will treat a zero as a valid response, and this can cause problems. For example, in the construction of a frequency distribution, treating zero as a valid value when it was meant to represent missing data will result in incorrect percents and cumulative percents in the resulting frequency distribution(s).

The scanning step also considers text entries. Perhaps a closed question includes six foils (possible answers), but allows the respondent to enter an additional item as the seventh, usually as

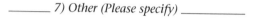
_____ 7) Other (Please specify) _____

These items must be analyzed as qualitative data before data entry can begin, assigning numbers to categories that emerge. In some cases unsolicited comments are entered; the investigator must decide whether they will be coded or ignored. Sometimes it is obvious that the respondent interpreted the question in a different way than was intended in spite of steps (such as pilot testing) that were completed to avoid this problem. In such a case the investigator, not the data entry clerk, needs to decide whether to devise a way to interpret the response or to code it as missing data. Missing data codes such as a 9 for items consisting of only five possible responses should be entered if it is not possible to interpret the intent of the subject accurately.

Quantitative data sets often contain categorical variables, such as gender or religion, in which the numbers assigned to each response are arbitrary. In designing a questionnaire these options should be numbered to facilitate easy data entry. For ordinal variables the responses should be displayed in ascending or descending order.

Qualitative Data. The preliminary data scanning in qualitative research (e.g., from interviews) is quite different. If the investigator is the sole data collector, consistency in establishing rapport, posing questions, and using probes can be maintained. However, if a team effort is involved, data screening is necessary even if careful, thorough training of interviewers was undertaken. Generally, recordings of the interviews or a sample of the interviews are reviewed early in the study to ensure that all interviewers are using reasonably consistent protocols. If substantial departures from accepted approaches are detected, the interview may need to be discarded.

The purpose of the study and the size of the data set should be considered in preparing the data for analysis. Qualitative data analysis usually has five broad purposes: instrument development, exploratory inquiry to identify variables and preliminary hypotheses in a little-known field, description, hypothesis testing, and theory development (Thomas, 1990). Instrument development and theory development are often at the extremes in size of the usual data set involved, with the other three kinds of studies falling somewhere in between. Whether statistics will be computed in the study is another essential consideration.

Based on the purpose of the study, the anticipated size of the data set, and whether statistical analyses are planned, two preliminary steps are usually necessary. First is selection of the unit of analysis. The purpose of the study will generally dictate the selection of words, themes, characters, items, or space and time as units of analysis (Berelson, 1981).

Themes and items are most frequently used in nursing research. In a study of nursing interventions perceived to be most helpful to families of patients in ICUs, a nurse researcher would probably use themes as the unit of analysis because *all* ideas from the subjects are of interest and must be included in comprehensive, mutually exclusive categories. In such a study, the investigator is not concerned about whether the data reflects responses of each subject equally. If one subject contributes one theme and another contributes nine themes, all 10 themes are coded and included in the data set.

Figure 26-2 illustrates the coding process using hypothetical data from eight subjects to clarify the use of themes as units of analysis. Coding a very large data set by themes using computer technology greatly increases the efficiency of the analysis.

In some studies the investigator needs to give equal weight to each response. In such a study, themes would be inappropriate because of the differences in numbers of themes contributed by the subjects in the sample. For example, a Delphi study question might be posed to Directors of Nursing in hospitals, "What practice in your hospital has been most effective in promoting utilization of appropriate research findings in nursing practice?" This question indicates that only the most important practice from each respondent is desired. Here the item should be the unit of analysis so that equal weight is given to each subject's response. The investigator would undoubtedly indicate that one and only one response is requested. If a subject includes more than one theme, the investigator attempts to determine from the wording of the response which is most important. In some cases this is impossible, and investigators adopt an arbitrary rule of coding the first response.

After the unit of analysis has been determined, the next step relates to coding, and two questions should be answered if possible. Although firm coding decisions may not be possible until data analysis is under way, the investigator should be able to make some preliminary decisions based on the study purpose and population. Will the coding be done at the latent or manifest level? Will the coding scheme require more than one level?

Looking ahead to data analysis and anticipated results is a necessary part of the planning process. For example, if the purpose is to develop a series of closed-ended questions about a topic, the open-ended questions will serve as an initial set of first-order categories. This set of classes may function well and serve as the set of comprehensive, mutually exclusive categories throughout the study. Actual responses to the questions, however, may reveal that the questions produced answers (categories) that were not mutually exclusive, and the coding scheme must be revised.

On the other hand, if an exploratory-descriptive study is launched to describe, for example, the needs of teenage, single mothers for parenting education, the categories will emerge from the data. The data may indicate promptly that a hierarchical coding system is most appropriate. For example, *safety* may be subdivided into settings such as the home, playground, or automobile. However, an initial set of categories may appear to be functioning well for much of the data, and the need to revise these categories may emerge relatively late in the study. The investigator must remain flexible and objective. The planning stage of the research process is as important as the planning stage of the nursing process. Provisions regarding data entry for computing frequencies of identified needs, as well as other descriptive sta-

Research question
How does preschool day care affect a child's health?

Sample
Convenience
34 mothers whose children attend one of two day care centers

Example of coded responses*
A two-level coding scheme was used: (1) reason, (2) positive/negative

[51]   [15]
01 - peer pressure to aid socializing . . . exposure to infectious diseases

[41]   [15]
02 - assurance of proper immunization status . . . exposed to more germs

[51]   [35]
03 - child learns to play with other children . . . exposure to accidents

[41]
04 - peer pressure & caretakers' influence to wash hands, brush teeth

[21]
05 - develop immunity to common infectious diseases before school

[35]   [52]   [41]
06 - accidents . . . more stimulation (other children) . . . health teaching

[51]   [51]
07 - learns consideration for other toddlers . . . increased socialization skills

[65]   [35]
08 - exposure to a child that bites . . . increased number of accidents

* Extraneous material has been eliminated from the responses.

Codes

Reasons | Positive/negative
1 exposed to more germs | 1 very positive
2 builds up immunity to infectious diseases | 2 positive
3 increased accidents | 3 neutral/ambiguous
4 health promotion, e.g., immunization & | 4 negative
  health habits such as hand washing | 5 very negative
5 improved socialization skills |
6 exposed to aggressive children/hurt |

Frequencies of reasons: 5(5), 3(3), 4(3), 1(2), 2(1), 6(1)
Frequencies of affect: 1(8), 2(1), 3(0), 4(0), 5(6)

Figure 26-2. Coding themes in qualitative data analysis.

tistics, will be considered when planning the data collection, coding, and subsequent analyses.

Data Entry, Storage, and Analysis

Quantitative Data. Many data sets consist wholly of numerical data that can be entered directly into a computer file. A computer file is simply a set of records entered in a computer and stored as a named file on a time-sharing computer's allocated disk space or on a microcomputer's floppy diskette or hard drive. (Magnetic tape can be used also, but this is uncommon.)

The arrangement of the data in the file is determined in advance so that the computer can be instructed to read the variables accurately. Commands result in each subject's age and other demographics, plus the responses to questions, being read in the same sequence. A word of caution is in order with respect to age. When dealing with infants and children, months may be preferable to years. For adults, age at the last birthday is usually requested so that fractions are avoided. In any event the researcher should give some thought to wording the question for a limited sort of "stimulus-response" so that only one response, the correct one, will be given to the stimulus.

The two formats in general use for keyboard-based data entry are called fixed format and free-field format. In fixed format, the investigator assigns certain variables to specific columns; each variable occupies a field consisting of one or more columns. The largest possible value of a variable determines the size of the field for that variable. For number of children, there may be a subject who has 10 or more children; therefore, two spaces are needed. Another concept, *right justification,* is important in relation to fixed format data entry. Right justification refers to placing the variable in the right part of the field if its digits do not occupy the entire field. If columns eight and nine are designated for number of children, both columns would be used for 10 or more. However, responses of one to nine should be placed in column nine. Column eight should be left blank, or a zero can be entered there. If a 2 were placed in column eight with column nine left blank by mistake, the computer would read the variable as 20 children!

Responses to closed-ended questions are easy to plan. If a subscale consists of 20 items, each having four possible responses, only one digit is needed for each item; hence 20 columns will be needed for the subscale. Choosing the number of digits for some variables is not so easy; if in doubt, use the largest possible field that might be needed. If income is requested in dollars, there is no need to enter the dollar sign, commas, or period. Note that six columns would allow for a maximum income of $999,999. If six columns are allotted and an income over $1 million is reported, most investigators would use 999999 for this entry.

Another potential problem area concerns items containing a number of answers or options, together with the instructions "Please check (✓) all that apply." In using fixed-field data entry, a column must be left for each option. Often the checks are coded "one" and the blanks are coded "zero". Using the zero for spaces left blank in such an item distinguishes the response from missing data and furnishes another reason for avoiding zero as a missing data code.

In free-field data entry, all data are entered in the same sequence for all subjects with separators such as blank spaces left after each variable. In this method the columns will not line up if differing numbers of digits have been entered for any variable in the data set. This method is not recommended for any but small data sets nor for any time-sharing statistical packages except MINITAB, because it is very easy to repeat or omit a variable, and the entries are difficult to check visually. Errors may not be detected, producing erroneous analyses.

In general, it is prudent to assign the first field of columns to the identification number of the subject and assign each variable to a specific set of columns for fixed format. Figure 26-3 displays a miniquestionnaire illustrating how the columns for data entry are generally incorporated into the questionnaire to facilitate data entry directly from the questionnaire. This coding scheme is designed for fixed format coding; the columns for the grade level will be 12 and 13 for all subjects. The lower part of Figure 26-3 shows how three hypothetical subjects' responses would be entered in both fixed format and free-field format. Note that no leading zeros are needed in free-field coding. This small data set is not particularly difficult to check, but with larger numbers of subjects and variables, visual checking of data that have been entered this way is very difficult.

Text editors have been available for many years on time-sharing computers. They were designed specifically for entering data into computer files and building job streams and are not as versatile as word processors. A job stream consists of a data set together with statements needed to access the computer and commands needed to use a statistical package program for analyzing the data set. Each line is limited to 80 columns, and each is generally numbered. Early text editors were *line editors,* meaning that the user could enter data one line at a time, pressing *Return* or *Enter* after each line to move the cursor to the spot for entering the next line. This is an efficient,

straightforward way to create a data set or job stream. An enhancement called a *full-screen editor* allows users to enter or modify an entire screen of data at one time. With either type, data entry creates a temporary file. This file resides in the computer's *active file,* meaning that the file is currently visible and useful.

The data set can be created, given a label, and stored. It can be modified, enlarged, and edited. Every text editor, like every word processor, has its own unique features, but learning one will help in learning another. There are general tasks to accomplish, just as there are with word processors.

Before beginning data entry for your study, it is a good idea to become thoroughly familiar with the text editor. Use of text may be easier at this stage than use of numbers. In any case, enter a few lines, and try to follow the manual's directions for the various tasks that might be needed during data entry:

1. Add new lines at the end, beginning, and middle of the file.
2. Renumber the file.
3. Replace a single character in a line with another.
4. Add a single character to the middle of a line.
5. Replace five characters with three.
6. Delete a line.
7. Delete three characters from a line.
8. Move a line from one spot to another.
9. Save the file.
10. Sign off; sign on and retrieve the file. Inspect it.
11. Print a hard copy of the file.
12. Delete the file and sign off again.

A few guidelines are in order regarding data entry. Each case should be started on a

A mini-questionnaire with coding guide included for fixed format coding

1-3 ___ ___ ___ ID
4 ___ Record number

Have you participated before in a parent training workshop about prevention of alcohol and other drug (AOD) use?
5 ___ (1) yes ___ (2) no

How important do you consider parent involvement in prevention of AOD use among youth? **Please circle your answer.**
6 **Extremely important   1   2   3   4   5   6   Extremely unimportant**

In this community, how serious do you consider each of the following problems to be?
Please use 1 for NOT SERIOUS up to 5 for VERY SERIOUS.
7 ___ a) drinking after driving
8 ___ b) frequent drinking by high school seniors
9 ___ c) regular smoking
10 ___ d) binge drinking (over 5 drinks/occasion)
11 ___ e) occasional use of marijuana

12-13 What is the grade level of your oldest child? ___

Please estimate your knowledge base about AOD using a scale of 1-12:
14-15 ___

Please rate your skills as Poor (1), Good (2), or Excellent (3)
16 ___ a) informing my child about alcohol's harmful effects
17 ___ b) informing my child about tobacco's harmful effects
18 ___ c) informing my child about the harmful effects of illicit drugs
19 ___ d) recognizing signs of alcohol use/abuse
20 ___ e) teaching my child peer refusal skills
21 ___ f) pointing out the false pictures displayed in alcohol ads
22 ___ g) successfully confronting my child if alcohol use is suspected

Fixed format coding	Free field coding
0011143423206083213221	1 1 1 4 3 4 2 3 2 6 8 3 2 1 3 2 2 1
0021265455412102331211	2 1 2 6 5 4 5 5 4 12 10 2 3 3 1 2 1 1
0031254533104043323111	3 1 2 5 4 5 3 3 1 4 4 3 3 2 3 1 1 1

Figure 26-3. Coding questionnaire responses into fixed and free field formats.

new line. The file should be saved frequently during data entry in case something goes wrong. Sometimes a computer can *go down* while you are working. Information on the screen disappears, and the computer is essentially out of order. In many time-sharing systems, when the problem has been corrected, something akin to this message will appear: "data saved from last session." In such cases the data can be recovered and data entry can continue. In other situations this does not occur and work can be lost. Use of surge protectors with microcomputers will prevent a surge of power from destroying work in progress. In other cases a local power failure or lightning can cause the loss of an active file. Since stored files are not affected, frequent saving while working is strongly recommended.

When all data have been entered, the file *must be saved.* On a time-sharing computer the SAVE command places the data set in the user's file and other users cannot access this file.

Entering data on several occasions is commonplace. After accessing the computer, the label assigned during the earlier session can be used to retrieve the file, and new data can be added to it. Saving the file is again necessary to preserve the new additions. *Caution: retrieval of an existing file is generally necessary to make additions to it.*

To illustrate, suppose that a user entered data for 35 subjects at one session, saved the data set as "THESIS," and signed off. At a later time, this same user signed on again to add another 25 cases to the data set. Instead of retrieving THESIS first, data entry was started immediately. After the twenty-fifth case had been entered, our hypothetical student entered the proper command to save THESIS. A text editor will generally respond as follows:

THESIS already on file. Replace?

If a "Yes" (or Y) is typed in, the new 25 cases will *replace* the earlier set of 35 cases! To update a file, users must retrieve it before adding to it. (Note: If you find yourself in such a quandary, ask for help before losing data or logging off. Sometimes the solution is fairly simple. The new data can be saved using a different name, such as "THESIS1". Then a COPY command can be used to add the THESIS file to this active file, thus combining the two data sets. After saving THESIS again, deletion of THESIS1 will prevent possible confusion later.)

Most text editors and statistical packages expect data to be entered in records not exceeding 80 columns. If your variables exceed 80 columns, the data can be continued onto the next line. It is a good idea to use the first few columns of each line for identification numbers and record numbers. Line one is record one and line two is record two, both from the same subject; the identification number will be the same on each line.

Figure 26-4 illustrates multiple records per subject entered in fixed format. In this illustration data have been entered for three records per subject for four subjects. Note the use of leading zeroes for the IDs. Variables such as years of experience may range from single-digit to double-digit answers. Thus two spaces are required for the *years of experience* field, and a leading zero would be required for all single-digit responses.

Fixed-field format is generally recommended. In large data sets its use does much for one's peace of mind regarding the accuracy of data entry. This practice also permits the user to scan the data visually for errors or omissions on the screen. Once a data set is complete, it should be stored twice, once for use as a working copy and a second time as a backup copy. When using microcomputers, it is a good idea to put the two files in different locations. Thus a file stored on a floppy diskette

The coding guide

Record 1			Record 2			Record 3		
Column	Variable	Value	Column	Variable	Value	Column	Variable	Value
1-3	ID #	ID	1-3	ID #	ID	1-3	ID #	ID
4	Record #	1	4	Record #	2	4	Record #	3
5-6	Age	age	5-14	Scl-It1/10	1 to 5	5/16	Sc4-It4/15	1 to 6
7	Ethnicity	1 to 5	15-24	Sc2-It1/10	1 to 4	17/26	Sc5-It1/10	1 to 4
8	Education	1 to 5	25-34	Sc3-It1/10	1 to 5	27/38	Sc6-It1/12	1 to 3

The data set

Four subjects, three records/subject

```
----------------------------------------------------------------------
Column numbers

1  1   2   2   3   3   4
1  5   0   5   0   5   0   5   0
----------------------------------------------------------------------
00113744
0012453221415433214443211225343224
0013654333421224342331224311232322312
00212933
0022223454332122341324315545332513
0023543443245122342341224221233221323 2
00312445
0032544322354124311224434533424353
0033564334332562122344342423323331222 31
00414245
0042134534432534423411234532234154
0043445632245321342343124213232231123 2
0051...
0052...
0053...
.......
```

Figure 26-4. Entering multiple records per subject in fixed format.

that is ruined one way or another may be lost, but its duplicate, stored on another floppy diskette, on a tape, or on the hard drive, remains intact.

Most experienced investigators check several aspects of the data by creating histograms and/or frequency distributions of the variables. First, these programs reveal *outliers,* values that fall outside the possible range for the variable. For example, in a sample of elderly subjects, defined as being age 65 or over, the histogram or frequency distribution reveals that one subject's age is 57. Either the subject's age was entered incorrectly or the subject should be eliminated from the data set. This preliminary work is sometimes called *data cleaning;* for efficiency, a computer-based approach is essential.

Another purpose served is to display the distributions of the variables. For many statistical tests a normal distribution of the variable in the population is required. You do not, of course, produce a histogram or frequency distribution of the population, but if the distribution of the sample is severely skewed or multimodal, it may be wise to consider using nonparametric (distribution-free) statistical tests. Another solution is the use of data transformations. For example, logarithms of the values may be normally distributed, and statistical tests can be performed on the *log transformations.*

Once the data are ready for analysis, several decisions are needed. One decision is the selection of statistical analyses to be performed. The primary considerations are the research questions or hypotheses, the level of the data, and the distributions of the variables. Another involves a choice between batch and interactive computing. A batch job simply refers to submitting a job stream (computer commands for all of the analyses required, along with the data) as a sort of package to be processed by the computer as a single job. In the other approach to computing, interactive, the investigator issues a command and the computer responds to that single command. The analysis continues as a series of commands and responses.

Commands used for data analysis will vary with the statistical package used and with the type of analysis required. All statistical programs require the investigator to identify the variable, its location, and usually its label.

Batch jobs are particularly useful for large jobs. An enormous number of analyses can be completed in a single run, and the printing is completed at the computing center, saving the investigator a great deal of time. Disadvantages must be recognized too. Any errors in the identification codes, location designations, commands, or data can cause the run to fail. Error messages are printed in the output. (Anyone who has not received an error message has not done much computing!) The investigator must make the corrections and submit the job again. However, a word of caution is needed here. If all codes and instructions are correct but the data contains an incorrect value or decimal point, erroneous results will be printed with no indication of the error(s). This last problem is equally applicable to interactive computing.

When these decisions have been made, it is time to describe the sample and proceed with analyses for the research questions or hypotheses. Procedures will depend entirely on the statistical programs selected. Figure 26-5 displays the input and output for a batch job using a popular program, SPSS, and the input and output for the same job in an interactive mode using another popular program, MINITAB. The same data set is used for all analyses illustrated. The output from SPSS and the input/output from MINITAB were printed directly from the printer that was used in the analyses. It should be noted that SPSS can also be used in an interactive mode; similarly, MINITAB can be used in a batch mode. In general, researchers use the batch mode on time-sharing computers for large jobs. When the data set is large and there are a lot of analyses to be performed, the tasks can be submitted as a single job and the time-sharing computer will complete the computing very quickly and print out the job rapidly.

Batch processing with SPSS   Interactive processing with MINITAB

Coding guides

SPSS:	ID	1-3
	Age	4-5
	Exp	6-7
	Educ	8
	It1-It10	9-18
	Yrrn	19

MINITAB:	ID	C1
	Age	C2
	Exp	C3
	Educ	C4
	It1-It10	C5-C14
	Yrrn	C15

Input

Data list file = D1
/ Age 4-5 Exp 6-7 Educ 8
It1 to It10 9-18 Yrrn 19
Frequencies variables = Educ It1
Correlations variables = Age Exp Educ

Input

Mtb > Tally C6-C9;
Subc > Counts;
Subc > Percents.

Output

Educ

Value label	Value	Frequency	Percent	Valid percent	Cum percent
	2	3	15.0	15.0	15.0
	3	17	85.0	85.0	100.0
	Total	20	100.0	100.0	

Valid cases 20   Missing cases   0

It1

Value label	Value	Frequency	Percent	Valid percent	Cum percent
	1	1	5.0	5.0	5.0
	2	9	45.0	45.0	50.0
	3	10	50.0	50.0	100.0
	Total	20	100.0	100.0	

Output

C6	Count	Percent	C7	Count	Percent
1	1	5.00	1	9	45.00
2	7	35.00	2	4	20.00
3	12	60.00	3	7	35.00
N =	20		N =	20	

C6	Count	Percent	C7	Count	Percent
1	9	45.00	1	2	10.00
2	9	45.00	2	11	55.00
3	2	10.00	3	7	35.00
N =	20		N =	20	

Input

Mtb > Corr Age Exp Educ

Output

	Age	Exp	Educ
Exp	0.950		
Educ	0.166	0.200	
Yrrn	0.527	0.573	0.0082

	Age	Exp	Educ
Age	1.0000 (20) P = .	.9498 (20) P = .000	.1664 (20) P = .242
Exp	.9498 (20) P = .000	1.0000 (20) P = .	.1996 (20) P = .199
Educ	.1664 (20) P = .242	.1996 (20) P = .199	1.0000 (20) P = .

Figure 26-5. Batch and interactive processing: input and output from SPSS and MINITAB.

Qualitative Data. To proceed with content analysis (or data reduction), the text from interviews and open-ended questions contained in questionnaires or notes from observations must be transcribed. In years past such data were typed, double- or triple-spaced with wide margins to allow investigators to delete extraneous information, identify units of analysis, and enter notes about emerging themes or their ideas concerning relationships among variables. Generally, the data were photocopied to provide a working copy while retaining the data set intact for future reference. Use of computers for data entry, coding, and data analysis will be addressed in subsequent sections.

The potential of the computer for facilitating data entry and storage lies in its ability to accept text as input, store it, allow for retrieval and movement of the text and, at the analysis stage, to permit the investigator to attach codes to various segments of the text. The most obvious computer application is simply word processing software. Norman (1989) described use of WordStar in storing and analyzing qualitative data in great detail. However, any word processing software with the capabilities listed above plus a *search feature* can be used.

For example, in the preliminary phase of managing interview data each interview is entered in a word processor's file. In many qualitative studies, data analysis begins with the first entry. Assuming that themes are the unit of analysis, the themes emerging from the first interview can be given preliminary codes. These are considered preliminary because the codes that represent categories may change in the course of analyzing additional data. It may be desirable fairly early in the data entry-analysis process to begin deleting extraneous material. Efficiency is served by eliminating useless material so that it will not be reviewed over and over again. However, these early decisions about coding and deletion of extraneous material may prove to be wrong during the process of constant comparative analysis. For this reason the data entered should be stored in two (or more) files. One or more serve as working file(s), while the other preserves the original data intact.

If problems of overlap or ambiguity occur, the *find feature* can be used to review a single category throughout the data set. In complex categories this simple on-screen review may be inadequate for dealing with the meanings and boundaries of the classes. In such cases the troublesome categories can each be copied into another file where review on screen or by printing out the file permits the investigator to resolve the problem(s). Clarification of what each category includes and what must be excluded from each is essential before work continues. Changes in one category may dictate review and changes in other categories.

Word processing software has several additional advantages for preliminary storage and management of qualitative data and its analysis. Interviews can be entered as soon as they are completed; obviously this task does not require the skills of the investigator. However, the investigator can review data on screen or in hard copy for indications that additional or different questions may be needed before proceeding with further interviewing. In addition, changes in a set of categories are common even in relatively small data sets. The word processor's ability to facilitate revisions in codes can be used in either the entire data set or in the separate file created from a single category when a division within this "single category" appears needed.

Another type of applications software, an indexing program, allows field notes and other kinds of text to be searched for specified words or phrases. First, the text must be entered or imported from a word processing file. Then the indexing software is used to process the file, making it ready to be searched. The actual search and retrieval is very rapid. Thomas and Schalk (1986) used ZyIndex to create an indexed, annotated bibliography of all literature concerning computing in nursing from 1974 through 1985. Although the purpose was retrieval of specialized information about computing in nursing, the search principles were identical. After the annotated bibliography was entered and indexed, searches were possible using key categories or Boolean logic. Figure 26-6 illustrates ZyIndex's potential for general searches and the two-level coding system used in this project. The same approach that was used in creating a computerized annotated bibliography can be applied to qualitative data analysis. As the analysis proceeds, single-, double-, or even triple-level codes can be devised to categorize emerging themes. Segments of text can be marked and printed out from different parts of the file, making it possible to create an outline of the themes with supporting documentation for each category displayed together. Review of each category then is simple and straightforward. Changes that may be necessary merely require electronic recording and rearrangement.

In general, data base systems are more useful than word processors for storing and managing qualitative data because of the many ways they can organize data for storage, retrieval, manipulation, and export to other systems. First, review of a little terminology is necessary to illustrate the use of a data base system.

Suppose that you are conducting a telephone survey. Each participant is identified in the data base by an identification number; this single piece of information is a *field*. In your brief interview you gather data about the subject's age, occupation, and opinions about the topic of interest to you. Each of these pieces of information occupies a field. Together, they form a *record*. Additional subjects are interviewed, producing additional records. Since information is gathered in a specific order for each participant, the data from the entire sample consist of records containing information in identical sequences. This combination of records constitutes a *file*. Since the order of information is the same for each subject, such a file structure is called a *sequential file*. However, the person entering the data may index each record so that the aggregate of any particular set of fields (for example, age) can be retrieved. This produces an *indexed file*. Think of an electronic filing system with the ability to access any field of the entire file and retrieve and manipulate these data as the user wishes in fractions of a second. A data base is a type of software that provides for this kind of high-level storage and manipulation of data.

Hypertext is a specialized application that gives users all of the features of a data base management system plus linkages and cross-referencing capabilities, allowing users to bring related topics to the screen. Nodes refer to each text entry, which can be marked by the user to connect it with one or more additional nodes (Hall & Marshall, 1992; Pfaffenberger, 1988; Brent & Anderson, 1990). Although such software takes some effort to learn, the savings in time and effort during the study are enormous. The larger the data set, the more likely it is that use of such software will also improve the rigor of the analysis.

The principles described for the use of word processors, indexing programs, data base systems, and hypertext have been used to design special software that is

Examples of operators in ZyIndex searches

Operator	General use	Examples
?	single character wild card	*wom?n* retrieves woman, women
*	multi-character wild card	*child** retrieves children, childish, childbirth, childhood, childbed
OR	enlarges search	*neonate or infant* retrieves files containing either word
AND	narrows search	*cancer and chemotherapy* retrieves only files containing both words
AND NOT	narrows search	*monitor and not fetal* retrieves files that contain monitor but not fetal
( )	combines operators	*(adolescent or teenager) and crime* retrieves files that contain either adolescent or teenager and also crime
W/n	delimits search for	*(old or elderly) W/15 (exercise or fitness)* retrieves files that contain either old or elderly within 15 spaces of either exercise or fitness
OR NOT	enlarges search	*adult or not (old or elderly)* retrieves files that contain adult but do not contain old or elderly

Coding scheme for ZyIndex-based annotated bibliography

First-level codes

A advocacy or position papers
B prescriptive or descriptive narrations
C informative articles about computer technology or computer literacy
D research and evaluation
E review articles
F software

Second-level codes

1 nursing administration
2 nursing practice-pediatrics
3 nursing practice-obstetrics
4 psychiatric nursing
5 nursing practice-medical surgical
6 community nursing
7 long-term care
8 nursing education

Figure 26-6. Using an indexing program: an example.

uniquely suited to data entry, management, and storage and that also completes the data analysis! Several books describing software such as ETHO, Text Analysis Package (TAP), QUALPRO, the ETHNOGRAPH, Textbase Alpha, and others should be consulted before selecting software for qualitative data analysis (Tesch, 1990; Fielding & Lee, 1991).

❧ OTHER COMPUTER APPLICATIONS

After discussing software for data collection, manipulation, storage, and analysis, it may seem strange to consider additional computer applications for nursing research. But there are more to consider and more being produced even as you read this! The technology is changing so fast that the reader is cautioned to consider the following material to be a mere sampling of what is available.

EXPERT SYSTEMS

Expert systems mimic human intelligence to help nurses make decisions in specialized areas. One of the earliest and best-known expert systems in nursing was called COMMES (Creighton On-Line Multiple Medical Education Services), programmed to respond to a user's request for information regarding patient care (Ryan, 1983). To develop this system, expert sources were consulted to form a knowledge base and to devise patterns of logic and decision making for accessing this information as a human expert would solve a problem. Thus a user may enter a query and receive an answer supplemented by the reasoning behind the decisions. Many people refer to expert systems as the most useful application of artificial intelligence (AI). Opinions differ however on what constitutes artificial intelligence.

One type of expert system of interest to nurse researchers guides the selection of statistical tests. For example, DYNA-COMP's *Statistical Consultant* (DATA SOURCES, 1994) asks the user a number of questions. Based on the user's answers, the program gives advice about appropriate statistical tests to be used. This program is PC-MS/DOS compatible. Another system, also for PC users, is called *Statistical Navigator Professional* (V 2.0) (DATA SOURCES, 1994) and responds to user's answers to a sequence of questions by recommending several statistical analyses, ranked in order of suitability. Explanations of how the recommended tests fit the research objectives and assumptions underlying the statistical tests are also given. Digital Equipment markets similar programs such as *RS/Explore Statistical Advisory Software* (V 2.1) in their BBN Software Products line for a variety of platforms, primarily time-sharing machines (hardware: DEC, VAX, DECStation, MicroVAX/VMS, MicroVMS, HP-HP-UX, IBMVM/CMS, and SUN). The cost of the PC software may be as little as $10. The cost of these expert systems for time-sharing computers may be as high as $24,000.

Another sort of expert system uses artificial intelligence strategies to guide the user's choice of data collection procedure. Depending on the situation and population, the program, *Data Collection Selection* from The Idea Works (DATA SOURCES, 1994), might recommend use of participant or nonparticipant observation, mailed questionnaires, face-to-face or telephone interviews, experiments, or simulations. It also generates reports.

Still another sort of expert system performs power analysis. *Design* is available in both PC-MS/DOS and Apple MacIntosh versions from SYSTAT, INC. (DATA SOURCES, 1994). This software will estimate needed sample sizes based on user-supplied effect sizes and significance levels. Another program that determines sample sizes and much more is marketed by The Idea Works, Inc.: *Ex-Sample* (V 3.0) and is PC-MS/DOS compatible (DATA SOURCES, 1994. This software performs traditional power analysis to determine sample sizes. In addition, it makes design recommendations about ways of reducing required sample sizes in the face of limited resources. *Sample Size Program* from New Alternatives, Inc. is also MS/DOS compatible and reports required sample sizes in response to user entries about the study variables.

COLLECTING PHYSIOLOGIC DATA

Mention has been made of analog computers and their usefulness as patient monitors in acute care settings. Analog computers are often connected to digital computers to perform data entry of physiologic variables on a continuous basis.

Martz and Beaumont (1982) described computer-based monitoring in an intensive care unit (ICU) as no more invasive than in other ICUs not using computers. Measurements are taken continuously from pressure lines, temperature probes, ECG leads, and a pneumotachograph and are reported every 10 minutes or on demand. Respiratory parameters include pressure, flow, pO_2 and PCO_2, breath-by-breath tidal volumes, and rates. Cardiac parameters are monitored from pressure lines and ECG leads. Any three variables can be plotted over a period of 1 to 24 hours providing graphic evidence of significant trends in the patient's condition. These data are accepted and processed by an analog computer and converted into numbers for transfer to a digital computer. The digital computer accepts and processes the numbers, comparing them to healthy ranges for each variable. Generally, in monitoring systems, if a problem occurs (i.e., if the actual value falls outside the healthy range), the output device notifies the nurse or physician. This is an analog-to-digital system. The digital computer accepts and processes information such as numbers or letters along with coded instructions that direct the computer's operations on the data. For research purposes the potential benefits of analog-to-digital computer analysis of physiologic data in time saved, accuracy, and nonintrusion relating to patient welfare are enormous.

PRESENTATION OF RESEARCH RESULTS

Programs are also available to produce presentation-quality graphics from statistical tests. (The Big Three have these capabilities, and other mainframe computer packages do as well.) This section deals only with products available for microcomputers. For Microsoft WINDOWS, STATSoft markets *CSS/3* (Release 3.1) for extensive statistical work plus *Quick CSS,* which includes presentation graphics along with statistical analyses. Extensive graphics options are available for Apple MacIntosh users too, for example, Abacus Concept's *Statview* (V 4.01) and *Statview SE + Graphics* (V 1.04).

An example of an expert system for helping investigators decide which type of graph to use for greatest impact and least distortion of results is called, appropriately enough, *Whichgraph* (V 1.0); it was designed for PC-MS/DOS microcomputers by The Idea Works, Inc.

SINGLE-PURPOSE APPLICATIONS

Finally, there are some single-purpose programs that do virtually everything for investigators engaged in surveys. For example, Apian Software's *Survey Pro* (V 1.3) integrates word processing and formatting options to produce surveys, structures a data base program to accept responses, analyzes results, and creates tables and bar charts. In addition, it can export data to spreadsheets, word processors, graphics software, data bases, and statistical programs in either ASCII or WK1 format (DATA SOURCES, 1994). Statpac, Inc. developed *Statpac Gold IV* (V 4.4) for total management of surveys from design through sample selection, telephone interviewing, data entry and management, basic statistical analyses, and presentation graphics. Persimmon Software's program, *Survey* (DATA SOURCES, 1994), is an editor and data collection and analysis system for surveys; either subjects or interviewers can enter the data. It can handle up to 100 questions, each with up to ten subject responses. Creative Research Systems' *Survey System* (V 5.0) takes care of the entire survey: data collection/analyses and presentation graphics. Data input can be from telephone or computer interviews, from scanners or from disk-by-mail (DATA SOURCES, 1994).

EVALUATING THE USE OF COMPUTER TECHNOLOGY

In many respects the evaluation of computer use in a study is an assessment of the computer literacy of the investigators. However, in reading a research report, this is often difficult because journal reviewers and editors request tight, sparsely described manuscripts, and a full description of ways in which computers were used may be considered nonessential. For example, use of a computer-based literature search is commonplace. Neither investigators nor journal editors are likely to want a description of the literature search included in a research report.

Many studies are reported without attention to the likelihood of type II error. That is, no power analysis is reported, and the sample size may be too small to detect significant differences or relationships even if they exist in the population. Thus in evaluating studies one would give high marks to an investigator who reported this information and even higher marks to one who used computer-based technology for the power analysis.

Data collection using computers is not always cost-effective. It is most appropriate for studies where data are collected from individuals one at a time. Telephone interviews were used earlier to illustrate the efficiency of using computers for this important part of a study. Use of notebook computers for face-to-face interviews *might* be appropriate. However, if investigator-subject rapport is an issue, the use of computers in the interview may be intrusive. In this case anonymous or confidential recording of the interview or even writing notes after the interview may be more desirable.

Questionnaires or Q sorts, if presented individually, for example, to patients on admission, are an example of appropriate use of computers. However, questionnaires administered to groups or by mail do not lend themselves to use of computer technology.

Sometimes, methods used for data analysis consist only of an explanation of the descriptive and inferential statistics selected for the study. Thus the reader may evaluate the appropriateness of the statistics chosen, but no mention is made of provisions used to ensure the accuracy of the data, the distributions of the data, or the statistical package used for the actual analysis. It is common practice to *assume* that careful data entry, data management, and data analyses were performed.

Regarding presentation of findings, most reviewers would not fault a report for

---

EVALUATING THE USE OF COMPUTER TECHNOLOGY IN RESEARCH

1. Do the investigators make clear their use of computer technology in relation to
   a. Sampling?
   b. Selection of data collection procedures?
   c. Data collection?
   d. Selection of statistics to be computed?
   e. Data entry and manipulation?
   f. Data analysis?

2. To what extent do the investigators' selections reveal their expertise in relation to state-of-the-art computer technology for each of the applications employed? That is, was the use of computers appropriate? To what extent were the decisions sound?

---

omitting a description of the way the graphics were produced. Such information is regarded in the same light as is preparation of the narrative portions of the manuscript, as a technical rather than a professional issue. The reader does not need to know what word processor was used either.

In summary, evaluation of an investigator's use of computer technology in a study is rather difficult because (1) information about its use is not often included in the report and (2) use of the technology is not always appropriate. Certainly, collection of data from 1000+ students in the alcohol and drug use survey that was described at the beginning of this chapter was better performed using paper-and-pencil measures and optical scanning rather than having each student enter his or her data at a PC. The one clear-cut issue relates to design considerations such as power analysis. The advent of computer technology makes this a simple task that should be performed routinely when inferential statistics are computed. Although current reports include mention of power analysis more often than was formerly the case, it is often neglected. This situation may change as nurses make greater use of computer technology in guiding their design decisions.

SUMMARY

- A typical computer system consists of an input device, the computer itself, and an output device. The computer itself consists of a central processing unit and storage devices.
- Computers may be classified according to what they do (digital versus analog), their size (mainframe, minicomputer, microcomputer), and their configuration (type of processor and operating system).
- Time-sharing computers (mainframe and minicomputers) allow many users simultaneous access and require IDs and passwords for access.
- Microcomputers (PCs) can now perform tasks formerly reserved for time-sharing machines.
- The most common use of computers in nursing research is for data analysis. Many options are available for both time-sharing computers and PCs.
- Preliminary steps in quantitative data analysis include scanning data for errors and omissions, examining the distributions of the variables, and making decisions about the handling of ambiguities.
- Preliminary steps in qualitative data analysis include data screening for consistency of interviewer communication and for missing/ambiguous data.

- Accurate coding and data entry are essential for both quantitative and qualitative studies. A variety of computer-based options are available to facilitate this step.
- Software for quantitative data analysis is available for both time-sharing computers and PCs; the scope and power of statistical package programs vary enormously.
- Software for qualitative data analysis includes word processors, data base systems, indexing programs, and hypertext; these programs speed up the analysis and generally improve its rigor.
- Expert systems are available to assist a nurse researcher in making decisions about sample size, approaches to data collection, and selection of statistics to be used.
- Analog computers can be used to collect data such as physiologic variables and feed the values directly into a digital computer for analysis.
- Word processors and graphics programs are in widespread use for producing research reports.
- Single-purpose programs (e.g., for surveys) do everything for the investigator from producing the survey instruments to analyzing the data and producing tables and graphs to display the results.
- Evaluation of investigators' use of computer technology is difficult because such use may not be reported in the manuscript; currently, data analysis is generally reported and its appropriateness to the study sample and questions/hypotheses can be judged.

FACILITATING CRITICAL THINKING

1. Student volunteers have entered survey data from a sample of 234 elderly women, defined as women age 62 and older. Assuming that all sorts of computer technology are available to you, what would you do to
   a. Check the accuracy of the data prior to data entry?
   b. Enter and store the data for analysis?
   c. Recheck the accuracy of the data?
   d. Examine the distributions of the variables?
   e. Confirm your own ideas about statistical tests to use?
   f. Select a statistical package for analyzing the data?
   g. Prepare a first draft of the narrative and tables of your research report?
   h. Prepare graphs?
2. As a school nurse in a small rural community, you have collected data about the health beliefs and health practices of the children in the elementary grades. To summarize these data for planning purposes and to inform school staff and parents about the current status, you wish to summarize the results of your survey and present findings, using graphs as much as possible. The school has both IBM-compatible and Apple MacIntosh computers with 60-MB hard drives. What programs would you select to perform needed tasks at the least cost?

References
SUBSTANTIVE
BRENT, E. E., & ANDERSON, R. E. (1990). *Computer applications in the social sciences.* New York: McGraw-Hill.

CHANG, B. (1991). Use of computers for Nursing Minimum Data Set and nursing home cost studies. *Western Journal of Nursing Research, 13,* 789-793.

COOK, M., & MAYERS, M. (1981). Computer assisted data base for nursing research. In H. Werley & M. Grier (Eds.), *Nursing information systems.* New York, Springer-Verlag.

DIXON, W., ET AL. (1981). *BMDP statistical software.* Berkeley, University of California Press.

FISHER, G. (ED.). (1994). *Data sources* (Vol. 13, No. 2). New York, Ziff Communications Company.

FOX, R., & VENTURA, M. (1984). Efficiency of automated literature search mechanisms. *Nursing Research, 33,* 172-177.

GRAVES, J., & FU, L. (1991). Researcher's workbench. *Computers in Nursing, 9,* 116-120.

HORN, C. E., & POIROT, J. L. (1981). *Computer literacy, Problem solving with computers.* Austin, TX, Sterling Swift.

KELLY, A., & SIME, A. (1990). Language as research data, Application of computer content analysis in nursing research. *Advances in Nursing Science, 12,* 32-34.

KOVNER, C. (1989). Using computerized databases for nursing research and quality assurance. *Computers in Nursing, 7,* 228-231.

LAUCHENBRUCH, P. (1989). Statistics for hospital epidemiology, On using microcomputers in statistical analysis. *Infection Control in Hospital Epidemiology, 10,* 422-426.

MARTZ, K. V., & BEAUMONT, J. O. (1982). Computer-based monitoring in an intensive care unit (ICU), Implications for nursing education. In R. D. Zielstorff (Ed.), *Computers in nursing.* Rockville, MD, Aspen.

MORSE, J. (1991). Subjects, respondents, informants and participants? *Qualitative Health Research, 1,* 403-406.

NORMAN, E. (1989). How to use word processing software to conduct content analysis. *Computers in Nursing, 7,* 127-128.

PFAFFENBERGER, B. (1988). *Microcomputer applications in qualitative research.* Newbury Park, CA, Sage.

SAS INSTITUTE (1991). *SAS user's guide.* Cary, NC, SAS Institute.

SPSS, INC. (1986). *SPSS user's guide.* Chicago, SPSS, Inc.

STEPHENS, L., SELIG, C., JONES, L., & GASTON-JOHANSSON, F. (1992). Research applications, Teaching staff nurses to use library search strategies. *Journal of Continuing Education in Nursing, 23,* 24-28.

TESCH, R. (1990). *Qualitative research, Analysis types and software tools.* New York, Falmer.

THOMAS, B., & SCHALK, L. (1986). Computers in nursing, A computer-based annotated bibliography. In B. Thomas & A. Leners (Eds.), *Instructional computing in nursing education.* Iowa City, IA, The University of Iowa Press.

CONCEPTUAL

BALL, M., HANNAH, K., JELGER, U., & PETERSON, H. (EDS.). (1988). *Nursing informatics, Where caring and technology meet.* New York, Springer-Verlag.

BARTON, A. (1990). What is the best personal computer system to use for research? *Florida Nurse, 38,* 20.

BERELSON, B. (1971). *Content analysis in communication research.* New York, Free Press.

CHARMIAK, E., & MCDERMOTT, D. (1986). *Artificial intelligence.* Reading, MA, Addison-Wesley.

GLEIT, C., & GRAHAM, B. (1988). Secondary data analysis, A valuable resource. *Nursing Research, 38,* 380-381.

HEYDEN, R. (1990). Database support for research. *Nursing Administration Quarterly, 14,* 74-75.

MCKEEHAN, N. (1989). Research databases, A new direction in collection development. *Bulletin of the Medical Librarians' Association, 77,* 252-255.

MELIA, K. (1989). Computer ethics . . . what data we should hold about people and who should have access to it. *Nursing Times, 85,* 62-63.

MORITZ, P. (1990). Information technology, A priority for nursing research. *Computers in Nursing, 8,* 111-115.

RYAN, S. (1983). Computers in nursing practice, COMMES, a national computer-based educational consultant. *Computers in Nursing, 1,* 1.

SIMPSON, R. (1991). Brainpower at your fingertips, The National Library of Medicine. *Nursing Management, 22,* 14,16.

SUMMERS, S. (1992). Using microcomputers to facilitate research studies. *Journal of Post Anesthesia Nursing, 7,* 48-53.

THOMAS, B. S. (1990). *Nursing research, An experiential approach.* St. Louis, Mosby.

VON WINTERFELDT, D., & EDWARDS, W. (1986). *Decision analysis and behavioral research.* Cambridge, Cambridge University Press.

YOUNGBLUT, J., LOVELAND-CHERRY, C., & HORAN, M. (1990). Data management issues in longitudinal research. *Nursing Research, 39,* 188-189.

ZIELSTORFF, R., JETTE, A., & BARNETT, G. (1990). Issues in designing an automated record system for clinical care and research. *Advances in Nursing Science, 13,* 75-88.

METHODOLOGICAL

BAKER, C. (1988). Computer applications in qualitative research. *Computers in Nursing, 6,* 211-214.

BARHYTE, D. (1989). Bar coding, A new tool for researchers. *Western Journal of Nursing Research, 11,* 347-351.

FIELDING, N. G., & LEE, R. M. (1991). *Using computers in qualitative research.* Newbury Park, CA, Sage.

HALL, L. D., & MARSHALL, K. P. (1992). *Computing for social research, Practical approaches.* Belmont, CA, Wadsworth.

HILLER, M., & BEYDA, V. (1981). Computers, medical records and the right to privacy. *Journal of Health, Politics, Policy and the Law, 6,* 463-487.

KOVNER, C. (1989). Using computerized databases for nursing research and quality assurance. *Computers in Nursing, 7,* 228-231.

McCARN, D. (1980). Medline, An introduction to on-line searching. *Journal of the American Society of Information Services, 31,* 181-192.

MORSE, J., & BOTTORFF, J. (1990). The use of ethology in clinical nursing research. *Advances in Nursing Science, 12,* 53-64.

MORSE, J., & MORSE, R. (1989). QUAL, A mainframe program for qualitative data analysis. *Nursing Research, 38,* 188-189.

MURPHY, J. (1979). Preparing research data for computerization. *American Journal of Nursing, 79,* 954-956.

RICE, C., GODKIN, M., & CATLIN, R. (1980). Methodological, technical and ethical issues of a computerized data system. *Journal of Family Practice, 10,* 1061-1067.

SEIDEL, J., KJOLSETH, R., & SEYMOUR, E. (1988). *The ethnograph, A user's guide (version 3.0).* Littleton, CO, Qualis Research Associates.

SMITH, M., & BARTON, J. (1992). Technologic enrichment of a community needs assessment. *Nursing Outlook, 40,* 33-37.

SNIDER, B. C., & THOMAS, B. S. (1971). *Selected statistical programs.* Iowa City, IA, University of Iowa Computing Center.

TENOPIR, C. (1991). Options for accessing databases. *Librarians' Journal, 116,* 73-75.

WALTZ, C., & BAUSELL, R. (1981). *Nursing research, Design, statistics and computer analysis.* Philadelphia, F.A. Davis.

HISTORICAL

ABDELLAH, F. (1966). Future directions of research in nursing. *American Journal of Nursing, 66,* 112-116.

BRYSON, D. (1991). The computer-literate nurse. *Computers in Nursing, 9,* 100-107.

GORTNER, S. (1980). Nursing research, Out of the past and into the future. *Nursing Research, 29,* 204-207.

HANNAH, K., & BALL, M. (1984). *Journal of Clinical Computing, 12,* 179-184.

HEFFERMAN, H. (Ed.). *Proceedings of the Fifth Annual Symposium on Computer Applications in Medical Care.* Silver Spring, MD, IEEE Computer Society Press.

NAISBITT, J. (1982). *Megatrends, Ten directions transforming our lives.* New York, Warner Books.

SABA, V., & McCORMICK, K. (1986). *Essentials of computers for nurses.* Philadelphia, J.B. Lippincott.

WERLEY, H. (1981). Nursing data accumulation, Historical perspective. In H. Werley & M. Grier (Eds.), *Nursing information systems.* New York, Springer-Verlag.

WERLEY, H., & GRIER, M. (1981). *Nursing information systems.* New York, Springer.

ZIELSTORFF, R. (1980). *Computers in nursing.* Rockville, MD, Aspen.

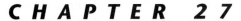

COMMUNICATING RESEARCH RESULTS

KAREN KELLY SCHUTZENHOFER

Two nurses attend graduate school in mental health nursing at the same time in different parts of the country. During their graduate studies both students read an article in an obscure journal describing an innovative intervention to improve the functioning of persons with chronic schizophrenia. Each develops a research project focusing on this intervention. In both studies the intervention is successful. One nurse presents her thesis project at several conferences, both as a paper and a poster, and eventually publishes a revised version of her thesis. She continues her research on schizophrenic persons and develops a research career around the topic. The second nurse successfully presents her study at the annual graduate student research day on campus and then sends her unrevised thesis to one research journal. It is rejected by the manuscript reviewers as inappropriate for that journal. She views her research as merely an academic requirement for completion of her degree. This nurse's research becomes little more than a book on a shelf, dusted once a year.

As this example demonstrates, research results that are not shared through the usual channels (e.g., oral presentations, posters, and publications) do little more than gather dust. Many excellent studies that focus on significant nursing issues line their authors' bookshelves and are never shared with the nursing community. Research that is not communicated to the nursing community benefits no one. Sharing one's research with others facilitates the expansion of nursing knowledge, creates change in nursing practice, and provides rewards to the researcher that are internal (e.g., sense of satisfaction, excitement of seeing one's name in print) or external (e.g., tenure and promotion in the academic setting, the award of research grants, travel to research conferences) (McCloskey & Swanson, 1985).

This chapter examines the structure and function of common types of research reports, provides guidelines for effective oral and poster presentations, discusses the process of publishing a research article, and presents a process for critiquing a research report.

⌒ *RESEARCH REPORTS*

Different kinds of research reports address different needs. Theses and dissertations serve to demonstrate the ability of students to conduct scholarly work and to communicate the processes and outcomes of a research project (Polit & Hungler, 1991). Research articles and conference presentations communicate the processes and outcomes of studies to encourage both replication and application. Research posters offer a highly visual method of presenting and sharing a study on a one-to-one or small-group basis. Abstracts summarize basic information about the methodology and outcomes of a project in order to facilitate the quick review of the study and to disseminate research information fast and efficiently.

Dissertations and theses are long, thorough documents, frequently 100 to 200 pages or more, that include exhaustive searches of the relevant literature. Although the development of the proposal and the conduct of the research are the work of the graduate or doctoral student, the process is closely monitored and supervised by the faculty advisor and other committee members. The finished product will reflect not only the efforts of the student but also the influences of the advisor and the committee.

Some graduate programs do not require a thesis (or, in rare situations, a dissertation) of every student. Some programs provide a nonthesis option, usually requiring the conduct of a clinical project. This project is then documented and evaluated in a written report that, like the thesis, documents the student's ability to conduct a scholarly project. Although these are not research studies, these projects usually require an extensive literature search in the proposal phase, like a thesis, and should reflect application of research findings.

KEY ELEMENTS OF A RESEARCH REPORT

Unlike theses and dissertations, research articles and paper presentations are concise and have greater potential to reach a wide audience. Page and time limits set the parameters for the length of articles and oral presentations, respectively. The specific format for a thesis or dissertation is usually detailed in the guidelines provided by the graduate or doctoral program. Most schools will require a format similar to that outlined in the box.

Just as each school determines the exact format of a thesis or dissertation, each journal provides information on its own editorial style in guidelines for authors that will be discussed later in this chapter. When abstracts are submitted for paper and poster presentations at research conferences, a required or recommended format is usually provided by the conference sponsor. The format of a paper or poster presentation will be influenced by the intended audience. Clarity is essential to all research reports. A well-developed research report is written to be understood by readers unfamiliar with the subject matter. Whatever the format of the report, all research reports include a core of essential information: the *title,* an *introduction* to the problem, an explanation of the research *methods* used, the *results* of the study, and a *discussion* of the significance and application of the findings.

Title

The title of a research study needs to be both meaningful and brief. Often the titles of theses and dissertations become lengthy because of the researcher's effort to make the title fully descriptive of the study. Scanning the recent theses or dissertations at any university may reveal some titles of 30 words or more. Inexperienced researchers may feel the need to title a study as soon as they begin to commit their ideas to paper.

TYPICAL FORMAT FOR THESES AND DISSERTATIONS

Preliminary pages
　Title page
　Required forms (e.g., signature sheet from committee)
　Acknowledgments
　Abstract
　Table of contents
　List of tables
　List of figures

Body of report
　Chapter I: Introduction
　Chapter II: Review of the literature
　Chapter III: Methods
　Chapter IV: Results
　Chapter V: Discussion, implications/application and summary
References/Bibliography
Appendices

Some may find it useful to postpone writing a title until at least the first draft of the proposal is written. The title should not exceed 15 words; an even shorter title is preferable. Avoid such superfluous phrases as "A Study of" or "An Investigation of" at the beginning of the title. Some grant programs will require that titles not exceed a certain number of characters (i.e., letters, numbers, and spaces) to facilitate computerization. Titles of abstracts submitted for research conferences must often fit onto the limited space provided on the abstract form. Finally, editors of journals may require that a title be more concise than the original title submitted.

Introduction

The introduction to any research study answers the question "why?". It emphasizes the importance of the study and provides an overview of the key concepts and questions of the study. The problem statement is an integral part of the introduction. The problem statement or the hypotheses indicate what the study attempts to investigate or resolve. A theoretical framework may be appropriate for some studies; for example, studies that examine aspects of human behavior or test models of nursing care delivery.

The literature review, which will proba-bly be a separate chapter in a thesis or dissertation, provides an overview of the current knowledge of the problem under study (APA, 1994). Theses and dissertations include exhaustive reviews of the literature. Such detail documents students' knowledge of the problem. Journal articles offer a much briefer review of the most salient literature related to the problem. Paper and poster presentations demand ever further distillation of the literature to meet time or space limits. These brief reviews provide the reader or listener with background information about the issue on which the current study builds. (See Chapter 7 for a discussion on how to conduct a literature review.)

Methods

This section of a research report is the most technical. The methods section explains the processes used in the research project. Sampling and subjects are key concepts examined in this section: who the subjects were, how they were recruited and selected, how many were included in the sampling, and why they were appropriate for this study. The sampling methodology (e.g., randomized, convenience, stratified) is detailed in this section of the research report.

The design of the study, including data collection techniques, is also outlined in the methods section. One of the key aspects of the design is the use of appropriate data collection instruments. Instruments used in data collection are described; discussion focuses on development, validity, and reliability of the research instrument. If a standardized, well-established instrument is used, this discussion will be brief. If the data collection instrument has been developed for this study, the discussion will detail the process of instrument development, including pilot testing. When an existing instrument has been adapted for use, the adaptation process must be discussed. In a research proposal, the plan for data analysis will be detailed in this section.

Results

The research subjects are described in the results section. In research on human subjects, the description of the subjects in the sample includes the number of subjects who actually participated and their relevant demographic characteristics, such as age, gender, marital status, years of work experience, and educational level. Much of this descriptive information may be included in tables, rather than in the narrative portion of this section (see Table 27-1). The use of tables reduces the verbiage, making the narrative more concise, and offers a precise and highly visual method of presenting the data.

In a research proposal, as previously noted, the proposed data analysis is usually included in the methods section. In the research report actual data analysis is detailed in the results section. When qualitative methodology is used, the narrative focuses on a summary of the thematic analysis of the interview content, journal entries, or other data. Quotations from the content are integrated throughout the analysis. When the study uses quantitative methods, descriptive statistics from the data are presented first, followed by the inferential statistics. When both qualitative and quantitative methods are used, usually the quantitative is described first. The qualitative data then may be used to explore or clarify the quantitative data, although this approach may not be appropriate to all such data.

The narrative portion of the results section can easily become confusing and difficult to follow as the writer explains the re-

Table 27-1
Sample Table of Demographic Characteristics From a Written Research Report (according to respondents' level of education)

	Tech. ($n = 55$)	BSN ($n = 42$)	MSN ($n = 37$)*	All ($n = 134$)
$\overline{X}$ years of work experience	14.99	13.26	19.97	14.16
$\overline{X}$ years since graduation	15.87	14.75	18.00	16.11
$\overline{X}$ age	41.24	39.89	42.43	41.13
Males	0(0%)	3(7.1%)	1(2.7%)	4(3%)
Females	55(100%)	39(92.2%)	36(97.7%)	130(97%)
Single	8(14.5%)	6(14.6%)	5(13.5%)	19(14.2%)
Married	35(63.3%)	28(68.3%)	27(73.0%)	90(67.7%)
Divorced/widowed/ separated	12(21.8%)	7(17.1%)	5(13.5%)	24(18.1%)

*One respondent did not answer all items.

Table 27-2
Sample Statistical Table

ANOVA (Scores by Basic/Highest Level of Education)

Source of variance	SS	df	MS	F
Between	6880.0	4	1720.20	5.069*
Within	43421.8	128	339.33	
Total	50302.6	132		

*$p < .01$.

search findings. Just as tables are useful in clarifying and making demographic data succinct, they are essential in bringing clarity to the data analysis. Tables allow the organized presentation of descriptive data to clarify the accompanying narrative description. Inferential data may require tables for the unambiguous and complete presentation of research findings. Chi-square and analysis of variance (ANOVA) are examples of two inferential statistics that may require the use of tables for appropriate presentation (see Table 27-2 for an example of an ANOVA table). The hypotheses noted earlier in the introduction section are also cited in this section. Hypotheses are neither proved nor disproved; they are supported or rejected by the data.

Discussion
The discussion brings the research report to closure. A well-developed discussion section "makes sense" of the research results. This is the most important section of any research report. The discussion section must be presented in precise and concise language, avoiding research jargon (Hayes, 1992; Wilson, 1985). This section must "sell" the research findings to the reader for application in practice or replication of the study (Wilson, 1985). For the reader who skips over the sections on methods and results and goes directly to the discussion, the merit of the study will rise or fall based on the reader's critique of the discussion.

The discussion identifies the limitations of the study and defends the validity of the findings in light of these limitations. Limitations include factors such as the inherent weaknesses in the sampling method (e.g., including only a random sample of registered nurses from one state because of limited funding for the research project) or the lack of generalizability of the findings (e.g., use of a convenience rather than a random sample or small sample size). Acknowledging the limitations of the study actually strengthens the presentation of the findings; the writer is prevented from drawing conclusions beyond what is reasonably supported by the data. Findings from relevant research cited in the literature review are compared and contrasted to the findings of the current study in the discussion section. This comparison supports the discussion of the application of the research findings and clarifies the significance of this study to the current body of knowledge (Morse, 1993). Recommendations for further study flow from this discussion. The researcher has the opportunity to recommend ways to minimize or eliminate the limitations of the current study, to offer alternative methodology or improvements of the methods of the study presented, to suggest new populations for study using the current methods, and to offer practical applications of the findings from the current study that provide a starting point for additional research.

Summary of the Key Elements
These guidelines for preparing a research report offer direction for the format of any type of research report. In the next sec-

tions, the special requirements of research paper presentations, posters, and published articles is presented.

RESEARCH PAPER PRESENTATIONS

The novice researcher is advised to attend one or more research conferences before presenting a research paper or poster to gain an appreciation for the processes of sharing research through presentations. Once the researcher is ready to share a study with the nursing community, a response to a call for abstracts starts the chain of events leading to the presentation of a research paper (or poster, as noted later in this chapter). Conference planners send out printed notices to members of research organizations and other professional associations and to schools of nursing and hospitals announcing an upcoming program. A call for abstracts, which invites researchers to submit the abstracts of their studies, notes the date, location, sponsor, and theme of the conference, and the format required for abstracts. The keynote speaker may also be listed in the call for abstracts.

The researcher's study must fit the theme of the conference in order to be appropriate for submission. If the researcher believes that the study fits the theme, the abstract can be submitted to the conference planners. Abstracts are subjected to a peer-review process. The peer-review process entails an anonymous review of an abstract (or, in other situations, a manuscript) by two or three reviewers, who are content experts, expert writers, or both. They evaluate the content, the technical merit of the work, and its relevance to the conference theme. The decision of the reviewers is returned to the submitter within a time frame of several weeks to several months. If accepted, the final version of the paper, in-

cluding appropriate audiovisual aids, can take days of work to prepare. The actual presentation usually takes no more than 15 to 30 minutes, including time for questions and answers. Acceptance of the abstract indicates the approbation of one's professional colleagues. Rejection of the abstract may reflect:

- A poorly written abstract
- The questionable quality of the research
- A poor fit with the conference theme
- A surplus of appropriate studies
- Failure to meet the guidelines for submission
- A missed deadline
- An overlong abstract

THE RESEARCH ABSTRACT

An abstract is a brief summary, usually no longer than one or two pages, of a larger body of work, in this case, a research project. The abstract can serve as the introduction of a written research report or as means of marketing and sharing one's research, as in response to a call for abstracts (Woods & Contazero, 1988). Some abstracts have word limitations, such as 100, 200, or 500 words. The use of the word count feature of a word-processing program can make the counting process both quick and easy. It is essential to stay within the page or word limits imposed on an abstract. An abstract that is too long may be rejected without review.

The abstract summarizes the key elements of a research report: problem statement (introduction), methods, results, and discussion. Abstracts are sometimes submitted for research in progress. Because the results of such a study are not available, the key elements may include information on the projected data analysis, omitting the results and discussion. When space limitations allow, the theoretical framework may

EXAMPLE OF A RESEARCH ABSTRACT

PROFESSIONAL AUTONOMY AND HIGHEST LEVEL OF NURSING EDUCATION

Research on the relationship between professional autonomy and level of nursing education has been inconclusive. A number of studies have used instruments originally designed to measure variables other than professional, such as personal or work autonomy.

This pilot study used the Professional Nursing Autonomy Scale (Schutzenhofer, 1987) to investigate the relationship between professional autonomy and highest level of nursing education. Members ($N = 250$) of a district nurses' association served as a convenience sample for the study, and 134 usable questionnaires were returned (53.6%). Subjects were classified by highest level of nursing education: 55 technical graduates (27 diplomas and 28 associate degrees), 42 baccalaureate graduates, and 37 master's degree graduates. Each subject completed a demographic questionnaire. An analysis of variance (ANOVA) yielded $F = 10.783$ ($p < .01$). Significant differences were found between technical and baccalaureate graduates ($F = 5.978$, $p < .01$) and between technical and master's degree graduates ($F = 9.659$, $p < .01$).

The findings of this study cannot be generalized to other nursing populations. However, they indicate a need for further study of the relationship between professional autonomy and level of nursing education using this scale.

Karen Kelly Schutzenhofer, EdD, RN, CNAA, 1988

also be identified in the abstract. The call for abstracts may include a form on which the abstract must be typed. Conference organizers may use a uniform format to allow the attractive and orderly presentation of a book of abstracts for the program. The abstract must be highly readable: a 10 or 12 character per inch (cpi) font is usually preferred. Using a very small font (e.g., 16 cpi) to meet space limitations may disqualify the abstract for review. Adhering to the guidelines for submission of an abstract is essential; disregard for the guidelines does not impress reviewers favorably. Such disregard reflects a careless attitude about the presentation of one's research. A sample of an abstract is provided in the box.

DEVELOPING THE VERBAL PRESENTATION

One of the main advantages of the verbal presentation is the relative speed with which one can disseminate research findings. The time between the initial call for abstracts and the actual presentation usually ranges between 4 and 10 months. The typical time frame for publishing an article, in comparison, is 12 to 24 months from submission of the manuscript to appearance of the article. In addition, interaction with an audience gives the researcher feedback on the study (Teel, 1990; Wilson, 1985). This feedback may enable the researcher to clarify, expand, or otherwise revise the theoretical framework, the data analysis, presentation of the results, the limitations, and the implications of the study.

Presentation of a paper at a conference should precede rather than follow publication of a study; many conferences will not consider previously published work for review. Paper (or poster) presentations may occur while the manuscript is under review or is pending publication, depending on conference guidelines. Presentation of a study at more than one conference is usually acceptable; multiple presentations of the same study in the same geographic region is not advisable.

Planning the Paper Presentation

The weeks or months between submission of the abstract and notification of acceptance (or rejection) is the time to begin developing the paper presentation from the original research report. Waiting until you are notified of acceptance may not leave enough time to complete the paper satisfactorily. For the novice presenter, ample time should be allowed for careful planning and revision before the presentation. Once the paper is accepted for presentation, the speaker can begin to tailor the presentation to the specific audience who will attend the conference. Take note of when the presentation will occur on the conference agenda. An early morning presentation usually indicates an alert audience at their peak of receptivity; presenting immediately after lunch offers the challenge of keeping an audience alert after a meal. If the presentation is scheduled late in the day, some of those attending will leave early for shopping, sightseeing, or dinner with friends. The last presentations of the conference are always subject to walkouts as some members of the audience hurry to catch planes, trains, and buses for the trip home (Selby, Tornquist, & Finerty, 1989a).

All presenters have their own styles of preparation and presentation. The following guidelines suggest ways to simplify the process of developing a presentation and to improve its quality.

Some writers work best from a written outline; others need only a mental outline to get them started. A novice speaker may find it helpful to write out the entire opening and closing statements, but do avoid writing out the full text of the rest of the paper (Wilson, 1985). It is tempting to read the paper verbatim when a full text is available. This can be very boring for listeners; members of the audience in a room with lights dimmed for slides may find it difficult to stay awake! Many experienced speakers use minimal notes, speaking from their slides or transparencies.

When using 8½- by 11-inch paper, develop an outline of phrases and facts. Many speakers prefer to use note cards with the essential content outlined. Larger size note cards, at least 4- by 6-inch cards, are easier to read in the light on the podium. Whether notes are typed or handwritten, the text should be adequately spaced to allow for revision during rehearsals. Mark the pages or cards in the margins to indicate when to change slides or transparencies. Rehearse the presentation several times, at least once in front of a mirror. Time the presentation during the rehearsal to make sure there is enough time for questions and answers. Mark the notes or outline for content to be cut if time runs short. Highlight words or phrases to be emphasized with a change in tone of voice or pace of speech. Practice not only the words to say and how to say them but also gestures and the use of audiovisual materials (Selby et al., 1989a).

Avoid the "five deadly sins" of research presentations as identified by Jackle (1992) and listed in the box. First, *ignoring the interests of the audience* can engender responses ranging from boredom to overt hostility (Jackle, 1992). Tailoring a presentation to the audience's needs holds their interest effectively (Selby et al., 1989a). The same study can be presented differently to a group of research-savvy PhDs than to a group of experienced staff nurses. Each presentation should include information relevant to that particular audience. A group of research methodologists will want more in-

---

THE "FIVE DEADLY SINS" OF RESEARCH PRESENTATIONS

1. Ignoring the interests of the audience
2. Impressing the audience with one's scholarly accomplishments
3. Overloading the audience with minutiae of the study
4. Burdening the audience with irrelevant handouts
5. Overloading the audience with slides and transparencies

---

formation on the design of the study than a group of clinicians; the clinicians will need more emphasis on the results and implications for clinical practice.

Second, *trying to impress the audience with one's scholarly accomplishments* usually leaves the speaker looking rather pompous (Jackle, 1992). The audience can determine the quality of the speaker's scholarly abilities on its own. Third, avoid *overloading the audience with the minutiae* of the study (Jackle, 1989, 1992). Plan the presentation to prevent spending too much time on the theoretical and methodologic aspects of the study. In a 25-minute presentation, allow 3 to 5 minutes to introduce the study and the theoretical framework, 5 minutes for the design, 10 minutes for the findings and application to practice, and another 5 minutes for questions and answers.

Fourth, never allow the audience to leave a presentation without written materials with the name and affiliation of the speaker, but do not *burden them with irrelevant handouts* (Jackle, 1989, 1992). Most conferences will provide a book of abstracts; some will also include handouts in these materials. Other conference organizers will expect speakers to bring their own handouts. If the letter of acceptance does not mention the handout issue, call the conference coordinator. If speakers are required to bring their own handouts, find out how many people are expected to at-

tend the session. Handouts of more than one page should be neatly stapled. The handout should clearly indicate the title of the conference and of the presentation, in addition to the name and affiliation of the speaker. Handouts of more than four pages may benefit from a cover sheet. Bring business cards to share with those attending the presentations and for networking during breaks, meals, and receptions.

Fifth, use slides or transparencies to add focus to a presentation, but avoid *overloading the audience with slides and transparencies* (Jackle, 1992). Multimedia exhibits are not essential for research presentations. Slides and transparencies are important adjuncts to successful research presentations and are useful in emphasizing or focusing attention on important points and clarifying data (Jackle, 1992). However, too many slides or transparencies can overload the audience. Use no more than one slide (or transparency) per minute of presentation. If the study received funding from an intramural or extramural source, use one of the first slides (or transparencies) to recognize the funding source.

Laser printers and personal computers can greatly simplify the process of creating the camera-ready text for slides. A typewriter or dry-transfer letters can also create highly readable slides. Do not use more than six words per line or eight lines for a text slide (Selby, Tornquist, & Finerty,

1989b). Tables of numbers can be effectively displayed on a slide to clarify statistical content. But no slide, including a text slide, should take more than a minute to read. Slides must be readable at the back of a conference room. Complex graphs, tables, or illustrations are not always readable. Consider using these materials as handouts or omitting them. Cartoons can often convey an idea very effectively; when one is scheduled to present after lunch or at the end of the day, judicious use of cartoons can enhance the attention of distracted members of the audience.

Photographs may also be appropriate to some presentations. Colorful slides are particularly useful in keeping the attention of the audience. Some presenters routinely use colorful photographs of scenery or flowers in between slides focusing on the content. Other presenters use black slides between the content slides when there is a gap of more than a minute between one content slide and the next. Many hospitals and colleges have media departments that make slides. Referrals from colleagues and the telephone directory are sources of businesses that can make slides.

The guidelines for slides also apply to transparencies. Transparencies are inexpensive and easily made (Hofland, 1987); typewritten or laser-printed pages can be photocopied onto transparency sheets. Cartoons or other illustrations can also be copied onto transparencies. Neatly handwritten materials or illustrations drawn by hand can also be copied onto transparencies. Transparencies should be stored with paper between each sheet. Cardboard frames make transparencies easier to handle. Transparencies are used most effectively in small conference rooms; images may not be clear enough or sufficiently large to be readable in more sizable conference rooms.

PRESENTING THE PAPER

A good night's sleep on the night before a presentation is essential. Avoid alcoholic or carbonated beverages at meals before the presentation (Winslow, 1991). Professional image is another important factor in successful presentations. Dress and grooming can create an image that will foster one's credibility as a professional or may detract from one's presentation (Winslow, 1991). A professional wardrobe does not have to be expensive; stylish men's and women's clothing can be purchased at reasonable prices at outlet and discount stores. Clothing should be congruent with the setting (Jader, 1991). Clothing may be more casual at a conference held at a beach resort than at a midtown hotel. Hats on women tend to take the focus off the presentation and put the focus on the presenter. Makeup should be subtle and appropriate to the harsh lighting of conference rooms. Facial hair on men must be neatly groomed.

Inspect the room in which the presentation will be given. This inspection can be done upon arrival at the conference or during the evening before or the morning of the presentation. If possible, do not wait until just before the presentation to check the room. Become familiar with the audiovisual equipment to be used. Avoid wasting your valuable presentation time learning to use the audiovisual equipment while you try to speak. Make sure that a glass of water will be available at the podium. Assess the arrangement of seats; determine how best to make eye contact with the audience (Rogers, 1990).

If you were not asked to send a biographic statement ahead of time, bring one to the conference. Give this statement to the session moderator to facilitate the introduction. When taking the podium after the introduction, greet your audience and relax! Take a few deep breaths before saying a word.

Be enthusiastic about the topic (Davidhizar & Cosgray, 1991). A speaker's tone of voice should reflect this enthusiasm without sounding melodramatic. The novice speaker needs to avoid being self-effacing. Sometimes novices tend to discredit themselves by making statements such as "I'm just a graduate student" (Roger, 1990; Wilson, 1985). Be confident in your ability to be an effective presenter.

During the course of the presentation, check the nonverbal feedback of the audience. If the audience seems not to understand, seek validation from them. Ask direct questions about the pace and complexity of the presentation (e.g., "Am I going too fast?" "Am I getting too detailed?"). Move away from the podium if the space is available; move closer to the audience. Involve your audience with frequent eye contact.

Most conferences build in time for questions and answers. Some speakers prefer to take questions during the course of their presentations; others prefer to take all questions at the end. The audience needs to know the speaker's preference. Some audiences are reluctant to ask questions. If questions are not raised by the audience, use the extra few minutes to discuss ethical or methodologic problems or to share serendipitous findings. Ask a colleague to raise a question to encourage others to ask questions. Pass out cards so the audience can write their questions out during the presentation. Admit when you cannot answer a question. Offer to provide the information by telephone or letter. If the session is being taped, repeat all questions and comments so that they will also be recorded (Wilson, 1985). Interaction with the audience can serve as a learning opportunity for you. Their questions may help you clarify the content for future presentations or publication of the research.

SUMMARY OF RESEARCH PAPER PRESENTATIONS

Paper presentations offer an interactive method of communicating research findings and allow for the quick communication of research findings, often within several weeks or months of the completion of the project. Poster presentations, discussed next, share this characteristic.

THE RESEARCH POSTER

The research poster offers novice presenters a relatively unintimidating vehicle for presenting their work. An effective way of learning to present posters is by observing the presentations of others. Note the design of the posters, the use of handouts and other supplemental materials, and the interaction styles of the presenters. The research poster presentation involves the preparation of the poster and a small-group discussion of the research. Posters can be used to present work in progress or completed studies. Like paper presentations, posters generally begin with a call for abstracts. Many calls will include both posters and papers. The author information form that accompanies the abstract may have a place to check off the author's preference for paper or poster presentation or no preference.

As with slides and transparencies, a personal computer and laser printer can ease the preparation of a poster. Graphic arts departments at colleges and universities and small graphic arts companies near college campuses may be able to do the preparation and layout of the poster. The personal computer allows the presenter to create a poster at a much lower cost. The poster boards and easel backs (for tabletop posters) are available at any art supply store. Colored poster board can create a visually engaging poster. Photographs, graphs, and tables are commonly used on posters in addition to text. Black print on white paper is most commonly used for the text, but color printers and colored paper can be used effectively.

The size of the poster is dictated by the available display area, whether the poster is to be wall mounted or displayed on a tabletop. The method of display will be identified in your letter of acceptance, along with size limitations and other information about the poster presentation session. A tabletop poster can be assembled in panels, usually two to four panels of poster board, measuring 20 by 30 inches. Wall-mounted posters can be assembled on panels, multiple sheets, or a single sheet of paper. Poster board panels can be transported in a portfolio carrier (available from business supply stores) or in a garment bag; paper posters can be rolled and transported in a tube. Most portfolio carriers will have to be checked with your luggage if you are flying to the conference site.

The research poster includes the same key elements as any other research report. The text, graphs, tables, and photographs should be concise; the poster should not take longer than five minutes to read. This will support the flow of those attending the poster session through display area. The size of font used is important; the text should be easily readable from 4 feet away.

The poster presentation is effectively supported, like verbal presentations, by handouts. Business cards should also be displayed. Copies of the data collection instrument and other relevant documents can be displayed. Poster presentations may also include videotapes or slides. However, you will generally need to pay a daily fee for electrical outlets and audiovisual equipment, if they are available at all for the poster session. Have a note pad available to get the names and addresses of those who do not have business cards and would like additional information or further opportunities for discussion (Lippman & Ponton, 1989; Lynn, 1989; Ryan, 1989).

Arrive at the poster display area plenty of time in advance to set up the poster before the viewing begins. Most poster sessions last at least 90 minutes. Some sessions may extend for several hours over 1 or 2 days, especially at those conferences where awards are conferred on selected presenters. Keep a beverage at hand; poster presenters spend much of their time talking about their research. Wear comfortable shoes (Ryan, 1989). Presenters may have a chair available, but it is awkward to sit in a chair and talk to those reviewing the poster. Plan to stand up throughout the presentation. Poster sessions are far less formal than paper presentations but are equally demanding.

SUMMARY OF POSTER PRESENTATIONS

Presenting a poster offers an opportunity to report one's research with individuals and small groups within the context of a large conference. The same key elements that are essential to other research reports are also part of the poster presentation. Poster sessions offer the novice researcher the opportunity to build skills and confidence in making research presentations.

PUBLISHING A RESEARCH REPORT

Swanson, McCloskey, and Bodensteiner (1992) reported on 92 journals that offered nurses publishing opportunities in the United States. This kind of information provides an excellent starting point for the researcher seeking to publish a study. Publishing a research report entails much more than typing a manuscript. Publishing requires a bit of additional research to ensure that the author, like a nurse giving medications, is sending the right manuscript in the right format to the right journal at the right time.

ETHICS AND ETIQUETTE

The first rule of publishing is that manuscripts are sent to one journal at a time. Mass marketing one's manuscript to several journals at once is not only unethical, but it can also put the author in the uncomfortable position of explaining to an editor that the manuscript cannot be published in the editor's journal because it has already been accepted by another journal. Editors will reject a manuscript when there is evidence that it is being submitted to more than one journal, such as the thesis submitted by a hopeful author who indicates in the cover letter that the manuscript has been submitted to several journals (Downs, 1991). It is also unethical to submit similar versions of the same manuscript to multiple journals. If both versions are published, the author's unethical behavior will be revealed. On the other hand, it is totally appropriate to break down a large study into smaller pieces and publish each as a separate article. In addition, a single, smaller study can also produce more than one article if each article focuses on a different aspect of the study. The manuscript submitted to a research journal can emphasize the methodology of the study, whereas the manuscript submitted to a clinical journal can focus on the practical application of the findings. Authors need to remember that the journal holding the copyright on their works owns the words, not the concepts (Blancett, 1986). Different words must be used in subsequent articles, but the basic concepts of the research can be addressed from a different perspective. Fraud and plagiarism can seriously discredit a writer (Blancett, 1991; Wilson, 1989).

Manuscripts must be submitted according to the guidelines for authors for that particular journal. Editors use peer reviewers who are volunteers, often members of the journal's editorial board, to evaluate manuscripts and recommend to the editor whether to publish a manuscript. Editors often receive manuscripts that were obviously prepared for another journal or are unrevised student papers. The manuscript may use the wrong editorial style, be too long, or fail to address other aspects of the journal's guidelines. Such disregard for the etiquette of publishing indicates a lack of attention to detail by the author and may result in a less favorable review or even rejection of the manuscript.

Timeliness is another issue of publishing etiquette, an issue that applies to both the author and the editor. When an author receives a conditional acceptance of the manuscript pending revision, the revised manuscript must be returned within the time frame stated by the editor. If the author cannot adhere to this schedule, the editor must be informed. A different time frame may be negotiated, although this means the article will appear in a later issue than originally planned. Likewise, editors and their reviewers have an obligation to make their evaluations of a manuscript's merit within a reasonable period of time. If the author has not received word of the manuscript's fate within a reasonable time, usually 3 to 4 months, a call to the editor is in order. Often this will break up any editorial logjam involving the manuscript (Gennaro & Vessey, 1990).

FIRST STEPS IN PUBLISHING

For the researcher the first step in publishing is to complete the study. Once the data analysis is completed and the findings are written in a rough draft, the next step is to select a journal. The nature of research itself will indicate a target audience. Some studies may be of greatest interest to those in a specific clinical specialty (e.g., community health or maternal-child nurses) or in a certain functional role (e.g., educators, administrators). Thus the choice of target journals will be narrowed first by the intended audience of the research. Check which journals the references from your study were published in. If certain journals dominate, consider them among those you wish to target. The level of complexity of the study is another good indicator of whether the target journal should be a research or practice publication. Even within the research publications, there are now journals directed at clinicians and devoted to the application of research findings. Read several journals, and read several issues of each journal to determine a possible fit between the study and the right journal. Other issues to consider include: circulation rate of the journal, rejection rate, the speed of turnaround from submission to acceptance to publication, and the prestige of the journal (refereed or nonrefereed) (Wilson, 1985). Articles, such as the one by Swanson et al. (1991), are very useful sources for this type of information.

Review recent issues of possible journals to determine if a similar study has been published recently; it is generally advisable to eliminate such journals from consideration. Narrow the journal choices to two or three, ranking them in the order in which the editors will be contacted. Read the most recent issues of these journals once again, this time to assess the writing style of the articles to ensure the good fit of the manuscript that will be submitted.

Query Letter

An optional next step may be the submission of a query letter to determine an editor's level of interest in a manuscript before submitting it. A query letter can save a writer time: considerable time can be lost by sending a manuscript to an editor who has no interest in the topic. Some journal editors prefer the query letter as the first contact from the author; a few do not want to receive query letters (Swanson et al., 1991). The query letter must be sent to the current editor (another publishing etiquette issue); check the most recent issue for the editor's name. The letter should identify the title of the study and provide information about the author (e.g., address and telephone number). An abstract of the study may accompany the letter or the study can be summarized in the body of the letter. If the editor sends no response to the query letter, send a follow-up letter or make a phone call to the editor in 4 to 6 weeks. A positive response from the editor should be acknowledged with a manuscript within a few weeks, not months later.

From Thesis to Manuscript

The next step is, of course, manuscript preparation. Although a thesis or dissertation constitutes a complete report of a research project, these require major revisions before submission. The chapter headings and the exhaustive literature reviews that characterize theses and dissertations are not appropriate in publishable manuscripts. Most journals have limits of 10 to 15 typewritten pages per manuscript; theses and dissertations tend to be much longer than this. Manuscripts that run longer than the journal's page limitations may be rejected without review or may receive a less favorable review. Members of your thesis or dissertation committee may be very helpful in the process of editing the text into a publishable form.

Guidelines for Authors

The journal's guidelines are the author's best friend. Although guidelines are often brief, they contain essential information about the editorial style, page limits, permissions, copyright, and the number of copies to be sent to the editor. The author also needs a good dictionary, a thesaurus, and the stylebook for the relevant editorial style. When word-processing software and a personal computer are used, the spell check, thesaurus, and word count features are invaluable. Software programs that format papers in selected editorial styles are also available to support writers. Editors and reviewers look much more favorably on the technical merits of a manuscript when the guidelines for authors have been followed. In addition, the writer must carefully observe the rules of grammar, syntax, and punctuation. A well-developed and well-implemented study may be rejected for publication if the manuscript is haphazardly written.

THE "WRITE" STUFF

Many journal editors take a strong stand on the use of sexist language (Blancett, 1989); avoid falling into the trap of sexist language without the use of awkward constructs like "she/he" and "her/him" throughout the manuscript. Using the plural form allows the use of neutral pronouns (e.g., "they," "them," and "their"). Other creative approaches to avoiding sexist language can be found in resource materials on writing (APA, 1994; Zorn, Smith, & Werley, 1991).

Good writing is not magic. Using language in an effective manner is a skill that comes with practice. Misuse of words (e.g., principle/principal, affect/effect); split infinitives (e.g., to carefully choose); the incorrect use of singular and plural nouns and verbs; the use of trendy language; wordiness; sentences that run too long; sentence fragments; the use of first person when the third person is preferred; and the use of passive, rather than active, voice are all examples of common writing problems

(Camilleri, 1987, 1988; Zorn et al., 1991). Attention to one's written work, peer review, and a good writer's manual can be important tools for good writing. Some writers may wish to hire an experienced editor or author to critique a manuscript. Computer programs are available to critique the structure of one's writing with recommendations for improvement. This may be an important investment for the novice writer. Manuscripts must always be typewritten and double-spaced. Copies must be legible (e.g., some dot matrix printers produce poor-quality copies).

A good manuscript will undergo several revisions. Good writing also requires critical review (Pagana, 1989). Share each draft with one or two colleagues, even former instructors. An experienced writer will generally be flattered if asked to review a work in process. However, do give reviewers ample time to read a draft. Do not expect overnight feedback; generally allow at least 3 to 5 days for colleagues to review a manuscript. Weigh the feedback carefully; pay particular attention to comments made in common by reviewers.

The manuscript should be readily understood by a reader who is not an expert in the field. It must not be so technical that the reader becomes lost in jargon with no way out except to put the article aside. When one becomes immersed in one's work, finding errors and evaluating the readability of the work become very difficult. The use of reviewers is important for keeping the manuscript reader friendly.

THE FINISHED WORK

The editorial manuscript reviews by colleagues are returned, the revisions of the manuscript are completed, and the final draft of the manuscript is complete. The manuscript is now ready to be sent to the editor after one more review. The writer must consult the guidelines for authors once again to determine how many copies of the manuscript are required. The manuscript should not include information about the identity of the author. Author information should only appear on the cover page and the cover letter. The address, telephone number, and fax or E-mail number (if applicable) of the contact author should be included in the cover letter and on the cover page. Make sure that the abstract is included. Are pages numbered and ordered sequentially? Are all the references listed on the reference pages cited in the text? Are tables and figures labeled clearly?

Before packaging the manuscript for mailing, consider sending a self-addressed, stamped postcard for the editor to return upon receipt of the manuscript. Although many editors send a letter of acknowledgment when a manuscript is received, some do not. The postcard provides a means of confirming that the editor has received the manuscript. Other options to consider would be registered mail, overnight delivery services, or other traceable couriers.

WAITING AND REVISING

The review process can take weeks to months. As noted, if the editor does not provide information on the status of a manuscript within a reasonable amount of time (usually about 3 months), a telephone call to the editor will generally clarify the reason for the delay and may break up the editorial logjam. If telephone contact is not possible, sending a letter may have the same effect.

Finally, you receive a letter from the editor announcing the fate of your manuscript. The usual outcomes of the review process are *publish as is, publish with major/minor revisions,* or *reject.* Rare is the manuscript that is published without revision. Even most of these will be subjected to some minor editorial changes. Most manuscripts are accepted conditionally and must be revised to some degree before final acceptance. Revisions must be made in a timely manner to ensure that the article will be published. A manuscript that is returned to the editor late may not be included in the planned issue of the journal. Some suggested revisions will be minor; some will entail a considerable amount of work (e.g., reducing the manuscript from 15 to 12 pages). Sometimes authors are directed to make revisions that they may view as inappropriate (e.g., deleting findings or discussion that some may find too controversial, altering the theoretical framework). Call the editor to discuss such revisions. Some editors will be willing to negotiate a mutually satisfactory alternative revision. Once the revisions are returned to the editor, sit back and enjoy this accomplishment, and then move on to the next project.

Submitting an unsolicited manuscript always leaves one open to rejection. If the manuscript is rejected, however, do not simply file the report and forget about it. More manuscripts are rejected because of poor writing than poor research (Swanson et al., 1991). Some are rejected because similar studies have recently been published in the journal or have already been accepted for future publication. Whatever the reason for rejection, the rejected manuscript can provide the writer with a learning opportunity. Once anger and disappointment have subsided, the letter outlining the reason(s) for rejection and the reviewers' comments (if provided) should be read again. Some editors may recommend another journal for consideration if the manuscript was rejected, sometimes in part, because it was inappropriate for that particular journal. Reframe the critique from the reviewers as a free editorial consultation (Gay & Edgli, 1989). Only after reviewing the comments carefully should the writer determine whether to discard the manuscript or to begin the process of revising the manuscript. If the writer decides to revise and submit to another journal, the process of review, revision, and waiting begins again.

SUMMARY OF THE PUBLICATION PROCESS

Once a research project is complete, researchers have an obligation to share their work with the professional community. Although presentations of research in the formats of papers and posters are valuable means of disseminating research quickly, the publication of a study provides a permanent record of the study that is available to a much wider audience (Wilson, 1985). Writing for publication is not a simple task but a complex skill that demands considerable practice.

EVALUATING A RESEARCH REPORT

This chapter has focused primarily on communicating one's own research. When research is shared with the professional community in any format, members of the profession are then obligated to evaluate the research for application to their practice as part of the continuing process of communicating research. Evaluating or critiquing a research report allows the research reader to determine the merit of the study and whether it is applicable to the individual's practice. The process of evaluating a research report requires breaking down the report into its component parts (Fleming & Hayter, 1974; Soeken, 1985). The factors listed in the box can assist in this evaluation process. (The reader is referred to Chapter 23.)

AUTHOR'S QUALIFICATIONS

Most journals give a brief biographic statement about authors. Conference proceedings will usually identify the credentials and affiliations of presenters. Do the reported credentials support the author's ability to conduct the study? The credibility of a single author holding only an associate degree or even a baccalaureate degree in nursing is questionable. Did the author rely on an unidentified collaborator? Are consultants or collaborators identified in an acknowledgment, although they are not listed as coauthors? Is there a citation of previous work by this author? On the other hand, few newly graduated MSNs or PhDs

---

EVALUATING THE RESEARCH REPORT

- Do the author's credentials support their ability to conduct the study?
- Is the journal a refereed (i.e., peer-reviewed) publication, or are articles selected by the editor?
- Does the abstract clearly and succinctly provide a summary of the study?
- Is the purpose of the study clearly stated?
- Is the literature review complete? Does it support the study's theoretical framework?

- Are the methods clearly stated so that they are understood by a reader who is not an expert?
- Are the results presented clearly?
- Is the relationship between the data and conclusions clear?
- Do recommendations for further study flow from the findings?
- Is the report easy to read?

conduct research without consultants, although they may have the appropriate educational credentials to be independent researchers.

QUALITY OF THE JOURNAL

The journal is also evaluated. Is the journal a refereed (i.e., peer-reviewed) publication, or are articles selected by the editor? Journals will usually provide this information in their published guidelines for authors or on the masthead. Publication in a peer-reviewed journal indicates that the report has already undergone a fairly rigorous review, but it does not mean that the study is without weakness.

ABSTRACT

Does the abstract clearly and succinctly provide a summary of the study? Are the major purposes and findings of the study clearly stated? In addition, does the title clearly tell you about the focus of the study?

PURPOSE OF THE STUDY

Why did the author carry out the study? The purpose needs to be clearly stated. Did the study seek to address a clinical problem or an administrative problem? Was the author trying to test an observation from the author's own practice? Did unmet patient needs stimulate the development and implementation of the study?

If the purpose is clearly stated, is it significant to the body of nursing knowledge? Operational definitions of significant terms must be clearly identified. If the study has an experimental design, are the hypotheses appropriately stated? If the design is historical or descriptive, for example, are the research questions adequately stated?

REVIEW OF THE LITERATURE

If the research is in a relatively new area of study, is literature on related research included? When appropriate, literature from disciplines outside of nursing must be included in the review. Are important references and seminal works included, or is the reference list studded with citations from obscure journals? Is the literature cited reviewed critically or just reported? Are all the publications noted in the reference list cited in the literature review? Are there gaps or inconsistencies in the literature, such as no recent publications or citations from only one journal? The author may not cite other current literature that takes a different view of the issue addressed by the author. Does the writing flow? Is the review just a series of summaries or an integrated review? The literature review should:

- Support the study's theoretical or conceptual framework
- Identify the underlying assumptions of the study
- Enable the researcher to avoid the mistakes made by others
- Clarify the research questions or hypotheses (Soeken, 1985).

DESCRIPTION OF METHODS AND PROCEDURES

The methods section must clarify whether the study is an original work or if it is a replication, extension, or modification of a previous work. The methods should be clearly stated so that they are understood by someone who is not an expert. Is the method of data collection appropriate to the problem being investigated? Are the data collection tools valid and reliable? In experimental designs, are independent and dependent variables clearly identified? The issue of human subjects must be addressed: how was informed consent gained from subjects?

Are the statistical tests appropriate to the data? Are descriptive statistics of the sample identified? If the data are reported in a narrative format, they must be presented in a manner that is understandable to the reader. If graphs and tables are used to report the data, are they easily interpreted by the reader? If inferential statistics are used, complete information must be provided (e.g., degrees of freedom, probability level).

DISCUSSION OF THE FINDINGS

The relationship between the data and the conclusions must be clear. One weakness of too many studies is that the conclusions are not firmly based on the data presented. If there is a previous body of research, how do the findings of this study compare? If the current findings are inconsistent with the existing body of research, are plausible explanations for the differences offered? Do recommendations for further research flow from the findings? For studies on clinical problems, are the implications for clinical practice noted and are they realistic for the clinician? Does the discussion focus on the original research questions or hypotheses, indicating whether the questions were satisfactorily answered or the hypotheses supported or rejected? Are the limitations identified and discussed in relation to the outcomes of the study? Are the recommendations for further study grounded in the findings of the study?

INTEGRATION OF THE REPORT

Is the report easily read? Is it so technical or so wordy that it was boring? Are the data presented in such a way that the reader is lost? Is there a logical flow of thought throughout the report?

SUMMARY OF RESEARCH REPORT EVALUATION

Evaluation of research reports is required before findings are integrated into practice or tested in replication studies. After reading and evaluating a research report, the reader needs to determine whether the work adds to the existing body of nursing knowledge and whether this new knowledge is applicable to the reader's clinical practice.

SUMMARY

- The major categories of research reports are theses, dissertations, paper presentations, posters, and articles.
- Theses and dissertations demonstrate a student's ability to conduct scholarly research and serve to communicate study findings.
- Paper presentations and posters enable researchers to communicate their work within weeks to months of completing a study.
- Although publishing a study in a journal may take longer than a year, the article is a lasting record of the research with broad circulation.
- The key elements of a research report are the *title*, an *introduction*, the *methods*, the *results*, and a *discussion*.
- An abstract is a brief summary of the key elements of a research project that introduces a written research report and facilitates sharing and marketing a study in research conferences.
- Paper and poster presentations should precede, not follow, publication of a study.
- A paper presentation requires significant preparation time, including rehearsal time.
- The judicious use of handouts, transparencies, and slides can enhance a paper presentation.
- Avoid the *five deadly sins* of paper presentations.
- Research posters include the basic elements of the research report in a highly visual format.
- The ethics of writing a research article demand that the article be submitted for review to one journal at a time.

- Systematically selecting the right journal speeds up the publication process.
- Adhering to the journal's guidelines for authors is essential to success in publishing.
- The rules of grammar, spelling, punctuation, and syntax are essential to effective writing, as is the process of revision.
- Even when the manuscript is accepted, more revisions are usually required.
- A rejected manuscript is often worth revising for resubmission to another journal.
- Evaluating a research report entails the critical review of the author's qualifications, quality of the journal, abstract, purpose of the study, review of the literature, description of methods and procedures, results of data analysis, discussion of the findings, and integration of the report.

FACILITATING CRITICAL THINKING

1. Select two or three articles from research journals. Identify the key elements of each research report.
2. Read a research article from a refereed journal, and then write an abstract of the article.
3. Ask a colleague to critique a paper you have written for school or for publication. Review the feedback with your colleague.
4. Attend a local research conference. Evaluate the presentations of two presenters. Note if they avoid the five deadly sins of paper presentations.
5. Review the poster presentations at the same research conference. Do the poster and the handouts adequately provide an overview of the study? Is the presenter well prepared to provide more detailed information when interacting with poster viewers?
6. Select a research article from a refereed journal. Evaluate the report using the criteria outlined in this chapter.

References

CONCEPTUAL

BLANCETT, S. S. (1991). The ethics of writing and publishing. *Journal of Nursing Administration, 21*(5), 31-36.

DOWNS, F. S. (1991). A construction report. *Nursing Research, 40,* 4.

GENNARO, S., & VESSEY, J. (1990). Waiting for Godot. *Nursing Research, 39,* 259.

HAYES, P. (1992). "De-jargonizing" research communication. *Clinical Nursing Research, 1,* 19-220.

MCCLOSKEY, J. C., & SWANSON, E. (1985). Publishing in practice journals: A responsibility of the researcher. *CNR Newsletter, 12*(3), 1-4.

MORSE, J. M. (1993). The perfect manuscript. *Qualitative Health Research, 3,* 3-5.

SWANSON, E. A., MCCLOSKEY, J. C., & BODENSTEINER, A. (1991). Publishing opportunities for nurses: A comparison of 92 U.S. journals. *IMAGE: Journal of Nursing Scholarship, 23,* 33-38.

WILSON, H. S. (1985). Disseminating research: The scholar's commitment. *Journal of Nursing Administration, 15*(3), 6-8.

METHODOLOGICAL

AMERICAN PSYCHOLOGICAL ASSOCIATION. (1994). *Publication manual of the American Psychological Association* (4th ed.). Washington, DC: The Association.

BLANCETT, S. S. (1986). Getting your research published. *Journal of Nursing Administration, 16*(2), 6.

BLANCETT, S. S. (1989). She is a man: Avoiding sexist language. *Journal of Nursing Administration, 19*(12), 5.

CAMILLERI, R. (1987). Six ways to write. *IMAGE: Journal of Nursing Scholarship, 19,* 210-212.

CAMILLERI, R. (1988). On elegant writing. *IMAGE: Journal of Nursing Scholarship, 20,* 169-171.

DAVIDHIZAR, R. & COSGRAY, R. (1991). Being an effective speaker. *Today's OR Nurse, 13*(8), 36-38.

FLEMING, J. W., & HAYTER, J. (1974). Reading research reports critically. *Nursing Outlook, 22,* 172-175.

GAY, J. T., & EDGLI, A. E. (1989). When your manuscript is rejected. *Nursing & Health Care, 10,* 459-461.

HOFLAND, S. L. (1987). Transparency design for effective oral presentations. *Journal of Continuing Education in Nursing, 18*(3), 83-88.

JACKLE, M. (1989). Presenting research to nurses in clinical practice. *Journal of Applied Nursing Research, 2,* 191-193.

JACKLE, M. (1992). Presenting research to perioperative audiences. *AORN Journal, 55,* 811-812, 814-815.

JADER, G. C. (1991). Ten tips for becoming a better public speaker. *Nurse Practitioner, 16*(9), 9-10.

LIPPMAN, D. T., & PONTON, K. S. (1989). Designing a research poster with impact. *Western Journal of Nursing Research, 11,* 477-485.

LYNN, M. R. (1989). Poster sessions: A good way to communicate research. *Journal of Pediatric Nursing, 4,* 211-213.

PAGANA, K. D. (1989). Writing strategies to demystify publishing. *Journal of Continuing Education in Nursing, 20*(2), 58, 63.

POLIT, D. F., & HUNGLER, B. P. (1991). *Nursing research: Principles and methods* (4th ed.). Philadelphia: J. B. Lippincott.

ROGERS, B. (1990). Research presentations. *AAOHN Journal, 38,* 191-192.

RYAN, N. M. (1989). Developing and presenting a research poster. *Applied Nursing Research, 2,* 52-55.

SELBY, M. L., TORNQUIST, E. M., & FINERTY, E. J. (1989a). How to present your research, part I. *Nursing Outlook, 37,* 172-175.

SELBY, M. L., TORNQUIST, E. M., & FINERTY, E. J. (1989b). How to present your research, part II. *Nursing Outlook, 37,* 236-238.

SOEKEN, K. L. (1985). Critiquing research: Steps for complete evaluation of an article. *AORN Journal, 41,* 882-893.

TEEL, C. S. (1990). Completing the research process: Presentations and publications. *Journal of Neuroscience Nursing, 22,* 125-127.

WILSON, H. S. (1989). *Research in nursing* (2nd ed.). Menlo Park, CA: Addison-Wesley.

WINSLOW, E. H. (1991). Overcome the fear of speaking in public. *American Journal of Nursing, 91*(5), 51-53.

WOODS, N. F., & CATANZARO, M. (Eds.). (1988). *Nursing research theory and practice.* St. Louis: Mosby.

ZORN, C. R., SMITH, M. C., & WERLEY, H. H. (1991). Watch your language. *Nursing Outlook, 39,* 183-185.

GLOSSARY

abstract Brief, comprehensive summary of a study.

accessible population Portion of target population available to the researcher.

active variable Characteristic investigated in a study. Also see *variable*.

aesthetic inquiry See *photography and aesthetic inquiry*.

aesthetics Appropriateness of the need for a qualitative study, including appropriateness of approach, construction, and implementation.

after-only design Experimental design with two randomly assigned groups—treatment and control. This design differs from the true experiment in that both groups are measured only after the experimental treatment.

alpha (α) Probability of type I error in research.

alternate hypothesis (H₁) Prediction that the independent variable will have an effect on the dependent variable.

analysis approach Strategy used in theory development in which concepts, statements, or theories are clarified or refined.

analysis of covariance (ANCOVA) Statistic that measures differences among group means; ANCOVA uses a statistical technique to equate the groups to an important variable.

analysis of variance (ANOVA) Parametric statistical test of mean differences among three or more populations.

analytical log Written summary of the theoretical notes, analytical memos, and researcher's conceptualizations over the course of a study.

anonymity Quality of being unknown or unidentified; in research, it is the fact that information from participants' responses in a study are protected from being linked to their identity by anyone, including the researcher.

applied research Scientific inquiry focused on generating, testing, and expanding knowledge for clinical practice.

assumption Overt and/or innate belief held about a phenomenon that is accepted as truth without proof or empirical evidence; unproven statement or principle whose accuracy is taken for granted on the basis of logical reasoning; an idea universally accepted as true.

attribute variable Preexisting characteristic or attribute of the population that cannot be manipulated.

autonomy Ethical principle of self-determination; freedom of an individual to make decisions independent of outside influences or coercion.

bar graph Frequency distribution graph reflecting a series of scores in which the height of the bar corresponds to the frequency of scores.

basic research Scientific inquiry focused on generating, testing, and expanding knowledge.

beneficence Ethical principle advocating doing good; in research, it is the researcher assuring research participants that benefits attained from participation in a study outweigh the risks of participation.

beta (β) probability of type II error in research.

bias Influences from various sources which may sway or distort the study outcome; difference between what an individual believes or observes about a phenomenon and the true phenomenon.

bimodal distribution Distribution with two peaks.

bivariate statistics Extended statistical analysis used to determine a relationship between two variables.

blinding Research technique used to minimize bias by withholding the study hypothesis or specific details of treatment from subjects until the study is completed. Also see *double-blinding*.

block design Incorporation of a potential confounding variable in the study design as an independent variable.

blocking See *block design*.

canonical correlation Measure of the strength of the relationship between two sets of variables.

case Singular observation, event, or participant that provides the data in a data set.

case-study method Detailed examination over time of a single setting, event, or subject to render in-depth descriptions of inherent dimensions and processes.

categorical/analytical scheme Researcher's chosen method of organizing, identifying, managing, and analyzing data.

categorical research data Information that represents qualitative features or properties of a variable; variables are identified or classified in descriptive terms.

causality Relationship between phenomena in which one phenomenon precedes and can be shown to influence another; causality often cannot be proven.

central tendency Descriptive statistical index used to describe a center of a set of scores—usually the mean, median, or mode.

chi-square test for goodness-of-fit Statistical test used to identify differences between the observed frequencies (data) and the expected frequencies (null hypothesis).

chi-square test for independence Statistical test using frequency data to test a hypothesis about the relationship between two variables; the frequency distribution is used to determine whether one variable is independent of another.

circumscribed conditions Defined boundaries or properties (physical or otherwise) of a research issue.

closed-ended question Question worded to elicit a limited response, such as yes or no. Also known as "fixed alternative question".

cluster analysis Research approach that uses a variety of techniques for data classification and reduction.

cluster sampling Probability sampling strategy that involves a successive random sampling of units; units sampled progress from large to small.

coding Process of identifying concepts and themes in raw data so patterns can be identified for further analysis.

common factors analysis Highly conceptual approach to factor analysis; this analysis is used when factors have been hypothesized and the researcher would like to estimate factors from available data. Also see *factor analysis*.

commonality Amount of variance one variable shares with another.

comparison Use of association and contrast to uncover conceptual similarities and differences in data.

complex hypothesis Statement of the causal or associative relationship between two or more independent variables and/or two or more dependent variables.

concept Abstract idea, mental image, or word picture of a phenomenon.

conceptual definition See *theoretical definition*.

conceptual framework Network of interrelated concepts and propositions that provide a structure for organizing and describing a phenomenon. Also see *metaparadigm*.

concurrent validity Truthfulness of the subject's current status in relation to the variable or standard.

confidentiality Assurance that information received from a research participant will not be given to a third party without the subject's permission.

confirmability Extent to which research findings, conclusions, and recommendations are supported by the data; extent to which three is internal agreement between the investigator's interpretations and the actual evidence.

constant Concept that does not change and has a single value.

constitutive patterns Relationships between themes.

construct Highly abstract concept which cannot be measured directly; only inferences can be made through less abstract indicators of the phenomenon.

contruct validity of putative causes and effects Extent to which the presumed causal relationship between two variables is indeed a relationship or is a result of a confounding variable.

content validity Assessment of an instrument's ability to measure what it purports to measure; degree to which the data collection tool reflects the body of knowledge pertaining to the concept being studied.

continuous variable Variable that has an infinite number of possible values ranging from positive to infinity, to negative to infinity; each value is capable of dividing into smaller and smaller units.

contrast question   Question worded to elicit a response which emphasizes differences of a phenomenon.

control   Screening out all extraneous influences on the dependent variable to avoid altering the true relationships between study variables.

control group   Group in an experimental investigation that does not receive an intervention or treatment; the comparison group.

convenience sampling   Nonprobability sampling strategy that uses the most readily accessible persons or objects as subjects in a study.

convergent validity principle   Different measures of the same trait should have a high correlation.

correlation   Bivariate statistical method used to indicate whether two variables are related and to measure the degree of that relationship; the direction of the relationship may be positive or negative.

correlation coefficient   Statistic that represents the degree of relationship between two variables.

correlational research   Examination of the strength of a relationship between two or more variables.

counterbalancing   Actively controlling extraneous forces by varying treatment orders to determine whether or not the order of presentation influences subject responses.

creative thinking   Thought processes that unite imaginative risk-taking with systematic scientific observation in the search for new ideas and the manipulation of knowledge and experience.

creativity   Ability to look at things differently than others; ability to produce something through imaginative skills or to bring something new into existence.

credibility   Believability of the findings and interpretations from the data; criterion used in evaluating qualitative studies.

criterion-referenced measurement   Comparison of the subject's score with a preset standard to determine whether or not the subject has acquired a set of target behaviors.

criterion-related validity   Multiple measures of the same concept; one instrument is compared to a second instrument which measures the same concept; this second instrument is the criterion by which the validity of the new instrument is checked.

criterion variable   See *dependent variable.*

critical thinking   Art of disciplined reasoning using various thought processes essential for assessing, integrating, and applying information.

critique   Unbiased and objective analysis of the strengths and weaknesses of a research report.

culture   System of beliefs, social forms, and material traits used by members of a group to interpret experiences and generate behavior.

data (sing. **datum**)   Pieces of information.

data analysis   Evaluation of information and its pertinence to the study variables.

data collection   Gathering of information from the sampling units.

data source triangulation   Collection of data over time from a variety of persons in a variety of contexts to validate the consistency of research results over time, place, and person.

deductive reasoning   Reasoning process which proceeds from generalized ideas to more specific ideas.

degrees of freedom   Number of quantities that are unknown minus the number of independent equations linking these unknowns; a function of the number in the sample.

Delphi survey technique   Data collection method which uses a panel of experts and multiple rounds of surveys to achieve consensus on a topic of interest.

dependability   Others can logically follow the processes and procedures used in the study and find the same or similar concepts, patterns, and themes as the researcher if given the same data, context, and perspective.

dependent variable   Outcome or criterion variable that is observed for changes to assess the possible effect of the treatment or manipulation.

derivation approach   Method of theory development in which metaphors or analogies are used to modify or refine a concept from one context for use in another context.

descriptive question   Broad question worded to elicit a picture of how the participant perceives a phenomenon.

descriptive research   Research studies which describe a phenomenon or examine relationships between variables through the use of questionnaires or structured observations.

descriptive statistics   Statistical methods which summarize, organize, and describe data, providing an organized visual representation of the data collected.

descriptive theory   A theory which classifies or describes specific dimensions or characteristics of individuals, groups, situations, or events by summarizing the commonalties found in discrete observations.

deterministic processes   Phenomena about which all identifying elements and their relative impact are known; processes that are devoid of randomness.

diachronic reliability   Stability of answers over time; assessment measure of similarity of responses in two qualitative studies done at separate times.

directional hypothesis Proposition which predicts the direction of the relationship between the dependent and the independent variable—for example, when a hypothesis states that one group's measure of central tendency will be greater than another's, rather than simply different.

discovery Scrutinization and examination of data to interpret the meaning of a phenomenon.

discrete variable Variable with a finite number of possible values.

discriminant analysis Alternate method for multiple regression used when the dependent variable is at a nominal level of measurement.

discriminant validity principle Principle asserting that instruments measuring different constructs should have low correlations with each other.

double-blinding Technique to eliminate bias by withholding the study hypotheses or specific details of treatments from both the subjects and the person(s) collecting and/or analyzing the data until the study is completed. Also see *blinding*.

effect size Statistical value that represents the magnitude of the results of a statistical analysis—for example, either the magnitude of a relationship between two variables or the magnitude of the difference between groups concerning a specific attribute.

eigenvalue Measure of how much variance can be explained by a linear combination of variables.

embedded review Review of literature that is included (embedded) in the research study; it is used to validate the approach or results of the study.

emic perspective Perspective of the phenomenon from the insider's point of view.

empirical findings Results that can be verified or disproved by experience or observation.

equivalence Assessment of reliability by using two versions of one instrument with one sample at one time.

error Difference between the measured value and the true value; inaccurate or false knowledge.

ethics Principles of conduct governing research which are reflected by the researcher's value of and concern for the participants in a study.

ethnographic research Method of examining cultures, subcultures, and ways of life within natural settings by a researcher who has been accepted by the cultural group. Also known as "ethnographic method" and "ethnographic study".

ethnography Qualitative study of a group of people including their language and their norms to collect, describe, and analyze the ways in which these people categorize the meaning of their world in a cultural context.

ethnoscience Qualitative method of describing cultural phenomena.

ethnoscience ethnography Taxonomic analysis of particular domains.

etic view Observer's perspective of the study and analysis of observed behavior.

ex post facto study Research in which the independent variable is a naturally occurring attribute, such as gender or age; groups are constituted "after the fact".

exhaustive When the selected intervals or categories include all possible values. Also see *mutually exclusive*.

experimental design Research design characterized by manipulation, control, and randomization; provides the strongest evidence for causality; also known as "true experimental design".

experimental group Group in an experimental investigation that receives the intervention or treatment.

experimental research Powerful, controlled examination of variables through manipulation of the independent variable, use of controls over the experimental conditions, use of control and experimental groups, and random assignment of subjects to the control or experimental group.

expert reviewers Evaluators with expertise in a particular field or subject.

explanatory theory Set of statements which conceptualize relationships among the dimensions or characteristics of individuals, groups, situations, or events.

exploratory research Flexible research approach used when little is known about the phenomenon under study.

external validity Extent to which an observed causal relationship can confidently be generalized to situations outside of the specific research setting.

extraneous variable Uncontrolled variable in the research environment that threatens the internal or external validity of the study.

face validity Determination through visual examination of the extent to which an instrument measures the domain of interest; face validity is an opinion, not a valid assessment.

factor analysis Data reduction, interdependence technique by which a large number of variables may be examined for interrelationships, combined into a smaller number of correlated variables, and then conceptually interpreted in terms of those correlations.

factors Commonalties or dimensions suggesting variable groupings.

fidelity Obligation to remain faithful to commitments.

field notes Detailed recordings of information collected in the field during a period of observation.

freestanding review Literature review conducted as an end to itself with new knowledge as a direct outcome.

frequency distribution Method of grouping data into categories and reporting the number of frequencies or occurrences in each category.

frequency polygon Line graph constructed from a frequency distribution to show the number of times each value occurs in a set of data.

generalizability Degree to which study findings from a sample can be related to a larger population.

grand theory Broad-scope theory representing concepts that are very abstract and not easily empirically tested.

grounded theory research Theory developed through an inductive approach in which theory is discovered or generated from data; simultaneous collection and analysis of data seek to develop and theoretically refine relevant categories, relationships are then hypothesized within and between categories forming a basis for emerging theory. Also known as "grounded theory development".

hermeneutics Study of the methodological principles of interpretation by using texts to explain a phenomenon.

histogram Diagram that represents the frequency of each class using vertical bars with no space between them, indicating the continuous nature of a variable; reflective of interval or ratio data.

historical approach Research method used to investigate past events.

historiography Science and art of reconstructing the past from a critical review of documents, artifacts, literature, and eyewitness or participant accounts of the event.

history (1) Threat to internal validity in which events occur between a pretest and a posttest that may affect the outcome of the treatment or response (2) part of the framework for qualitative research that records and explains past events.

humanistic/holistic paradigm World view that assumes multiple realities by which people create a value based on perceptions and experiences and recognize the unique context from which these experiences arise. Also known as "nursing scientific paradigm".

hypothesis Prediction of the expected relationship between the independent and dependent variables. Also see *alternate hypothesis, complex hypothesis, directional hypothesis, nondirectional hypothesis, null hypothesis, research hypothesis, simple hypothesis.*

independent variable Variable believed to influence the dependent variable; in experimental study, it is the variable that is manipulated and controlled by the researcher. Also known as "predictor variable".

inductive analysis Process of identifying patterns by drawing inferences through the examination of specific events.

inductive reasoning Reasoning process which proceeds from specific ideas to more generalized ideas.

inferential statistics Statistical techniques used to estimate or predict a population parameter from a sample statistic. Also see *nonparametric statistical tests, parametric statistical tests.*

informants Members of the population under study, they provide information and help interpret the setting and situational occurrences for the researcher. Also known as "respondents."

informed consent The obligation of the researcher to obtain voluntary consent for participation in a research project after informing the participants of potential risks and benefits.

institutional review board Board established to review biomedical and behavioral research involving human subjects within an agency or in agency-sponsored programs.

internal validity Degree to which the outcome can be attributed to the experimental treatment and not extraneous variables; determination of whether an observed relationship between variables is indeed causal.

intrarater reliability Reliability based on two or more raters using the same instrumentation or plan independently and concurrently rating the same event.

intervening variable Type of extraneous variable that cannot be controlled, is innate to the participant, and whose effect on the study cannot be measured.

interview Data collection method that uses verbal communication between researcher and respondent to elicit information about a given topic through direct questioning; interviews can be "structured" or "unstructured".

intrarater reliability Reliability based on the use of one rater to rate the same observation or instrument on two or more occasions.

inverse relationship Relationship between variables where an increase in one variable is associated with a decrease in the other variable.

investigator triangulation Using multiple observers and analysts to evaluate raw data from both the same and a different perspectives.

justice Ethical principle asserting that individuals should be treated equally.

key informant Person of significant influence or leadership in a culture being studied who is willing to provide information to the researcher.

Kruskal-Wallis test Nonparametric alternative to the parametric analysis of variance with no assumption about normal distribution or homogeneity of variance; requires quantitative data collected or converted into ranks from three or more independent groups.

Kuder-Richardson formula Technique for estimating internal consistency of a data collection instrument.

level of significance (alpha level) The risk of making a type I error, that is, of incorrectly rejecting the null hypothesis; the level is set by the researcher before the study begins.

Likert scale Summated rating scale used to ascertain opinions or attitudes; each item contains a range or scaled response on a particular question stemming from "strongly agree" to "strongly disagree."

limitations Weaknesses in a study, such as uncontrolled variables, that restrict the generalizability of the findings.

literature review Systematic search of published works to gain information about a research topic.

longitudinal study Nonexperimental research design in which a researcher collects data from the same group at different points in time.

manipulation Active initiation, implementation, and termination of procedures within the specifications of a given research design.

Mann-Whitney U test Nonparametric test used to determine whether two groups are significantly different when scores from two sets of data are ranked and compared; alternate to the independent sample t-test when parametric assumptions for t-test cannot be met.

matching Control method using one or more extraneous variables (usually up to three) that attempts to find subject(s) from the first control group who have the specific matching variable.

maturation Changes in research subjects over time that can affect study results.

mean Arithmetic average of all the scores in a distribution; sum of all scores divided by the total number of scores.

measurement (1) In quantitative research, the process of assigning numbers to objects in which the number represents the quantity of the attribute being studied (2) In qualitative research, the assignment of words, phrases, or concepts into categories that represent the characteristics possessed by the phenomena under study. Also see *interval measurement, nominal measurement, ordinal measurement, ratio measurement.*

median Midpoint or middle value of a distribution of scores; half the measure are above the median and half the measures are below.

metaanalysis Research method that compiles the findings of multiple studies in a specific area to make conclusions about that particular area.

metaparadigm Philosophy which provides structure for theories of a discipline; constructs and relational statements single out concerns unique to a particular discipline.

methodologic Systematic approach to techniques, procedures, or modes of inquiry.

methodological notes Personal directions, appraisals of the researcher's approach or style, comments regarding the study design and implementation, and methodological reminders for future plans or points of clarification.

methodological triangulation Using different data collection techniques in the same study to counterbalance their respective strengths and weaknesses. Also see *triangulation.*

middle-range theory Theory limited in number of concepts and scope that attempts to explain a smaller part of the universe than does a grand theory; testable due to specificity.

modality Number of peaks in a frequency distribution.

mode Value occurring most frequently in a set of data.

multimodal distribution Curve representing a distribution of numbers that has more than one peak.

multiple analysis of covariance (MANCOVA) Statistical test that uses metric covariates to determine the effect of independent variables on dependent variables. Also see *analysis of variance (ANOVA).*

multiple regression analysis Statistical technique of predicting changes in the dependent variable resulting from changes in the independent variables, determining which independent variables are useful predictors of the dependent variable, and ascertaining the proportion of change in the dependent variable attributable to each independent variable. Also known as "multiple regression".

mutually exclusive Single score, case, or concept that fits appropriately into only one category or group.

naturalistic inquiry Qualitative research conducted in the natural setting working with (rather than on) people.

network sampling (snowballing) Nonprobability sampling strategy used for locating samples which are difficult to find. It uses social networks—the fact that friends tend to have characteristics in common; subjects who meet the eligibility criteria are asked to help locate others who meet the same criteria.

nominal measurement Level of measurement in which observations are categorized or sorted based on defined properties; each category is distinct, mutually exclusive, and exhaustive.

nondirectional hypothesis Propositional statement that does not specify the direction of the relationship between the independent and dependent variable. For example, when a hypothesis states there is a difference in one group's measure of central tendency but does not state the direction of that difference. See *two-tailed statistical test*.

nonexperimental design Study that does not involve the manipulation, control, or randomization of a variable but instead attempts to describe an already existing situation.

nonmaleficence Ethical principle of a researcher asserting that a subject will not be harmed as a result of participation in research.

nonparametric tests Statistical tests which require fewer assumptions about the characteristics of the population distribution, i.e., do not require a normal distribution for the population data; these tests may be performed on qualitative data.

nonprobability sampling Sample selection method in which random selection is not used, therefore each element or participant in the study does not have an independent and equal chance of being included in the study. Nonprobability methods are convenience sampling, quota sampling, purposive sampling, and snowball sampling.

nonrefereed journal Periodical in which the editor makes the decisions regarding publication of manuscripts.

normal distribution Frequency distribution of a set of variables usually represented by a bell-shaped curve. A symmetrical distribution in which 68.26% of all scores fall between one standard deviation above and one standard deviation below the mean (mean = mode = median).

norm-referenced measures Method of evaluating performance of an individual relative to the performance of other individuals or established norms based on comparison or normative group.

null hypothesis (H_0) Prediction that the independent variable will not have an effect on the dependent variable; predicts there will be no difference, no change, or no effect on the dependent variable for the populations that are being compared.

one-tailed statistical test Test used when the research hypothesis is directional. See *directional hypothesis*.

open coding Categorizing (tagging) data to identify underlying patterns.

open-ended question Question that allows a respondent to qualify an answer.

operational definition Specification of how a concept will be measured in terms of the research protocol or instrument to be used.

ordinal measurement Level of measurement in which scores or observations are ranked in order without equal distance between individual data.

paradigm Unique view of the world that prescribes the nature and direction of science within a discipline. Also see *humanistic/holistic paradigm, symbolic interactionist paradigm*.

parameter Measurement which describes population values; estimated from statistics.

parametric statistical tests Statistical tests which make inferences about a specific population parameter; these tests require assumptions about characteristics of the population distribution.

Pearson product-moment correlation coefficient Parametric statistical test for correlation in which interval level data are used to determine the strength of the relationship between the variables.

personal/methodological journal Compilation of the personal and methodological notes taken during an inquiry. See *methodological notes, personal notes*.

personal notes Researcher's personal reflections feelings, experiences, preconceived ideas, assumptions, and reactions.

phenomenological research A descriptive qualitative research methodology in which the essence of the phenomena under study is interpreted through the "lived experience" of individuals. Also see *phenomenology*.

phenomenology Defined as a method, phenomenology is a theoretical, long-term study of the meaning or essence of a human experience; defined as a philosophy, phenomenology is a concern for the meaning of human experience rather than scientific measurements of human behavior.

photography and aesthetic inquiry Use of visuals as research tools to validate a researcher's objective recollection; context of time, place, artist's motivation, nature of content, and depiction of a phenomenon should be evaluated.

physiologic measure Method of assessing a respondent's biophysical, biochemical, or microbiologic status.

pilot study Preliminary research conducted to test elements of experimental design before an actual full-scale study begins.

point estimation Statistical technique that allows an investigator to use information from a random sample to determine a single numerical value that would be a good indicator of the value of an underlying parameter.

population Entire set of individuals, events, places, or objects that possess the specific characteristics or attributes being studied. Also see *accessible population, target population*.

posttest Procedure in which data are collected after the administration of an experimental treatment.

power Probability that a statistical test will reject the null hypothesis (H_0) when the null hypothesis (H_0) is in fact false.

power analysis Procedure for estimating the likelihood that a type II error has been committed in a reported study; procedure for examining power prospectively for the purpose of determining the necessary sample size.

predictive theory Set of statements which express precise relationships among the dimensions or characteristics of a phenomenon in which a specific outcome can be predicted. Also known as "practice theory".

predictive validity Type of criterion-related validity which determines if test scores measuring the predictor variable can predict future standing, status, or performance.

predictor variable See *dependent variable*.

pretest Collection of data before administration of an experimental treatment; also, preliminary trials with data collection instruments.

pretest-posttest design Experimental design in which data are collected both before and after administration of treatment.

primary source The original work of a theorist or researcher; in historical research it is a person, book, document, or artifact that provides first-hand information. Primary sources include eyewitness accounts of historic events provided by original documents, films, letters, diaries, records, artifacts, periodicals, or tapes.

privacy Ethical principle advocating protection of all information to maintain confidentiality between the participant and the researcher.

probability sampling Randomized method of selecting subjects for a research study that promotes optimum representation of the target population; each subject has an equal and independent chance (or probability greater than zero) of being included in the study.

problem statement Statement or question describing the subject that will be under investigation.

proposition General statement about the relationship(s) among concepts in a theory.

prospective study Nonexperimental study that begins with an exploration of assumed causes and then moves forward in time to the presumed effect.

purpose Specific aim of the research study.

purposive sampling Nonprobability sampling strategy in which the researcher selects subjects who are considered to be typical of the population.

Q-sort Data collection method in which the subject sorts statements into specified piles based on the investigator's instruction—for example, piles categorized as agree, neither agree nor disagree, and disagree.

qualitative analysis Organization, summarization, and interpretation of communications that are not numerical by nature.

qualitative approach Systematic inquiry into the understanding of human beings and the nature and meaning of their transactions with themselves and their surroundings; a method which develops a theory related to a phenomenon.

qualitative design Collection, integration, and synthesis of narrative, nonnumerical data; this design is also used for theory generation and formulation of hypotheses. Also see *quantitative design*.

qualitative research Exploration of little-known phenomena that are not easily quantified or categorized using inductive reasoning to develop generalizations or theories from specific observations or interviews. Also see *quantitative research*.

quantitative analysis Manipulation of data through various mathematical procedures designed to produce descriptive or inferential information.

quantitative design Collection, integration, and analysis of numerical data. Also see *qualitative research*.

quantitative research Rigorous, systematic, objective examination of specific concepts and their relationships to test theory by focusing on numerical data, statistical analysis, and controls to eliminate bias. Also see *qualitative research*.

quasi-experimental research Research in which causal relationships between selected variables are examined through manipulation of the independent variable but without the control group and random assignment of subjects used in experimental research.

questionnaire Participant self-reporting measurement instrument used to obtain information about attitudes, knowledge, feelings, and other reactions that cannot easily be observed or measured physiologically.

quixotic reliability Type of reliability characteristic of circumstances in which a single method of observation continually yields an unvarying measurement.

quota sampling Nonprobability sampling strategy which identifies the strata of the population and proportionately represents the strata in the sample.

random assignment Allocation of sampling units to treatment and control conditions in a nonsystematic way using a random decision method.

random error Error caused by chance factors that influence the measurement of phenomena, such as changing conditions relative to the subject, the environment, or the instrument.

random processes Probabilistic processes about which nothing is known.

random selection Sampling method in which every member of the study population has an equal chance of being selected into the sample.

range Measure of variability derived by subtracting the lowest score from the highest score.

rating scales Measurement of an ordered set of categorical items representative of a variable. Numbers are assigned to each categorical item representing more or less of the variable.

ratio measurement Level of measurement which possesses all properties of interval measurement (equal numerical distance between scores with mutually exclusive and exhaustive categories) plus an absolute zero point.

refereed journal Periodical that uses expert reviewers to determine whether or not an article is to be published.

reflection Contemplation, dialogue, and critical appraisal focused on the data.

regression variance Percentage of variation in the dependent variable that can be explained by the independent variable.

reliability Ability of a instrument to consistently measure what it purports to measure; the extent to which random variation influences consistency, stability, and dependability of results. Also see *diachronic reliability, quixotic reliability, synchronic reliability*.

reliable Quality of research results to be replicated.

replication Repetition of a study using different samples conducted in different settings.

representativeness How well the sample represents the variables of interest in the target population.

research Scientific process of inquiry involving purposeful, systematic, and rigorous collection, analysis, and interpretation of data. Also see *applied research, basic research, correlational research, descriptive research, ethnographic research, experimental research, explanatory research, exploratory research, grounded theory research, historical research, phenomenological research, qualitative research, quantitative research, quasi-experimental research*.

research design Structural framework for study implementation, including selection of design, data collection methods, sampling framework, and data entry/analysis plan.

research problem Specific area of interest and general description of the problem to be solved.

research problem statement Delineation of specifically what is being studied.

research process Systematic method of examining a problem.

research purpose Specific statement of why the problem is being studied; purpose flows deductively from the problem statement.

research question Question or statement used to establish associations between variables; this is used when there is limited knowledge about a phenomenon and the research is descriptive in nature.

research utilization Systematic method of implementing sound, research-based innovations in clinical practice, evaluating outcomes, and sharing knowledge through research dissemination.

research variable Operationalized concept being examined in a research study.

residual variable Percentage of variation in the dependent variable that cannot be explained by the independent variable.

response rate Rate of participation in a study.

retrospective study Nonexperimental research design that begins with the phenomenon of interest (dependent variable) in the present and examines its relationship to another variable (independent variable) in the past.

risk-benefit ratio Extent to which the benefits of the study are maximized and the risks are minimized to protect subjects from harm during the study.

sample Subset or portion selected to represent the population of interest.

sample statistics Statistical characteristics of a sample, e.g., mode, median variance, standard distribution.

sampling Process of selecting a subset of the population in which the entire population is represented.

sampling distribution Distribution of statistics constructed to allow a study of the relationship between the characteristics of a sample (sample statistics) and the population parameters.

sampling error Amount of error that can be anticipated if the sample measure (mean, standard deviation) is used to estimate the population measure (even when samples are randomly drawn from the same population); the difference between the sample statistics and the corresponding population parameters.

sampling frame Comprehensive list of all the sampling elements (subjects) in the target population.

sampling method Process by which subsets of a population are selected for a research study.

scale Self-report inventory that provides a set of response symbols for each item. A rating or score is assigned to each response.

scientific approach Logical, orderly, and objective means of generating and testing ideas.

scientific method Systematic method of questioning and challenging the validity of scientific assumptions.

secondary source Scholarly material written about a theory or research by a person or persons other than the individual(s) who developed the theory or conducted the research. A secondary sources often represent summaries and critiques of a theorist's or researcher's work.

selective coding Clustering codes to create categories.

self-report Data collection instrument in which subjects are asked directly about the study variables.

semantic differential scale Measurement of attitudes toward a concept by asking the respondent to rate qualities on a point scale anchored by bipolar adjectives (happy, sad; hard, easy).

sensitivity Measurement ability of a data collection technique or instrument to discriminate individual differences of a measured attribute.

significance level Probability that the investigator will mistakenly reject the null hypothesis when it is true, that is, will conclude that a statistically significant difference or association exists when it does not.

simple hypothesis Statement of an associative or causal relationship between one independent variable and one dependent variable.

simple random sampling Probability sampling strategy in which the population is defined, sampling frame is listed, and members are randomly selected into the study period.

skewness Property of asymmetry.

snowballing See *network sampling*.

Solomon four-group design Experimental design with four randomly assigned groups—the pretest-posttest intervention group, the pretest-posttest control group, an intervention group with only the posttest measurement, and a control group with only the post-test meaurement.

standard deviation Square root of the variance. Also see *variance*.

standard error Measurement of the standard distance (deviation) between a sample measure and the population measure.

statistic Data collected from a sample used to estimate population parameters.

statistical conclusion validity Extent to which covariation is present between the independent and dependent variables at the statistical level.

statistical significance Extent to which results are unlikely to be attributable to chance.

story line Main theme in an analytical memo.

stratified random sampling Probability sampling strategy in which the population is divided into strata or subgroups. An appropriate number of elements from each subgroup are randomly selected based on their proportion in the population.

stratum (pl. **strata**) Grouping of mutually exclusive variables such as ethnicity, gender, age, and education level.

structural question Question formulated to evaluate how people order or categorize information.

subject Single member (individual, object, event, group, or place) of the population under study.

symbolic interaction Theoretical orientation to qualitative research. Also see *symbolic interactionist paradigm*.

symbolic interactionist paradigm Belief in the concept that people negotiate their reality in interactions with others; explanation of human behavior in terms of meaning and perceptions.

synchronic reliability Similarity of qualitative measurements within the same time period.

synthesis approach Method of theory development in which information from a variety of sources is used to construct a new concept.

systematic error Error that is a fundamental or integral part of the measuring device.

systematic sampling Probability sampling strategy that involves the selection of subjects who are randomly drawn from a population list at fixed intervals.

target population Set of individuals or objects to which a researcher wishes to generalize research findings.

test-retest reliability Assessment of the stability of a measure, determined by repeating measurements twice under the same testing conditions within a prescribed time interval and comparing the paired scores.

thematic analysis Process of categorizing and re-categorizing data until a satisfactory system is established.

theoretical Hypothetical or speculative; abstract.

theoretical coding Proposing relationships and actively validating them in the data.

theoretical definition Definition of concepts created from the theoretical framework and defined in abstract terms using other concepts from the theory.

theoretical framework Concepts and the relational statements to be examined or tested in a particular research study.

theoretical notes Researcher's initial interpretations, inferences, and speculations about emerging patterns and themes.

theoretical sensitivity Extent to which researcher has insight, an ability to give meaning to data, and the capability to identify pertinent information.

theoretical triangulation Combining multiple perspectives and hypotheses into a single study.

theory Set of interrelated constructs (concepts), definitions, and propositions that present a systematic view of a phenomenon by specifying proposed relationships among variables.

theory derivation Process of adapting a theory from another discipline to add insight into some phenomenon.

time series design Quasi-experimental design used to determine trends before and after treatment; general measurements are taken before the treatment and at the specified times after the treatment.

transferability Extent to which a study's findings would be similar in another context; criterion for evaluating qualitative research.

triangulation Validation of findings by utilization of two or more research methods that show similar or noncontradictory results. Also known as "triangulation of methods".

true experimental design See *experimental design.*

trustworthiness Degree to which the research findings can be believed; criterion for evaluating qualitative research studies.

t-test Parametric statistical method that uses data to test a hypothesis about the difference in population means.

two-tailed statistical test Test used when the research hypothesis is nondirectional.

type I error Rejection of the null hypothesis when it should be accepted.

type II error Acceptance of the null hypothesis when it should be rejected.

unit of analysis Sample; in qualitative research, the individual, group, event, process, or phenomenon to be explored.

validity (1) In quantitative research, the extent to which an instrument measures what it purports to measure. (2) In qualitative research, the extent to which the research findings represent reality. Also see *concurrent validity, content validity, construct validity, criterion-related validity, external validity, internal validity, predictive validity.*

variable Characteristic being measured that varies among the subjects being studied. Also see *active variable, attribute variable, continuous variable, dependent variable, discrete variable, extraneous variable, independent variable, intervening variable, research variable.*

variance Average squared standard deviation or average squared distance from the mean.

veracity Truthfulness; specifically, in informing others about the nature of the study.

visual analogue scale Self-reporting measure of physical stimuli (pain, shortness of breath) on a linear scale anchored by two words or phrases (no pain, extreme pain; worst, best).

Wilcoxon signed-rank test Nonparametric statistical method used to test the differences between two treatments of a single sample; a basic assumption is that the dependent variable is continuous.

Z score Used to compare measurements in standard units; examines the relative distance of the scores from the mean.

Areas Under the Normal Curve (Z-scores)

Proportion of Total Area Under the Normal Curve Between Mean Ordinate and Ordinate at Given z Distance from the Mean

$\frac{x}{\sigma}$ or z	Second Decimal Place in z									
	.00	.01	.02	.03	.04	.05	.06	.07	.08	.09
.0	.0000	.0040	.0080	.0120	.0160	.0199	.0239	.0279	.0319	.0359
.1	.0398	.0438	.0478	.0517	.0557	.0596	.0636	.0675	.0714	.0753
.2	.0793	.0832	.0871	.0910	.0948	.0987	.1026	.1064	.1103	.1141
.3	.1179	.1217	.1255	.1293	.1331	.1368	.1406	.1443	.1480	.1517
.4	.1554	.1591	.1628	.1664	.1700	.1736	.1722	.1808	.1844	.1879
.5	.1915	.1950	.1985	.2019	.2054	.2088	.2123	.2157	.2190	.2224
.6	.2257	.2291	.2324	.2357	.2389	.2422	.2454	.2486	.2517	.2549
.7	.2580	.2611	.2642	.2673	.2704	.2734	.2764	.2794	.2823	.2852
.8	.2881	.2910	.2939	.2967	.2995	.3023	.3051	.3078	.3106	.3133
.9	.3159	.3186	.3212	.3238	.3264	.3289	.3315	.3340	.3365	.3389
1.0	.3413	.3438	.3461	.3485	.3508	.3531	.3554	.3577	.3599	.3621
1.1	.3643	.3665	.3686	.3708	.3729	.3749	.3770	.3790	.3810	.3830
1.2	.3849	.3869	.3888	.3907	.3925	.3944	.3962	.3980	.3997	.4015
1.3	.4032	.4049	.4066	.4082	.4099	.4115	.4131	.4147	.4162	.4177
1.4	.4192	.4207	.4222	.4236	.4251	.4265	.4279	.4292	.4306	.4319
1.5	.4332	.4345	.4357	.4370	.4382	.4394	.4406	.4418	.4429	.4441
1.6	.4452	.4463	.4474	.4484	.4495	.4505	.4515	.4525	.4535	.4545
1.7	.4554	.4564	.4573	.4582	.4591	.4599	.4608	.4616	.4625	.4633
1.8	.4641	.4649	.4656	.4664	.4671	.4678	.4686	.4693	.4699	.4706
1.9	.4713	.4719	.4726	.4732	.4738	.4744	.4750	.4756	.4761	.4767
2.0	.4772	.4778	.4783	.4788	.4793	.4798	.4803	.4808	.4812	.4817
2.1	.4821	.4826	.4830	.4834	.4838	.4842	.4846	.4850	.4854	.4857
2.2	.4861	.4864	.4868	.4871	.4875	.4878	.4881	.4884	.4887	.4890
2.3	.4893	.4896	.4898	.4901	.4904	.4906	.4909	.4911	.4913	.4916
2.4	.4918	.4920	.4922	.4925	.4927	.4929	.4931	.4932	.4934	.4936
2.5	.4938	.4940	.4941	.4943	.4945	.4946	.4948	.4949	.4951	.4952
2.6	.4953	.4955	.4956	.4957	.4959	.4960	.4961	.4962	.4963	.4964
2.7	.4965	.4966	.4967	.4968	.4969	.4970	.4971	.4972	.4973	.4974
2.8	.4974	.4975	.4976	.4977	.4977	.4978	.4979	.4979	.4980	.4981
2.9	.4981	.4982	.4982	.4983	.4984	.4984	.4985	.4985	.4986	.4986
3.0	.4987	.4987	.4987	.4988	.4988	.4989	.4989	.4989	.4990	.4990
3.1	.4990	.4991	.4991	.4991	.4992	.4992	.4992	.4992	.4993	.4993
3.2	.4993	.4993	.4994	.4994	.4994	.4994	.4994	.4995	.4995	.4995
3.3	.4995	.4995	.4995	.4996	.4996	.4996	.4996	.4996	.4996	.4997
3.4	.4997	.4997	.4997	.4997	.4997	.4997	.4997	.4997	.4997	.4998
3.5	.4998									
4.0	.49997									
4.5	.499997									
5.0	.4999997									

From Roscoe, J. T. (1975). *Fundamental research statistics for the behavioral sciences* (2nd ed.). New York: Holt, Rinehart, and Winston.

Appendix B

Distribution of *t* for Given Probability Levels

df	Level of Significance for One-Tailed Test					
	.10	.05	.025	.01	.005	.0005
	Level of Significance for Two-Tailed Test					
	.20	.10	.05	.02	.01	.001
1	3.078	6.314	12.706	31.821	63.657	636.619
2	1.886	2.920	4.303	6.965	9.925	31.598
3	1.638	2.353	3.182	4.541	5.841	12.941
4	1.533	2.132	2.776	3.747	4.604	8.610
5	1.476	2.015	2.571	3.365	4.032	6.859
6	1.440	1.943	2.447	3.143	3.707	5.959
7	1.415	1.895	2.365	2.998	3.499	5.405
8	1.397	1.860	2.306	2.896	3.355	5.041
9	1.383	1.833	2.262	2.821	3.250	4.781
10	1.372	1.812	2.228	2.764	3.169	4.587
11	1.363	1.796	2.201	2.718	3.106	4.437
12	1.356	1.782	2.179	2.681	3.055	4.318
13	1.350	1.771	2.160	2.650	3.012	4.221
14	1.345	1.761	2.145	2.624	2.977	4.140
15	1.341	1.753	2.131	2.602	2.947	4.073
16	1.337	1.746	2.120	2.583	2.921	4.015
17	1.333	1.740	2.110	2.567	2.898	3.965
18	1.330	1.734	2.101	2.552	2.878	3.992
19	1.328	1.729	2.093	2.539	2.861	3.883
20	1.325	1.725	2.086	2.528	2.845	3.850
21	1.323	1.721	2.080	2.518	2.831	3.819
22	1.321	1.717	2.074	3.508	2.819	3.792
23	1.319	1.714	2.069	2.500	2.807	3.767
24	1.318	1.711	2.064	2.492	2.797	3.745
25	1.316	1.708	2.060	2.485	2.787	3.725
26	1.315	1.706	2.056	2.479	2.779	3.707
27	1.314	1.703	2.052	2.473	2.771	3.690
28	1.313	1.701	2.048	2.467	2.763	3.674
29	1.311	1.699	2.045	2.462	2.756	3.659
30	1.310	1.697	2.042	2.457	2.750	3.646
40	1.303	1.684	2.021	2.423	2.704	3.551
60	1.296	1.671	2.000	2.390	2.660	3.460
120	1.289	1.658	1.980	2.358	2.617	3.373
∞	1.282	1.645	1.960	2.326	2.576	3.291

*This table is abridged from Table III of R. A. Fisher and F. Yates, *Statistical tables for biological agricultural, and medical research*, published by Oliver and Boyd, Ltd., Edinburgh, by permission of the authors and publishers. In Roscoe, J. T. (1975). *Fundamental research statistics for the behavioral sciences* (2nd ed.). New York; Holt, Rinehart, and Winston.

Mann-Whitney *U*

One-Tailed Test at .05 Level; Two-Tailed Test at .10 Level

m	n=1	2	3	4	5	6	7	8	9	10	11	12	13	14	15	16	17	18	19	20
1	—																			
2	—	—																		
3	—	—	0																	
4	—	—	0	1																
5	—	0	1	2	4															
6	—	0	2	3	5	7														
7	—	0	2	4	6	8	11													
8	—	1	3	5	8	10	13	15												
9	—	1	4	6	9	12	15	18	21											
10	—	1	4	7	11	14	17	20	24	27										
11	—	1	5	8	12	16	19	23	27	31	34									
12	—	2	5	9	13	17	21	26	30	34	38	42								
13	—	2	6	10	15	19	24	28	33	37	42	47	51							
14	—	3	7	11	16	21	26	31	36	41	46	51	56	61						
15	—	3	7	12	18	23	28	33	39	44	50	55	61	66	72					
16	—	3	8	14	19	25	30	36	42	48	54	60	65	71	77	83				
17	—	3	9	15	20	26	33	39	45	51	57	64	70	77	83	89	96			
18	—	4	9	16	22	28	35	41	48	55	61	68	75	82	88	95	102	109		
19	0	4	10	17	23	30	37	44	51	58	65	72	80	87	94	101	109	116	123	
20	0	4	11	18	25	32	39	47	54	62	69	77	84	92	100	107	115	123	130	138
21	0	5	11	19	26	34	41	49	57	65	73	81	89	97	105	113	121	130	138	146
22	0	5	12	20	28	36	44	52	60	68	77	85	94	102	111	119	128	136	145	154
23	0	5	13	21	29	37	46	54	63	72	81	90	98	107	116	125	134	143	152	161
24	0	6	13	22	30	39	48	57	66	75	85	94	103	113	122	131	141	150	160	162
25	0	6	14	23	32	41	50	60	69	79	89	98	108	118	128	137	147	157	167	177
26	0	6	15	24	33	43	53	62	72	82	92	103	113	123	133	143	154	164	174	185
27	0	7	15	25	35	45	55	65	75	86	96	107	117	128	139	149	160	171	182	192
28	0	7	16	26	36	46	57	68	78	89	100	111	122	133	144	156	167	178	189	200
29	0	7	17	27	38	48	59	70	82	93	104	116	127	138	150	162	173	185	196	208
30	0	7	17	28	39	50	61	73	85	96	108	120	132	144	156	168	180	192	204	216
31	0	8	18	29	40	52	64	76	88	100	112	124	136	149	161	174	186	199	211	224
32	0	8	19	30	42	54	66	78	91	103	116	128	141	154	167	180	193	206	218	231
33	0	8	19	31	43	56	68	81	94	107	120	133	146	159	172	186	199	212	226	239
34	0	9	20	32	45	57	70	84	97	110	124	137	151	164	178	192	206	219	233	247
35	0	9	21	33	46	59	73	86	100	114	128	141	156	170	184	198	212	226	241	255
36	0	9	21	34	48	61	75	89	103	117	131	146	160	175	189	204	219	233	248	263
37	0	10	22	35	49	63	77	91	106	121	135	150	165	180	195	210	225	240	255	271
38	0	10	23	36	50	65	79	94	109	124	139	154	170	185	201	216	232	247	263	278
39	1	10	23	38	52	67	82	97	112	128	143	159	175	190	206	222	238	254	270	286
40	1	11	24	39	53	68	84	99	115	131	147	163	179	196	212	228	245	261	278	294

Continued.

This table is reprinted from *American Statistical Association Journal* (September 1964), pp. 927-932.

Mann-Whitney *U*—cont'd
One-Tailed Test at .025 Level; Two-Tailed Test at .05 Level

m	1	2	3	4	5	6	7	8	9	10	11	12	13	14	15	16	17	18	19	20
1	—																			
2	—	—																		
3	—	—	—																	
4	—	—	—	0																
5	—	—	0	1	2															
6	—	—	1	2	3	5														
7	—	—	1	3	5	6	8													
8	—	0	2	4	6	8	10	13												
9	—	0	2	4	7	10	12	15	17											
10	—	0	3	5	8	11	14	17	20	23										
11	—	0	3	6	9	13	16	19	23	26	30									
12	—	1	4	7	11	14	18	22	26	29	33	37								
13	—	1	4	8	12	16	20	24	28	33	37	41	45							
14	—	1	5	9	13	17	22	26	31	36	40	45	50	55						
15	—	1	5	10	14	19	24	29	34	39	44	49	54	59	64					
16	—	1	6	11	15	21	26	31	37	42	47	53	59	64	70	75				
17	—	2	6	11	17	22	28	34	39	45	51	57	63	69	75	81	87			
18	—	2	7	12	18	24	30	36	42	48	55	61	67	74	80	86	93	99		
19	—	2	7	13	19	25	32	38	45	52	58	65	72	78	85	92	99	106	113	
20	—	2	8	14	20	27	34	41	48	55	62	69	76	83	90	98	105	112	119	127
21	—	3	8	15	22	29	36	43	50	58	65	73	80	88	96	103	111	119	126	134
22	—	3	9	16	23	30	38	45	53	61	69	77	85	93	101	109	117	125	133	141
23	—	3	9	17	24	32	40	48	56	64	73	81	89	98	106	115	123	132	140	149
24	—	3	10	17	25	33	42	50	59	67	76	85	94	102	111	120	129	138	147	156
25	—	3	10	18	27	35	44	53	62	71	80	89	98	107	117	126	135	145	154	163
26	—	4	11	19	28	37	46	55	64	74	83	93	102	112	122	132	141	151	161	171
27	—	4	11	20	29	38	48	57	67	77	87	97	107	117	127	137	147	158	168	178
28	—	4	12	21	30	40	50	60	70	80	90	101	111	122	132	143	154	164	175	186
29	—	4	13	22	32	42	52	62	73	83	94	105	116	127	138	149	160	171	182	193
30	—	5	13	23	33	43	54	65	76	87	98	109	120	131	143	154	166	177	189	200
31	—	5	14	24	34	45	56	67	78	90	101	113	125	136	148	160	172	184	196	208
32	—	5	14	24	35	46	58	69	81	93	105	117	129	141	153	166	178	190	203	215
33	—	5	15	25	37	48	60	72	84	96	108	121	133	146	159	171	184	197	210	222
34	—	5	15	26	38	50	62	74	87	99	112	125	138	151	164	177	190	203	217	230
35	—	6	16	27	39	51	64	77	89	103	116	129	142	156	169	183	196	210	224	237
36	—	6	16	28	40	53	66	79	92	106	119	133	147	161	174	188	202	216	231	245
37	—	6	17	29	41	55	68	81	95	109	123	137	151	165	180	194	209	223	238	252
38	—	6	17	30	43	56	70	84	98	112	127	141	156	170	185	200	215	230	245	259
39	0	7	18	31	44	58	72	86	101	115	130	145	160	175	190	206	321	236	252	267
40	0	7	18	31	45	59	74	89	103	119	134	149	165	180	196	211	227	243	258	274

Mann-Whitney *U*—cont'd
One-Tailed Test at .01 Level; Two-Tailed Test at .02 Level

m	1	2	3	4	5	6	7	8	9	10	11	12	13	14	15	16	17	18	19	20
1	—																			
2	—	—																		
3	—	—	—																	
4	—	—	—	—																
5	—	—	—	0	1															
6	—	—	—	1	2	3														
7	—	—	0	1	3	4	6													
8	—	—	0	2	4	6	7	9												
9	—	—	1	3	5	7	9	11	14											
10	—	—	1	3	6	8	11	13	16	19										
11	—	—	1	4	7	9	12	15	18	22	25									
12	—	—	2	5	8	11	14	17	21	24	28	31								
13	—	0	2	5	9	12	16	20	23	27	31	35	39							
14	—	0	2	6	10	13	17	22	26	30	34	38	43	47						
15	—	0	3	7	11	15	19	24	28	33	37	42	47	51	56					
16	—	0	3	7	12	16	21	26	31	36	41	46	51	56	61	66				
17	—	0	4	8	13	18	23	28	33	38	44	49	55	60	66	71	77			
18	—	0	4	9	14	19	24	30	36	41	47	53	59	65	70	76	82	88		
19	—	1	4	9	15	20	26	32	38	44	50	56	63	69	75	82	88	94	101	
20	—	1	5	10	16	22	28	34	40	47	53	60	67	73	80	87	93	100	107	114
21	—	1	5	11	17	23	30	36	43	50	57	64	71	78	85	92	99	106	113	121
22	—	1	6	11	18	24	31	38	45	53	60	67	75	82	90	97	105	112	120	127
23	—	1	6	12	19	26	33	40	48	55	63	71	79	87	94	102	110	118	126	134
24	—	1	6	13	20	27	35	42	50	58	66	75	83	91	99	108	116	124	133	141
25	—	1	7	13	21	29	36	45	53	61	70	78	87	95	104	113	122	130	139	148
26	—	1	7	14	22	30	38	47	55	64	73	82	91	100	109	118	127	136	146	155
27	—	2	7	15	23	31	40	49	58	67	76	85	95	104	114	123	133	142	152	162
28	—	2	8	16	24	33	42	51	60	70	79	89	99	109	119	129	139	149	159	169
29	—	2	8	16	25	34	43	53	63	73	83	93	103	113	123	134	144	155	165	176
30	—	2	9	17	26	35	45	55	65	76	86	96	107	118	128	139	150	161	172	182
31	—	2	9	18	27	37	47	57	68	78	89	100	111	122	133	144	156	167	178	189
32	—	2	9	18	28	38	49	59	70	81	92	104	115	127	138	150	161	173	185	196
33	—	2	10	19	29	40	50	61	73	84	96	107	119	131	143	155	167	179	191	203
34	—	3	10	20	30	41	52	64	75	87	99	111	123	135	148	160	173	185	198	210
35	—	3	11	20	31	42	54	66	78	90	102	115	127	140	153	165	178	191	204	217
36	—	3	11	21	32	44	56	68	80	93	106	118	131	144	158	171	184	197	211	224
37	—	3	11	22	33	45	57	70	83	96	109	122	135	149	162	176	190	203	217	231
38	—	3	12	22	34	46	59	72	85	99	112	126	139	153	167	181	195	209	224	238
39	—	3	12	23	35	48	61	74	88	101	115	129	144	158	172	187	201	216	230	245
40	—	3	13	24	36	49	63	76	90	104	119	133	148	162	177	192	207	222	237	252

Continued.

Mann-Whitney *U*—cont'd

One-Tailed Test at .005 Level; Two-Tailed Test at .01 Level

m	1	2	3	4	5	6	7	8	9	10	11	12	13	14	15	16	17	18	19	20
1	—																			
2	—	—																		
3	—	—	—																	
4	—	—	—	—																
5	—	—	—	—	0															
6	—	—	—	0	1	2														
7	—	—	—	0	1	2	4													
8	—	—	—	1	2	4	6	7												
9	—	—	0	1	3	5	7	9	11											
10	—	—	0	2	4	6	9	11	13	16										
11	—	—	0	2	5	7	10	13	16	18	21									
12	—	—	1	3	6	9	12	15	18	21	24	27								
13	—	—	1	3	7	10	13	17	20	24	27	31	34							
14	—	—	1	4	7	11	15	18	22	26	30	34	38	42						
15	—	—	2	5	8	12	16	20	24	29	33	37	42	46	51					
16	—	—	2	5	9	13	18	22	27	31	36	41	45	50	55	60				
17	—	—	2	6	10	15	19	24	29	34	39	44	49	54	60	65	70			
18	—	—	2	6	11	16	21	26	31	37	42	47	53	58	64	70	75	81		
19	—	0	3	7	12	17	22	28	33	39	45	51	57	63	69	74	81	87	93	
20	—	0	3	8	13	18	24	30	36	42	48	54	60	67	73	79	86	92	99	105
21	—	0	3	8	14	19	25	32	38	44	51	58	64	71	78	84	91	98	105	112
22	—	0	4	9	14	21	27	34	40	47	54	61	68	75	82	89	96	104	111	118
23	—	0	4	9	15	22	29	35	43	50	57	64	72	79	87	94	102	109	117	125
24	—	0	4	10	16	23	30	37	45	52	60	68	75	83	91	99	107	115	123	131
25	—	0	5	10	17	24	32	39	47	55	63	71	79	87	96	104	112	121	129	138
26	—	0	5	11	18	25	33	41	49	58	66	74	83	92	100	109	118	127	135	144
27	—	1	5	12	19	27	35	43	52	60	69	78	87	96	105	114	123	132	142	151
28	—	1	5	12	20	28	36	45	54	63	72	81	91	100	109	119	128	138	148	157
29	—	1	6	13	21	29	38	47	56	66	75	85	94	104	114	124	134	144	154	164
30	—	1	6	13	22	30	40	49	58	68	78	88	98	108	119	129	139	150	160	170
31	—	1	6	14	22	32	41	51	61	71	81	92	102	113	123	134	145	155	166	177
32	—	1	7	14	23	33	43	53	63	74	84	95	106	117	128	139	150	161	172	184
33	—	1	7	15	24	34	44	55	65	76	87	98	110	121	132	144	155	167	179	190
34	—	1	7	16	25	35	46	57	68	79	90	102	113	125	137	149	161	173	185	197
35	—	1	8	16	26	37	47	59	70	82	93	105	117	129	142	154	166	179	191	203
36	—	1	8	17	27	38	49	60	72	84	96	109	121	134	146	159	172	184	197	210
37	—	1	8	17	28	39	51	62	75	87	99	112	125	138	151	164	177	190	203	217
38	—	1	9	18	29	40	52	64	77	90	102	116	129	142	155	169	182	196	210	223
39	—	2	9	19	30	41	54	66	79	92	106	119	133	146	160	174	188	202	216	230
40	—	2	9	19	31	43	55	68	81	95	109	122	136	150	165	179	193	208	222	237

Wilcoxon Matched-Pairs Signed-Ranks Test*

N	Level of Significance for One-Tailed Test		
	.025	**.01**	**.005**
	Level of Significance for Two-Tailed Test		
	.05	**.02**	**.01**
6	0	–	–
7	2	0	–
8	4	2	0
9	6	3	2
10	8	5	3
11	11	7	5
12	14	10	7
13	17	13	10
14	21	16	13
15	25	20	16
16	30	24	20
17	35	28	23
18	40	33	28
19	46	38	32
20	52	43	38
21	59	49	43
22	66	56	49
23	73	62	55
24	81	69	61
25	89	77	68

*Adapted from Table I of F. Wilcoxon, *Some rapid approximate statistical procedures,* p. 13, American Cyanamid Company, New York, 1949, with their kind permission. In Roscoe, J. T. (1975). *Fundamental research statistics for the behavioral sciences* (2nd ed.). New York: Holt, Rinehart, and Winston.

Appendix E

Distribution of Chi-Square for Given Probability Levels

df	.99	.98	.95	.90	.80	.70	.50	.30	.20	.10	.05	.02	.01	.001
1	.00016	.00663	.00393	.0158	.0642	.148	.455	1.074	1.642	2.706	3.841	5.412	6.635	10.827
2	.0201	.0404	.103	.211	.446	.713	1.386	2.408	3.219	4.605	5.991	7.824	9.210	13.815
3	.115	.185	.352	.584	1.005	1.424	2.366	3.665	4.642	6.251	7.815	9.837	11.345	16.266
4	.297	.429	.711	1.064	1.649	2.195	3.357	4.878	3.989	7.779	9.488	11.668	13.277	18.467
5	.554	.752	1.145	1.610	2.343	3.000	4.351	6.064	7.289	9.236	11.070	13.388	15.086	20.515
6	.872	1.134	1.635	2.204	3.070	3.828	5.348	7.231	8.558	10.645	12.592	15.033	16.812	22.457
7	1.239	1.564	2.167	2.833	3.822	4.671	6.346	8.383	9.803	12.017	14.067	16.622	18.475	24.322
8	1.646	2.032	2.733	3.490	4.594	5.527	7.344	9.524	11.030	13.362	15.507	18.168	20.090	26.125
9	2.088	2.532	3.325	4.168	5.380	6.393	8.343	10.656	12.242	14.684	16.919	19.679	21.666	27.877
10	2.558	3.059	3.940	4.865	6.179	7.267	9.342	11.781	13.442	15.987	18.307	21.161	23.209	29.588
11	3.053	3.609	4.575	5.578	6.989	8.148	10.341	12.899	14.631	17.275	19.675	22.618	24.725	31.264
12	3.571	4.178	5.226	6.304	7.807	9.034	11.340	14.011	15.812	18.549	21.026	24.054	26.217	32.909
13	4.107	4.765	5.892	7.042	8.634	9.926	12.340	15.119	16.985	19.812	22.362	25.472	27.688	34.528
14	4.660	5.368	6.571	7.790	9.467	10.821	13.339	16.222	18.151	21.064	23.685	26.873	29.141	36.123
15	5.229	5.985	7.261	8.547	10.307	11.721	14.339	17.322	19.311	22.307	24.996	28.259	30.578	37.697
16	5.812	6.614	7.962	9.312	11.152	12.624	15.338	18.418	20.465	23.542	26.296	29.633	32.000	39.252
17	6.408	7.255	8.672	10.085	12.002	13.531	16.338	19.511	21.615	24.769	27.587	30.995	33.409	40.790
18	7.015	7.906	9.390	10.865	12.857	14.440	17.338	20.601	22.760	25.989	28.869	32.346	34.805	42.312
19	7.633	8.567	10.117	11.651	13.716	15.352	18.338	21.689	23.900	27.204	30.144	33.687	36.191	43.820
20	8.260	9.237	10.851	12.443	14.578	16.266	19.337	22.775	25.038	28.412	31.410	35.030	37.566	45.315
21	8.897	9.915	11.591	13.240	15.445	17.182	20.337	23.858	26.171	29.615	32.671	36.343	38.932	46.797
22	9.542	10.600	12.338	14.041	16.314	18.101	21.337	24.939	27.301	30.813	33.924	37.659	40.289	48.268
23	10.196	11.293	13.091	14.848	17.187	19.021	22.337	26.018	28.429	32.007	35.172	38.968	41.638	49.728
24	10.856	11.992	13.848	15.659	18.062	19.943	23.337	27.096	29.553	33.196	36.415	40.270	42.980	51.179
25	11.524	12.697	14.611	16.473	18.940	20.867	24.337	28.172	30.675	34.382	37.652	41.566	44.314	52.620

df														
26	12.198	13.409	15.379	17.292	19.820	21.792	25.336	29.246	31.795	35.563	38.885	42.856	45.642	54.052
27	12.879	14.125	16.151	18.114	20.703	22.719	26336	30.319	32.912	36.741	40.113	44.140	46.963	55.476
28	13.565	14.847	16.928	18.939	21.588	23.647	27.336	31.391	34.027	37.916	41.337	45.419	48.278	56.893
29	14.256	15.574	17.708	19.768	22.475	24.577	28.336	32.461	35.139	39.087	42.557	46.693	49.588	58.302
30	14.953	16.306	18.493	20.599	23.364	25.508	29.336	33.530	36.250	40.256	43.773	47.962	50.892	59.703
32	16.362	17.783	20.072	22.271	25.148	27.373	31.336	35.665	38.466	42.585	46.194	50.487	53.486	62.487
34	17.789	19.275	21.664	23.952	26.938	29.242	33.336	37.795	40.676	44.903	48.602	52.995	56.061	65.247
36	19.233	20.783	23.269	25.643	28.735	31.115	35.336	39.922	42.879	47.212	50.999	55.489	58.619	67.985
38	20.691	22.304	24.884	27.343	30.537	32.992	37.335	42.045	45.076	49.513	53.384	57.969	61.162	70.703
40	22.164	23.838	26.509	29.051	32.345	34.872	39.335	44.165	47.269	51.805	55.769	60.436	63.691	73.402
42	23.650	25.383	28.144	30.765	34.157	36.755	41.335	46.282	49.456	54.090	58.124	62.892	66.206	76.084
44	25.148	26.939	29.787	32.487	35.974	38.641	43.335	48.396	51.369	60.481	65.337	68.710	78.750	51.639
46	26.657	28.504	31.439	34.215	37.795	40.529	45.335	50.507	53.818	58.641	62.830	67.771	71.201	81.400
48	28.177	30.080	33.098	35.959	39.621	42.420	47.335	52.616	55.993	60.907	65.171	70.197	73.683	84.037
50	29.707	31.664	34.764	37.689	41.449	44.313	49.335	54.723	58.164	63.167	67.505	72.613	76.154	86.661
52	31.246	33.256	36.437	39.433	43.281	46.209	51.335	56.827	60.332	65.422	69.832	75.021	78.616	89.272
54	32.793	34.856	38.116	41.183	45.117	48.106	53.335	58.930	62.496	67.673	72.153	77.422	81.069	91.872
56	34.350	36.464	39.801	42.937	46.955	50.005	55.335	61.031	64.658	69.919	74.468	79.815	83.513	94.461
58	35.913	38.078	41.492	44.696	48.797	51.906	57.335	63.129	66.816	72.160	76.778	82.201	85.950	97.039
60	37.485	39.699	43.188	46.459	50.641	53.809	59.335	65.227	68.972	74.397	79.082	84.580	88.379	99.607
62	39.063	41.327	44.889	48.226	52.487	55.714	61.335	67.322	71.125	76.630	81.381	86.953	90.802	102.166
64	40.649	42.960	46.595	49.996	54.336	57.620	63.335	69.416	73.276	78.860	83.675	89.320	93.217	104.716
66	42.240	44.599	48.305	51.770	56.188	59.527	65.335	71.508	75.424	81.085	85.965	91.681	95.626	107.258
68	43.838	46.244	50.020	53.548	58.042	61.436	67.335	73.600	77.571	83.308	88.250	94.037	98.208	109.791
70	45.442	47.893	51.739	55.329	59.898	63.346	69.334	75.689	79.715	85.527	90.531	96.388	100.425	112.317

For larger values of *df*, the expression $\sqrt{2X^2} - \sqrt{2df - 1}$ may be used as a normal deviate with unit variance, remembering that the probability for x^2 corresponds with that of a single tail of the normal curve.

This table is adapted from R. A. Fisher and F. Yates, *Statistical tables for biological, agricultural and medical research*, Oliver and Boyd, Ltd., Edinburgh, by permission of the authors and publishers. In Roscoe, J. T. (1975). *Fundamental research statistics for the behavioral sciences* (2nd ed.). New York: Holt, Rinehart, and Winston.

Appendix F

Transformation of r to Z

r	z	r	z	r	z	r	z	r	z
.000	.000	.200	.203	.400	.424	.600	.693	.800	1.099
.005	.005	.205	.208	.405	.430	.605	.701	.805	1.113
.010	.010	.210	.213	.410	.436	.610	.709	.810	1.127
.015	.015	.215	.218	.415	.442	.615	.717	.815	1.142
.020	.020	.220	.224	.420	.448	.620	.725	.820	1.157
.025	.025	.225	.229	.425	.454	.625	.733	.825	1.172
.030	.030	.230	.234	.430	.460	.630	.741	.830	1.188
.035	.035	.235	.239	.435	.466	.635	.750	.835	1.204
.040	.040	.240	.245	.440	.472	.640	.758	.840	1.221
.045	.045	.245	.250	.445	.478	.645	.767	.845	1.238
.050	.050	.250	.255	.450	.485	.650	.775	.850	1.256
.055	.055	.255	.261	.455	.491	.655	.784	.855	1.274
.060	.060	.260	.266	.460	.497	.660	.793	.860	1.293
.065	.065	.265	.271	.465	.504	.665	.802	.865	1.313
.070	.070	.270	.277	.470	.510	.670	.811	.870	1.333
.075	.075	.275	.282	.475	.517	.675	.820	.875	1.354
.080	.080	.280	.288	.480	.523	.680	.829	.880	1.376
.085	.085	.285	.293	.485	.530	.685	.838	.885	1.398
.090	.090	.290	.299	.490	.536	.690	.848	.890	1.422
.095	.095	.295	.304	.495	.543	.695	.858	.895	1.447
.100	.100	.300	.310	.500	.549	.700	.867	.900	1.472
.105	.105	.305	.315	.505	.556	.705	.877	.905	1.499
.110	.110	.310	.321	.510	.563	.710	.887	.910	1.528
.115	.116	.315	.326	.515	.570	.715	.897	.915	1.557
.120	.121	.320	.332	.520	.576	.720	.908	.920	1.589
.125	.126	.325	.337	.525	.583	.725	.918	.925	1.623
.130	.131	.330	.343	.530	.590	.730	.929	.930	1.658
.135	.136	.335	.348	.535	.597	.735	.940	.935	1.697
.140	.141	.340	.354	.540	.604	.740	.950	.940	1.738
.145	.146	.345	.360	.545	.611	.745	.962	.945	1.783
.150	.151	.350	.365	.550	.618	.750	.973	.950	1.832
.155	.156	.355	.371	.555	.626	.755	.984	.955	1.886
.160	.161	.360	.377	.560	.633	.760	.996	.960	1.946
.165	.167	.365	.383	.565	.640	.765	1.008	.965	2.014
.170	.172	.370	.388	.570	.648	.770	1.020	.970	2.092
.175	.177	.375	.394	.575	.655	.775	1.033	.975	2.185
.180	.182	.380	.400	.580	.662	.780	1.045	.980	2.298
.185	.187	.385	.406	.585	.670	.785	1.058	.985	2.443
.190	.192	.390	.412	.590	.678	.790	1.071	.990	2.647
.195	.198	.395	.418	.595	.685	.795	1.085	.995	2.994

This table was constructed by F. P. Kilpatrick and D. A. Buchanan.
This table is reprinted from Edwards, A. L. (1967). *Statistical methods* (2nd ed.). New York: Holt, Rinehart and Winston.

Critical Values of the Pearson Correlation Coefficient*

N − 2 = df	**Level of Significance for One-Tailed Test**			
	.05	.025	.01	.005
	Level of Significance for Two-Tailed Test			
	.10	.05	.02	.01
1	.988	.997	.9995	.9999
2	.900	.950	.980	.990
3	.805	.878	.934	.959
4	.729	.811	.882	.917
5	.669	.754	.833	.874
6	.622	.707	.789	.834
7	.582	.666	.750	.798
8	.549	.632	.716	.765
9	.521	.602	.685	.735
10	.497	.576	.658	.708
11	.576	.553	.634	.684
12	.458	.532	.612	.661
13	.441	.514	.592	.641
14	.426	.497	.574	.623
15	.412	.482	.558	.606
16	.400	.468	.542	.590
17	.389	.456	.528	.575
18	.378	.444	.516	.561
19	.369	.433	.503	.549
20	.360	.423	.492	.537

Continued.

*Abridged from R. A. Fisher and F. Yates, *Statistical tables for biological, agricultural, and medical research,* Oliver Boyd, Ltd., Edinburgh, by permission of the authors and publishers. In Roscoe, J. T. (1975). *Fundamental research statistics for the behavioral sciences* (2nd ed.). New York: Holt, Rinehart, and Winston.

Critical Values of the Pearson Correlation Coefficient—cont'd

N − 2 = df	Level of Significance for One-Tailed Test			
	.05	.025	.01	.005
	Level of Significance for Two-Tailed Test			
	.10	.05	.02	.01
21	.352	.413	.482	.526
22	.344	.404	.472	.515
23	.337	.396	.462	.505
24	.330	.388	.453	.496
25	.323	.381	.445	.487
26	.317	.374	.437	.479
27	.311	.367	.430	.471
28	.306	.361	.423	.463
29	.301	.355	.416	.486
30	.296	.349	.409	.449
35	.275	.325	.381	.418
40	.257	.304	.358	.393
45	.243	.288	.338	.372
50	.231	.273	.322	.354
60	.211	.250	.295	.325
70	.195	.232	.274	.303
80	.183	.217	.256	.283
90	.173	.205	.242	.267
100	.164	.195	.230	.254

Critical Values of the Spearman Correlation Coefficient

N	Level of Significance for a One-Tailed Test			
	.05	**.025**	**.01**	**.005**
	Level of Significance for a Two-Tailed Test			
	.10	**.05**	**.02**	**.01**
4	1.000			
5	.900	1.000	1.000	
6	.829	.886	.943	1.000
7	.714	.786	.893	.929
8	.643	.738	.833	.881
9	.600	.683	.783	.833
10	.564	.648	.746	.794
12	.506	.591	.712	.777
14	.456	.544	.645	.715
16	.425	.506	.601	.665
18	.399	.475	.564	.625
20	.377	.450	.534	.591
22	.359	.428	.508	.562
24	.343	.409	.485	.537
26	.329	.392	.465	.515
28	.317	.377	.448	.496
30	.306	.364	.432	.478

From Roscoe, J. T. (1975). *Fundamental research statistics for the behavioral sciences* (2nd ed.). New York: Holt, Rinehart, and Winston.

Appendix I

The *F*-Distribution* (.05 Level)

df₁df₂	1	2	3	4	5	6	7	8	9
1	161.4	199.5	215.7	224.6	230.0	234.0	236.8	238.9	240.5
2	18.51	19.00	19.16	19.25	19.30	19.33	19.35	19.37	19.38
3	10.13	9.55	9.28	9.12	9.01	8.94	8.89	8.85	8.81
4	7.71	6.94	6.59	6.39	6.26	6.16	6.09	6.04	6.00
5	6.61	5.79	5.41	5.19	5.05	4.95	4.88	4.82	4.77
6	5.99	5.14	4.76	4.53	4.39	4.28	4.21	4.15	4.10
7	5.59	4.74	4.35	4.12	3.97	3.87	3.79	3.73	3.68
8	5.32	4.46	4.07	3.84	3.69	3.58	3.50	3.44	3.39
9	5.12	4.26	3.86	3.63	3.48	3.37	3.29	3.23	3.18
10	4.96	4.10	3.71	3.48	3.33	3.22	3.14	3.07	3.02
11	4.84	3.98	3.59	3.36	3.20	3.09	3.01	2.95	2.90
12	4.75	3.89	3.49	3.26	3.11	3.00	2.91	2.85	2.80
13	4.67	3.81	3.41	3.18	3.03	2.92	2.83	2.77	2.71
14	4.60	3.74	3.34	3.11	2.96	2.85	2.76	2.70	2.65
15	4.54	3.68	3.29	3.06	2.90	2.79	2.71	2.64	2.59
16	4.49	3.63	3.24	3.01	2.85	2.74	2.66	2.59	2.54
17	4.45	3.59	3.20	2.96	2.81	2.70	2.61	2.55	2.49
18	4.41	3.55	3.16	2.93	2.77	2.66	2.58	2.51	2.46
19	4.38	3.52	3.13	2.90	2.74	2.63	2.54	2.48	2.42
20	4.35	3.49	3.10	2.87	2.71	2.60	2.51	2.45	2.39
21	4.32	3.47	3.07	2.84	2.68	2.57	2.49	2.42	2.37
22	4.30	3.44	3.05	2.82	2.66	2.55	2.46	2.40	2.34
23	4.28	3.42	3.03	2.80	2.64	2.53	2.44	2.37	2.32
24	4.26	3.40	3.01	2.78	2.62	2.51	2.42	2.36	2.30
25	4.24	3.39	2.99	2.76	2.60	2.49	2.40	2.34	2.28
26	4.23	3.37	2.98	2.74	2.59	2.47	2.39	2.32	2.27
27	4.21	3.35	2.96	2.73	2.57	2.46	2.37	2.31	2.25
28	4.20	3.34	2.95	2.71	2.56	2.45	2.36	2.29	2.24
29	4.18	3.33	2.93	2.70	2.55	2.43	2.35	2.28	2.22
30	4.17	3.32	2.92	2.69	2.53	2.42	2.33	2.27	2.21
40	4.08	3.23	2.84	2.61	2.45	2.34	2.25	2.18	2.12
60	4.00	3.15	2.76	2.53	2.37	2.25	2.17	2.10	2.04
120	3.92	3.07	2.68	2.45	2.29	2.17	2.09	2.02	1.96
∞	3.84	3.00	2.60	2.37	2.21	2.10	2.01	1.94	1.88

This table is abridged from Table 18 of the *Biometrika Tables for Statisticians,* Vol. 1 (ed. 1), edited by E. S. Pearson and H. O. Hartley. Reproduced by the kind permission of E. S. Pearson and the trustees of *Biometrika.*
In Roscoe J. T. (1975). *Fundamental research statistics for the behavioral sciences* (2nd ed.). New York: Holt, Rinehart, and Winston.

10	12	15	20	24	30	40	60	120	∞
241.9	243.9	245.9	248.0	249.1	250.1	251.1	252.2	2.53.3	254.3
19.40	19.41	19.43	19.45	19.45	19.46	19.47	19.48	19.49	19.50
8.79	8.74	8.70	8.66	8.64	8.62	8.59	8.57	8.55	8.53
5.96	5.91	5.86	5.80	5.77	5.75	5.72	5.69	5.66	5.63
4.74	4.68	4.62	4.56	4.53	4.50	4.46	4.43	4.40	4.36
4.06	4.00	3.94	3.87	3.84	3.81	3.77	3.74	3.70	3.67
3.64	3.57	3.51	3.44	3.41	3.38	3.34	3.30	3.27	3.23
3.35	3.28	3.22	3.15	3.12	3.08	3.04	3.01	2.97	2.93
3.14	3.07	3.01	2.94	2.90	2.86	2.83	2.79	2.75	2.71
2.98	2.91	2.85	2.77	2.74	2.70	2.66	2.62	2.58	2.54
2.85	2.79	2.72	2.65	2.61	2.57	2.53	2.49	2.45	2.40
2.75	2.69	2.62	2.54	2.51	2.47	2.43	2.38	2.34	2.30
2.67	2.60	2.53	2.46	2.42	2.38	2.34	2.30	2.25	2.21
2.60	2.53	2.46	2.39	2.35	2.31	2.27	2.22	2.18	2.13
2.54	2.48	2.40	2.33	2.29	2.25	2.20	2.16	2.11	2.07
2.42	2.35	2.28	2.24	2.19	2.15	2.11	2.06	2.01	
2.45	2.38	2.31	2.23	2.19	2.15	2.10	2.06	2.01	1.96
2.41	2.34	2.27	2.19	2.15	2.11	2.06	2.02	1.97	1.92
2.38	2.31	2.23	2.16	2.11	2.07	2.03	1.98	1.93	1.88
2.35	2.28	2.20	2.12	2.08	2.04	1.99	1.95	1.90	1.84
2.32	2.25	2.18	2.10	2.05	2.01	1.96	1.92	1.87	1.81
2.30	2.23	2.15	2.07	2.03	1.98	1.94	1.89	1.84	1.78
2.27	2.20	2.13	2.05	2.01	1.96	1.91	1.86	1.81	1.76
2.25	2.18	2.11	2.03	1.98	1.94	1.89	1.84	1.79	1.73
2.24	2.16	2.09	2.01	1.96	1.92	1.87	1.82	1.77	1.71
2.22	2.15	2.07	1.99	1.95	1.90	1.85	1.80	1.75	1.69
2.20	2.13	2.06	1.97	1.93	1.88	1.84	1.79	1.73	1.67
2.19	2.12	2.04	1.96	1.91	1.87	1.82	1.77	1.71	1.65
2.18	2.10	2.03	1.94	1.90	1.85	1.81	1.75	1.70	1.64
2.16	2.09	2.01	1.93	1.89	1.84	1.79	1.74	1.68	1.62
2.08	2.00	1.92	1.84	1.79	1.74	1.69	1.64	1.58	1.51
1.99	1.92	1.84	1.75	1.70	1.65	1.59	1.53	1.47	1.39
1.91	1.83	1.75	1.66	1.61	1.55	1.50	1.43	1.35	1.25
1.83	1.75	1.67	1.57	1.52	1.46	1.39	1.32	1.22	1.00

Continued.

The _F_-Distribution* (.05 Level)—cont'd

df₁df₂	1	2	3	4	5	6	7	8	9
1	4052	4999.5	5403	5625	5764	5859	5928	5982	6022
2	98.5	99.00	99.17	99.25	99.30	99.33	99.36	99.37	99.39
3	34.12	30.82	29.46	28.71	28.24	27.91	27.67	27.49	27.35
4	21.20	18.00	16.69	15.98	15.52	15.21	14.98	14.80	14.66
5	16.26	13.27	12.06	11.39	10.97	10.67	10.46	10.29	10.16
6	13.75	10.92	9.78	9.15	8.75	8.47	8.26	8.10	7.98
7	12.25	9.55	8.45	7.85	7.46	7.19	6.99	6.81	6.72
8	11.26	8.65	7.59	7.01	6.63	6.37	6.18	6.03	5.91
9	10.56	8.02	6.99	6.42	6.06	5.80	5.61	5.47	5.35
10	10.04	7.56	6.55	5.99	5.64	5.39	5.20	5.06	4.94
11	9.65	7.21	6.22	5.67	5.32	5.07	4.89	4.74	4.63
12	9.33	6.93	5.95	5.41	5.06	4.82	4.64	4.50	4.39
13	9.07	6.70	5.74	5.21	4.86	4.62	4.44	4.30	4.19
14	8.86	6.51	5.56	5.04	4.69	4.46	4.28	4.14	4.03
15	8.68	6.36	5.42	4.89	4.56	4.32	4.14	4.00	3.89
16	8.53	6.23	5.29	4.77	4.44	4.20	4.03	3.89	3.78
17	8.40	6.11	5.18	4.67	4.34	4.10	3.93	3.79	3.68
18	8.29	6.01	5.09	4.58	4.25	4.01	3.84	3.71	3.60
19	8.18	5.93	5.01	4.50	4.17	3.94	3.77	3.63	3.52
20	8.10	5.85	4.94	4.43	4.10	3.87	3.70	3.56	3.46
21	8.02	5.78	4.87	4.37	4.04	3.81	3.64	3.51	3.40
22	7.95	5.72	4.82	4.31	3.99	3.76	3.59	3.45	3.35
23	7.88	5.66	4.76	4.26	3.94	3.71	3.54	3.41	3.30
24	7.82	5.61	4.72	4.22	3.90	3.67	3.50	3.36	3.26
25	7.77	5.57	4.68	4.18	3.85	3.63	3.46	3.32	3.22
26	7.72	5.53	4.64	4.14	3.82	3.59	3.42	3.29	3.18
27	7.68	5.49	4.60	4.11	3.78	3.56	3.39	3.26	3.15
28	7.64	5.45	4.57	4.07	3.75	3.53	3.36	3.23	3.12
29	7.60	5.42	4.54	4.04	3.73	3.50	3.33	3.20	3.09
30	7.56	5.39	4.51	4.02	3.70	3.47	3.30	3.17	3.07
40	7.31	5.18	4.31	3.83	3.51	3.29	3.12	2.99	2.89
60	7.08	4.98	4.13	3.65	3.34	3.12	2.95	2.82	2.72
120	6.85	4.79	3.95	3.48	3.17	2.96	2.79	2.66	2.56
∞	6.63	4.61	3.78	3.32	3.02	2.80	2.64	2.51	2.41

10	12	15	20	24	30	40	60	120	∞
6056	6106	6157	6209	6235	6261	6287	6313	6339	6366
99.40	99.42	99.43	99.45	99.46	99.47	99.47	99.48	99.49	99.50
27.23	27.05	26.87	26.69	26.60	26.50	26.41	26.32	.26.22	26.13
14.55	14.37	14.20	14.02	13.93	13.84	13.75	13.65	13.56	13.46
10.05	9.89	9.72	9.55	9.47	9.38	9.29	9.20	9.11	9.02
7.87	7.72	7.56	7.40	7.31	7.23	7.14	7.06	6.97	6.88
6.62	6.47	6.31	6.16	6.07	5.99	5.91	5.82	5.74	5.65
5.81	5.67	5.52	5.36	5.28	5.20	5.12	5.03	4.95	4.86
5.26	5.11	4.96	4.81	4.73	4.65	4.57	4.48	4.40	4.31
4.85	4.71	4.56	4.41	4.33	4.25	4.17	4.08	4.00	3.91
4.54	4.40	4.25	4.10	4.02	3.94	3.86	3.78	3.69	3.60
4.30	4.16	4.01	3.86	3.78	3.70	3.62	3.54	3.45	3.36
4.10	3.96	3.82	3.66	3.59	3.51	3.43	3.34	3.25	3.17
3.94	3.80	3.66	3.51	3.43	3.35	3.27	3.18	3.09	3.00
3.80	3.67	3.52	3.37	3.29	3.21	3.13	3.05	2.96	2.87
3.69	3.55	3.41	3.26	3.18	3.10	3.02	2.93	2.84	2.75
3.59	3.46	3.31	3.16	3.08	3.00	2.92	2.83	2.75	2.65
3.51	3.37	3.23	3.08	3.00	2.92	2.84	2.75	2.66	2.57
3.43	3.30	3.15	3.00	2.92	2.84	2.76	2.67	2.58	2.49
3.37	3.23	3.09	2.94	2.86	2.78	2.69	2.61	2.52	2.42
3.31	3.17	3.03	2.88	2.80	2.72	2.64	2.55	2.46	2.36
3.26	3.12	2.98	2.83	2.75	2.67	2.58	2.50	2.40	2.31
3.21	3.07	2.93	2.78	2.70	2.62	2.54	2.45	2.35	2.26
3.17	3.03	2.89	2.74	2.66	2.58	2.49	2.40	2.31	2.21
3.13	2.99	2.85	2.70	2.62	2.54	2.45	2.36	2.27	2.17
3.09	2.96	2.81	2.66	2.58	2.50	2.42	2.33	2.23	2.13
3.06	2.93	2.78	2.63	2.55	2.47	2.38	2.29	2.20	2.10
3.03	2.90	2.75	2.60	2.52	2.44	2.35	2.26	2.17	2.06
3.00	2.87	2.73	2.57	2.49	2.41	2.33	2.23	2.14	2.03
2.98	2.84	2.70	2.55	2.47	2.39	2.30	2.21	2.11	2.01
2.80	2.66	2.52	2.37	2.29	2.20	2.11	2.02	1.92	1.80
2.63	2.50	2.35	2.20	2.12	2.03	1.94	1.84	1.73	1.60
2.47	2.34	2.19	2.03	1.95	1.86	1.76	1.66	1.53	1.38
2.32	2.18	2.04	1.88	1.79	1.70	1.59	1.47	1.32	1.00

INDEX